Workshop Conference Hoechst Werk Kalle-Albert

ARTICULAR CARTILAGE AND OSTEOARTHRITIS

Workshop Conference Hoechst Werk Kalle-Albert
Wiesbaden
May 12–16, 1991
co-sponsored by the World Health Organization

Articular Cartilage and Osteoarthritis

Editors

Klaus E. Kuettner, Ph.D.
*Departments of Biochemistry
and Orthopedic Surgery
Rush-Presbyterian-St. Luke's Medical Center
Chicago, Illinois*

Rudolf Schleyerbach, D.V.M.
*Department of Pharmacological
Research
Hoechst Werk Kalle-Albert
Wiesbaden, Federal Republic
of Germany*

Jacques G. Peyron, M.D.
*Rhumatologue Qualifie
Neuilly sur Seine
France*

Vincent C. Hascall, Ph.D.
*Bone Research Branch
National Institute of
Dental Research
Bethesda, Maryland*

Raven Press New York

Raven Press, Ltd., 1185 Avenue of Americas, New York, New York 10036

Made in the United States of America

Library of Congress Cataloging-in-Publication Data
Articular cartilage and osteoarthritis/editors, Klaus E. Kuettner . . . [et al.].
   p. cm.
  Based on the International Workshop on Articular Cartilage and
Osteoarthritis, held in Wiesbaden, Germany in May 1991.
  Includes bibliographical references and index.
  ISBN 0-88167-862-7
  1. Osteoarthritis—Congresses. 2. Articular cartilage—Congresses. I. Kuettner, Klaus E. II. International Workshop on Articular Cartilage and Osteoarthritis (1991: Wiesbaden, Germany) [DNLM: 1. Cartilage, Articular—physiology— congresses. 2. Osteoarthritis—congresses. WE 300 A7912 1991]
RC931.067A78 1991
616.7'223—dc20
DNLM/DLC
for Library of Congress   91-32639
                                        CIP

9 8 7 6 5 4 3 2 1

Contents

Part I: Structural Components of Cartilage: Proteoglycans

Part II: Structural Components of Cartilage: Matrix Biology

Part IX: Experimental Osteoarthritis: Animal Models

Part X: Pharmacology in Osteoarthritis

Part XI: Drug Evaluation in Osteoarthritis

Contributing Authors

K. Abendroth
Department of Rheumatology
University of Jena
0-6902 Jena, Federal Republic of
  Germany

Nina Ahmad
Jefferson Institute of Molecular
  Medicine
Jefferson Medical College
Thomas Jefferson University
Philadelphia, Pennsylvania 19107

T. Aigner
Max-Planck-Society
Clinical Research Units for
  Rheumatology
University of Erlangen-Nürnberg
Schwabachanlage 10
8520 Erlangen, Federal Republic of
  Germany

Leena Ala-Kokko
Jefferson Institute of Molecular
  Medicine
Jefferson Medical College
Thomas Jefferson University
Philadelphia, Pennsylvania 19107

T. P. Andriacchi
Departments of Biochemistry and
  Orthopedic Surgery
Rush-Presbyterian-St. Luke's Medical
  Center
Chicago, Illinois 60612

J. Arokoski
Department of Anatomy
University of Kuopio
SF-70211 Kuopio, Finland

R. Atkins
Department of Pathology
University of Bristol
Bristol BS8 1TD, United Kingdom

Margaret B. Aydelotte
Department of Biochemistry
Rush Medical College
Rush-Presbyterian-St. Luke's Medical
  Center
1653 West Congress Parkway
Chicago, Illinois 60612

B. Bach, Jr.
Department of Internal Medicine
Rush Medical College
Rush-Presbyterian-St. Luke's Medical
  Center
Chicago, Illinois 60612

Mark S. Baker
Division of Clinical Sciences
John Curtin School of Medical Research
Australian National University
Canberra 2601, Australia

Clinton Baldwin
Jefferson Institute of Molecular
  Medicine
Jefferson Medical College
Thomas Jefferson University
Philadelphia, Pennsylvania 19107

Frank P. Barry
Department of Biochemistry and
  Molecular Biology
University of South Florida Medical
  School
Tampa, Florida 33612

Robert R. Bartlett
Pharmacologic Research
  Vasotherapeutics/Antirheumatics
Hoechst AG Kalle-Albert
6200 Wiesbaden, Federal Republic of
  Germany

Michael T. Bayliss
Department of Biochemistry
Kennedy Institute of Rheumatology
6 Bute Gardens
Hammersmith, London W67DW
United Kingdom

Paul D. Benya
Department of Orthopaedics
University of Southern California
Orthopaedic Hospital
2400 South Flower Street
Los Angeles, California 90007-2697

Shirley Bolis
Department of Tissue Physiology
Strangeways Research Laboratory
Worts Causeway
Cambridge CB1 4RN, United Kingdom

Kenneth D. Brandt
Department of Medicine
Rheumatology Division
Indiana University Medical Center
1100 West Michigan Street
Indianapolis, Indiana 46223

Peter Bruckner
Laboratorium für Biochemie I
Eidgenössische Technische Hochschule
8092 Zurich, Switzerland

Kay Brune
Institut für Pharmakologie und
  Toxikologie
der Universität Erlangen-Nürnberg
Universitatsstrasse 22
8520 Erlangen, Federal Republic of
  Germany

J. C. Buckland-Wright
Division of Anatomy and Cell Biology
United Medical and Dental Schools of
  Guy's and St. Thomas's Hospitals
London Bridge
London SE1 9RT, United Kingdom

Joseph A. Buckwalter
Department of Orthopaedics
University of Iowa Hospital
Iowa City, Iowa 52242

Renate Bürgin
Laboratorium für Biochemie I
Eidgenössische Technische Hochschule
8092 Zurich, Switzerland

Nancy Burton-Wurster
James A. Baker Institute for Animal
  Health
Cornell University
Ithaca, New York 14853

E. Buzás
Institute of Anatomy
University of Medicine
Debrecen, Hungary

Giles V. Campion
Section of Rheumatology
Clinical Research
Hoechst AG Werk Kalle-Albert
P.O. Box 3540
D-6200 Wiesbaden 12, Federal Republic
  of Germany

T. A. Carpenter
University of Cambridge
School of Clinical Medicine
Cambridge CB2 2PZ, United Kingdom

Bruce Caterson
Division of Orthopaedic Surgery
University of North Carolina at Chapel
  Hill
CB# 7055
266 Burnett-Womack Building
Chapel Hill, North Carolina 27599

F. Chaminade
CNRS URA. 584
Hopital des Enfants-Malades
Paris, France

L. Chandrasekaran
Department of BioStructure and
    Function
School of Dental Medicine
University of Connecticut Health Center
Farmington, Connecticut 06030

H. U. Choi
Orthopedic Research
Montefiore Medical Center
Bronx, New York 10467

C. Collins
Department of Pathology
University of Bristol, Bristol BS8 1TD,
United Kingdom

T. Derek V. Cooke
Department of Surgery
Queen's University
Kingston Ontario
Kingston, Ontario, Canada

G. Cs-Szabó
Biochemistry Division
Kennedy Institute of Rheumatology
London, United Kingdom

Janet Cushnaghan
Rheumatology Unit
Bristol Royal Infirmary
Marlborough Street
Bristol BS2 8HW, United Kingdom

Ben J. de Vries
Department of Rheumatology
University Hospital Nijmegen
6525 GA Nijmegen, The Netherlands

Rita Dharmavaram
Departments of Medicine and
    Biochemistry and Molecular Biology
Jefferson Medical College
Thomas Jefferson University
Philadelphia, Pennsylvania 19107

Paul A. Dieppe
Rheumatology Unit
Bristol Royal Infirmary
Marlborough Street
Bristol BS2 8HW, United Kingdom

John T. Dingle
Department of Physiology
Strangeways Research Laboratory
Worts Causeway
Cambridge CB1 4RN, United Kingdom

T. Do
CNRS URA. 584
Hopital des Enfants-Malades
Paris, France

D. A. Dossing
Department of Biochemistry
Rush-Presbyterian-St. Luke's Medical
    Center
Chicago, Illinois 60612

Jayesh Dudhia
Biochemistry Division
Kennedy Institute of Rheumatology
Bute Gardens
Hammersmith, London W6 7DW,
    United Kingdom

Eric F. Eikenberry
Department of Pathology
Robert Wood Johnson Medical School
UMDNJ
Piscataway, New Jersey 08854

C. J. Elson
Department of Pathology and
    Microbiology
University of Bristol
Bristol BS8 1TD, United Kingdom

R. G. Evans
Department of Pathology
University of Bristol, Bristol BS8 1TD,
United Kingdom

David R. Eyre
Department of Orthopaedics
University of Washington
RK-10
Seattle, Washington 98195

Amanda J. Fosang
Department of Medicine
University of Melbourne
Royal Melbourne Hospital
Royal Parade
Parkville 3050, Australia

C. Franzelius
Institute fur Pharmakologie und
*   Toxikologie*
Universitat Erlangen-Nürnberg
Universitatssrasse 22
8520 Erlangen, Federal Republic of
*   Germany*

P. M. Freeman
Departments of Biochemistry and
*   Orthopedic Surgery*
Rush-Presbyterian-St. Luke's Medical
*   Center*
Chicago, Illinois 60612

Kanji Fukuda
Department of Biochemistry
Rush Medical College
Rush-Presbyterian-St. Luke's Medical
*   Center*
1653 West Congress Parkway
Chicago, Illinois 60612

Cs. Fülöp
Department of Biochemistry
Rush-Presbyterian-St. Luke's Medical
*   Center*
Chicago, Illinois 60612, and
Institute of Anatomy
University of Medicine
Debrecen, Hungary

Suresh J. Gadher
Department of Arthritis Research
Roussel Research Laboratories
Kingfisher Drive
Swindon, Wiltshire SN3 5BZ, United
*   Kingdom*

C. R. Gardner
Department of Biological Research
Roussel Laboratories
Kingfisher Drive
Covingham
Swindon, Wiltshire SN3 532, United
*   Kingdom*

P. Garred
Institute of Immunology and
*   Rheumatology*
Rikshospitalet
Oslo, Norway

Robert Garrone
Laboratoire de Cytologie Moleculaire
UPR CNRS 412
Institut de Biologie et Chimie des
*   Proteines*
69622 Villeurbanne Cedex, France

Steven H. Gitelis
Department of Orthopedic Surgery
Rush Medical College
Rush-Presbyterian-St. Luke's Medical
*   Center*
Chicago, Illinois 60612

Tibor T. Glant
Departments of Biochemistry and
*   Orthopedic Surgery*
Rush-Presbyterian-St. Luke's Medical
*   Center*
1653 West Congress Parkway
Chicago, Illinois 60612

Daphne C. L. Goh
Department of Biochemistry
Charing Cross and Westminster
*   Medical School*
Fulham Palace Road
London W6 8RF, United Kingdom

Mary B. Goldring
Massachusetts General Hospital and
Harvard University Medical School
Boston, Massachusetts 02129

Alan J. Grodzinsky
Department of Electrical Engineering
    and Computer Science
Massachusetts Institute of Technology
Harvard-MIT Division of Health
    Sciences and Technology
MIT Room 38-377
Cambridge, Massachusetts 02139

Andrew Hall
University Laboratory of Physiology
Oxford University
Parks Road
Oxford OX1 3PT, United Kingdom

Laurance D. Hall
School of Clinical Medicine
University of Cambridge
Robinson Way
Cambridge CB2 2PZ, United Kingdom

Christopher J. Handley
Department of Biochemistry
Monash University
Clayton, Victoria 3168, Australia

Timothy E. Hardingham
Biochemistry Division
Kennedy Institute of Rheumatology
Bute Gardens
Hammersmith, London W67DW,
    United Kingdom

Vincent C. Hascall
Bone Research Branch
National Institute of Dental Research
National Institutes of Health
Building 30
Room 106
Bethesda, Maryland 20892

Hans J. Häuselmann
Department of Biochemistry
Rush Medical College
Rush-Presbyterian-St. Luke's Medical
    Center
1653 West Congress Parkway
Chicago, Illinois 60612

Heinz Hausser
Institute of Physiological Chemistry and
    Pathophysiology
Westfälische Wilhelms-Universität
Waldeyerstr. 15
D-4400 Münster, Federal Republic of
    Germany

Taro Hayakawa
Department of Biochemistry
School of Dentistry
Aichi-Gakuin University
Chikusa-ku
Nagoya, Aichi, 464 Japan

Hans-Hubert Heilmann
Department of Orthopedic Surgery
Medical School Charite
Humboldt University of Berlin
Scharnhorststr. 3
0-1040 Berlin, Federal Republic of
    Germany

Dick K. Heinegård
Department of Medical and
    Physiological Chemistry
Lund University
P.O. Box 94
S-22100 Lund, Sweden

H. J. Helminen
Department of Anatomy
University of Kuopio
SF-70211 Kuopio, Finland

G. Hetland
Institute of Immunology and
    Rheumatology
Rikshospitalet
Oslo, Norway

R. J. Hodgson
University of Cambridge
School of Clinical Medicine
Cambridge CB2 2PZ, United Kingdom

David C. Howell
Arthritis Division
Department of Medicine
University of Miami
School of Medicine
1600 West 10th Avenue
Miami, Florida 33101

Clare E. Hughes
Department of Surgery
University of North Carolina at Chapel
* Hill*
CB# 7055 Burnett-Womack Building
Chapel Hill, North Carolina 27599

Ernst B. Hunziker
M. E. Müller Institute for Biomechanics
University of Bern
Murtenstrasse 35
3010 Bern, Switzerland

Mirna Z. Ilic
Department of Biochemistry
Monash University
Clayton, Victoria 3168, Australia

Yasuaki Inamori
Department of Orthopaedic Surgery
National Defense Medical College
3-2 Namiki
Tokorozawa, Saitama, 359 Japan

S. Ismaiel
Department of Pathology
University of Bristol
Bristol BS8 1TD, United Kingdom

Petr Issaev
Institute of Rheumatology Branch
USSR-AMS
Volgograd, Russia

M. K. Jasani
Ciba-Geigy
556 Morris Avenue
Summit, New Jersey 07901

Sergio A. Jimenez
Departments of Medicine and
* Rheumatology Research*
Jefferson Medical College
Thomas Jefferson University
233 South 10th Street
Room 509
Bluemle Life Sciences Building
Philadelphia, Pennsylvania 19107

C. Johnson
Department of Biochemistry
Rush Medical College
Rush-Presbyterian-St. Luke's Medical
* Center*
Chicago, Illinois 60612

T. Johnson
Orthopedic Research
Montefiore Medical Center
Bronx, New York 10467

Brian Johnstone
Department of Surgery
University of North Carolina at Chapel
* Hill*
CB# 7055 Burnett-Womack Building
Chapel Hill, North Carolina 27599

Leo A. B. Joosten
Department of Rheumatology
University Hospital Nijmegen
6525 GA Nijmegen, The Netherlands

Jukka S. Jurvelin
Department of Anatomy
University of Kuopio
P.O. Box 1627
SF-70211 Kuopio, Finland

Alfred Karbowski
Orthopedic University Hospital
Westfälische Wilhelms-Universität
Albert-Schweitzer
Str. 33
D-4400 Münster, Federal Republic of
  Germany

R. Kierse
Anatomische Anstalt
Ludwig-Maximilians-Universität
8000 München 2, Federal Republic of
  Germany

Toshiyuki Kikuchi
Department of Orthopaedic Surgery
National Defense Medical College
3-2 Namiki
Tokorozawa, Saitama, 359 Japan

Koji Kimata
Institute for Molecular Science of
  Medicine
Aichi Medical University
Yazako, Nagakute
Aichi 480-11, Japan

James H. Kimura
Breech Research Laboratory
Bone and Joint Center
Henry Ford Hospital
2799 West Grand Boulevard
Detroit, Michigan 48202

T. Kirsch
Max-Planck-Society
Clinical Research Units for
  Rheumatology
University of Erlangen-Nürnberg
Schwabachanlage 10
8520 Erlangen, Federal Republic of
  Germany

Ilkka Kiviranta
Departments of Anatomy and Surgery
University of Kuopio
P.O. Box 1627
SF-70211 Kuopio, Finland

Robert Knowlton
Jefferson Institute of Molecular
  Medicine
Jefferson Medical College
Thomas Jefferson University
Philadelphia, Pennsylvania 19107

Hans Kresse
Institute of Physiological Chemistry and
  Pathophysiology
Westfälische Wilhelms-Universität
Waldeyerstrasse 15
D-4400 Münster, Federal Republic of
  Germany

Klaus E. Kuettner
Departments of Biochemistry and
  Orthopedic Surgery
Rush Medical College
Rush-Presbyterian-St. Luke's Medical
  Center
1653 West Congress Parkway
Chicago, Illinois 60612

T. M. Laue
Department of Biochemistry
University of New Hampshire
Durham, New Hampshire 03824

Mary Ellen Lenz
Department of Biochemistry
Rush Medical College
Rush-Presbyterian-St. Luke's Medical
  Center
1653 West Congress Parkway
Chicago, Illinois 60612

J. Rodney Levick
Department of Physiology
St. George's Hospital Medical School
University of London
Granmer Terrace, Tooting
London SW17 ORE, United Kingdom

Klaus Lindenhayn
Department of Orthopedic Surgery
Humboldt University of Berlin
Medical School Charite
Berlin, Federal Republic of Germany

L. Stefan Lohmander
Department of Orthopedics
University Hospital
University of Lund
S-22185 Lund, Sweden

Dennis A. Lowther
Department of Biochemistry
Monash University
Wellington Road
Clayton, Victoria 3168, Australia

George Lust
James A. Baker Institute for Animal
   Health
Cornell University
Ithaca, New York 14853

J. A. Lynch
Division of Anatomy
UMDS
Guy's Hospital
London, United Kingdom

D. Lyons
Department of Biochemistry
University of New Hampshire
Durham, New Hampshire 03824

D. G. Macfarlane
Department of Rheumatology
Kent & Sussex Hospital
Tunbridge Wells
Kent, United Kingdom

Frédéric Mallein-Gerin
Laboratoire de Cytologie Moleculaire
UPR CNRS 412
Institut de Biologie et Chimie des
   Proteines
69622 Villeurbanne Cedex, France

Daniel H. Manicourt
Department of Internal Medicine
Rheumatology Unit
St. Luc University Hospital
Louvain University
Avenue Hippocrate 10 UCL 5390
1200 Brussels, Belgium

P. Maroteaux
CNRS URA. 584
Hopital des Enfants-Malades
Paris, France

Alice Maroudas
Department of Biomedical Engineering
Julius Silver Institutes
Technion-Israel Institute of Technology
Kiryat Technion
Haifa 32000, Israel

Vladislav F. Martemjanow
Institute of Rheumatology Branch
USSR-AMS
Volgograd, Russia

Roger M. Mason
Department of Biochemistry
Charing Cross and Westminster
   Medical School
London W6 8RF, United Kingdom

Tim McAlindon
Rheumatology Unit
Bristol Royal Infirmary
Malborough Street
Bristol BS2, 8HW, United Kingdom

F. McCrae
Rheumatology Unit
Bristol Royal Infirmary
Bristol BS2 8HW, United Kingdom

Alison M. McLaren
Rowett Research Institute
Bucksburn, Aberdeen, United Kingdom

Markus Mendler
Laboratorium für Biochemie I
Eidgenössiche Technische Hochschule
8092 Zurich, Switzerland

James F. S. Middleton
Strangeway's Research Laboratory
Worts Causeway
Cambridge CB1 4RN, United Kingdom

K. Mikecz
Departments of Biochemistry and
  Orthopedic Surgery
Rush-Presbyterian-St. Luke's Medical
  Center
Chicago, Illinois 60612

Peter Miller
Roussel Laboratories
Kingfisher Drive
Covingham, Swindon
Wiltshire SN3 5B2, United Kingdom

Meng Tuck Mok
Department of Biochemistry
Monash University
Clayton, Victoria 3168, Australia

J. Mollenhauer
Institute für Pharmakologie und
  Toxikologie
Universitat Erlangen-Nürnberg
8520 Erlangen, Federal Republic of
  Germany

Teresa I. Morales
Bone Research Branch
National Institute of Dental Research
National Institutes of Health
Bethesda, Maryland 20892

John S. Mort
Shriners Hospital for Crippled Children
1529 Cedar Avenue
Montreal, Quebec, H3G 1A6 Canada

Helen M. Muir
Department of Biochemistry
Charing Cross Hospital
Hammersmith
London W68RF, England

Francisco J. Müller
Department of Medicine
Miami University
School of Medicine
P.O. Box 016960
Coral Gables, Florida 33101

Magdalena Müller-Gerbl
Department of Anatomy
Ludwig Maximilian-Universität
  München
Pettenkoferstr 11
8000 Munchen 2, Federal Republic of
  Germany

R. N. Natarajan
Departments of Biochemistry and
  Orthopedic Surgery
Rush-Presbyterian-St. Luke's Medical
  Center
Chicago, Illinois 60612

A. Nerlich
Institute of Pathology
University of Munich
8000 München 2, Federal Republic of
  Germany

Quang Nguyen
Joint Diseases Laboratory
Shriners Hospital for Crippled Children
1529 Cedar Avenue
Montreal, Quebec H3G 1AG, Canada

Phyllis Nicol
Rowett Research Institute
Bucksburn, Aberdeen, United Kingdom

Yoshihiro Nishida
Nagoya University
School of Medicine
Chikusa
Nagoya, Aichi, 466 Japan

Birgit Ober
Institute of Physiological Chemistry and
  Pathophysiology
Westfälische Wilhelms-Universität
Waldeyerstr. 15
D-4400 Münster, Federal Republic of
  Germany

Theodore R. Oegema, Jr.
Department of Orthopaedic Surgery
University of Minnesota
Box 310 UMHC
420 Delaware Street, SE
Minneapolis, Minnesota 55455

Monika Oestensen
Department of Rheumatology
University Hospital of Trondheim
Olav Kyrresgate 17
7006 Trondheim, Norway

R. Oettmeier
Department of Orthopaedics
University of Jena
0-6900 Jena, Federal Republic of
    Germany

Bjorn R. Olsen
Department of Anatomy and Cellular
    Biology
Harvard Medical School
220 Longwood Avenue
Boston, Massachusetts 02115

Dennis R. Ongchi
Department of Internal Medicine
Section of Rheumatology
Rush Medical College
Rush-Presbyterian-St. Luke's Medical
    Center
1653 West Congress Parkway
Chicago, Illinois 60612

Babatunde O. Oyajobi
Department of Human Metabolism and
    Clinical Biochemistry
University of Sheffield Medical School
Beech Hill Road
Sheffield, South Yorkshire S10 2RX,
    United Kingdom

M. F. Pearse
Department of Pathology
University of Bristol
Bristol BS8 1TD, United Kingdom

Jacques G. Peyron
Centre de Rhumatologie
Hopital de la Pitie
75013 Paris, France

Edson Rosa Pimentel
Department of Medical and
    Physiological Chemistry
P.O. Box 94
S-221 00 Lund, Sweden

Julio C. Pita
Department of Medicine
University of Miami
School of Medicine
P.O. Box 016960
Coral Gables, Florida 33101

Anna H. K. Plaas
Department of Orthopaedic Research
Shriner's Hospital for Crippled Children
12502 North Pine Drive
Tampa, Florida 33612-9499

F. M. Ponsford
Department of Pathology
University of Bristol, Bristol BS8 1TD,
    United Kingdom

C. Anthony Poole
Department of Anatomy
School of Medicine
University of Auckland
Auckland, New Zealand

Orna Popper
Department of Biomedical Engineering
Julius Silver Institutes
Technion-Israel Institute of Technology
Kiryat Technion
Haifa, 32000, Israel

Kenneth P. H. Pritzker
Departments of Pathology and Surgery
Mount Sinai Hospital
University of Toronto
600 University Avenue
Toronto, Ontario M5G 1X5, Canada

Darwin J. Prockop
Departments of Medicine and Molecular
  Biology
Jefferson Institute of Molecular
  Medicine
Jefferson Medical College
Thomas Jefferson University
Philadelphia, Pennsylvania 19107

Wolfhart Puhl
Orthopädische Klinik
Akademisches Krankenhaus der
  Universität Ulm
Oberer Eselsberg 45
7900 Ulm, Federal Rebublic of
  Germany

R. Putz
Anatomische Anstalt
Ludwig-Maximilians-Universität
8000 Munchen 2, Federal Republic of
  Germany

Ruth X. Raiss
Pharmacologic Research
Hoechst AG Werk Kalle-Albert
P.O. Box 3540
D-6200 Wiesbaden, Federal Republic of
  Germany

Anthony Ratcliffe
Department of Orthopaedic Surgery
Columbia University
College of Physicians and Surgeons
630 West 168th Street
New York, New York 10032

Anthony Reginato
Departments of Medicine and
  Biochemistry and Molecular Biology
Jefferson Medical College
Thomas Jefferson University
Philadelphia, Pennsylvania 19107

E. Reichenberger
Max-Planck-Society
Clinical Research Units for
  Rheumatology
University of Erlangen-Nürnberg
Schwabachanlage 10
8520 Erlangen, Federal Republic of
  Germany

Simon P. Robins
Biochemical Sciences Division
Rowett Research Institute
Greenburn Road
Bucksburn, Aberdeen AB295B, United
  Kingdom

H. Clem Robinson
Department of Biochemistry
Monash University
Clayton, Victoria 3168, Australia

Lawrence C. Rosenberg
Orthopaedic Research Laboratory
Montefiore Medical Center
111 East 210th Street
Bronx, New York 10467

A. J. Roth
Department of Orthopaedics
University of Jena,
0-6900 Jena, Federal Republic of
  Germany

Peter J. Roughley
Genetics Unit
Shriner's Hospital for Crippled Children
1529 Cedar Avenue
Montreal, Quebec, Canada H3G 1RG

R. G. G. Russell
Departments of Human Metabolism and
  Clinical Biochemistry
University of Sheffield Medical School
Beech Hill Road
Sheffield S10 2RX, United Kingdom

Anna-Marja Säämänen
Department of Anatomy
University of Kuopio
P.O. Box 6
SF-70211 Kuopio, Finland

Robert L.-Y. Sah
Harvard-MIT Division of Health
  Sciences and Technology
77 Massachusetts Avenue
Room 38-377
Cambridge, Massachusetts 02139

Linda J. Sandell
Departments of Orthopaedics and
  Biochemistry
University of Washington and Veterans
  Administration Medical Center
1660 South Columbian Way
Seattle, Washington 98108

John D. Sandy
Department of Biochemistry and
  Molecular Biology
University of South Florida
Shriner's Hospital for Crippled Children
12502 North Pine Drive
Tampa, Florida 33612

Shinichi Satsuma
Department of Surgery
Orthopaedic Division
Queen's University
Kingston, Ontario, Canada K7L 3N6

Ryuichi Saura
Department of Orthopaedic Surgery
Kobe University School of Medicine
Chuo-ku, Kobe 650, Japan

Rudolf Schleyerbach
Department of Pharmacological
  Research
Hoechst AG Werk Kalle-Albert
6200 Weisbaden 12
Wiesbaden, Federal Republic of
  Germany

T. M. Schmid
Department of Biochemistry
Rush Medical College
Rush-Presbyterian-St. Luke's Medical
  Center
Chicago, Illinois 60612

Rosa Schneiderman
Department of Biomedical Engineering
Julius Silver Institutes
Technion-Israel Institute of Technology
Kiryat Technion
Haifa 32000, Israel

Thomas J. Schnitzer
Department of Internal Medicine
Section of Rheumatology
Rush-Presbyterian-St. Luke's Medical
  Center
1653 West Congress Parkway
Chicago, Illinois 60612

A. Schulmeister
Institute für Pharmakologie und
  Toxikologie
Universität Erlangen-Nürnberg
Universitatssrasse 22
8520 Erlangen, Federal Republic of
  Germany

Barbara L. Schumacher
Department of Biochemistry
Rush Medical College
Rush-Presbyterian-St. Luke's Medical
  Center
1653 West Congress Parkway
Chicago, Illinois 60612

Allan Scudamore
Department of Surgery
Orthopaedic Division
Queen's University
Kingston, Ontario, Canada K7L 3N6

M. P. Seed
Roussel Laboratories
Kingfisher Drive
Swindon, Wiltshire SN3 532, United
  Kingdom

Markus J. Seibel
Department of Internal Medicine
Bone Research Laboratories
University of Heidelberg, Federal
  Republic of Germany

Masayuki Shinmei
Department of Orthopaedic Surgery
National Defense Medical College
3-2 Namiki
Tokorozawa, Saitman, Japan 359

Tamayuki Shinomura
Institute for Molecular Science of
  Medicine
Aichi Medical University
Yazako
Nagakute, Aichi, 480-11 Japan

Absorn Sriratana
Department of Biochemistry
Monash University
Wellington Road
Clayton, Victoria 3168, Australia

Ritta Stanescu
URA 584, CNRS
Hopital des Enfants Malades
149, Rue de Sevres
75015 Paris, France

Victor Stanescu
URA 584, CNRS
Hopital des Enfants Malades
149, Rue de Sevres
75015 Paris, France

Juergen Steinmeyer
Department of Pharmacology and
  Toxicology
University of Bonn
5300 Bonn, Federal Republic of
  Germany

R. Stiansen
Institute of Immunology and
  Rheumatology
Rikshospitalet
Oslo, Norway

H. Stöß
Institute of Pathology
University of Erlangen-Nürnberg
Krankenhausstr. 8–10
8520 Erlangen, Federal Republic of
  Germany

Barry M. E. Sweet
Department of Orthopaedic Surgery
Medical School
University of the Witwatersrand
Parktown, Johannesburg, South Africa

Markku I. Tammi
Department of Anatomy
University of Kuopio
P.O. Box 1627
SF-70211 Kuopio, Finland

L.-H. Tang
Montefiore Medical Center
Bronx, New York and
University of New Hampshire
Durham, New Hampshire 27710

Marvin L. Tanzer
Department of BioStructure and
  Function
University of Connecticut Health Center
263 Farmington Avenue
Farmington, Connecticut 06030

Roby C. Thompson, Jr.
Department of Orthopaedic Surgery
University of Minnesota
Box 492 UMHC
420 Delaware Street, SE
Minneapolis, Minnesota 55455

T. A. Thomson
Roussel Laboratories
Kingfisher Drive
Swindon, Wiltshire SN3 532, United
  Kingdom

Eugene J-M. A. Thonar
*Departments of Biochemistry and
    Internal Medicine
Section of Rheumatology
Rush Medical College
Rush-Presbyterian-St. Luke's Medical
    Center
1653 West Congress Parkway
Chicago, Illinois 60612*

Jenny A. Tyler
*Department of Tissue Physiology
Strangeways Research Laboratory
Worts Causeway
Cambridge CB1 4RN, United Kingdom*

Daniel Uebelhart
*Departments of Biochemistry and
    Internal Medicine
Section of Rheumatology
Rush Medical College
Rush-Presbyterian-St. Luke's Medical
    Center
1653 West Congress Parkway
Chicago, Illinois 60612*

Jill Urban
*University Laboratory of Physiology
Oxford University
Parks Road
Oxford OX1 3PT, United Kingdom*

Martin A. F. J. van de Laar
*Research Laboratory
Jan van Breemen Institute
Dr. J. van Breemenstraat 2
1056 AB Amsterdam, The Netherlands*

Fons A. J. van de Loo
*Department of Rheumatology
University Hospital Nijmegen
6525 GA Nijmegen, The Netherlands*

Wim B. van den Berg
*Department of Rheumatology
University Hospital
Geert Grooteplein Zuid
6525 GA Nijmegen, The Netherlands*

Jan K. van der Korst
*Research Laboratory
Jan van Breemen Institute
Dr. J. van Breemenstraat 2
1056 AB Amsterdam, The Netherlands*

Peter M. van der Kraan
*Department of Rheumatology
University Hospital Nijmegen
6525 GA Nijmegen, The Netherlands*

Michel van der Rest
*Laboratoire de Cytologie Moleculaire
UPR CNRS 412
Institut de Biologie et Chimie des
    Proteines
69622 Villeurbanne Cedex, France*

Robert J. van de Stadt
*Research Laboratory
Jan van Breemen Institute
Dr. J. van Breemenstraat 2
1056 AB Amsterdam, The Netherlands*

G. P. Jos van Kampen
*Research Laboratory
Jan ven Breemen Institute
Dr. J. van Breemenstraat 2
1056 AB Amsterdam, The Netherlands*

Eric Vignon
*Department of Rhumatologie
Hopital Edouard Herriot
Pavillon F
Place d'Arsonval
69437 Lyon, Cedex 03, France*

Elly L. Vitters
Department of Rheumatology
University Hospital Nijmegen
6525 GA Nijmegen, The Netherlands

Klaus von der Mark
Max-Planck-Society
Clinical Research Groups for
* Rheumatology*
University of Erlangen-Nürnberg
Schwabachanlage 10
8520 Erlangen, Federal Republic of
* Germany*

Zena Werb
Laboratory of Radiobiology and
* Environmental Health*
University of California
LR102
San Francisco, California 94143

G. Weseloh
Orthopedical Clinics
University of Erlangen-Nürnberg
Rathsbergerstr. 57
8520 Erlangen, Federal Republic of
* Germany*

Kaspar H. Winterhalter
Laboratorium für Biochemie I
Eidgenössiche Technische Hochschule
8092 Zurich, Switzerland

James M. Williams
Departments of Anatomy, Biochemistry,
* and Internal Medicine*
Rush Medical College
Rush-Presbyterian-St. Luke's Medical
* Center*
1653 West Congress Parkway
Chicago, Illinois 60612

Petra Witsch-Prehm
Institute of Physiological Chemistry and
* Pathophysiology*
Westfälische Wilhelms-Universität
Waldeyerstr. 15
D-4400 Münster, Federal Republic of
* Germany*

Shirley Wong-Palms
Department of Biochemistry and
* Molecular Biology*
University of South Florida Medical
* School*
Tampa, Florida 33612

P. Woods
Department of Orthopaedics
University of Washington
RK-10
Seattle, Washington 98195

D. E. Woolley
University Hospital of South Manchester
Manchester, United Kingdom

S. F. Wotton
A.F.R.C. Institute of Food Research
Bristol, United Kingdom

Jiangtao Wu
Departments of Orthopaedics and
* Biochemistry*
University of Washington and Veterans
* Administration Medical Center*
Seattle, Washington 98108

Jiann-Jiu Wu
Department of Orthopaedics
University of Washington
RK-10
Seattle, Washington 98195

Rina Yamin
Massachusetts General Hospital and
Harvard University Medical School
Boston, Massachusetts 02129

Yasuo Yoshihara
Department of Orthopedic Surgery
National Defense Medical College
3-2 Namiki
Tokorozawa, Saitama 359, Japan

Oliver Zamparo
Departments of Orthopaedics and
   Biochemistry
University of Washington and Veterans
   Administration Medical Center
Seattle, Washington 98108

Alexander Zborovsky
Department of Internal Diseases
Institute of Rheumatology Branch
Academy of Medical Sciences
Volgograd State Medical Institute
76 Zemliachki Street
Volgograd, Russia

Opening Address

It is an honor and a pleasure for me as a representative of Pharmaceutical Research of Hoechst to welcome so many distinguished scientists from all over the world to the International Workshop on Articular Cartilage and Osteoarthritis.

The 1985 International Workshop on Articular Cartilage Biochemistry is a stepping stone to this present meeting, which has a much wider scope with the introduction of pathophysiological, pharmacological, and clinical aspects of articular cartilage and joint physiology. One important result of the 1985 meeting was that many contacts at the basic research level between ourselves and other research groups were strengthened and new investigative directions were initiated. In drug development research, it is necessary to attack complex disease processes such as osteoarthritis with a multi-disciplinary approach; but it is also clear that we require the interaction of the specialists from university and clinical settings to realize the final goal, therapeutic success. The interactions can only occur through a workshop of this kind, which is probably unique in that it covers osteoarthritis from molecular biology to clinical research. We are sponsoring this workshop with Roussel Laboratories (Swindon, England), which is novel in the history of the Hoechst workshops. It reflects the beginning of fruitful research cooperation in the field of rheumatology which we are now conducting with our colleagues from Roussel.

I would like to take the opportunity to thank Klaus Kuettner, Vincent Hascall, and Jacques Peyron for their initiative and efforts in planning and organizing this meeting; Dr. Ruth Raiss who took much of the weight and responsibility from my shoulders in order to organize the Hoechst part of the workshop; Albert Roussel, Pharma Wiesbaden, Roussel Uclaf Paris, and Roussel Laboratories Swindon for their support, without which this workshop would simply not have taken place. Finally, I appreciate the co-sponsorship of the World Health Organization.

It remains for me to wish you a fruitful and intellectually stimulating time in Wiesbaden.

Dr. Rudolf Schleyerbach
Hoechst Werk Kalle-Albert
Wiesbaden, Federal Republic of Germany

Opening Address

I am greatly honored to be invited to address the International Workshop on Articular Cartilage and Osteoarthritis on behalf of the Director General of the World Health Organization (WHO). This workshop focuses on basic mechanisms of osteoarthritis, the most prevalent rheumatic disease among musculoskeletal disorders. In the United States, about one-third of the adult population suffers from various musculoskeletal signs or symptoms, and rheumatic diseases had cost approximately 21 billion dollars in 1980, an amount equal to 1% of the United States gross national product. These conditions are responsible for 5% of all hospital discharges, 10% of all hospital procedures, and 9% of all physician calls. Chronic rheumatic conditions are not only a burden to developed countries; they equally affect developing countries. For example, the World Health Organization/International League Against Rheumatism Joint Community-Oriented Program for the Control of Rheumatic Diseases has found that the prevalence of rheumatic complaints is similar in Indonesia and Australia. The present situation regarding prevention and control of osteoarthritis is unsatisfactory due to a lack of appropriate knowledge of the etiology and pathogenesis of the disease, especially in the field of cartilage metabolism which plays a key role in understanding osteoarthritis.

Without understanding of the mechanisms of disease development and progression, no effective preventive strategy can be elaborated. To stimulate research in the field of cartilage metabolism and other etiopathological aspects of osteoarthritis, WHO is in the process of designing a new collaborating center in the field of osteoarthritis at the Department of Biochemistry, Rush-Presbyterian-St. Luke's Medical Center, Chicago, Illinois, USA. This center will collaborate with WHO in the development and improvement of biochemical predictors of osteoarthritis and in the development of cartilage metabolic markers for the possible subclassification of the disease's entities. It will allow WHO to organize a prospective epidemiological study for the early detection of degenerative joint diseases, for the selection of high risk groups, and the effective prevention of osteoarthritis. This is in accordance with the aim of the WHO rheumatic diseases program: to reduce the incidence, prevalence, morbidity, mortality, and disability of these diseases.

Allow me to express my hope that this particular workshop, in which the advances in fundamental research will be reviewed, will contribute to a better understanding of the problems mentioned above. I am confident that the outcome will be of great value to biomedical researchers and to health care workers throughout the world.

Dr. Nicolai G. Khaltaev
Acting Chief
Diabetes and other Noncommunical Diseases
World Health Organization, Geneva, Switzerland

Opening Address

I am glad to convey greetings to this distinguished audience on behalf of Dr. Heinz Riesenhuber, the General Minister for Research and Technology. In particular, I am pleased to welcome Dr. Khaltaev of the World Health Organization. The Federal Ministry for Research and Technology is very grateful to HOECHST and Roussel UCLAF for cosponsoring this international workshop.

Let me say some words on the ministry's view of the subject matter of this workshop. Many people suffer from degenerative deformation of the joints; about 25% of patients 50 years of age or older experience great pain and are often severely handicapped. These facts alone reveal the major importance of this disease in view of health policy. In addition, there is a tremendous financial burden on the national economy to be considered, as merely in the Federal Republic of Germany, this disease accounts for approximately 20 billion Deutschmarks per year. Despite these facts, the importance of arthrosis in relation to diseases with a more dramatic course such as cancer, diabetes, or inflammatory rheumatic diseases is generally underestimated by the public. In addition to this lack of awareness, relevant research occupies a comparatively modest position among research priorities. It should be noted that with regard to research promotion by the Federal Ministry for Research and Technology, to date requests for funds for research on arthrosis have been extremely few in comparison with the number of requests for funds to support research on inflammatory rheumatic diseases. The major importance of arthrosis in view of health policy combined with the urgent need for improved clinical methods, equipment for disease prevention, early diagnosis, and treatment of this disease make the development of innovative strategies for research in the field an imperative goal. This seems a promising approach, because relevant activities in recent years have shown that research in this complex field is possible and that new methods lead to fresh and highly satisfactory achievements by involving a variety of disciplines. By adopting a comprehensive approach and choosing excellent speakers, the International Workshop on Articular Cartilage and Osteoarthritis provides an outstanding opportunity for the discussion of existing approaches and experience as a basis for international and interdisciplinary communication and for the elaboration of concepts for arthrosis research. The workshop is, therefore, also a challenge whose acceptance entails a great deal of effort. I wish you every success for the completion of your chosen task.

Dr. Hermann Strub
Ministerialdirigent
Federal Ministry for Research and Technology
Bonn, Federal Republic of Germany

Preface

In 1985 our hosts sponsored the first workshop, entitled Articular Cartilage Biochemistry, which resulted in a book with the same name published by Raven Press in early 1986. At that time we decided to mix different disciplines, but keep as the main focus the biochemistry of articular cartilage and its components. Since then, there has been an explosion of information in the field. It is now time to share, in a larger group, the current state of our knowledge at both the basic science and the clinical levels. Cartilage in health and disease remains the center of our discussion.

Articular cartilage covers the ends of long bones and is a shock-absorbing tissue that protects the more rigid underlying bone and provides smooth articulation and bending of the joints during load-bearing and physical activity. The ability of this tissue to change shape rapidly and reversibly, is directly attributable to a resilient, elastic matrix with a high content of highly soluble molecules of large size (proteoglycans), which are entrapped in an insoluble network of fibers (collagen). Proteoglycans, collagens, and other molecules in the tissue are produced by cartilage cells, the chondrocytes. These cells also control, through mechanisms that are not well understood, the synchronized maintenance of the matrix by replacing molecules that are degraded and have lost functionality.

Arthritic diseases, which affect more people than any other ailment, are a major cause of human suffering. Although precise definitions of osteoarthritis are frequently debated, everyone agrees that it involves loss of function of cartilage. Osteoarthritis affects most people in late middle age. In this disease, articular cartilage undergoes a slow progressive degeneration (self destruction), often in many joints. In contrast to rheumatoid arthritis (a chronic inflammatory joint disease) osteoarthritis is a non-inflammatory disease with intermittent inflammatory episodes. Since articular cartilage does not contain nerve endings, the degradation of cartilage in osteoarthritis does not cause pain and thus may progress for some time before it is detected. Even rapidly advancing imaging techniques can only detect pronounced losses of cartilage mass. Therefore, new methods are being developed that permit the detection of cartilage changes in body fluids such as synovial fluid, serum, and urine.

Since articular cartilage can no longer repair itself once the arrangement of the supporting fibers has been disrupted, early detection of abnormal tissue changes is a prerequisite for successful therapeutic intervention. We have to learn more about this complex, fascinating tissue, for with understanding will come those insights and new developments required to begin to prevent or reverse the disease. This book, based on a Workshop held in Wiesbaden, Federal Republic of Germany in May, 1991, provides new knowledge to stimulate all of us to intensify our efforts in understanding normal and abnormal processes as they occur in the articular cartilage.

The cooperation and interdependence between biochemistry, medicine, and pharmacology are crucial for progress, especially in the development of new drugs. Scientific medicine and clinical investigation have opened new avenues to understand the etiopathology of osteoarthritis and point ways for the biochemist and biologist to address new, pressing questions. Answers to these inquiries on the articular cartilage will lead to further expansion in our search for understanding the progression of the disease. With the birth of new knowledge, a part of human suffering may well be alleviated in the future. The goal of this book is to provide investigators with timely new information to follow paths with trail markers through this knowledge, always keeping in mind the patient who is waiting for successful treatment.

Klaus E. Kuettner, Ph.D.
Vincent C. Hascall, Ph.D.

Acknowledgments

The scientific organizers of the Articular Cartilage Biochemistry workshop would like to thank Hoechst Werk Kalle-Albert for providing the supportive "matrix" within which the various scientists were able to interact so effectively and naturally. Our hosts introduced that element of fun and culture surrounding the intensity of the scientific discussions which created a feeling and esprit for the workshop that all who attended will remember. We only hope that the workshop provided our hosts with the background and information that they sought in originally agreeing to sponsor it.

The editors also thank Ms. Jozefa Boros, Kongressagentur, Leverkusen, for the excellent transcription of the workshop presentations.

This acknowledgment for the first Workshop, written in October, 1985, at Hotel Hirschen, Glottertal in the Black Forest, is even more appropriate for the second Workshop. We need only to note that the second Workshop was titled Articular Cartilage and Osteoarthritis, that Ms. Jozefa Boros has renamed her company VICOM (Visual-Communication), that Dr. Ruth Raiss was essential to the scientific organization of the meeting, and that Dr. Jacques Peyron was vital for coordinating the Discussion–Impact of Basic Research on Diagnosis, Understanding and Treatment of Osteoarthritis.

It has indeed been a pleasure to work with Ms. Boros and her outstanding staff as we distilled transcripts of the extensive and stimulating dialogues and debates at the Workshop into the discussion sections of this book. We hope we have preserved the flavor and spontaneity of the originals in the distillation process, and that the participants will forgive us if we "put words in their mouths" that were not exactly what they intended. As in the first workshop we truly feel that these discussions were perhaps the most important part of our scientific "matrix" and hope that the reader will agree.

In closing we want to express our warmest thanks, not only in behalf of ourselves, but also from the organizing committee and all contributors to the workshop, to Dr. Erhard Wolf who gave unprecedented support to this endeavor, which reflects his lifelong commitment to research in arthritis.

Glottertal
Klaus E. Kuettner, Ph.D.
Vince C. Hascall, Ph.D.

Workshop Conference Hoechst Werk Kalle-Albert

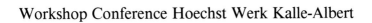

ARTICULAR CARTILAGE AND OSTEOARTHRITIS

Articular Cartilage and Osteoarthritis,
edited by K. Kuettner et al.
Raven Press, Ltd., New York © 1992.

Part I: Structural Components of Cartilage: Proteoglycans

Introduction

Hans Kresse

*Institute of Physiological Chemistry and Pathobiochemistry, University of Münster,
Waldeyerstrasse 15, D-W-4400 Münster, Germany*

Cartilage certainly represents the classic source of proteoglycans; and aggrecan, the most abundant proteoglycan species in cartilage, is the only proteoglycan that has been given detailed attention in modern textbooks on biochemistry and cell biology. In spite of the wealth of investigations on cartilage proteoglycans, the inventory of chondroitin/dermatan sulfate proteoglycans that are components of this tissue still needs to be completed. In addition to aggrecan, two members of the small proteoglycan family, biglycan and decorin, are present (1). Type IX collagen is considered a minor collagen but also is a part-time minor proteoglycan. Further, immunochemical evidence indicates that cartilage contains another member of the small proteoglycan family. This proteoglycan was first found in the secretions of osteosarcoma cells and has tentatively been named centoglycan after the size of its glycosylated core protein (2). A large heterodimeric proteoglycan, bis-derman, is a further candidate as a cartilage proteoglycan (3).

Two chapters here report on the domain structure of aggrecan. While it is evident from rotary-shadowing images that only the N-terminal globular G1 domain binds aggrecan to hyaluronan and link protein, the events that convert the G1 domain from a low to a high affinity hyaluronan-binding form are not yet known. A distinct function of the homologous G2 domain for matrix assembly or proteoglycan metabolism has not yet been elucidated. A functional role of the C-terminal globular G3 domain also has not yet been established, although it consists of a lectin-homologous segment, an EGF-like sequence, and a sequence related to a complement regulatory protein. Most interesting is the observation of alternate usage of exons encoding parts of the G3 domain (4). The C-terminal G3 as well as the G1 domains are often proteolytically removed. Therefore, it will be of great importance to be able to distinguish between aggrecan molecules with or without these domains. Exon-specific marker peptides developed by Dr.

John Sandy will certainly be of great help in approaching these problems. Further unresolved questions concern the regulation of aggrecan expression on the transcriptional and translational level. Furthermore, we are a long way from understanding the factors that regulate the biosynthesis of the glycosaminoglycan moiety; the number, size, and composition of the chains; their changes during development and aging; the local factors responsible for the production of site-specific proteoglycans; and the sequence of events leading to aggrecan fragmentation during the development of osteoarthritis.

Other large proteoglycans play a role in cartilage differentiation. At prechondrogenic stages, chick limb mesenchyme synthesizes a large chondroitin sulfate proteoglycan which is intimately related, and possibly identical, to versican (1). Versican is expressed in most human tissues. It is also a hyaluronan-binding proteoglycan and is composed of domains that suggest the possibility for interactions with growth factors and carbohydrate ligands. Work by Dr. Koji Kimata suggests an important function for this proteoglycan in mesenchymal cell condensation, an event that must take place prior to the onset of chondrogenesis.

A further contribution is a report on the functions of the small dermatan sulfate proteoglycans, biglycan and decorin, in articular cartilage. It has been shown recently that important differences in the expression of these proteoglycans occur in articular regions of developing bones. Some regions, such as subperichondral bone, were rich in biglycan-mRNA whereas other regions were rich in decorin-mRNA and vice versa. Immunolocalization indicated that the interterritorial matrix stained for decorin, and biglycan was found in territorial capsules of chondrocytes (5). It should be noted that the function of biglycan is not yet known, although its core protein is highly homologous to decorin core protein. Decorin, on the other hand binds to interstitial collagen types I and II, thereby influencing collagen fibrillogenesis and/or fibrial organization. It has also been shown that one of the consequences of the interaction of decorin with fibronectin may be an inhibition of fibroblast adhesion to a fibronectin substrate. There is still some controversy about whether the core protein of decorin alone or the intact proteoglycan is responsible for this effect (6). Recently, a role of decorin in the control of cell proliferation has been suggested, possibly because of its ability to bind transforming growth factor-β (1). It will be of great interest to see whether these small proteoglycans are responsible for the observation that superficial defects of articular cartilage do not heal.

REFERENCES

1. Ruoslahti E. Proteoglycans in cell regulation. *J Biol Chem* 1989;264:13369–13372.
2. Schwarz K, Breuer, B, Kresse H. Biosynthesis and properties of a further member of the small chondroitin/dermatan sulfate proteoglycan family. *J Biol Chem* 1990;265:22023–22028.

3. Breuer R, Quentin-Hoffmann E, Cully Z, Götte M, Kresse H. A novel large dermatan sulfate proteoglycan from human fibroblasts. *J Biol Chem* 1991;226:13224–13232.
4. Baldwin CT, Reginato AM, Prockop DJ. A new epidermal growth factor-like domain in the human core protein for the large cartilage-specific proteoglycan. Evidence for alternative splicing of the domain. *J Biol Chem* 1989;264:15747–15750.
5. Bianco P, Fisher LW, Young MF, Termine JD, Gehron Robey P. Expression and localization of the two small proteoglycans biglycan and decorin in developing human skeletal and non-skeletal tissues. *J Histochem Cytochem* 1990;38:1549–1563.
6. Winnemöller M, Schmidt G, Kresse H. Influence of decorin on fibroblast adhesion to fibronectin. *Eur J Cell Biol* 1991;54:10–17.

Articular Cartilage and Osteoarthritis,
edited by K. Kuettner et al.
Raven Press, Ltd., New York © 1992.

1

Aggrecan, the Chondroitin Sulfate/Keratan Sulfate Proteoglycan from Cartilage

Timothy E. Hardingham,* Amanda J. Fosang,†
and Jayesh Dudhia*

**Kennedy Institute of Rheumatology, Hammersmith,
London W6 7DW, United Kingdom;
†Department of Medicine, University of Melbourne,
Royal Melbourne Hospital, Parkville, Victoria, Australia*

Cartilage such as in the articular surface of diarthroidal joints is a highly specialized connective tissue with a biomechanical function which is particularly suited to bearing compressive load (1). It is also the site for the growth and development of all the major long bones of the body. Articular cartilage is not innervated and contains no blood vessels. It consists of a large, highly expanded extracellular matrix that is laid down and maintained by a sparse population of cells, the chondrocytes. The properties of the tissue depend on the structure and organization of the macromolecules in the extracellular matrix. They can largely be understood in terms of the roles of the two major constituents, collagens and proteoglycan. The collagen, principally type II, but also type IX and XI, forms a dense fibrillar network that is embedded in a high concentration of proteoglycan (up to 100 mg/ml). The proteoglycan, because of its polyanionic glycosaminoglycan chains, creates a large osmotic pressure that draws water into the tissue and expands the collagen network. It is the balance between the osmotic swelling pressure of the proteoglycans and the tension in the collagen fibers that results in the compressive properties characteristic of the tissue. Cartilage is thus a fiber-reinforced composite, solid matrix swollen with water. Its biomechanical properties are critically dependent on the integrity of the collagen network and on maintenance of a high concentration of proteoglycans within the matrix. The maintenance of the tissue depends on the continued activity of the chondrocytes. Proteoglycans are slowly turned over even in mature cartilage, and there must be coordinate control of their synthesis and secretion by chondrocytes and their extracellular degradation and turnover in the matrix.

   The most abundant proteoglycan in cartilage is aggrecan, the large aggregating proteoglycan, which contains several features which appear to have evolved for its specialized biomechanical role in cartilage (Fig. 1). The structure consists of

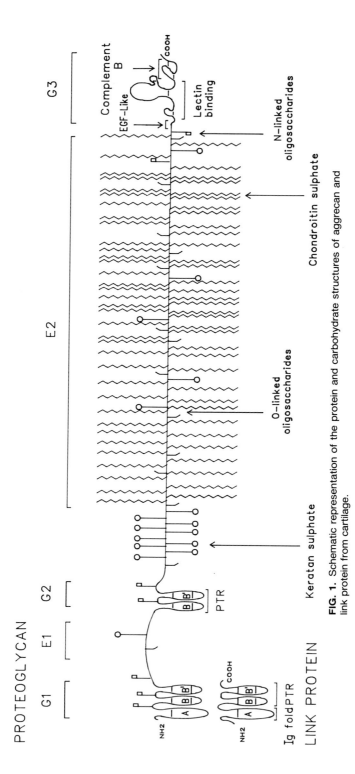

FIG. 1. Schematic representation of the protein and carbohydrate structures of aggrecan and link protein from cartilage.

an extended protein core to which many chondroitin sulfate and keratan sulfate chains (up to 150) are attached. This densely substituted protein with a branched or "bottle brush" structure provides a highly focused concentration of polyanion which is fully hydrated and space-filling. But it has a much lower viscosity and a smaller excluded volume than a long chain unbranched polyanion, such as hyaluronan, of comparable mol. wt. The proteoglycan product when newly secreted by the chondrocyte thus remains to a reasonable extent mobile within the matrix. However, its ability to aggregate by specifically binding to hyaluronan (2) provides an extracellular mechanism for helping to immobilize the proteoglycan within the matrix, and this is assisted by the participation of a separate globular link protein which binds to both proteoglycan and hyaluronan (3,4). Although all the components of the aggregate, proteoglycan, link protein, and hyaluronan are synthesized by the chondrocytes within cartilage, only proteoglycan and link protein become mixed within any intracellular compartments. Whereas proteoglycan and link protein follow the pathways of biosynthesis of other secretory proteins through compartments of the rough (RER) and smooth (Golgi) endoplasmic reticulum, there is evidence that hyaluronan is synthesized at the plasma membrane (5). This is also apparent in chondrocytes, where hyaluronan synthesis is unaffected by monensin at a concentration where the late stages in proteoglycan synthesis are highly inhibited (6). Thus proteoglycan and link protein only have the opportunity to interact with hyaluronan after their secretion by the chondrocyte. There also appears to be a mechanism which limits the initial avidity of proteoglycan-hyaluronan binding following secretion which changes over 1 to 2 days as some structural maturation process occurs (7,8).

For "mature" proteoglycans extracted from cartilage, the affinity for hyaluronan has $K \sim 2 \times 10^{-8}$ M (9), but in the presence of link protein, which forms link protein-proteoglycan and link protein-hyaluronan bonds, the dissociation of proteoglycan from a link stabilized aggregate is not experimentally detectable (4). The dissociation constant must thus be below 1×10^{-11} M. The size of proteoglycan aggregates is determined by a number of parameters (Table 1). Hyaluronan chains can be of very great length, up to mol. wt. 5 to 6×10^6 and 10 μ long. However, most in articular cartilage are in the mol. wt. range 3×10^5

TABLE 1. *Size of proteoglycan aggregates formed with varying amounts of hyaluronan of different chain lengths*

Hyaluronan % (w/w) of proteoglycan	Hyaluronan mol. wt.		
	0.5×10^6	1.0×10^6	5.0×10^6
0.5	50 (11 $\times$ 10^8)[a]	100 (2 $\times$ 10^8)	500 (1 $\times$ 10^9)
1	25 (5 $\times$ 10^7)	50 (1 $\times$ 10^8)	250 (5 $\times$ 10^8)
3	8 (1.6 $\times$ 10^7)	17 (3.4 $\times$ 10^7)	83 (1.75 $\times$ 10^8)
10	2–3 (5 $\times$ 10^6)	5 (1 $\times$ 10^7)	25 (5 $\times$ 10^7)

[a] Average number of proteoglycans bound to each hyaluronan chain and the mass of the aggregate in parentheses.

to 6×10^5 (10), although newly synthesized chains even in mature tissue are considerably larger. The length of the hyaluronan chain determines the number of proteoglycans that can bind to it, but this is also limited by the proximity of adjacent proteoglycans. Steric restrictions separate proteoglycans such that each occupies a length of hyaluronan of about mol. wt. 7,000 at maximum packing density (11). This is seen only when there is an excess of proteoglycan. However, in most tissues there is sufficient hyaluronan to bind all the proteoglycans, and lower packing densities with more space between proteoglycans bound to aggregates are commonly seen in most aggregate preparations reformed from tissue extracts. The size of proteoglycan aggregates thus varies from very small (2–5 proteoglycans) when there is a large excess of hyaluronan and/or it is of low mol. wt., up to exceedingly large (400–800 proteoglycans) when the hyaluronan is of particularly high mol. wt. and there is an excess of proteoglycan (Table 1). These aggregates by criteria such as gel chromatography on Sepharose 2B would all be excluded from the column and therefore appear similar. It requires techniques such as rate zonal sedimentation or quasi-elastic light scattering to distinguish them (12,13). They also have very different rheological flow properties and viscoelastic behavior (14).

AGGRECAN PROTEIN STRUCTURE

Investigation of the protein core structure has shown it to be the product of a single gene copy. It has an interesting multidomain structure (Fig. 1) which, by rotary shadowing electron microscopy, appears as three globular and two extended segments (15). The complete sequence from two species, rat chondrosarcoma (16) and human cartilage (17), have been determined, but partial sequences from several other species are known. The N-terminal region of the protein core contains two globular domains G1 and G2 separated by a 21 nm extended segment (Fig. 2). The major extended region bearing much of the keratan sulfate and all of the chondroitin sulfate appears to be about 260 nm long by rotary shadowing and joins G2 to the C-terminal globular domain G3.

$\longrightarrow$

FIG. 2. Rotary shadowing electron micrograph of the interaction of proteoglycan G1-G2 fragment with hyaluronan and with and without link protein. Proteoglycan G1-G2 fragment (19) was mixed with hyaluronan (**A**) and with hyaluronan and link protein (**B**) in molar ratios G1-G2:HA segment; 1:0.33 and G1-G2:LP:HA segment; 1:0.33:3. The presence of link protein increases the mass density along the central HA filament. The G2 domain remains unbound to the HA in the presence or absence of link protein. *Arrows* indicate possible superhelical regions in the complexes. The segments marked **a** and **b** are compared at high magnification in (**a**) and (**b**) G2 domains extend off the main axis in both preparations. The arrow marks a visible interglobular connection. Scale bars are 100 nm. (From Mörgelin et al., ref. 21, with permission.)

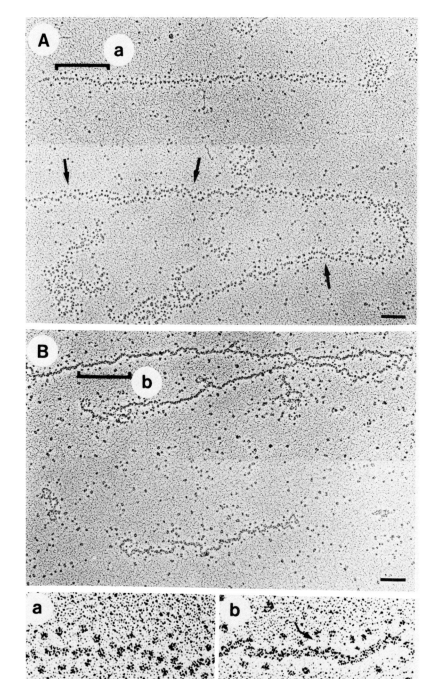

G1 AND G2 DOMAINS

The N-terminal globular G1 and G2 domains have been prepared from pig laryngeal cartilage proteoglycan by proteolytic digestion (18–20). Extensive tryptic digestion of proteoglycan aggregate leaves the G1 domain and link protein largely intact and still bound to hyaluronan. Both the G1 domain and link protein retain their functional properties when prepared in this way (18), although link protein loses a short N-terminal peptide under these conditions. The G1 fragment isolated in this way contains about 25% carbohydrate, some keratan sulfate as well as oligosaccharides, and migrates on SDS polyacrylamide gel electrophoresis (PAGE) with M_r 65 kDa. However, it still appears as a single globular domain by rotary shadowing, binds noncooperatively to hyaluronan, and also interacts with link protein (20).

When proteoglycan aggregates are digested with trypsin under more gentle conditions, a larger fragment can be isolated which contains both G1 and G2 domains (19). This appears as a double globe structure by rotary shadowing electron microscopy, and interaction experiments show that only one domain (G1) is active in binding to hyaluronan and to link protein (21) (Fig. 2). The G2 domain was isolated from the G1-G2 preparation by digestion with V8 proteinase under nondenaturing conditions (19). It contained even more keratan sulfate than the G1 domain and migrated on SDS-PAGE as a broad band of 110 kDa, which is sharpened to 70 kDa after keratanase digestion. Removal of a major part of the keratan sulfate was also necessary for the detection of a protein epitope detected by a monoclonal antibody 1-C-6 (22). The isolated G2 domain also showed no properties of interaction with hyaluronan, link protein, or other soluble matrix proteins.

Investigation of the protein structures of the G1, G2 domains and link protein has shown them to be closely related (23). Both the G1 domain and link protein contain two structural motifs, an N-terminal immunoglobulin-fold (Ig fold) and a tandem repeat sequence characterized by a disulfide bonded double loop structure) (Fig. 2). The G2 domain was also shown to contain a similar tandem repeat sequence, but no Ig fold (Fig. 3).

The Ig-fold motifs of G1 domain and link protein were compared using consensus sequence methods and structure prediction. A pattern of β sheet structure was identified in variable region Ig folds for which the crystal structure was known (24). This established that both contained the basic structural framework of an Ig fold and that they were members of a broad family of proteins containing related Ig-fold motifs. The analysis also showed that the regions in which the Ig folds of G1 domain and link protein with the greatest differences were in sequences comparable to the hypervariable loop regions. These form part of the Ig-fold motif that may be involved in protein-protein interactions and thus might provide the site for binding between G1 domain and link protein (Fig. 3).

No comparable crystal structures are available for the tandem repeat structure. However, a related sequence has been identified in a lymphocyte homing receptor

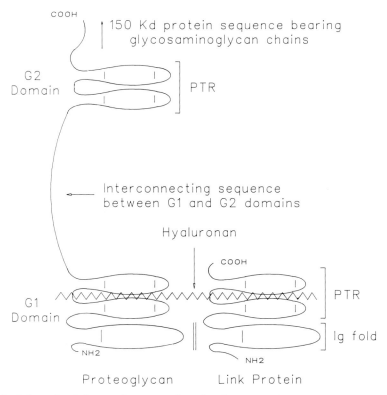

FIG. 3. Schematic of the protein structural motifs of aggrecan G1 and G2 domains and link protein. Tentative assignment of interaction between proteoglycan tandem repeat (PTR) motifs and hyaluronan and between the Ig folds of link protein and the aggrecan G1 domain are also shown.

CD-44, and this has been shown to be a cell-surface receptor for hyaluronan (25) (Fig. 3). The observations support the results from experiments which showed that hyaluronan binding of link protein was associated with the C-terminal tandem repeat region (26) (Fig. 3). The sequence in CD-44 contains only a single loop structure (PR in Fig. 4) and has specificity for hexasaccharide lengths of hyaluronan, whereas G1 domain and link protein both have specificity for decasaccharide lengths. The double loop structure found in G1 domain and link protein may thus be necessary to provide a binding site extending over a longer segment of hyaluronan. This may offer greater stability and/or greater specificity of binding.

The G1 domain of proteoglycan is a "tough" structure (27). It generally resists proteinase attack and thermal denaturation ($t\frac{1}{2}$ 80°C 120 min) and it survives exposure to most solvents, ethanol, acetone, ether, and chaotropic agents such as guanidine HCl, KSCN, and urea. Even after reduction of its disulfide bonds, it renatures under oxidizing conditions with considerable efficiency. The native

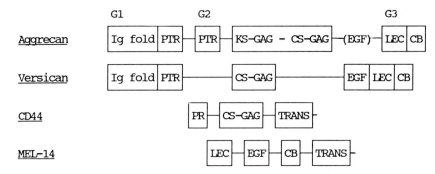

FIG. 4. Comparison of the modular protein structures of aggrecan with the fibroblast proteoglycan versican and cell surface molecules CD44 and MEL-14. Ig fold, immunoglobulin fold; PTR, proteoglycan tandem repeat; PR, single proteoglycan repeat; KS-GAG, keratan sulfate region; CS-GAG, chondroitin sulfate region; EGF, epidermal growth factor-like region; CB, complement B component sequence; TRANS, trans-transmembrane sequence; LEC, lectin-like sequence.

state of the G1 domain is thus very stable and thermodynamically preferred, and perhaps these are appropriate qualities for a matrix protein with a lifetime that may extend to several years within the cartilage matrix.

G3 DOMAIN

The C-terminal G3 domain of aggrecan was only identified when the first cDNA sequences were determined for the protein core (28) and independently at the same time by the use of rotary shadowing electron microscopy to visualize proteoglycans (20,21). The failure to detect it prior to these investigations resulted largely from the difficulty in detecting small differences in protein core size/composition among the heterogenous population of proteoglycans extracted from cartilage, and also because only a fraction of the molecules extracted from cartilage appear to retain an intact G3 domain (21). Many proteoglycans in the tissue appear to have lost some part of their C-terminal structure including the G3 domain, together with varying proportions of the chondroitin sulfate-rich region, presumably as a result of proteolytic action in the matrix. Accurate figures have not yet been published on the content of G3 in purified proteoglycans from different sources, but estimates from rotary shadowing electron microscopy suggest that only 10 to 50% of proteoglycans extracted from cartilage have an intact G3 domain.

The amino acid sequence of the G3 domain has been determined in five different species. It is entirely unrelated to the G1 and G2 domains, but contains elements with sequence similarities to two other protein families (Fig. 3). The first of these is a family of cell surface carbohydrate receptors, a notable member of which is the hepatic asialoglycoprotein receptor, and the second is related to complement B component. However, it has been reported that for human cartilage proteoglycan, an alternatively spliced form lacking the complement B component is the most common (17). There are ten cysteine residues in the G3 domain, and the amino acid sequence is highly conserved (>90%) among cartilage proteoglycans from different species (29). There is also considerable similarity in sequence (~65%) with the corresponding C-terminal domain of the fibroblast proteoglycan, versican (30) (Fig. 3). The G3 domain has been expressed from cDNA and showed weak carbohydrate binding with some specificity for fucose and galactose (31). The G3 domain may thus have some binding specificity itself with a role in matrix organization. Alternatively, it may have a function of importance during the synthesis, intracellular translocation, glycosylation, and secretion of proteoglycan, rather than during its lifetime in the matrix.

The sequence similarity to complement B components is low and was established by consensus sequence methods (32). There is a large family of other proteins, many of which contain repetitive copies of this sequence, including complement proteins, other serum proteins, and cell surface molecules such as the cell adhesion molecule Mel-14 (Fig. 3). This is particularly interesting because Mel-14 also contains a lectin-like region and an EGF-like sequence. The cDNA for human G3 has been shown to have a splicing variant with an EGF-like sequence next to its lectin-like region (33). The structural elements in G3 can thus be similar to those in Mel-14, although lacking a transmembrane and cytoplasmic domain. Specific functions of the complement B region or EGF-like sequences have not been separately tested.

CHONDROITIN SULFATE- AND KERATAN SULFATE-RICH REGIONS

The substitution of chondroitin sulfate on the protein core is entirely restricted to the regions between the G2 and G3 domains, whereas keratan sulfate (KS) is found much closer to the N-terminus of the protein core, including on the G1 domain, as well as in a more specific KS-rich region on the C-terminal side of the G2 domain (Fig. 1, Table 2). This KS-rich region was absent from the cDNA of rat chondrosarcoma proteoglycan, but was present in different lengths in bovine and human sequences (29,34). The bovine KS-rich region contained 23 consecutive 6 amino acid repeats of similar but not identical sequence, whereas the human had only 11 such repeats. The long chondroitin sulfate (CS) attachment region was interesting in that it consisted of two regions, each with distinct repeating sequence patterns within them, but these were part of the same large, single exon in the DNA sequence. The human sequence also contained a long repeating string (19 repeats) of 19 amino acids in the first part of the CS attachment region. This was longer than in the rat sequence, such that it contained 77 Ser-Gly sequences compared with 49 in the rat (29). The second region of CS attachment was more similar in both species.

The limited number of available sequences from different species so far shows that the structures of the globular protein domains are highly conserved, whereas

TABLE 2. *Domain structure of cartilage aggregating proteoglycan and link protein*

Protein domain	Protein mol. mass (kDa)	Carbohydrate	Structural motifs	Functions
Link protein	39	N-linked	Ig fold PTR	G1 binding HA binding
Proteoglycan				
G1	38	N- and O-linked KS chains	Ig fold PTR	LP binding HA binding
E1	12	KS chains	—	No HA
G2	25	N- and O-linked	PTR	binding?
KS ⎫	5–10	KS chains		
⎬ E2				
CS ⎭	125	CS chains		GAG
	~110	KS chains O-linked		attachment
G3	25	N-linked	(EGF) Lectin Complement B	Gal/Fuc binding Protein interaction?

KS chains, keratan sulfate chains; CS chains, chondroitin sulfate chains; N-, O-, N- or O-linked oligosaccharides; LP, link protein; Lectin, hepatocyte cell surface glycoprotein receptor-like domain; GAG, glycosaminoglycan; PTR, proteoglycan tandem repeat; HA, hyaluronan; Gal, galactose; Fuc, fucose.

the extended, highly glycosylated regions are more variable. The CS-attachment regions all contain a high content of Ser-Gly residues, but there is considerable variation in their number and in their spatial distribution. The conserved sequences in globular domains may be associated with the greater constraints placed upon amino acid side chains in globular structures compared with extended sequences. However, it is clear that the lack of conservation of the detailed distribution of CS chains suggests that this is unlikely to be crucial in determining their function on proteoglycans in the matrix.

VARIATIONS IN GLYCOSYLATION

Cartilage proteoglycans have for a long time been characterized as showing great variation in carbohydrate composition, and this was a severe handicap in the elucidation of their structure (11). Cartilage proteoglycans contain chondroitin sulfate, keratan sulfate, and O-linked and N-linked oligosaccharides. The number, size, sulfation pattern, and charge density of these substituents are known to change with development and aging and to vary from site to site, but few proteoglycans have been studied in any precise molecular detail. Some of the changes apparent in proteoglycans extracted from cartilage may reflect matrix degradation processes, which, for example, can create protein-rich and keratan sulfate-rich proteoglycan fragments that are of relatively small size. Some changes in biosynthetic glycosylation may thus be obscured by structural changes within the extracellular matrix, and few details of the changes in the pattern of glycosylation during biosynthesis have been investigated. The factors which influence and control glycosylation of proteoglycans are poorly understood.

Some aspects of chondroitin sulfate biosynthesis can be modulated in chondrocytes *in vitro.* The addition of xyloside acceptor to chondrocytes stimulates the synthesis of more chains, but most of these are on the free xyloside and are of shorter average length (35). At the same time, fewer but similarly shortened chains are made on the proteoglycan. In contrast, if the supply of protein core is limited by inhibiting protein synthesis, there is less net synthesis, but the chains are much longer (36,37). This also occurs if the temperature is dropped; a smaller number of longer chains is synthesized. In relatively short experiments it is thus possible to perturb chain synthesis nonphysiologically with results which show that the rate of chain synthesis and chain length are inversely correlated (35,38). However, if chain synthesis is perturbed by more physiological methods, such as by stimulating it with growth factors (in fetal calf serum) or inhibiting it with cytokines, such as interleukin (IL)-1, the rate of synthesis is changed, but there is no change in chain length (35). Under these circumstances it appears that the enzymes and mechanism of chain synthesis are all up-regulated or down-regulated coordinately with protein core synthesis, such that chain characteristics are maintained in spite of changes in the synthesis rate.

Several factors now suggest that many details of chondroitin sulfate structure are in fact closely controlled during biosynthesis. Comparison of the chondroitin sulfate chains on aggrecan and on decorin (small CS-PG) in pig laryngeal cartilage showed the chains to differ in size and also in disaccharide composition (Table 3) (39). Since they were apparently made by the same cells within the same tissue, this implies that the chondroitin sulfate synthesized on aggrecan was made differently from that synthesized on decorin. This suggests that the protein core was able to influence glycosylation and sulfation, even on these long, extended glycosaminoglycan chains. This comparison of chondroitin sulfate chains on different proteoglycans in human articular cartilage was even more revealing (Table 3) (39), as not only were there differences in chain length and disaccharide composition for aggrecan and decorin, but those attached to aggrecan were chondroitin sulfate, whereas those attached to decorin were dermatan sulfate, with considerable epimerization of glucuronate to iduronate. Again a differential

TABLE 3. *Disaccharide composition of chondroitin/dermatan sulfate chains of large aggregating proteoglycans (aggrecan) and small CS/DS proteoglycans (decorin)*

| | Pig laryngeal and human articular cartilage | | | | | |
	Human C4S	C6S	COS	Pig C4S	C6S	COS
Aggrecan	10	86	4	75	20	5
Decorin	66	34	<1	93	6	1

From Sampaio et al., ref. 39.

chain synthesis distinguishes one proteoglycan from another and apparently is made within the same biosynthetic system.

Further details of chondroitin sulfate chain structure and its biological modulation are being investigated in two different ways. First, a series of monoclonal antibodies have been prepared which recognize specific epitopes within chondroitin sulfate chain structures. They are therefore able to provide techniques that distinguish between chondroitin sulfate with a low or high epitope content. The epitopes involve chain terminal structures or particular patterns of sulfation within the chains. Application of these monoclonals has been used to show developmentally regulated changes in chondroitin sulfate structure associated with cell differentiation and morphogenesis of cartilaginous and noncartilaginous tissues (40,41). Second, in mature articular cartilage they have been shown to detect changes in chondroitin sulfate structure associated with an experimentally induced model of osteoarthritis in canines (41). Chondroitin sulfate chain synthesis was therefore being modulated by chondrocytes in response to the early changes associated with articular cartilage pathology.

A second and complementary approach to investigating chondroitin sulfate chain structure has focused on determining the changes in the pattern of disaccharide sulfation from the nonreducing terminal of a chondroitin sulfate chain to its linkage with the protein core. This was carried out by analyzing partial chondroitinase ABC digests of cartilage proteoglycans (42). By determining the disaccharide composition of the released digest products at each stage of digestion, and comparing them with the disaccharide composition of the shortened chondroitin sulfate chain remaining attached to the proteoglycan, the results reveal the average composition of chains as their length is shortened. For a pig laryngeal proteoglycan preparation, some characteristics of the chain were revealed by this technique. The proportion of 6-sulfated relative to 4-sulfated disaccharides increased as the chains were shortened except in the region immediately adjacent to the neutral sugar linkage to protein, where a nonsulfated disaccharide was most abundant. Additional experiments are necessary to determine if there are general patterns common to aggrecan in all cartilages, or if they vary with anatomical site and in 4-, 6-sulfate ratios, and also how the pattern of chain structure is modulated in chondrocytes in response to growth factors or cytokines. Changes in chain structure may be part of the mechanisms by which the chondrocyte can control the properties of the cartilage extracellular matrix that surrounds it.

How have the many investigations of aggrecan equipped us to understand more about the health and diseases that affect articular cartilage? First, there is a clear understanding that any failure to maintain the proteoglycan content of articular cartilage will adversely affect its biomechanical properties. Even if this does not lead to direct damage, it may bring about unsatisfactory adaptive responses in other joint components that may eventually prejudice joint function.

A fall in proteoglycan content of the tissue may result from a suppression of synthesis or from an increase in matrix degradation. A study of the proteoglycan fragments released from cartilage *in vitro* into culture medium or *in vivo* into synovial fluid gives important information about the degradative activities that produce them. Proteoglycans are particularly vulnerable to proteinase attack and therefore provide a sensitive reporter of matrix proteinase action, and if specific cleavage sequences are determined, this will also enable the type of enzyme(s) concerned to be identified.

Studies of the protein core structure and investigation of its separate domains will enable a clearer understanding of the reasons for its complex origin and will identify the roles played by the different component parts. The cartilage proteoglycan also provides an excellent opportunity to investigate the control of glycosaminoglycan chain synthesis and to ascertain both the importance of sulfation patterns within the chains and whether they carry specific sequences that may have special functions in the matrix.

ACKNOWLEDGMENT

This work was carried out with the support of the Arthritis and Rheumatism Council (United Kingdom) and the Medical Research Council (United Kingdom).

REFERENCES

1. Hardingham TE, Bayliss MT. Proteoglycans of articular cartilage: changes in aging and joint disease. *Semin Arthritis Rheum* 1990;20:12–33.
2. Hardingham TE, Muir H. The specific interaction of hyaluronic acid with cartilage proteoglycans. *Biochim Biophys Acta* 1972;279:401–405.
3. Heinegård D, Hascall VC. Aggregation of cartilage proteoglycans. III. Characterization of the proteins isolated from trypsin digests of aggregates. *J Biol Chem* 1974;249:4250–4256.
4. Hardingham TE. The role of link protein in the structure of cartilage proteoglycan aggregates. *Biochem J* 1979;177:237–247.
5. Prehm P. Synthesis of hyaluronate in differentiated teratocarcinoma cells. Characterization of the synthetase. *Biochem J* 1983;211:181–189.
6. Mitchell D, Hardingham T. Monensin inhibits synthesis of proteoglycan, but not hyaluronate, in chondrocytes. *Biochem J* 1982;202:249–254.
7. Bayliss MT, Ridgeway GD, Ali SY. Delayed aggregation of proteoglycans in adult human articular cartilage. *Biosci Reps* 1984;4:827–833.
8. Sandy JD, O'Neill, Ratzlaff LC. Acquisition of hyaluronate-binding affinity in vivo by newly synthesized proteoglycans. *Biochem J* 1989;258:875–880.
9. Nieduszynski IA, Sheehan JK, Phelps CF, Hardingham TE, Muir H. Equilibrium binding studies of pig laryngeal proteoglycans with hyaluronate oligosaccharide fractions. *Biochem J* 1980;185:104–114.
10. Holmes MWA, Bayliss MT, Muir H. Hyaluronic acid in human articular cartilage. *Biochem J* 1988;250:435–441.
11. Hardingham TE. Proteoglycans: their structure, interactions and molecular organization in cartilage. *Biochem Soc Trans* 1981;9:489–497.
12. Pita J, Muller F, Morales S, Alarcon E. Ultracentrifugal characterization of proteoglycans from rat growth cartilage. *J Biol Chem* 1979;254:10313–10320.
13. Ohno H, Blackwell J, Jamieson AM, Carrino DA, Caplan AI. Calibration of the relative molecular mass of proteoglycan subunit by column chromatography on Sepharose CL-2B. *Biochem J* 1986;235:553–557.

14. Hardingham TE, Muir H, Kwan MK et al. Viscoelastic properties of proteoglycan solutions with varying properties present as aggregates. *J Orthop Res* 1987;5:36–46.
15. Paulsson M, Morgelin M, Wiedemann H, et al. Extended and globular protein domains in cartilage proteoglycans. *Biochem J* 1987;245:763–772.
16. Doege KJ, Sasaki M, Horigan E, Hassel JR, Yamada Y. Complete primary structure of the rat cartilage proteoglycan core protein deduced from cDNA clones. *J Biol Chem* 1987;262:17757–17767.
17. Doege KJ, Sasaki M, Kimura T, Yamada Y. Complete coding sequence deduced primary structure of the human cartilage large aggregating proteoglycan, aggrecan. *J Biol Chem* 1991;266:894–902.
18. Bonnet F, Dunham D, Hardingham TE. Structure and interactions of cartilage proteoglycan binding region and link protein. *Biochem J* 1985;228:77–85.
19. Fosang AJ, Hardingham TE. Isolation of the N-terminal globular domains from cartilage proteoglycans. *Biochem J* 1989;261:801–809.
20. Hardingham TE, Beardmore-Gray M, Dunham DG, Ratcliffe A. Cartilage proteoglycans. In: Evered D, Whelan J, eds. *Function of the proteoglycans.* Ciba Foundation Symposium, 1986;24: 30–39.
21. Morgelin M, Paulsson M, Hardingham TE, Heinegård D, Engel J. Cartilage proteoglycans: assembly with hyaluronate and link protein as studied by electron microscopy. *Biochem J* 1988;253: 175–185.
22. Fosang AJ, Hardingham TE. 1-C-6 epitope in cartilage proteoglycan G2 domain is masked by keratan sulphate. *Biochem J* 1991;273:369–373.
23. Neame PJ, Christner JE, Baker JR. Cartilage proteoglycan aggregates. The link protein and proteoglycan amino-terminal globular domains have similar structure. *J Biol Chem* 1987;262: 17768–17778.
24. Perkins SJ, Nealis AS, Dudhia J, Hardingham TE. Immunoglobulin fold tandem repeat structures in proteoglycan N-terminal domains and link protein. *J Mol Biol* 1989;206:737–753.
25. Aruffo A, Stamenkovic I, Melnick M, Underhill CB, Seed B. CD44 is the principle cell surface receptor for hyaluronate. *Cell* 1990;61:1303–1313.
26. Goetinck PF, Stirpe NS, Tsonis PA, Carlone D. The tandemly repeated sequence of cartilage link protein contains the site for interaction with hyaluronic acid. *Cell* 1987;105:2403–2408.
27. Hardingham TE, Ewins RJF, Muir H. Cartilage proteoglycans. Structure and heterogeneity of the protein core and the effects of specific protein modifications on the binding to hyaluronate. *Biochem J* 1976;157:127–143.
28. Sai S, Tanaka T, Kosher RA, Tanzer ML. Cloning and sequence analysis of a partial cDNA for chicken cartilage proteoglycan core protein. *Proc Natl Acad Sci USA* 1986;83:5081–5085.
29. Hardingham TE, Fosang AJ, Dudhia J. Domain structure in aggregating proteoglycans from cartilage. *Biochem Soc Trans* 1990:18:794–796.
30. Zimmerman DR, Ruoslahti E. Multiple domains of the large fibroblast proteoglycan, versican. *EMBO* 1989;8:2975–2981.
31. Halberg DH, Proulx G, Doege K, Yamada Y, Drickamer K. A segment of the cartilage proteoglycan core protein has lectin-like activity. *J Biol Chem* 1988;263:9486–9490.
32. Patthy L. Detecting homology of distantly related proteins with consensus sequences. *J Mol Biol* 1987;198:567–577.
33. Baldwin CT, Reginato AM, Prockop DJ. A new epidermal growth factor-like domain in the human core protein for the large cartilage specific proteoglycan. *J Biol Chem* 1989;264:15747–15750.
34. Antonsson P, Heinegård D, Oldberg Å. The keratan sulfate-enriched region of bovine cartilage proteoglycan consists of consecutively repeated hexapeptide motif. *J Biol Chem* 1989;264:16170–16173.
35. Mitchell DC, Hardingham TE. The control of chondroitin sulphate biosynthesis and its influence on the structure of cartilage proteoglycans. *Biochem J* 1982;202:387–395.
36. Mitchell D, Hardingham TE. The effects of cycloheximide on the biosynthesis and secretion by chondrocytes in culture. *Biochem J* 1981;196:521–529.
37. Kimura J, Caputo C, Hascall V. The effect of cycloheximide on synthesis of proteoglycans by cultured chondrocytes from the Swarm rat chondrosarcoma. *J Biol Chem* 1981;256:4368–4376.
38. Lohmander LS, Hascall VC, Yanagishita M, Kuettner KE, Kimura JH. Post translational events in proteoglycan synthesis: kinetics of synthesis of chondroitin sulfate and oligosaccharides on the core protein. *Arch Biochem Biophys* 1986;250:211–227.

39. Sampaio L, Bayliss MT, Hardingham TE. Dermatan sulphate proteoglycan from human articular cartilage. *Biochem J* 1988;254:757–764.
40. Sorrell JM, Mahmoodian F, Schafer IA, Davis B, Caterson B. Identification of monoclonal antibodies that recognise novel epitopes in native chondroitin/dermatan sulphate glycosaminoglycan chains: their use in mapping functionally distinct domains of human skin. *J Histochem Cytochem* 1990;38:393–402.
41. Caterson B, Mahmoodian F, Sorrell JM, et al. Modulation of native chondroitin sulphate structure in tissue development and in disease. *J Cell Sci* 1990;97:411–417.
42. Hardingham TE, Fosang AJ, Ewins RJF. Sequence structure in chondroitin sulphate chains. *37th Trans Orthop Res Soc USA* 1991;4.

DISCUSSION

Kresse: It is quite clear how important the cDNA-derived sequence data are for an evaluation of potential functional domains of aggrecan. However, it is surprising how little data have been added since we have learned that the core protein contains globular domains such as the G2 domain and the G3 lectin and complement B-like regions. Could you comment on the functionality of the aggrecan G2 domain, for example?

Hardingham: The G2 domain shows no strong interaction with other cartilage matrix components, but that was tested under conditions where quite strong interactions are needed to pick them up. In processes like turnover, G2 seems to be a region where there is easy proteolytic attack. When we digest proteoglycan with stromelysin, about half the total G2 domain detected with an immunoassay is lost, even when there is only modest cleavage of the protein core. So I think the G2 domain is a particularly easy area for attack of proteinases. And this is quite an important site for cleavage of the proteoglycan, because it separates the G1 domain that helps anchor the proteoglycans in an aggregate structure from the major chondroitin sulfate-bearing region, which provides the main physical properties of the proteoglycans in the tissue.

Lowther: It is possible that there are feedback mechanisms between the extracellular concentration of the proteoglycans and the chondrocytes. Do we know which region of the molecule will interact with the chondrocyte surface?

Hardingham: I don't know if any region interacts specifically. Mike Dean and Harry Martin at the Kennedy Institute did an interesting experiment looking at intact proteoglycans and showed that they were taken up by human monocytic cells by a normal process and transferred to lyosomes. If the proteoglycans were partly degraded, they were handled quite differently. This raises the question about cleavage of matrix macromolecules and what may be exposed when this happens. Maybe some sites are revealed that are not available on the intact molecules, and these may be recognized by cell receptors.

Hascall: What possible roles will alternate splicing, such as the presence or absence of the EGF domain, have?

Hardingham: In Kurt Doege's last paper he commented that the most abundant mRNA for human aggrecan from young individuals was the form that had a lectin domain, but no adjacent EGF sequence and no complement-related sequence. I don't know of any evidence as to how much of the different forms are present in the expressed protein. It remains an interesting possibility that in the chondrocyte response to matrix damage, it may switch in alternative elements, such as an EGF-like sequence, that would carry some message out into the matrix.

Plaas: Do you think that all molecules that are synthesized carry the G3 domain and that it is subsequently lost outside the cell, or do you think that there are two populations of core proteins synthesized, one with and one without G3?

Hardingham: It would be my prejudice that most molecules are made with an intact G3 domain, but that some molecules lose it very early in their lives. It has a highly conserved structure, which suggests that it does have an important function, but this function may be inside the cell during synthesis and not out in the matrix.

Mason: The EM pictures of monomers would be typical for proteoglycans in free solution. What would they look like in the tissue?

Hardingham: Proteoglycans exist in cartilage at very high concentrations where they are forced to occupy much less space than they do in free solution. If you put them into small volumes, there has to be a lot of overlap of their domains or the domain of each molecule must get smaller. Barry Preston's experiments have shown that there is contraction of the overall domain, which reduces the extent to which they interdigitate. I imagine proteoglycans exist in cartilage as a partly interdigitated network. I would suggest that most of them are not bound to the fibrillar matrix, although some may be.

Mason: Aggregan and decorin made in the same cells have strikingly different disaccharide composition. How is that achieved within the Golgi complex?

Hardingham: There is not very much data concerning different subcompartments in Golgi for making different types of carbohydrate chains. In localization experiments we showed that all the medial and trans-Golgi compartments in chondrocytes contain chondroitin sulfate proteoglycans, whereas the cis-Golgi did not. So if there is segregation of chain synthesis, it probably occurs within common compartments. There may be organization of the synthetic enzymes into multienzyme complexes specialized for each type of proteoglycan. Perhaps each contains a receptor for the specific types of protein cores that allow the synthetic machinery to add the appropriate glycosaminoglycan chains. The multienzyme complexes may be organized in two-dimensional arrays similar to those proposed by Ulf Lindahl for heparin and heparan sulfate biosynthesis.

Kresse: In this context one should also consider the observation that the disaccharide composition of xyloside-induced glycosaminoglycan chains depends on the concentration of the added xylosides, and in this case, the xyloside does not contain any core protein information.

Articular Cartilage and Osteoarthritis,
edited by K. Kuettner et al.
Raven Press, Ltd., New York © 1992.

2

Extracellular Metabolism of Aggrecan

John D. Sandy

*Shriners Hospital for Crippled Children, Tampa Unit, and Department of Biochemistry
and Molecular Biology, University of South Florida, Tampa, Florida 33612*

The major space-filling matrix macromolecule of cartilage is the large chondroitin sulfate/keratan sulfate proteoglycan (1), now commonly referred to as aggrecan (2). Aggrecan is a multidomain molecule, with a core protein of about 220 kDa encoded by 16 exons, the boundaries of which correspond closely to the distinct structural elements of the aggrecan core protein (2). Thus the G1 domain at the N-terminal is composed of three subdomains which are encoded by exons 3, 4, and 5, respectively. The interglobular domain (IGD) is encoded by exon 6, the G2 domain by exons 7 and 8, and the glycosaminoglycan-bearing domains [keratan sulfate (KS) and chondroitin sulfate (CS)] by exons 9 and 10. At the C-terminal, exons 11 thru 16 encode the five regions of the G3 domain which includes an EGF-like sequence (exon 11), a lectin-like sequence (exons 12–14), and a complement regulatory protein (CRP)-like sequence (exon 15). In developing human cartilage, there are multiple mRNA transcripts for aggrecan which have been shown to be generated by alternate usage of exons 11 and 15 (3).

The G1 domain binds aggrecan to hyaluronate and link protein, interactions which organize aggregates and retain aggrecan monomers in the tissue. Specific functions for the interglobular domain, G2 domain, and KS domain are yet to be identified, and while the G3 domain is composed of three discrete elements (EGF, lectin, complement regulatory protein), which have also been found together in a number of cell adhesion molecules (4), a role for this chimeric structure in aggrecan is unclear at present. At the tissue level, the major functional domain of aggrecan is the CS-attachment region, since it is substitution of this extended central region of the core protein with polyanionic CS chains which renders aggrecan osmotically active, and which thereby confers on cartilage an ability to reversibly deform under load.

In this chapter, experiments will be described which show that the extracellular metabolism and turnover of aggrecan is markedly influenced by critical processing events which occur at both the N-terminal (G1-IGD-G2) and C-terminal (G3) regions of the core protein (Fig. 1). A major research challenge in this area of cartilage biology is to describe these events at the protein structural level, and to identify the nature and the mode of action of the processing enzymes involved.

BACKGROUND

A diagrammatic view of what appear to be the major events in the extracellular processing of aggrecan is shown in Fig. 1. Processing of the N-terminal G1 domain during biosynthesis and secretion of aggrecan is indicated by marked variation in the capacity of newly synthesized molecules to bind to hyaluronan. Thus, there is extensive evidence (see ref. 5 for review) for a pool of aggrecan (shown as Pool A, Fig. 1) which exhibits a low affinity for hyaluronan. This population appears to have a half-life of about 24 hr *in vivo* (6) and probably represents a very small percentage of the total matrix aggrecan. This transient biosynthetic form is converted in the matrix into a form with a high affinity for binding of hyaluronan, and the end-product of this assembly process is the proteoglycan aggregate composed of many monomers bound in a link protein-stabilized form to hyaluronan (shown as Pool B, Fig. 1). These two pools may also represent the metabolically active (Pool A) and inactive (Pool B) turnover pools found

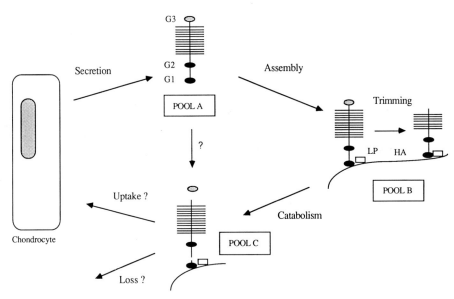

FIG. 1. Extracellular metabolism of aggrecan. Aggrecan monomers are secreted by chondrocytes and enter a transient biosynthetic pool with a low affinity of binding for hyaluronan (*Pool A*). The majority of Pool A molecules undergo assembly into link-stabilized aggregates (*Pool B*) and acquire a high binding affinity for hyaluronan. Pool B molecules undergo trimming at the C-terminal and N-terminal proteolysis, which includes cleavage of a glutamate-alanine bond within the interglobular domain (22). The nonaggregating fragments formed (*Pool C*) may be removed by chondrocyte uptake or loss by diffusion. G1, G2, and G3 refer to the three globular domains of aggrecan; LP, link protein; HA, hyaluronan.

both *in vivo* (6) and in cartilage explant studies (11) of mature cartilage. Molecules in the inactive pool B may have an *in vivo* half-life of up to 300 days in mature animals (7) and this must therefore constitute the major pool of extractable aggrecan in mature cartilages.

Processing of the C-terminal region of molecules in this pool apparently takes the form of a slowly progressive "trimming" which removes the G3 domain and regions of the CS-attachment region. Such C-terminal processing is suggested by analysis of extracted aggrecan which reveals molecules of varying size under the microscope (8) and subpopulations with distinct electrophoretic properties (9). The large hyaluronan-bound product of such "trimming" must remain in Pool B (see Fig. 1); however, the fate of the small fragments released from the C-terminal region is unknown.

A proportion of the molecules in Pool B will subsequently undergo proteolysis near the N-terminal to generate large CS-bearing fragments which have lost the ability to bind hyaluronan. This population (Pool C, Fig. 1) also represents a very small percentage of the total tissue aggrecan, since molecules which can no longer bind to hyaluronan appear to be freely diffusible in cartilage and are therefore rapidly lost from the matrix. It is not yet clear whether this loss is entirely by diffusion out of the tissue or whether endocytosis by chondrocytes is also involved. In this regard, explants studies with 35-S-labeled rabbit cartilage (18) indicated that less than 10% of degraded molecules enter the lysosomes and result in the liberation of inorganic sulfate. It does appear (10) that there is a coordinated removal of hyaluronan and chondroitin sulfate from this catabolic pool. However, the metabolic fate of this hyaluronan and the other byproducts of this process, that is link protein and the N-terminal regions of aggrecan, remains to be clearly established.

In summary, it appears that the half-life of aggrecan in cartilage is largely determined by the rate at which individual molecules undergo cleavage near the N-terminal and so lose the capacity to bind hyaluronan. Thus, molecules for which proteolytic processing is confined to the extreme C-terminal regions of the molecule will exhibit a long matrix half-life, probably in excess of 100 days, whereas molecules which undergo N-terminal cleavage soon after secretion will have a correspondingly short half-life. In this regard there is evidence from both explant (11) and *in vivo* labeling studies (6) for a proportion of newly secreted molecules with a half-life of only 1 to 2 days. These molecules appear to be rapidly degraded soon after secretion and as a result they lose the capacity to bind to hyaluronan and thereby enter the short half-life pool (Pool C) directly from the biosynthetic pool (Pool A).

VARIATION IN HYALURONATE BINDING AFFINITY
OF NEWLY SYNTHESIZED MOLECULES

Whereas aggrecan purified from cartilage binds to hyaluronan with a Kd of about 50 nM, newly synthesized molecules have a lower affinity, and a period of extracellular processing is necessary to convert this "precursor" form to the mature matrix form. Such a delay in acquisition of high affinity binding might be necessary to allow newly secreted molecules to diffuse to proteoglycan-deficient regions of the matrix distant from the cell. A number of studies have shown that the binding affinity of proteoglycans formed during pulse labeling in human cartilage explants increases during chase periods in the tissue (ref. 12, among others). We examined the hyaluronate binding properties of aggrecan synthesized over a 24 hr labeling period and released into the medium of chondrocyte cultures (5). Such a radiolabeled product bound very poorly to hyaluronan relative to the tissue aggrecan which was used as carrier in these studies. Interestingly, this low affinity could be markedly improved simply by incubating samples under mildly alkaline conditions; thus after 24 hr at pH 8.6, the newly synthesized aggrecan exhibited a markedly higher affinity than the tissue aggrecan which was essentially unaffected by the treatment (13).

These results supported the idea that variable affinity may be due to variation in the arrangement of disulfides in the G1 domain; thus disulfide rearrangement in proteins generally proceeds more rapidly in alkaline than in neutral pH since the thiol groups involved have pK values of about 9. A controlling effect of matrix pH on this process was also supported by explant studies (14) in which the rate of conversion to the high affinity form was shown to be promoted by a pH increase within the physiologic range; thus the half-life for the affinity change was 10.6 hr at pH 6.99 but only 5.7 hr at pH 7.45 (see ref. 14 for details). In addition, the process of conversion was found to be age-dependent *in vivo* (6) where the half-life was estimated at 12 hr in developing cartilages but greater than 24 hr in mature articular cartilage.

To investigate further the possible involvement of disulfide rearrangements in this process, we have developed a method for the isolation and characterization of disulfide-bonded peptides from aggrecan (15). This method has established the disulfide pattern for all three globular domains (Fig. 2). By an exhaustive sequence analysis of all disulfide-bonded species which could be detected by a sensitive fluorescence assay of tryptic maps, we demonstrated directly that the pattern shown here for the G1 domain is the quantitatively predominant form in extracted bovine aggrecan; thus no evidence for pairings other than those shown in Fig. 2 was obtained.

It has recently been suggested (3) on the basis of sequence similarities between the aggrecan G1 loop B (the central loop of the G1 domain shown on Fig. 2), link protein loop B, and the Hermes lymphocyte homing receptor, that the hyaluronan binding activity of these proteins is largely dependent on this loop B structure. Studies in which synthetic peptides from the tandem repeat loops were found to inhibit the binding of link protein to hyaluronan (16) would also accommodate this view. If this is the case, then experiments which assess the disulfide arrangements in G1 loop B of biosynthetically labeled aggrecan of low and high affinity should indicate whether variable affinity is related to altered disulfide bonding arrangements. In this regard it may be helpful that the G1

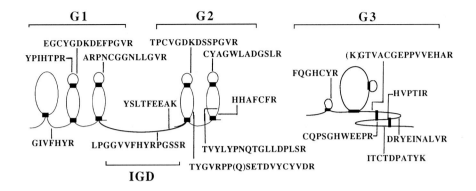

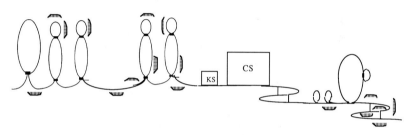

FIG. 2. Location of marker peptides isolated from aggrecan. **Top:** The location and complete sequence of marker peptides from the G1, IGD, G2, and G3 domains of bovine aggrecan. The positions of the disulfide bonds are indicated (*heavy lines*). **Bottom:** The position of these markers (*combs*) in relation to the KS and CS-rich domains of aggrecan. The three disulfide bonds shown between the CS domain and the G3 domain indicate the position of the variably expressed EGF-like sequence. IGD, interglobular domain; KS, Keratan sulfate; CS, chondroitin sulfate; EGF, epidermal growth factor. (From Sandy et al., ref. 17, with permission.)

loop B of aggrecan can be isolated from trypsin digests as a peptide triplet containing both the disulfide bonds normally present in this tandem repeat loop structure (15).

VARIATION IN CONTENT OF THE G3 DOMAIN OF AGGRECAN

The presence of a C-terminal globular domain on aggrecan, containing a cysteine-rich, lectin-like sequence, was first indicated from cDNAs corresponding to the 3' end of protein core mRNA from rat, chick, and bovine sources (see ref. 3). More recently, it has also been shown from cDNA clones for the human core protein (3) that the C-terminal region of aggrecan is a complex structure which may include an EGF-like sequence, a lectin-like sequence, and a complement regulatory protein (CRP) sequence. In addition, it has been found that there are alternatively spliced forms of human aggrecan core transcripts, some of which lack the EGF and CRP sequences.

Direct evidence for the presence of the G3 domain on tissue aggrecan was first obtained from electron microscopy after rotary shadowing (8). Interestingly, these studies detected the G3 domain on only about 30% of molecules from mature bovine nasal cartilage, and it was suggested that this is due to slow C-terminal "trimming" of aggrecan during prolonged periods in the matrix. On the other hand, the same authors showed that only about 50% of the aggrecan isolated from the rapidly growing rat chondrosarcoma carried the G3 domain, suggesting that a deficiency of G3 may be a common feature of aggrecan, even in "immature" cartilages.

In order to investigate questions regarding the expression and turnover of the G3 domain, we have developed a peptide mapping procedure (17) which can be used to determine directly the G3 domain content of different aggrecan preparations. The method involves the production, isolation, and quantitation of marker peptides from the three globular domains (G1, G2, and G3) and the interglobular domain (IGD) (see Fig. 2 for marker locations). Tryptic peptides are separated by sequential anion exchange, cation exchange, and reversed phase HPLC, and are quantitated by absorbance at 220 nm. The values obtained (peak area per μg core protein) are found to be a function of the molar yield and also the size and aromatic residue content of individual peptides.

To examine the reproducibility of this method for all markers, seven separate analyses of calf articular aggrecan were done. The peptide content data showed good agreement between assays, and clearly illustrated the effect of peptide structure on the absorbance values obtained. For example, peptides from the G2 domain gave values from as low as 2569 area units per μg core protein (for HHAFCFR) to as high as 13,760 area units per μg core protein (for TYGVRPPSETDVYCYVDR). Since these G2 peptides were isolated in similar molar yields, this difference must be largely due to the enhancing effects of size and aromatic residue content (particularly tyrosine) on the molar absorptivity of peptides at 220 nm; this makes good sense in the present comparison since HHAF (see above) is a heptapeptide with one phenylalanine residue, whereas TYGV is an octadecapeptide with three tyrosine residues.

To develop a method of assessing the relative content of any one peptide in different samples, we normalized the peak area values to the value obtained in each assay for the G2 peptide TYGV. This peptide was chosen because it is derived from the G2 domain, an essentially invariant structure in most aggrecan samples we have examined, and also because the peak area values for TYGV always showed very good agreement in multiple assays of a single sample.

The normalized data for each of seven assays was then used to calculate a mean normalized value for each peptide; this is shown on Fig. 3. Peptides of similar size and aromaticity from the G1, IGD, and G2 domains gave similar normalized values; for example, the markers YPIH (G1), YSLT (IGD), and CYAG (G2) are each small peptides containing one tyrosine residue, and their

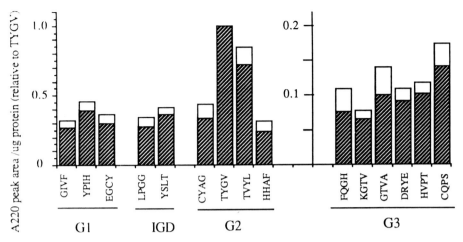

FIG. 3. Quantitation of marker peptides from the globular domains of aggrecan. The peptide content values [peak area (A220) per µg core protein] for seven separate assays of calf aggrecan were each normalized to the value obtained in the identical assay for the G2 peptide TYGV. The histogram shows the mean of these normalized values for each peptide, and the error box (*unfilled*) shows the standard deviation of the mean. Note that the G3 peptides are plotted on an expanded scale. It should be noted that the values shown are a function of both peptide structure and abundance. The four N-terminal residues only of each peptide are given. (From Sandy et al., ref. 17, with permission.)

mean values were 0.40, 0.36, and 0.35 units, respectively (Fig. 3). In contrast, all G3 peptides gave consistently low values (note expanded scale for G3 peptides on Fig. 3), and this did not appear to be simply explainable in terms of peptide structure. For example, the G3 peptide FQGHCYR and the G1 peptide GIVFHYR are both heptapeptides with one phenylalanine and one tyrosine residue; however, the mean normalized value for FQGHCYR (0.081) was only 31% of the value obtained for GIVFHYR (0.265).

These data therefore support the idea (8) that many tissue aggrecan molecules lack G3, and further suggest that maybe as few as 30% of the G1/G2-bearing aggrecan molecules in newborn calf cartilage carry the G3 domain. To investigate this further, we analyzed the domain content of aggrecan secreted by newborn calf chondrocytes over days 2 through 10 in high density monolayer culture. A direct comparative analysis of calf tissue A1D1 and cell product A1D1 (Fig. 4) showed clearly that the two preparations had almost identical contents of G1, IGD, and G2 domain but that the cell culture product carried a 2- to 2.5-fold higher content of all G3 domain marker peptides. It appears, therefore, that calf chondrocytes in culture secrete aggrecan with an approximate 1:1:1 molar ratio of the three globular domains (G1, G2, and G3), whereas aggrecan isolated from calf cartilage has a domain ratio of about 1:1:0.3.

It remains to be determined whether the apparent deficiency of the G3 domain on extracted calf molecules is the result of proteolysis soon after secretion, or of

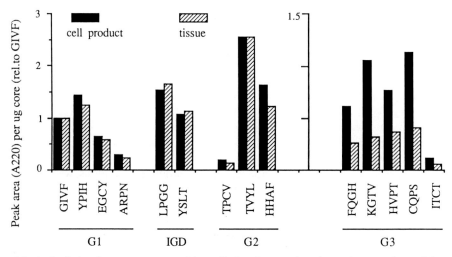

FIG. 4. Analysis of aggrecan secreted by calf chondrocytes in culture. A comparison of the domain content of aggrecan from calf cartilage (*hatched columns*) and from calf chondrocyte cultures (*filled columns*) is shown. In both cases the peptide content values [peak area (A220) per μg core protein] have been normalized to the value obtained for the G1 peptide GIVF. It can be seen that the cell product is markedly enriched in G3 domain relative to aggrecan from the tissue.

alterations in the abundance of alternative mRNA transcripts which might affect the level of G3 expression.

PROTEOLYSIS WITHIN THE N-TERMINAL DOMAINS OF AGGRECAN

Our early observation (18) that aggrecan degradation in cartilage explants appears to be initiated by proteolytic cleavage within or near N-terminal domains, with the release of large nonaggregating products, has been widely confirmed in cultures of bovine and porcine cartilage (see ref. 17 for review), and also in human cartilage (19). As details of the sequence and globular domain structure of the N-terminal region of bovine and human aggrecan have become available, it has become possible to design experiments to examine precise points of cleavage involved in such N-terminal processing.

We have taken the approach that determination of the cleavage point(s) involved in normal or stimulated catabolism of aggrecan in cartilage is best made on "natural" catabolic products isolated from fresh cartilage or from cartilage explant cultures. We therefore set out to isolate and characterize the large nonaggregating molecules present in extracts of calf and steer articular cartilage. Following isolation by CsCl gradient centrifugation, A1D1 preparations were separated into aggregating and nonaggregating pools by isokinetic cesium sulfate gradient centrifugation in the presence of excess hyaluronan. The nonaggregated species, which represented about 25% of the total aggrecan present in most samples, were further purified by a second cesium sulfate gradient separation in the presence of excess hyaluronan; again a major proportion formed aggregates so that after two such steps, less than 8% of the starting material could be identified as nonaggregating. It therefore appears that little, if any, of the hydrodynamically large, high bouyant density molecules present in fresh extracts of bovine articular cartilages are truly nonaggregating. This is consistent with the idea (see Fig. 1) that nonaggregating fragments of aggrecan are rapidly lost from the cartilage matrix *in vivo*.

In order to generate sufficient nonaggregating product for analysis, we therefore isolated large CS-rich product(s) from calf articular cartilage explant cultures. In one set of experiments (17), explants were maintained for 15 days in a basal medium [Hams F-12 supplemented with 20 mM HEPES, 44 mM sodium bicarbonate, 2 mM glutamine, 0.1% (w/v) BSA] to which was added, with each daily medium change, 20 U/ml interleukin 1α. The aggrecan released into the medium over this period, which accounted for about 65% of the starting tissue content, was isolated by CsCl gradient centrifugation and shown to comprise about 20% aggregating and 80% nonaggregating species.

Quantitative peptide mapping of this explant catabolic product directly demonstrated a marked reduction in the content of the G1 marker peptides GIVF, YPIH, and EGCY relative to tissue aggrecan. The low but measurable content of G1 markers on the medium product was also consistent with the low but measurable aggregability of these samples. In addition, this analysis showed that the catabolic product(s) carried a high content of the interglobular domain and G2 markers, and an apparently reduced content of G3 markers. These results (17) therefore supported and extended earlier immunological data showing a reduction in the G1 content of pig (20) and rabbit (21) explant medium aggrecan. The peptide analysis also showed that aggrecan catabolism in explants involves the proteolytic separation of G1 from the remainder of the molecule, as opposed to a process involving fragmentation of G1 with loss of its antigenicity and of hyaluronan-binding activity.

Since the explant product was deficient in G1 markers but rich in markers from the COOH-terminal region of the interglobular domain and the G2 domain (see Fig. 2 for marker locations), the results indicated that a major cleavage generated during explant catabolism was within the N-terminal region of the interglobular domain. To investigate this further, we prepared the medium product (days 2–15 combined) from calf articular cartilage explants which had been prelabeled at day 2 with tritiated proline and maintained in the presence of interleukin 1α. This D1 preparation, which contained greater than 86% of the glycosaminoglycan recovered from the gradient and which showed 12% aggregability with hyaluronan, was prepared for N-terminal analysis. The method of preparation (see ref. 22) involved deglycosylation by sequential digestion with chondroitinase ABC and keratanase and removal of digestion products by filtration on an Ultrafree-MC filter unit with a nominal exclusion limit of 100 kDa. The recovery of tritium-labeled aggrecan core protein through this procedure was always greater than 72%, and 10 μg (about 50 pmol) of aggrecan core protein was taken for sequencing.

N-terminal analysis (22) showed only one major (at about 30 pmol yield) and one minor (at about 5 pmol yield) sequence. The major sequence, ARGxx-ILxAKPDF, was sufficiently similar to a sequence toward the N-terminal end of the rat and human interglobular domain (3) to identify a new N-terminal on the degraded aggrecan molecules (Fig. 5). In the human protein, the N-terminal alanine residue of this species is located 45 residues from the most C-terminal cysteine of the G1 domain and 101 residues from the most N-terminal cysteine of the G2 domain. Specific cleavage at this site was also entirely consistent with the data from quantitative peptide mapping and would appear to explain the observation that cartilage explants from many species (see ref. 17 for review) release large nonaggregating fragments of aggrecan in culture. The minor product isolated after deglycosylation showed an N-terminal sequence of VEVS, and this is the expected N-terminal for the small proportion of aggregating molecules in these samples.

Similar analyses were also done on reduced and carboxymethylated products, and the same N-terminal sequences were obtained. This suggests that catabolic processing under these conditions is not accompanied by proteolytic cleavage within the G2 domain. It is also interesting to note that the recovery of tritiated core protein through the preparative steps for N-terminal analysis was reproducibly high at about 75%. Since this procedure involved isolation of deglycosylated core species on a 100 kDa molecular weight cut-off filter, it seems that few, if any, of the core species were of low molecular weight. When taken together with the detection of only one new N-terminal, it seems reasonable to conclude that aggrecan catabolism under these conditions involves primarily, or maybe exclusively, the single proteolytic cleavage identified in Fig. 5.

To determine whether cleavage of aggrecan at this site also occurs during turnover *in vivo*, it will be necessary to characterize the normal end-product of this catabolic process, that is, the globular domain protein from the N-terminal

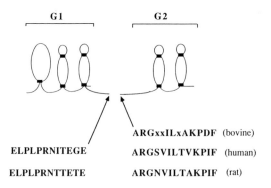

FIG. 5. Location of a cleavage site within the interglobular domain of aggrecan. A major product of the catabolism of aggrecan in bovine explant cultures bears the N-terminal sequence given here (bovine). The location of the cleavage site was made by comparison of the determined bovine sequence with the established sequences shown here for human and rat interglobular domain (3).

G1   G2

ELPLPRNITEGE   ARGxxILxAKPDF (bovine)

ELPLPRNTTETE   ARGSVILTVKPIF (human)

                      ARGNVILTAKPIF (rat)

of aggrecan. Such a product appears to be abundant in aged human articular cartilages, where it retains the ability to bind hyaluronan (23). Our preliminary analysis of similar material from steer cartilage A1D4 samples indicates that it has the expected N-terminal of VEVS and contains all three loops of the G1 domain (see Fig. 2). Identification of the C-terminal sequence of this species should soon provide definitive answers as to the importance of specific interglobular domain cleavage points in normal aggrecan turnover *in vivo*.

FUTURE WORK AND CONCLUDING REMARKS

Some of the major unsolved research problems in this area can be summarized as follows:

1. What is the nature of the N-terminal processing which converts molecules of low hyaluronan binding affinity into a high affinity form? Is this accompanied by disulfide bond rearrangements or possibly by changes in the tertiary structure of the G1 domain which do not involve alterations in covalent bonding?

2. What is the nature of the C-terminal processing which generates molecules of varying core protein size? Is the absence of the G3 domain from some molecules simply a result of extracellular proteolysis, or could alternate G3 exon usage be involved? If a specific protease is involved, what is the cleavage site and does this protease act inside the cell, at the cell surface, or in the interterritorial matrix?

3. What is the nature of the N-terminal proteolysis which appears to initiate aggrecan catabolism *in vivo?* Does it involve cleavage at the glutamate-alanine bond suggested from the bovine explant studies? Which protease(s) are involved and what determines the susceptibility of aggrecan molecules to such directed proteolysis? What is the metabolic fate of the hyaluronan, the hyaluronan-bound G1 domain, and the link protein, which are byproducts of such processing?

In relation to catabolism, the glutamate-alanine cleavage (Fig. 5) does not clearly indicate the nature of the protease(s) involved. Thus, a neutral metalloproteinase from human cartilage explants (24) has been shown to cleave a histidine-isoleucine bond near the N-terminus of link protein, and human fibroblast stromelysin, which appears closely related to the cartilage enzyme, very specifically cleaves a glutamine-phenylalanine bond in substance P and its analogs (25).

Answers to the questions posed should continue to emerge as we obtain more information on the structure-function relationships of the G2 and G3 domains of aggrecan. In this regard, it may be that the kinetics and tissue location of the turnover events summarized above might, to some degree, be controlled by protein-protein or protein-carbohydrate interactions involving these two globular domains.

Finally, the peptide mapping methods described in this article represent a new and potentially useful tool for future research directed toward improving the treatment of joint diseases such as osteoarthritis. For example, since the majority of the marker peptides described here are found in human aggrecan, it should be possible to use these methods to examine synovial fluids for evidence of aggrecan-core specific markers. Such information might then be used to develop a highly specific immunoassay to monitor disease activity.

ACKNOWLEDGMENTS

I wish to thank my collaborators at the Shriners Hospital, Tampa Unit, for their continuing support in the work described in this article. In particular, I wish to acknowledge contributions made by Carl Flannery, Ray Boynton, John Gordy, Peter Neame, and Carmen Young. Financial support for this work came from The Shriners Hospitals of North America and grant AR 38580 from the National Institutes of Health.

REFERENCES

1. Hascall VC. Proteoglycans: the chondroitin sulfate/keratan sulfate proteoglycans of cartilage. *ISI atlas of science: biochemistry.* 1988;1:189–198.
2. Doege K, Sasaki M, Yamada Y. Rat and human cartilage proteoglycan (aggrecan) gene structure. *Biochem Soc Trans* 1990;18:200–202.
3. Doege K, Sasaki M, Kimura T, Yamada Y. Complete coding sequence and deduced primary structure of the human cartilage large aggregating proteoglycan, aggrecan. *J Biol Chem* 1991;266: 894–902.
4. Stoolman LM. Adhesion molecules controlling lymphocyte migration. *Cell* 1989;56:907–910.
5. Sandy JD, Plaas AHK. Studies on the hyaluronate binding affinity of newly synthesised proteo- glycans in chondrocyte cultures. *Arch Biochem Biophys* 1989;271:300–314.
6. Sandy JD, O Neill JO, Ratzlaff L. Acquisition of hyaluronate binding affinity by newly synthesized proteoglycans in vivo. *Biochem J* 1989;258:875–880.
7. Maroudas A. Metabolism of cartilagenous tissues: a quantitative approach. In: Maroudas A, Holborrow EJ, eds. *Studies in joint disease, vol. 1.* England: Pitman Medical, 1980;59–86.
8. Paulsson M, Morgelin M, Wiedemann H, et al. Extended and globular protein domains in cartilage proteoglycans. *Biochem J* 1987;245:763–772.
9. Stanescu V. Analytical and preparative electrophoresis of proteoglycan monomers in agarose submerged gels. In: Maroudas A, Kuettner KE, eds. *Methods in cartilage research.* Academic Press, San Diego, 1990;44–46.
10. Morales II, Hascall VC. Correlated metabolism of proteoglycans and hyaluronic acid in bovine cartilage organ cultures. *J Biol Chem* 1988;263:3632–3638.
11. Sandy JD, Plaas AHK. Age-related changes in the kinetics of release of proteoglycans from normal rabbit cartilage explants. *J Ortho Res* 1986;4:263–272.
12. Oegema TR, Jr. Delayed formation of proteoglycan aggregate structures in human articular cartilage disease states. *Nature* 1980;288:583–585.
13. Plaas AHK, Sandy JD. The affinity of newly synthesised proteoglycan for hyaluronic acid can be enhanced by exposure to mild alkali. *Biochem J* 1986;234:221–223.
14. Sah RL, Grodzinsky AJ, Plaas AHK, Sandy JD. Effects of tissue compression on the hyaluronate binding properties of newly synthesised proteoglycans in cartilage explants. *Biochem J* 1990;267: 803–808.
15. Sandy J, Flannery C, Boynton R, Neame P. Isolation and characterization of disulfide-bonded peptides from the three globular domains of aggregating cartilage proteoglycan. *J Biol Chem* 1990;265:21108–21113.
16. Goetinck PF, Stirpe NS, Tsonis PA, Carlone D. The tandemly repeated sequences of cartilage link protein contain the sites for interaction with hyaluronic acid. *J Cell Biol* 1987;105:2403– 2408.
17. Sandy JD, Boynton RE, Flannery CR. Analysis of the catabolism of aggrecan in cartilage explants by quantitation of peptides from the three globular domains. *J Biol Chem* 1991;266:8198–8205.

18. Sandy JD, Brown H, Lowther DA. Degradation of proteoglycan in articular cartilage. *Biochim Biophys Acta* 1978;543:536–544.
19. Campbell IK, Roughley PJ, Mort JS. The action of human articular cartilage metalloproteinase on proteoglycan and link protein. *Biochem J* 1986;237:117–122.
20. Ratcliffe A, Tyler J, Hardingham T. Articular cartilage cultured with interleukin 1 *Biochem J* 1986;238:571–580.
21. Sandy JD, Flannery CR, Plaas AHK. Structural studies on proteoglycan catabolism in rabbit articular cartilage explant cultures. *Biochim Biophys Acta* 1987;931:255–261.
22. Sandy JD, Neame PJ, Boynton RE, Flannery CR. Catabolism of aggrecan in cartilage explants. Identification of a major cleavage site within the interglobular domain. *J Biol Chem* 1991;266: 8683–8685.
23. Roughley PJ. Changes in cartilage proteoglycan structure during ageing: origins and effects—a review. *Agents and Actions Supplements* 1986;18:19–29.
24. Nguyen Q, Murphy G, Roughley PJ, Mort JS. Degradation of proteoglycan aggregate by a cartilage metalloproteinase. *Biochem J* 1989;259:61–67.
25. Teahan J, Harrison R, Izquierdo M, Stein R. Substrate specificity of human fibroblast stromelysin. Hydrolysis of substance P and its analogues. *Biochemistry* 1989;28:8497–8501.

DISCUSSION

Handley: In explant cultures, we have also shown that the core protein of aggrecan is cleaved between glutamate and alanine in the sequence NITEGEAR between the G1 and G2 domains. Further, we found two other cleavage sites between glutamate-alanine and glutamate-leucine which are in the chondroitin sulfate attachment region. This suggests that there may be a particular protease involved in the cleavage of the core protein at specific sites. Furthermore, the synovial fluid and serum of animals that we get cartilage from appear to contain similar peptides. This suggests that after proteolytic cleavage, the core protein fragments make their way into the synovial fluid and then into the plasma. These core protein fragments are then probably taken up by the liver.

Sandy: Yes, I think that this is an important issue. If one is able to find products (specific N-terminal sequences) in synovial fluid, this would identify important cleavage points in normal aggrecan turnover. Another issue which arises from our work is to determine which protease is responsible for the glutamate-alanine cleavage. We have been unable to generate that clip with stromelysin in solution studies, but this needs further work. On the other hand, a proportion of the residual G1 domain molecules which are present in human cartilage has C-termini which are identical to that derived by stromelysin digestion of human aggrecan in solution, and this is not the glutamate-alanine cleavage in the interglobular domain.

Kuettner: Did you ever stimulate your chondrocytes or explants with retinol to see if you get different cleavage fragments than with interleukin-1?

Sandy: No, the only other experiments we have done are with basal cultures in which tissue is explanted in medium without serum, with or without recombinant interleukin-1. In both cases the major released product carried the N-terminal ARG-sequence.

Bayliss: Have you looked at the G1 domain that accumulates with aging in human cartilage to see if the C-terminal sequence is similar or dissimilar to that generated in your stromelysin enzyme studies?

Sandy: The data on the C-terminal of the G1 domain can be reproduced with immature and mature human cartilage, and also in osteoarthritic cartilage. In all these sources we can isolate that C-terminal peptide. Therefore, it does seem to be a very characteristic cleavage point for aggrecan *in vivo* at all ages. These data do not, however, exclude the possibility of there being other cleavage points in the interglobular domain of human aggrecan *in vivo*.

Articular Cartilage and Osteoarthritis,
edited by K. Kuettner et al.
Raven Press, Ltd., New York © 1992.

3

A Large Chondroitin Sulfate Proteoglycan (PG-M) and Cartilage Differentiation

Tamayuki Shinomura,* Yoshihiro Nishida,† and Koji Kimata*

*Institute for Molecular Science of Medicine, Aichi Medical University, Yazako, Nagakute, Aichi 480-11, Japan; †Nagoya University School of Medicine, Chikusa, Nagoya 466, Japan

In vivo, cartilage development in chick limb buds begins at stage 24. One of the main features of the development is earlier formation of mesenchymal cell condensations at stage 23. The formation of these condensations is considered to be essential for subsequent chondrogenesis and a key step in determining the formation of correct skeletal patterns. Therefore, this cell condensation should be associated with highly organized molecular events which occur with spatiotemporal regulation. A series of recent studies suggests that interactions between receptors on the cell surface and extracellular matrix molecules play a major role in this regulation (1,2). It is important, then, to investigate the extracellular matrix molecules, particularly those present in the condensing mesenchymes, to help understand the mechanisms that control mesenchymal cell condensation as an initial step of cartilage development.

PG-M, a large chondroitin sulfate proteoglycan, is one of the major extracellular matrix components in chick embryonic limb buds at stage 23 (Fig. 1). This proteoglycan has a molecular mass of more than 1,000 kDa and differs from PG-H, another large chondroitin sulfate proteoglycan characteristically found in cartilage (3). An important role for PG-M in the condensation process has been suggested by its unique distribution in limb buds as shown below. In addition, PG-M can bind to fibronectin, hyaluronic acid, and type I collagen, which were other major matrix molecules in the condensing mesenchyme (4). It is likely, therefore, that PG-M may modulate interactions between cells and these molecules, thereby participating in regulation of the condensation event.

This chapter will review molecular aspects of extracellular matrix components characteristic of precartilage cell condensation in chick limb buds, especially

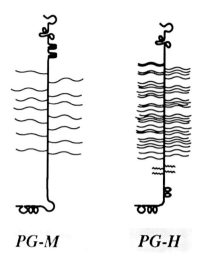

FIG. 1. Postulated structures of PG-M and PG-H. The partial structure of PG-M (the one-third from the carboxy terminal) was predicted by cDNA analysis. The other two-thirds is postulated assuming that PG-M is identical in molecular structure to the human fibroblast proteoglycan, versican (8). The structure of PG-H is based on the sequence analysis for the rat cartilage proteoglycan, aggrecan (9).

PG-M   *PG-H*

properties of PG-M, and discuss possible roles these molecules have in mesenchymal condensation and subsequent chondrogenesis.

PG-M A MAJOR EXTRACELLULAR MATRIX PROTEOGLYCAN IN LIMB BUDS

Limb buds obtained from chick embryos at stage 22/23 were metabolically labeled with [^{35}S]sulfate. Tissues were then subjected to a conventional extraction for proteoglycans using 4M guanidine HCl dissociative conditions. Proteoglycans in the extract consist of two populations that differ in molecular size. The large one, which is excluded from Sepharose CL-4B, contains only chondroitin sulfate chains and represents approximately 60% of the labeled proteoglycans (Fig. 2). The smaller one consists of at least two different proteoglycans bearing heparan sulfate or chondroitin sulfate chains, respectively. Further characterization has shown that the heparan sulfate proteoglycans can be separated into two fractions having different buoyant densities. Heparan sulfate proteoglycans of low and high density probably correspond to a basement membrane heparan sulfate proteoglycan and a plasma membrane-intercalated heparan sulfate proteoglycan, respectively, since both of these types are found by immunohistochemical localization in the limb buds (5,6). The large and major chondroitin sulfate proteoglycan appeared to correspond to PG-M which we previously purified and characterized (3), since anti-PG-M antibodies immunoprecipitated this proteoglycan completely (Fig. 2). We have thus concluded that PG-M is a major proteoglycan in the extracellular matrix of limb buds at prechondrogenic stages.

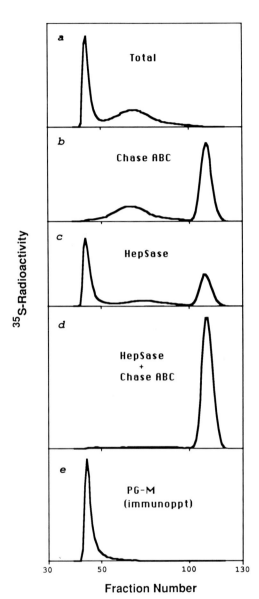

FIG. 2. Sepharose CL-4B column chromatography of proteoglycans isolated from chick limb buds at stage 22/23. LImb buds were metabolically labeled with [^{35}S]sulfate. After incubation for 5 hr, tissues were subjected to a conventional procedure for the extraction of proteoglycans in 4M guanidine-HCl dissociative conditions. Aliquots were treated with chondroitinase ABC (*b*), heparitinase (*c*), and chondroitinase ABC plus heparitinase (*d*), as described previously (3). Proteoglycans were immunoprecipitated with rabbit anti-PG-M antibodies from the other aliquot (*e*). The nontreated sample (*a*) and treated samples were applied to the Sepharose CL-4B column under dissociative conditions.

LOCALIZATION OF PG-M IN MESENCHYMAL CELL CONDENSATIONS

Distributions of PG-M in the limb buds at various stages were examined by immunohistochemical localization. This proteoglycan was rather uniformly distributed throughout the mesoderm before condensation. However, when condensation occurs at stage 23, the concentration in the condensation area is preferentially increased (5). With maturation of cartilage, PG-M gradually disappears from the matrix, in contrast to a dramatic increase of PG-H (aggrecan) (3). Other extracellular matrix molecules such as fibronectin, type I collagen, type III collagen, hyaluronic acid, laminin, and type IV collagen were distributed rather uniformly throughout the limb bud, although some of these molecules showed somewhat increased or decreased concentrations in the condensation area (2). These observations strongly suggest a unique role of PG-M in the mesenchymal cell condensation.

MODIFICATION OF CELL ADHESION BY PG-M

One way to evaluate PG-M's suggested unique role in the mesenchymal cell condensation is to determine whether PG-M can modify interactions between cells and fibronectin or type I collagen, two other major molecules in the condensing mesenchyme matrix. We therefore examined the effects of PG-M on cell attachment to dishes coated with these molecules. PG-M inhibited cell attachment to fibronectin or type I collagen in a dose-dependent manner, irrespective of cell origin (7). Interestingly, treatment of the proteoglycan with either proteolytic enzymes or chondroitinase abolished its inhibitory effects on the cell adhesion. In addition, blocking the immobilization of added PG-M to plastic surfaces of coated dishes by pretreating the dishes with serum albumin also abolished the inhibitory activity of PG-M. The results suggest that only the proteoglycan form was responsible for the activity and the immobilized fraction of PG-M could act as a cell adhesion inhibitor. Since immobilization of proteoglycan *in vitro* presumably corresponds to formation of proteoglycan aggregates with other matrix molecules *in vivo,* the ability of PG-M to bind to fibronectin and type I collagen appears to be important for PG-M functions. It is also interesting that the active site for the interaction between cells and PG-M is on the chondroitin sulfate chains (7).

Solursh has explored *in vitro* the conditions necessary for mesenchymal cells to differentiate into chondrocytes, and found that cell shape influences the differentiation via changes in cytoskeletal elements (1). It is now well-known that the shape of a cell can be regulated by interactions between matrix substrate molecules and receptors on the cell surface. Since PG-M can modify these interactions, it was worthwhile to determine the effects of exogenously added PG-M on the differentiation of precartilage cells *in vitro.*

Mesenchymal cells were prepared from chick limb buds at stage 22/23 and cultured on dishes coated with fibronectin or type I collagen in a serum-free, BGJb medium. Cell aggregation and subsequent chondrogenic differentiation *in vitro* were examined with or without exogenous addition of PG-M (Fig. 3). Cells on coated dishes without PG-M became attached to the substrates and

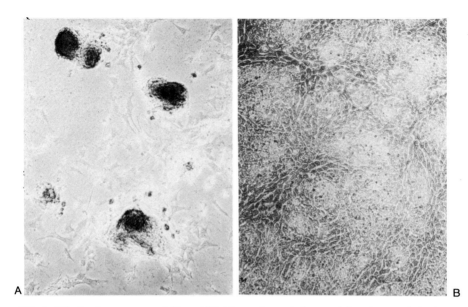

FIG. 3. Effects of exogenous addition of PG-M on cell morphology and chondrogenesis *in vitro*. Mesenchymal cells prepared from chick limb buds at prechondrogenic stages were cultured on fibronectin- or type I collagen-coated dishes in a serum-free, BGJb medium. PG-M with the final concentration of 5 g/ml was added to some of the dishes after the innoculation of cells. Cells without PG-M attached to the dishes spread well. However, cells with PG-M did not spread and formed cell aggregates within 3 hr. Cell aggregates thus formed showed a positive staining with Alcian blue after 1 day of culturing (**A**). In contrast, cells without PG-M did not show the staining until 4 days of culturing (**B**). Further confirmation for cartilage phenotype expression was also performed by the positive reactivity with anti-PG-H antibodies (data not shown).

then spread, and 5 or 6 days were required for the cells to form nodules and matrix with cartilage phenotypic molecules such as PG-H and type II collagen. When cells were placed on coated dishes with PG-M, or on the coated dishes that had been treated with PG-M, they attached to the substrates but did not spread, and they formed nodules and matrix with cartilage phenotypic molecules within 1 day.

We therefore suggest that modification of cell-matrix molecule interactions by PG-M plays an important role in the formation of mesenchymal cell condensations and subsequent chondrogenesis.

cDNA CLONING AND DEDUCED AMINO ACID SEQUENCE OF PG-M CORE PROTEIN

Two overlapping cDNA clones (λMa and λMb) approximately 3.2 Kb in length were selected by the reaction with rabbit antibodies to PG-M in a λgt11 cDNA expression library constructed from chick limb bud poly (A⁺) RNA. After reinsertion into pGEM-3zf(−), Sau3AI or BamHI fragments were subcloned into M13mp18, and PCR methods were used to obtain smaller fragments of the cDNA clones. Nucleotide sequences were determined by the dideoxynucleotide termination method. λMa was 3243 nucleotides long, including 819 nucleotides of 3'-noncoding sequence. It encoded 808 amino acids from a carboxy terminus of a polypeptide, corresponding to one-third of the total amino acid residues. Homology analysis of the deduced amino acid sequence (Fig. 4) revealed a complement regulatory protein-like domain (residues 704–764), a lectin-like domain (residues 575–703), and two EGF-like domains (residues 498–536 and 537–574) from the carboxy terminal. The same set of domain elements has been identified in the carboxy-terminal portion of versican, a large chondroitin sulfate proteoglycan expressed by human fibroblasts (residues 2306–2366, 2179–2305, and 2103–2178) (8). The homologies are high: 93% for the complement regulatory protein-like domain, 96% for the lectin-like domain, and 68 and 84% for the two EGF-like domains. Because of this high homology, we tentatively concluded that PG-M is the chick equivalent of versican. However, the amino acid sequence of the remaining N-terminal side, which contains seven potential glycosaminoglycan attachment sites, differed considerably from the comparable region of

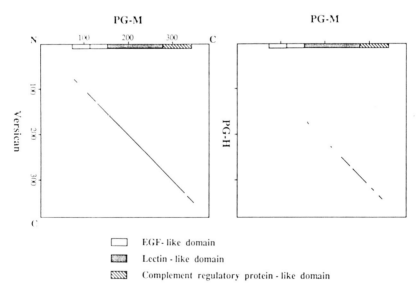

FIG. 4. Protein homology plots (>80%) of PG-M to versican **(left)** and PG-H **(right)**. Deduced amino acid sequence based on the analysis for λMa cDNA clone was compared with sequences of the corresponding parts of versican and PG-H using a DNASIS program (Hitachi Co., Tokyo).

the glycosaminoglycan attachment domain of versican. Therefore the entire primary structure must be determined to verify this conclusion.

DISCUSSION AND SOME PROSPECTS

The predicted amino acid sequence of the obtained cDNA clone indicates that the chick PG-M core protein contains three domains in the carboxy terminal with an extremely high homology to a human fibroblast versican, particularly in the lectin-like domain where only five of 115 amino acid residues were different (Fig. 5). The occurrence of domains with such evolutionarily conserved primary

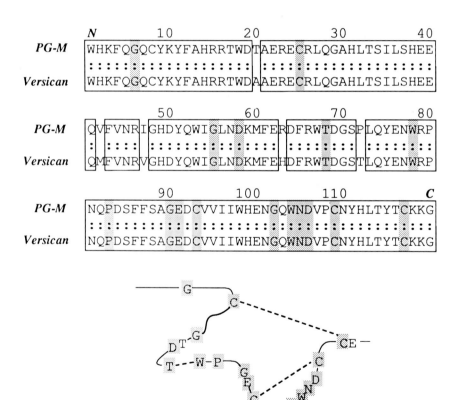

FIG. 5. Comparison of amino acid sequences for lectin-like domains between PG-M and versican. Amino acid residues marked by shadow correspond to those which are consensus structural features of carbohydrate-recognition domains in C-type animal lectins (*inserted diagram*) shown by Drickamer (ref. 13, with permission).

sequences suggests that they have important biological roles. A lectin-like domain is also found in cartilage-derived large chondroitin sulfate proteoglycan (9). Interestingly, it has been shown, in this case, that the domain actually shows weak binding activity to galactose and fucose residues (10). Aulthouse and Solursh (11) have reported that a β-galactose–specific lectin, peanut agglutinin (PNA), specifically reacts with the condensing mesenchyme *in vivo* and with precartilage cell aggregates *in vitro*. This suggests that the condensing mesenchyme contains molecule(s) with β-galactose residues at nonreducing ends. It is possible that these PNA-binding molecule(s) may be actual ligand(s) for PG-M.

From the above observations, we tentatively propose molecular mechanisms for mesenchymal cell condensation and subsequent chondrogenesis in which interactions between extracellular matrix molecules and their cell surface receptors are involved. The preferential expression or accumulation of PG-M in the mesenchymal cell condensing area may modify interactions of the cells with surrounding matrix molecules, thereby inducing changes in the cell shape or cytoskeletal elements which are related to chondrogenic differentiation. Selective expression of PNA-binding molecules on the cells and their interaction with a β-galactose lectin might enhance or induce formation of mesenchymal cell aggregates apparently involved in determining skeletal patterns.

There are many questions raised against this hypothesis. For example, PG-M is also distributed on basement membranes lying under the ectoderm and in mesenchymes at the distal end of the limb, although the concentration appears to be low. What functions can we expect for PG-M in these tissues? Also, there is no evidence for the participation of interactions between galactose lectin-like molecules and PNA-binding molecules in the cell aggregation. Furthermore, another type of β-galactose lectin of low molecular weight (12) shows uniform distribution throughout the mesenchyme (unpublished observation).

Recent advances in molecular biological techniques will help us gain insight into functions of PG-M. We now have cDNA clones for PG-M, and it may be possible to enhance or suppress PG-M synthesis *in vitro* or even *in vivo* by introducing sense or antisense PG-M DNA into the cells and see the effects on differentiation of mesenchymal cells into chondrocytes. If we choose the DNA fragment, it is possible to investigate functions of the encoded polypeptide as well.

Cartilage-derived large chondroitin sulfate proteoglycan (PG-H) also has the same inhibitory activity for cell attachment to matrix substrate molecules as does PG-M (7). It is likely that this cartilage proteoglycan also functions in cartilage to regulate interactions between cells and cartilage matrix molecules. As discussed above and also pointed out by Solursh (1), the interaction may greatly affect the shape of a chondrocyte and thereby influence the maintenance and maturation of chondrocyte functions. Studies from this perspective may help us understand not only cartilage differentiation, but also some cartilage diseases.

REFERENCES

1. Solursh M. Environmental regulation of limb chondrogenesis. In: Kuettner KE, Schleyerbach R, Hascall VC, eds. *Articular cartilage biochemistry.* New York: Raven Press, 1985;145–161.
2. Shinomura T, Kimata K. Precartilage condensation during skeletal pattern formation. *Develop Growth Differ* 1990;32:243–248.
3. Kimata K, Oike Y, Tani K, et al. A large chondroitin sulfate proteoglycan (PG-M) synthesized before chondrogenesis in the limb bud of chick embryo. *J Biol Chem* 1986;261:13517–13525.
4. Yamagata M, Yamada KM, Yoneda M, Suzuki S, Kimata K. Chondroitin sulfate proteoglycan (PG-M-like proteoglycan) is involved in the binding of hyaluronic acid to cellular fibronectin. *J Biol Chem* 1986;261:13526–13535.
5. Shinomura T, Jensen KL, Yamagata M, Kimata K, Solursh M. The distribution of mesenchyme proteoglycan (PG-M) during wing bud outgrowth. *Anat Embryol* 1990;181:227–233.
6. Solursh M, Reiter RS, Jensen KL, Kato M, Bernfield M. Transient expression of a cell surface heparan sulfate proteoglycan (syndecan) during limb development. *Dev Biol* 1990;140:83–92.
7. Yamagata M, Suzuki, S, Akiyama SK, Yamada KM, Kimata K. Regulation of cell-substrate adhesion by proteoglycans-immobilized on extracellular substrates. *J Biol Chem* 1989;264:8012–8018.
8. Zimmermann DR, Ruoslahti E. Multiple domains of the large fibroblast proteoglycan, versican. *EMBO J* 1989;8:2975–2981.
9. Doege K, Sasaki M, Horigan E, Hassell JR, Yamada Y. Complete primary structure of the rat cartilage proteoglycan core protein deduced from cDNA clones. *J Biol Chem* 1987;262:17757–17767.
10. Halberg DF, Proulx G, Doege K, Yamada Y, Drickamer K. A segment of the cartilage proteoglycan core protein has lectin-like activity. *J Biol Chem* 1988;263:9486–9490.
11. Aulthouse AL, Solursh M. The detection of a precartilage, blastema-specific marker. *Dev Biol* 1987;120:377–384.
12. Sakakura Y, Hirabayashi J, Oda Y, Ohyama Y, Kasai K. Structure of chicken 16-KDa β-galactoside-binding lectin. *J Biol Chem* 1990;265:21573–21579.
13. Drickamer K. Two distinct classes of carbohydrate-recognition domains in animal lectins. *J Biol Chem* 1988;263:9557–9560.

DISCUSSION

Plaas: Do you know whether the fibronectin in your embryonic system carries poly-lactosamine? Maybe this might be involved in the binding of PG-M to fibronectin. This glycosylation has been reported for fibronectin extracted from embryonic tissue.

Kimata: I don't know. But, as far as we examined, PG-M binds to any types of fibronectin such as human plasma fibronectin. So, I don't think this kind of glycosylation could be involved in the binding.

Tanzer: Tenascin has been shown to interfere with fibronectin modulation of cell binding. Would you compare those results with yours?

Kimata: We have observed the same effect of tenascin in our culture system (chick limb bud cells). However, we doubt that the effect is due to tenascin itself, because we found that PG-M firmly associated with tenascin and pure tenascin was very difficult to obtain. In relation to this, Edelman's (1) group also reports the presence of cytotactin/tenascin-associated proteoglycan which may correspond to PG-M.

Kimura: Can PG-M form link protein-stabilized aggregates with hyaluronic acid; and why is PG-M replaced in cartilage by aggrecan?

Kimata: PG-M interacts with hyaluronic acid but link proteins are not involved. I don't know the reason. Aggrecan plays an important role in stabilizing cartilage structure. In contrast, in limb buds, PG-M temporarily appears to give some signals to the cells just before the mesenchymal cell condensation occurs. After cartilage is formed, it disappears. Its metabolism must be very rapid, thus it may not be necessary to stabilize the binding of PG-M to hyaluronic acid. That may be the reason link proteins are not involved.

Kresse: Decorin shares two functional properties with PG-M. It inhibits cell adhesion and it interacts with collagen. Would there be an effect on cartilage condensation if you culture the mesenchymal cells on decorin?

Kimata: We have evidence that the activity of PG-M depends on the presence of chondroitin sulfate chains. Since decorin has a chondroitin sulfate chain, it might give similar results in our culture system. The proteoglycan form is essential since we do not get the condensation when we just add chondroitin sulfate chains to the system. We suspect there may be some important functions in the core protein.

Hascall: Is there any evidence that PG-M or versican might reappear in events associated with osteoarthritis such as osteophyte formation?

Kimata: We are now making antibodies to recognize human PG-M/versican and these may help answer your question in the future.

Muir: To follow up, in advanced human osteoarthritis, cell condensation in clusters is seen. Do you think the PG-M could be involved in this abnormal process?

Kimata: This is also an interesting question to answer, when the antibodies become available. So far we can only say, "It is likely."

REFERENCE

1. Hoffman S, Crossin KL, Edelman GM. *J. Cell Biol.* 1988;106:519–532.

Articular Cartilage and Osteoarthritis,
edited by K. Kuettner et al.
Raven Press, Ltd., New York © 1992.

4

Structure and Function of Dermatan Sulfate Proteoglycans in Articular Cartilage

Lawrence C. Rosenberg

Orthopaedic Research Laboratory, Montefiore Medical Center,
New York, New York 10467

Articular cartilage contains two forms of dermatan sulfate proteoglycans called DSPG I, or biglycan, and DSPG II, or decorin. The DSPGs are multifunctional macromolecules that bind to collagens, fibronectin, growth factors, heparin cofactor II, and a variety of other macromolecules. The DSPGs bind to the surfaces of collagen fibrils and inhibit collagen fibrillogenesis (1–7). They bind to fibronectin and inhibit cell adhesion (8–11). The DSPGs bind to TGFβ and inhibit the mitogenic activity of TGFβ (12). Iduronic acid-rich dermatan sulfate chains of the DSPGs bind to heparin cofactor II and inhibit thrombin activity and clot formation (13). Thus the DSPGs inhibit processes which are involved in tissue repair.

These inhibitory properties of the DSPGs have only recently been described, and the precise biologic functions and significance of these properties in normal mature articular cartilage are not yet understood. However, it may be that at some stage during the formation of a connective tissue such as articular cartilage, when the composition and architecture of the tissue are satisfactory, DSPGs are then synthesized and secreted into extracellular matrix where they bind to fibronectin and collagens, and prevent further cell migration or structural alterations in the tissue. The DSPGs may provide a mechanism for preventing further alterations in the structure of a satisfactorily formed normal mature connective tissue.

Whatever are the actual biologic functions of the DSPGs in normal mature connective tissues, the capacity of the DSPGs to inhibit processes involved in tissue repair appears to be directly involved in the pathogenesis of the articular cartilage degeneration that occurs in early human osteoarthritis. Specifically, the capacity of the DSPGs to inhibit processes involved in tissue repair may help explain why lesions restricted to the substance of articular cartilage, i.e., *superficial lesions* of the kind seen in early human osteoarthritis, do not heal.

CHARACTERISTICS OF THE EARLY HUMAN
OSTEOARTHRITIC LESION

The histopathologic hallmarks of the articular cartilage degeneration which occurs in early human osteoarthritis are well-known (14,15). These characteristic gross and microscopic changes consist of disruption of the collagen fibril bundles in the superficial tangential zone; the formation of vertical clefts and fissures and the development of overt fibrillation; the loss of proteoglycans and of metachromatic staining from the extracellular matrix of the fibrillated cartilage; the formation of chondrocyte clusters or brood capsules; the absence of repair within the clefts and fissures of the fibrillated cartilage; and a progressive decrease in the thickness of the cartilage. These changes have been called "open" chondromalacia (15).

However, even prior to the development of fissures, clefts, and overt fibrillation, important pathologic changes occur in the superficial regions of articular cartilage where the surface is still intact. Ohno *et al.* (15) have studied biopsy specimens obtained at operations from young patients with knee pain due to clear-cut mechanical derangements, who had extensive pathologic changes characteristic of open chondromalacia. Articular cartilage tissue samples taken adjacent to open chondromalacic lesions revealed early pathologic changes which precede and lead to the development of open chondromalacia. In these areas, the articular cartilage was soft, boggy, and swollen, but the surface was intact and without fibrillation. There was a loss of metachromatic staining in the pericellular matrix of chondrocytes just below the superficial tangential zone. This phenomenon has been called *chondrocytic chondrolysis* by Hirohata (15). In the pericellular regions with chondrocytic chondrolysis, *matrix streaks* frequently appeared which radiated from the chondrocyte lacunae and pericellular regions out into the surrounding extracellular matrix. Ultrastructurally, these matrix streaks appeared to represent collagen fibril bundle disruptions which originated from pericellular regions with chondrocytic chondrolysis. These early pathologic changes were called closed chondromalacia. Ohno *et al.* suggested that when these collagen fibril disruptions or matrix streaks which radiate from chondrocytes of chondrocyte clusters eventually extend to the cartilage surface, an open fissure is formed, and closed chondromalacia is transformed into open chondromalacia. The article by Ohno *et al.* (15) is important because it focuses in a coherent, integrated fashion on the initial early changes which occur in articular cartilage degeneration and lead to the well-known lesions with overt fibrillation.

With the development of overt fibrillation, deep vertical clefts and fissures are formed. There is a loss of the large aggregating proteoglycans from matrix and the elastic properties of the cartilage are diminished. In response to these degenerative changes, chondrocyte clusters are formed which synthesize increased amounts of proteoglycan. In contrast to injury and tissue loss in other locations, the chondrocytes within these clusters do not migrate into the clefts or fissures.

No fibrin clot is present in the clefts or fissures. Depending on the size of the superficial defect, there may or may not be some abortive proliferation of cells in the superficial tangential zone, and some of these cells may begin to migrate over the edges of the surface of the defect. However, most of the defect remains uncovered by cells, and there is no cell migration into the defects. Thus, the defects are not filled by a reparative tissue.

The same picture is seen in small, superficial lesions in rabbit articular cartilage (16,17). The appearance is essentially the same when the defects are examined at 24 hr, 3 months or 1 year following injury. There is no cell migration into the defects. Examination of the joint in the experimental animal dramatically demonstrates the failure of fibrin clot to attach to the surfaces of the defects, compared with synovial membrane. When animals are examined at 24 hr after arthrotomy, there is fibrin clot within the joint which is attached to synovial membrane, but it does not adhere to the articular cartilage and there is no clot within the superficial cartilage defects.

For years scientists have wondered why superficial lesions restricted to the substance of articular cartilage do not heal. Why do the fibrillated lesions of articular cartilage grow larger and deeper during the development of human osteoarthritis and never undergo repair? Why do undifferentiated mesenchymal cells or fibroblasts not grow into the clefts and fissures of fibrillated cartilage and fill these defects with reparative tissue? Until recently, we were unable to begin to answer these questions.

We used to think that superficial lesions do not heal because they do not have access to the macrophages, endothelial cells, and mesenchymal cells which reside in marrow. Recent observations indicate that this hypothesis is incorrect. Superficial lesions do not need access to cells in marrow for repair. The problems to be solved in eliciting the repair of superficial defects are not related to a potential source of reparative cells. The problem lies elsewhere. Articular cartilage contains DSPGs that inhibit clot formation and the attachment of fibrin clot to the surfaces of superficial cartilage defects; the DSPGs also inhibit the adhesion and migration of mesenchymal cells over the surfaces of superficial defects. In superficial defects of articular cartilage, analogous to the early human osteoarthritic lesion, it may be necessary to degrade and remove DSPGs from the surfaces of superficial defects to allow cell attachment and cell migration into the defects, and to elicit the first step in the process of articular cartilage repair.

STRUCTURES OF DERMATAN SULFATE PROTEOGLYCANS

Two forms of dermatan sulfate proteoglycans, *biglycan* (DSPG I) and *decorin* (DSPG II), are present in the extracellular matrix of articular cartilage (18–20). The same types of proteoglycans have been found in a variety of other connective tissues (21–35). Biglycan and decorin have different core proteins. The amino acid sequences of human and bovine biglycan and decorin have been determined (36–40). The identification and classification of a small interstitial proteoglycan from a particular connective tissue such as biglycan or decorin are based on the primary structure of its core protein. Dermatan sulfate is a hybrid glycosaminoglycan (41–50). It contains two types of disaccharide repeating units [IdoA(α1→3)GalNAc and GlcA(β1→3)GalNac] within the same glycosaminoglycan chain. According to one system of nomenclature, a glycosaminoglycan chain is called a dermatan sulfate chain if it contains some iduronate-containing disaccharide repeating units (41–50). Biglycan and decorin from most connective tissues contain dermatan sulfate chains, but the percentage of iduronate-containing disaccharide repeating units and their arrangement in the glycosaminoglycan chains vary greatly from tissue to tissue. Thus, the dermatan sulfate chains of biglycan and decorin from skin and articular cartilage contain approximately 80% and 40% iduronate, respectively (18,20). The glycosaminoglycan chains of biglycan and decorin from bone and bovine nasal cartilage contain no iduronate (31–35) and are, therefore, chondroitin sulfate chains.

Figure 1 presents a diagram of the structures of biglycan and decorin. Biglycan and decorin from bovine articular cartilage have true monomeric molecular weights of approximately 100,000 and 70,000, respectively, based on sedimentation equilibrium studies in 4 M guanidine HCl. The core proteins of biglycan and decorin both have molecular weights of approximately 37,000, and the articular cartilage proteoglycans contain glycosaminoglycan chains approximately 30,000 in molecular weight.

The primary structure of the core proteins of biglycan and decorin are of special interest. Except for the NH_2-terminus, the primary structures of bovine and human biglycan are highly homologous with those of bovine and human decorin (36–40). The amino acid sequences of biglycan and decorin are approximately 55% homologous. However, the amino acid sequences of the first 20 amino acids at the NH_2-terminal regions of biglycan and decorin are completely different. Biglycan contains two glycosaminoglycan chains (Fig. 1) attached

---

→

FIG. 1. The structures of selected members of the family of small interstitial proteoglycans. Biglycan and decorin have different core proteins. Biglycan contains two glycosaminoglycan chains attached to Ser[5] and Ser[11]. Decorin contains one glycosaminoglycan chain attached to Ser[4]. Dermatan sulfate is a hybrid glycosaminoglycan that contains two kinds of disaccharide repeating units (41–50). One is composed of iduronate and N-acetylgalactosamine. The other is composed of glucuronate and N-acetylgalactosamine, the same as that present in chondroitin sulfate chains. However, chondroitin sulfate chains contain only glucuronate and no iduronate. Biglycan and decorin from different tissues each possess a core protein with the same primary structure, yet contain glycosaminoglycan chains that differ greatly in iduronic acid content and structure. In the diagram, iduronate is shown by the *black hexagons*. Glucuronate, N-acetylgalactosamine and linkage region xylose and galactose are shown by *white hexagons*. The dermatan sulfate chains of both biglycan and decorin from skin contain approximately 80% iduronate, and the iduronate-containing disaccharide repeating units are arranged as large block oligosaccharides. The dermatan sulfate chains of biglycan and decorin from articular cartilage contain approximately 40% iduronate. Biglycan and decorin from bone contain chondroitin sulfate chains.

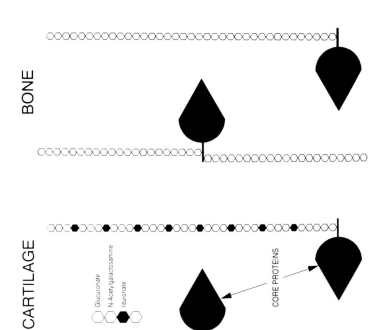

SKIN　　　CARTILAGE　　　BONE

Glucuronate
N-Acetylgalactosamine
Iduronate

CORE PROTEINS

```
                                                              LxxLx
DEEASGAETTSGI-PDLDSLPPTYSAMCPFGCHCHLRVVQCSDLGLKA--VPKEISPDTTLLD    60
D    -IGPEEHF EVPEIE MGP-V   R Q          EK--   DLP   A          58
          HPI EVSKVASHLE N DKRN T --L -DLPK        I H             39
          A G  AP S AGTL D GRR  TWASL TAFPV    E V                 39
          VTLSPKD QVFRSD GSSIS QPPAEIPGYL ----A  VH A              39


LxxNxLSxL           LxxLxLxxNxLSxL              LxxLxLxxNxLSxL
LQNNDISELRKDDFKGLQHLYALVLVNNKISKIHEKAFSPLRKLQKLYISKNHLVEIPPN      120
   K T IKDG N KN  T I I           SPG  A  V  ER  L  Q K L EK       118
  SE LLYTFSLATLMPYTR TQ N DRCELT LQVDGT-- PV GT DL H Q QSL LL      97
  TG N TA PPGLLDA P---------------------------------------·       57
  VEFFNLTH PANLLQ ASK QE H SS GLESLSPEFLRPVPQ RV DLTR A TGL  GLF   101


    LxxLxLxxNxLSxL           LxxLxLxxNxLSxL             LxxLxLx
-LPSSLVELRIHDNRIRKVPKGVFSGLRNMNEIEMGGNPLENSGFEPGAFDGLK-LNYLRIS    180
-M KT Q    VEET  R S  N   NQ IVV LT    KS  I N   QMKS I  A        179
GQTLPALTVLDSF RLTSL LGALR  GELQ LYLK  E KTLPPGLLT--PTPK EKLSLA    157
---------------------------------------------------------------
QASAT DT VLKE QLEVLEVSWLH  KALGHLDLS  R RKLPPGLLA--NFTL RT DLG    161


xNxLSxL            LxxLxLxxNxLSxL          LxxLxLxxNxLSxL
EAKLTGIPKDL---PETLNELHLDHNKIQAIELEDLLRYSKLYRLGLGHNQIRMIENGSLSFL  240
DTNI T  QG --- PS T    G   TKVDAAS KGLNN AK   SF S SAVD    ANT    239
NN    EL AG LNGL N DT L QE SLYT PKGFF-------------------------   193
---------------------------------------------------------------
ENQ ETL P  LRG LQ ER    EG  L VLGKDL  PQPD RY F NG KLARVAAGAFQGL  224


  LxxLxLxxNxLSxL           LxxLxLxxNxLSxL
PTLRELHLDNNKLSRVPAGLPDLKLLQVVYLHTNNITKVGVNDF-CPVGFGVKRAYYNGIS    300
  H       N    AK  G VA H YI   N  SAI S    -  P YNT K S S V       299
----------------------GSH  PFAF HG PWLCN------ EILYFRRWLQDNAENVYV  230
----------------------A RTAH GA PWRCD------ RLVPLRAWLAGRPER       91
RQ DM D SN S AS  E   WASLGQPNWDMRDGFDISGNPWI-- DQNLSDLYRWLQAQ-    282


LFNNPVPYWEVQPATFRCVTDRLAIQFGNYY                PG I (BIGLYCAN)
  S   Q   I  S      VV A V  L                  PGII (DECORIN)
KQGVD KAMTSNV SVQ DNSDKFPVYKYPGKGCPTLGDEGDTDLYDYYPEE-- GP1B ALPHA
APYR----------DLR  APP RGRLLP LAEDELRAACAPGPLCWGAIAA-- GP1B BETA
------KDKMFSQNDTR AGPEAVKGQTLLAVAKSQ           LRG
```

FIG. 2. Comparison of the primary structures of bovine biglycan, decorin, platelet glycoprotein 1B (GP1B), and the leucine-rich α_2-glycoprotein (LRG). The sequences of bovine PG I (biglycan) and PG II (decorin) are aligned with each other. The human equivalents differ from the bovine sequence in the 22 NH$_2$-terminal amino acids. In the remainder of the sequence, comprising the leucine-rich repeats and the COOH-terminal disulfide bond-containing region, only seven residues differ between human and bovine PG I and 16 residues differ between human and bovine PG II.

The consensus sequence for a leucine-rich repeat is shown above the proteoglycan sequences. Numbers on the right refer to the residue number starting at the NH$_2$-terminal of the intact protein. Disulfide bonds are shown by lines.

The sequences of the NH$_2$-terminal (extracellular) regions of platelet proteins GP1b alpha and beta are also shown for comparison and have been aligned with the proteoglycans using the NH$_2$-terminal disulfide bond-defined loop, the leucine-rich repeats, and the less conserved COOH-terminal disulfide bond-defined loop. The lowest of the five sequences is the leucine-rich alpha-2 glycoprotein (LRG).

Blanks indicate identity with PG I. Some gaps (−) have been inserted to improve the alignment. Modified from Neame et al., (ref. 40).

to serine residues at positions 5 and 11 at the NH_2-terminus, whereas decorin contains a single glycosaminoglycan chain attached to the serine residue at position 4. The core proteins of biglycan and decorin are composed of four distinct domains. Domain 1 at the NH_2-terminus consists of 20 to 23 amino acids and contains the glycosaminoglycan chain attachment sites described above. Domain 2 is adjacent to domain 1 near the NH_2-terminus. It contains a disulfide bond between Cys^{27} and Cys^{40}, and contains a cysteine pattern similar to a domain in mouse metallothioneine.

Domain 3 is a large domain consisting of approximately 230 amino acids, which comprises most of the core protein. As shown in Fig. 2, domain 3 of both biglycan and decorin contains a series of ten leucine-rich repeats, each 14 residues in length, characterized by the consensus sequence LxxLxLxxNxLSxL in which leucine is present at positions 1, 4, 6, 11, and 14 of the 14 residue amino acid sequence (40). Leucine-rich repeats with the same consensus sequence are present in other proteins, including the leucine-rich α_2-glycoprotein (LRG), and platelet membrane glycoprotein (GPIb) that binds von Willebrand's factor and is involved in platelet aggregation (36–40, 51). Domain 4 consists of 49 amino acids and contains an amino acid sequence unique to biglycan and decorin.

Figure 1 shows only a few selected members of the family of small interstitial proteoglycans whose core proteins show significant homology. Schwarz *et al.* (52) have isolated from the medium of cultured human MG-63 osteosarcoma cells and human skin fibroblasts another small interstitial proteoglycan called PG-100, based on the 100 kDa molecular mass of the proteoglycan core protein. An antiserum against PG-100 showed partial cross-reactivity with decorin. PG-100 contained a single chondroitin sulfate chain of average molecular mass 29 kDa. PG-100 did not bind to type I collagen fibrils or TGFβ.

BIOCHEMICAL PROPERTIES OF THE DSPGs

Studies of the effects of biglycan and decorin on cell adhesion to fibronectin described below have required that biglycan and decorin be isolated to homogeneity in amounts sufficient for these studies. The procedure used for the isolation of the individual species to homogeneity involves six basic steps (20). The identification of biglycan and decorin in fractions from sequential chromatographic procedures used for their isolation has been facilitated by their distinctive appearance and complete separation on SDS-polyacrylamide gel electrophoresis (PAGE) (18–20). Biglycan and decorin from calf articular cartilage have true monomeric molecular weights of 100,000 and 70,000 in 4 M guanidine HCl, based on sedimentation equilibrium studies. However, in other solvents, biglycan forms higher oligomers and on SDS-PAGE, both biglycan and decorin have relatively slow mobilities compared with protein standards. Because of this, biglycan and decorin have apparent average molecular weight of approximately 300,000 and 120,000 on SDS-PAGE (20). Biglycan and decorin separate completely on SDS-PAGE and form two distinct broad bands that stain intensely

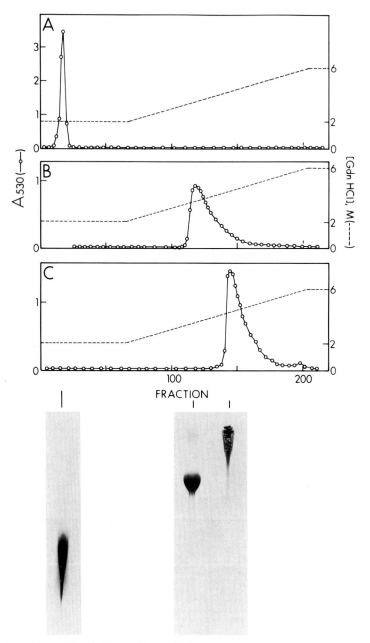

FIG. 3. Comparison of the binding affinities of the homogeneous, individual species, biglycan and decorin, on octyl-Sepharose. Forty mg of homogeneous biglycan or decorin, or 20 mg of dermatan sulfate chains prepared from the mixture of DS-PGs from articular cartilage, were applied to a 2.7 × 50 cm octyl-Sepharose column at 25°C, and allowed to bind to the column for 2 hr before elution was begun. The column was eluted with three column volumes of 2 M GdnHCl, then with a 2 M to 6 M GdnHCl linear gradient. Fractions were monitored for uronate. Biglycan and decorin and chains eluted from the columns were then examined by SDS-PAGE on the same toluidine blue-stained 4–20% gradient slab gel. **A:** Dermatan sulfate chains; **B:** decorin; **C:** biglycan.

with toluidine blue (Fig. 5). This greatly facilitates their identification during the isolation of the individual species to homogeneity. The first five steps in the isolation procedure involve the extraction and separation of the mixture of the DSPGs from all other contaminating macromolecules. The sixth and final step involves the use of hydrophobic chromatography on octyl-Sepharose to separate biglycan and decorin from each other and isolate the individual species to homogeneity. Figure 3 shows the elution of dermatan sulfate chains, and of purified

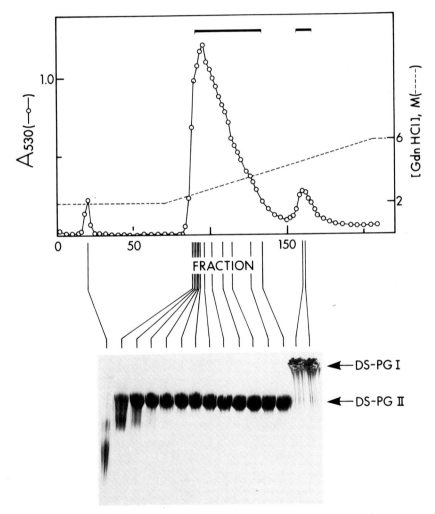

FIG. 4. Isolation of biglycan (DSPG I) and decorin (DSPG II) from bovine fetal skin by octyl-Sepharose chromatography. DSPGs (130 mg in 44 ml) were applied to a 2.7 × 50 cm octyl-Sepharose column in 2 M GdnHCl, 0.15 M sodium acetate, pH 6.3 at 25°C. The column was washed with three column volumes of 2 M GdnHCl, then eluted with a 2 to 6 M GdnHCl linear gradient. Fractions (13.8 ml) collected at a flow rate of 120 ml/hr were analyzed for uronate and by SDS-PAGE. (From Choi et al., ref. 20, with permission).

decorin and biglycan which have been applied individually to octyl-Sepharose columns in three different experiments. Dermatan sulfate chains do not bind to octyl-Sepharose. Decorin and biglycan have different affinities related to differences in the hydrophobicity of their core proteins.

A stringent test of the capacity of octyl-Sepharose chromatography to separate free dermatan sulfate chains, decorin, and biglycan is seen when fractions from bovine fetal skin, which contain free chains, mainly decorin and relatively small amounts of biglycan, are subjected to octyl-Sepharose chromatography using a 2 M to 6 M guanidine HCl gradient (Fig. 4). Free chains do not bind and are eluted in the 2 M guanidine HCl wash. Decorin is eluted at 2.8 to 3.9 M guanidine HCl. Bovine fetal skin contains very small amounts of biglycan which are concentrated and eluted at approximately 4.5 M guanidine HCl. Figure 5 shows the appearance on SDS-PAGE of biglycan and decorin isolated from calf articular cartilage and bovine fetal skin isolated by this procedure.

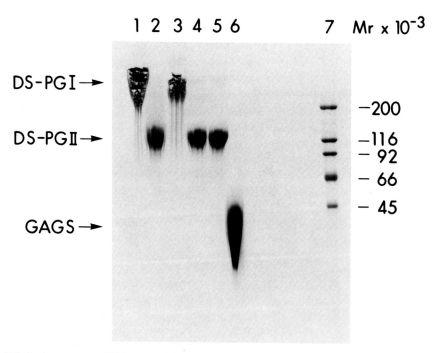

FIG. 5. Appearance of biglycan and decorin on toluidine blue-stained 4–20% gradient slab gel, following SDS-PAGE in 0.375 M Tris. **Lanes 1 and 2:** Biglycan and decorin from calf articular cartilage, respectively; **Lane 3:** biglycan from bovine fetal skin; **Lanes 4 and 5:** two different preparations of decorin from bovine fetal skin; **Lane 6:** glycosaminoglycan chains prepared from the mixture of DSPGs from articular cartilage; **Lane 7:** M_r standards. (From Choi et al., ref. 20, with permission).

STUDIES OF THE BINDING OF DSPGs TO FIBRONECTIN

Results from three different laboratories have shown that decorin, biglycan, and their core proteins bind to intact fibronectin (8–11,53). Lewandowska *et al.* (9) demonstrated the binding of DSPGs from bovine articular cartilage to intact fibronectin by affinity chromatography using fibronectin-Sepharose columns. Schmidt *et al.* (8) demonstrated the binding of decorin from human skin fibroblasts and its core protein to fibronectin using a solid phase assay. Lebaron *et al.* (11) examined the binding of decorin, biglycan, and their core proteins to fibronectin in the following studies.

Decorin and biglycan were prepared from bovine articular cartilage and characterized as previously described (20). The proteoglycans were iodinated using the chloramine-T method. Immulon plates were coated with either intact fibronectin or the 105 kDa cell binding domain of fibronectin. Nonspecific sites were blocked with bovine serum albumin. ^{125}I-DSPG was incubated for 3 hr in fibronectin-coated wells, or fibronectin-coated wells that had been preincubated for 1 hr with unlabeled cold DSPG, DSPG core proteins, or glycosaminoglycan chains prepared from the DSPGs. Unbound DSPGs were removed, the wells were rinsed, and the bound ^{125}I-DSPGs were determined in a gamma counter. ^{125}I-decorin or ^{125}I-biglycan alone bound avidly to intact fibronectin or the 105 kDa cell binding domain (CBD) of fibronectin. Unlabeled cold DSPG or the DSPG core protein strongly inhibited this binding, whereas dermatan sulfate chains were only weakly inhibitory. These results indicate that intact DSPGs bind to intact fibronectin and that the binding is mediated predominantly by the proteoglycan core protein. However, the weak effect of the dermatan sulfate chains in these competitive inhibition experiments, and additional observations described below, suggest that the dermatan sulfate chains may under some conditions also interact with fibronectin, affect its conformation and binding properties, and play a role in the capacity of the DSPGs to bind to fibronectin and inhibit cell adhesion. For example, Schmidt *et al.* (8) made the following observations.

Preincubation of fibronectin with dermatan sulfate or heparin chains had no effect on the subsequent binding of decorin or its core protein to fibronectin. However, when dermatan sulfate chains or heparin were incubated simultaneously with decorin or its core protein, the binding of decorin or its core protein to fibronectin was greatly decreased.

Studies were also carried out to identify the fibronectin fragments and domains within fibronectin to which decorin and biglycan bind. Following the digestion of fibronectin with chymotrypsin, Lewandowska *et al.* (9) prepared a 120 kDa cell-binding fragment (CBF) which contained RGD-mediated cell-binding activity, but no heparin- or collagen-binding activity when assayed as a soluble ligand. Fibronectin or CBF were adsorbed to tissue culture wells, incubated with DSPGs, rinsed, and the amounts of bound DSPGs determined by ELISA. The DSPGs bound avidly to fibronectin and CBF. Indeed, twice as much DSPG bound to CBF as to intact fibronectin, suggesting that the binding affinity of DSPGs for CBF might be higher than that for intact fibronectin. Similar observations have been made by Lebaron et al. (11).

Lebaron et al. (11) examined the binding of intact decorin, biglycan, and their core proteins to the 105 kDa cell-binding domain (CBD) of fibronectin, using ^{125}I-DSPG and competitive inhibition studies with unlabeled DSPG, DSPG core proteins, and dermatan sulfate chains. The studies demonstrated that the intact DSPG bound to CBD, and that the binding was strongly inhibited by the intact DSPG or its core protein. The authors concluded that DSPGs bind to the CBD of fibronectin via the DSPG core proteins. However, Schmidt et al. (8) obtained different results. Fibronectin peptides that contained the CBD NH_2-terminal, or COOH-terminal heparin-binding domain, or collagen-binding domain were prepared by digestion with cathepsin D, trypsin, or chymotrypsin, and isolated by affinity chromatography using heparin-Sepharose, gelatin-Sepharose, and gel chromatography. The homogeneity of the peptides was assessed by chromatography and SDS-PAGE. Decorin and its core protein bound strongly to peptides that contained the COOH-terminal heparin-binding domain. They bound weakly to peptides containing the NH_2-terminal heparin-binding domain.

Under the conditions used in these earlier studies (8), binding of decorin core protein to the CBD of fibronectin could not be demonstrated. However, in subsequent studies by Winnemoller et al. (53), the binding of decorin core protein to the CBD of fibronectin was clearly demonstrated. Thus, the binding of decorin and biglycan to fibronectin is mediated predominantly by the binding of the proteoglycan core protein to the CBD of fibronectin. However, the dermatan sulfate proteoglycans also appear to bind to other fibronectin domains.

DSPGs INHIBIT CELL ADHESION TO FIBRONECTIN

Several studies have also shown that decorin and biglycan inhibit the attachment of cells to fibronectin or its fragments. Lewandowska et al. (9) examined the effect of articular cartilage DSPGs on cell adhesion to intact fibronectin and to its 120 kDa CBF. BALB/3T3 cells were labeled with [³H]thymidine and added to fibronectin or CBF-coated substrata that had been pretreated with the mixture of DSPGs from bovine articular cartilage. Pretreatment with the mixture of *decorin and biglycan* from articular cartilage strongly inhibited the attachment and spreading of the 3T3 cells on either fibronectin or CBF. Pretreatment of the *cells* with DSPGs did not inhibit adhesion, suggesting that the binding of the DSPGs to cell surface receptors is not involved in the mechanism by which cell adhesion is inhibited. Dermatan sulfate chains or core proteins prepared from the DSPGs did not inhibit cell attachment. The intact proteoglycan with its glycosaminoglycan chains was necessary for inhibition.

One possible interpretation of the results described above is that an intact DSPG such as biglycan binds via its core protein to or near the CBD of fibronectin, the glycosaminoglycan chains of the DSPG then block the binding of cell surface receptors (integrins) to RGD-containing cell-binding sites of fibronectin, and this prevents cell attachment. However, additional observations by Lewandowska *et al.* (9) could not be reconciled with this hypothesis. Cell attachment could also be inhibited with high concentrations of heparin (>500 μg/ml). Fragments from cellular fibronectin (44 and 47 kDa) which contained the COOH-terminal heparin-binding domain and the "extra" domain, EDa, but no RGD-containing CBD supported cell attachment which was completely inhibited by the DSPGs. Based on these observations, Lewandowska *et al.* (9) suggested that the mechanism of inhibition involved the binding of the DSPGs to a cryptic glycosaminoglycan-binding domain present in the 120 kDa CBF. Lewandowska *et al.* (9) presented evidence that this cryptic GAG-binding domain was active and supported the binding of DSPGs only in substratum-bound CBF or intact fibronectin and was not observed in soluble CBF or fibronectin. Thus, Lewandowska *et al.* (9) suggested that the DSPGs bind to fibronectin via their GAG chains and the DSPGs either sterically hinder the binding of cell surface receptors (integrins), or the binding of the DSPGs results in a conformational change in fibronectin which decreases the binding affinity of the cell surface receptors for fibronectin RGD-containing binding sites.

Bidanset *et al.* (11) examined the capacity of decorin and biglycan from bovine articular cartilage to inhibit the attachment of CHO cells or rat embryo fibroblasts to intact fibronectin. Cells were labeled with ^{3}H-thymidine, and endogenous protein synthesis was inhibited with cycloheximide. Tissue culture wells were coated with fibronectin or CBD. The fibronectin or CBD on the wells was then preincubated with decorin or biglycan for 1 hr prior to the addition of cells. Labeled cells were then added and allowed to attach for 90 min in the presence of decorin or biglycan. Unattached cells were removed and the percentage of attached cells was determined. Both decorin and biglycan were potent inhibitors of cell attachment to CBD. At 20 μg/ml, cell attachment was decreased by 80%, and at 50 μg/ml, cell attachment was almost completely inhibited. However, the results with intact fibronectin were surprising. Under the conditions used by Bidanset *et al.,* neither decorin nor biglycan had a significant effect on the attachment of CHO cells or rat embryo fibroblasts to intact fibronectin. Lewandowska *et al.* (9) and Bidanset *et al.* (11) all found that articular cartilage DSPGs strongly inhibit the attachment of cells to the CBD *fragment* of fibronectin. However, Lewandowska *et al.* found that 3T3 cell attachment to intact fibronectin is also strongly inhibited, while Lebaron *et al.* (11) found that CHO cell and rat embryo fibroblast attachment to intact fibronectin is not inhibited. The reason for these different results is not known.

Bidanset *et al.* (11) studied the mechanism of inhibition of CHO cell attachment to the CBD of fibronectin. Studies were carried out to determine if the inhibitory effect of the DSPGs was due to an interaction between the proteoglycans and the CHO cells, or the binding of proteoglycan to the CBD. Cells were incubated with decorin or biglycan, rinsed, then seeded on CBD-coated wells. Pretreatment of CHO cells did not inhibit attachment. However, when CBD-coated wells were pretreated with proteoglycan and rinsed, cell attachment was inhibited, almost to the same extent as when proteoglycan was added to CBD-coated wells and remained present through the incubation.

As noted above, Bidanset *et al.* (11) have provided evidence that the core proteins of decorin and biglycan bind avidly to CBD. Experiments were carried out to determine whether the binding of decorin or biglycan *core protein* to CBD would inhibit the attachment of CHO cells to CBD. Wells were coated with CBD and preincubated with either intact decorin, biglycan, their core proteins, or their GAG chains. Preincubation of substrates with the core proteins or GAG chains did not inhibit the attachment of CHO cells to CBD. Intact decorin or biglycan was essential to inhibit the attachment of CHO cells to CBD. However, preincubation of CBD with DSPG core protein will block the binding of intact DSPG to CBD, and abolish the capacity of the intact DSPG to inhibit attachment.

Winnemoller *et al.* (53) have shown that human fibroblast decorin and its core protein inhibit the adhesion of fibroblasts to intact fibronectin and its CBD. Decorin was isolated directly from the medium of cultured human fibroblasts under nondenaturing conditions. Other studies have involved the use of decorin and biglycan initially extracted from cartilage in 4 M guanidine HCl (9,11). Winnemoller *et al.* (53) noted that to demonstrate the inhibition by decorin of cell adhesion to intact fibronectin, it was essential to avoid denaturing conditions. Exposure to guanidine, repeated freezing and thawing, etc. resulted in a loss of biologic activity. In the presence of decorin, there was a 30 to 40% inhibition of cell adhesion to intact fibronectin, compared to over 90% inhibition in the studies of Lewandowska *et al.* (9). Decorin core protein also inhibited cell adhesion to intact fibronectin, but in most experiments, it was less effective than intact decorin. Dermatan sulfate, heparan sulfate, and heparin had no effect. Similar results were obtained when the fibronectin CBD, rather than intact fibronectin, was used.

The binding of decorin core protein to fibronectin and its CBD was carefully reexamined using polyclonal antibodies to decorin core protein in a solid phase immunoassay, or ^{35}S-methionine-labeled decorin or decorin core protein. Both methods clearly demonstrated that decorin and its core protein bind to fibronectin and its CBD.

In summary, the binding of the DSPGs to fibronectin and the capacity of the DSPGs to inhibit cell adhesion to fibronectin have now been examined in several laboratories. The present state of knowledge is summarized in Fig. 6. These studies have shown that DSPGs bind to fibronectin and inhibit cell attachment to fibronectin or its fragments. The core proteins of biglycan and decorin bind strongly to fibronectin and appear to mediate the binding of the proteoglycan to fibronectin. However, to obtain a maximal inhibitory effect on cell attachment, an intact proteoglycan with its glycosaminoglycan chains was required in the majority of these studies.

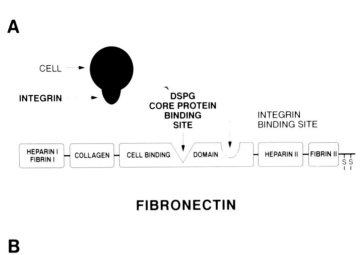

FIBRONECTIN

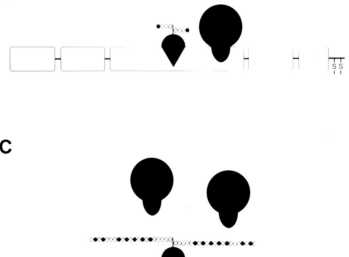

FIG. 6. The binding of a small interstitial dermatan sulfate proteoglycan to fibronectin and its inhibitory effect on cell adhesion. **A:** Decorin and biglycan bind via their core proteins to the cell-binding domain of fibronectin. **B:** In the studies of Lewandowska *et al.* (9) and Lebaron *et al.* (11), the binding of the DSPG core protein to the cell-binding domain of fibronectin did not inhibit cell adhesion. **C:** In these studies (9,11), intact biglycan or decorin with its glycosaminoglycan chains was required for a strong inhibitory effect on cell adhesion.

This suggests that the glycosaminoglycan chains of the proteoglycan may interact with fibronectin and affect its conformation and interactions with cells, or that the proteoglycan glycosaminoglycan chains may interact with the cells themselves during the process of cell attachment in a way that is not presently understood. The biochemical mechanisms involved in the inhibition of cell adhesion to fibronectin by decorin and biglycan are not yet clear.

ACKNOWLEDGMENTS

This work was supported by United States Public Health Service grants AR34614 and AR21498.

REFERENCES

1. Scott JE, Orford CR. Dermatan sulphate-rich proteoglycan associates with rat tail tendon collagen at the d band in the gap region. *Biochem J* 1981;195:213–216.
2. Scott JE. The periphery of the developing collagen fibril. Quantitative relationships with dermatan sulphate and other surface-associated species. *Biochem J* 1984;218:229–233.
3. Scott JE, Hughes EW. Proteoglycan-collagen relationships in developing chick and bovine tendons. Influence of the physiological environment. *Connect Tissue Res* 1986;14:267–278.
4. Scott JE. Proteoglycan-fibrillar collagen interactions. *Biochem J* 1988;252:313–323.
5. Vogel KG, Paulsson M, Heinegard D. Specific inhibition of type I and type II collagen fibrillogenesis by the small proteoglycan of tendon. *Biochem J* 1984;223:587–597.
6. Vogel KG, Trotter JA. The effect of proteoglycans on the morphology of collagen fibrils formed in vitro. *Coll Rel Res* 1987;7:105–114.
7. Brown DC, Vogel KG. Characteristics of the in vitro interaction of a small proteoglycan (PGII) of bovine tendon with type I collagen. *Matrix* 1989;9:468–478.
8. Schmidt G, Robenek H, Harrach B, Glossl J, Nolte V, Hormann H, Richter H, Kresse H. Interaction of small dermatan sulfate proteoglycan from fibroblasts with fibronectin. *J Cell Biol* 1987;104:1,683–691.
9. Lewandowska K, Choi HU, Rosenberg LC, Zardi L, Culp LA. Fibronectin-mediated adhesion of fibroblasts: inhibition by dermatan sulfate proteoglycan and evidence for a cryptic glycosaminoglycan-binding domain. *J Cell Biol* 1987;105:1,443–454.
10. Rosenberg LC, Choi HU, Poole AR, Lewandowska K, Culp LA. Biological roles of dermatan sulphate proteoglycans. In: *Functions of the proteoglycans.* Ciba Foundation Symposium 124. Chichester, England: John Wiley, 1986;47–68.
11. Bidanset DJ, Lebaron, R, Rosenberg L, Murphy-Ullrich JE, Hook M. Regulation of cell substrate adhesion: effects of small galactosaminoglycan-containing proteoglycans. (submitted).
12. Yamaguchi Y, Mann DM, Ruoslahti E. Negative regulation of transforming growth factor-β by the proteoglycan decorin. *Nature* 1990;346:281–284.
13. Tollefsen DM, Peacock ME, Monafo WJ. Molecular size of dermatan sulfate oligosaccharides required to bind and activate heparin cofactor II. *J Biol Chem* 1986;261:8854–8858.
14. Mankin HJ. The reaction of articular cartilage to injury and osteoarthritis. *N Engl J Med* 1974;291:1285–1292.
15. Ohno O, Naito J, Iguchi T, Ishikawa H, Hirohata K, Cooke T. An electron microscopic study of early pathology in chondromalacia of the patella. *J Bone Joint Surg* 1988;70-A:883–899.
16. Meachim G. The effects of scarification on articular cartilage of the rabbit. *J Bone Joint Surg* 1963;45-B:150–161.
17. Moscowitz RW, Davis W, Sammarco J, Martens M, Baker J, Mayor M, Burstein AH, Frankel VH. Experimentally induced degenerative joint lesions following partial meniscectomy in the rabbit. *Arthritis Rheum* 1973;16:397–405.

18. Rosenberg LC, Choi HU, Tang L-H, Johnson TL, Pal S, Webber C, Reiner A, Poole AR. Isolation of dermatan sulfate proteoglycans from mature bovine articular cartilages. *J Biol Chem* 1985;260: 6304–6313.

19. Sampaio LDeO, Bayliss MT, Hardingham TE, Muir H. Dermatan sulphate proteoglycan from human articular cartilage. Variation in its content with age and its structural comparison with a small chondroitin sulphate proteoglycan from pig laryngeal cartilage. *Biochem J* 1988;254: 757–764.

20. Choi HU, Johnson TL, Pal S, Tang L-H, Rosenberg L, Neame PJ. Characterization of the dermatan sulfate proteoglycans, DS-PGI and DS-PGII, from bovine articular cartilage and skin isolated by octyl-Sepharose chromatography. *J Biol Chem* 1989;264:2876–2884.

21. Vogel KG, Heinegard D. Characterization of proteoglycans from adult bovine tendon. *J Biol Chem* 1985;260:9298–9306.

22. Vogel KG, Evanko SP. Proteoglycans of fetal bovine tendon. *J Biol Chem* 1987;262:13,607–613.

23. Vogel KG, Fisher LW. Comparisons of antibody reactivity and enzyme sensitivity between small proteoglycans from bovine tendon, bone and cartilage. *J Biol Chem* 1986;261:11,334–340.

24. Miyamoto I, Nagase S. Isolation and characterization of proteodermatan sulfate from rat skin. *J Biochem (Tokyo)* 1980;88:1,793–803.

25. Fujii N, Nagai Y. Isolation and characterization of proteodermatan sulfate from calf skin. *J Biochem (Tokyo)* 1981;90:1249–1258.

26. Damle SP, Coster L, Gregory JD. Proteodermatan sulfate isolated from pig skin. *J Biol Chem* 1982;257:5,523–5,527.

27. Pearson CH, Winterbottom N, Fackre DS, Scott PG, Carpenter MR. The NH_2-terminal amino acid sequence of bovine skin proteodermatan sulfate. *J Biol Chem* 1983;258:15,101–104.

28. Coster L, Fransson LA. Isolation and characterization of dermatan sulphate proteoglycans from bovine sclera. *Biochem J* 1981;193:143–153.

29. Coster L, Fransson LA, Sheehan J, Nieduszynski IA, Phelps CF. Self-association of dermatan sulphate proteoglycans from bovine sclera. *Biochem J* 1981;197:483–490.

30. Coster L, Rosenberg LC, van der Rest M, Poole AR. The dermatan sulfate proteoglycans of bovine sclera and their relationship to those of articular cartilage. An immunological and biochemical study. *J Biol Chem* 1987;262:3809–3812.

31. Fisher LW, Termine JD, Dejter SW Jr, Shitson SW, Yanagishita M, Kimura JH, Hascall VC, Kleinman HK, Hassell JR, Nilsson B. Proteoglycans of developing bone. *J Biol Chem* 1983;258: 6,588–594.

32. Franzen A, Heinegard D. Extraction and purification of proteoglycans from mature bovine bone. *Biochem J* 1984;224:47–58.

33. Fisher LW. The nature of proteoglycans of bone. In: Butler WT, ed. *The chemistry and biology of mineralized tissues.* Birmingham: EBSCO Media, 1985;188–196.

34. Fisher LW, Hawkins GR, Tuross N, Termine JD. Purification and partial characterization of small proteoglycans I and II, bone sialoproteins I and II, and osteonectin from the mineral component of developing human bone. *J Biol Chem* 1987;262:9,702–708.

35. Heinegard D, Paulsson M, Inerot S, Carlstrom C. A novel low-molecular weight chondroitin sulphate proteoglycan isolated from cartilage. *Biochem J* 1981;197:355–366.

36. Krusius T, Ruoslahti E. Primary structure of an extracellular matrix proteoglycan core protein deduced from cloned cDNA. *Proc Natl Acad Sci USA* 1986;83:7,683–687.

37. Day AA, Ramis CI, Fisher LW, Gehron-Robey P, Termine JD, Young MF. Characterization of bone PG II cDNA and its relationship to PG II mRNA from other connective tissues. *Nucleic Acids Res* 1986;14:9861–9876.

38. Day AA, McQuillan CI, Termine JD, Young MF. Molecular cloning and sequence analysis of the cDNA for small proteoglycan II of bovine bone. *Biochem J* 1987;248:801–805.

39. Fisher LW, Termine JD, Young MF. Deduced protein sequence of bone small proteoglycan I (biglycan) shows homology with proteoglycan II (decorin) and several nonconnective tissue proteins in a variety of species. *J Biol Chem* 1989;264:4,571–576.

40. Neame PJ, Choi HU, Rosenberg LC. The primary structure of the core protein of the small, leucine-rich proteoglycan (PG I) from bovine articular cartilage. *J Biol Chem* 1989;264:8,653–661.

41. Fransson LA, Roden L. Structure of dermatan sulfate. I. Degradation by testicular hyaluronidase. *J Biol Chem* 1967;242:4,161–169.

42. Fransson LA, Roden L. Structure of dermatan sulfate. II. Characterization of products obtained by hyaluronidase digestion of dermatan sulfate. *J Biol Chem* 1967;242:4,170–175.
43. Fransson LA. Structure of dermatan sulfate. III. The hybrid structure of dermatan sulfate from umbilical cord. *J Biol Chem* 1968;243:1,504–510.
44. Fransson LA, Malmstrom A. Structure of pig skin dermatan sulfate. I. Distribution of D-glucuronic acid residues. *Eur J Biochem* 1971;18:422–430.
45. Coster L, Malmstrom A, Sjoberg I, Fransson LA. The co-polymeric structure of pig skin dermatan sulphate. Distribution of L-iduronic acid sulphate residues in co-polymeric chains. *Biochem J* 1975;145:379–389.
46. Malmstrom A, Carlstedt I, Aberg L, Fransson LA. The co-polymeric structure of dermatan sulphate produced by cultured human fibroblasts. Different distribution of iduronic acid- and glucuronic acid-containing units in soluble and cell-associated glycans. *Biochem J.* 1975;151: 477–489.
47. Fransson LA. Interaction between dermatan sulphate chains. I. Affinity chromatography of co-polymeric galactosaminoglycans on dermatan sulphate-substituted agarose. *Biochim Biophys Acta* 1976;437:106–115.
48. Fransson LA, Coster L. Interaction between dermatan sulphate chains. II. Structural studies on aggregating glycan chains and oligosaccharides with affinity for dermatan sulphate-substituted agarose. *Biochim Biophys Acta* 1979;582:132–144.
49. Fransson LA, Nieduszynski IA, Phelps CF, Sheenan JK. Interactions between dermatan sulphate chains. III. Light-scattering and viscometry studies of self-association. *Biochim Biophys Acta* 1979;586:179–188.
50. Fransson LA, Coster L, Malmstrom A, Sheenan JK. Self-association of scleral proteodermatan sulfate. Evidence for interaction via the dermatan sulfate side chains. *J Biol Chem* 1982;257: 6,333–338.
51. Patthy L. Detecting homology of distantly related proteins with consensus sequences. *J Mol Biol* 1987;198:567–577.
52. Schwarz K, Breuer B, Kresse H. Biosynthesis and properties of a further member of the small chondroitin/dermatan sulfate proteoglycan family. *J Biol Chem* 1990;265:22023–22028.
53. Winnemoller M, Schmidt G, Kresse H. Influence of decorin on fibroblast adhesion to fibronectin. *Eur J Cell Biol* 1991;54:10–17.

DISCUSSION

Hascall: There are differences between the functions of biglycan and decorin. Most evidence indicates that biglycan does not interact well with collagen and that this is not its particular function. There is some very interesting work now coming out on the relationship of biglycan to skeletal growth. Ule Vetter and collaborators at the National Institutes of Health have shown a correlation between biglycan synthesis in fibroblasts from patients with Turner's and Klinefelter's syndromes and skeletal growth. In cartilage the localization of these two proteoglycans appears to be quite different, with the biglycan being more cell- and cell matrix-associated, while decorin is more concentrated in the matrix, consistent with its binding function to collagen.

Rosenberg: I agree with the clear difference in immunohistochemical localization. However, with regard to biglycan interacting with collagen, some work indicates that biglycan can bind to collagen under somewhat different experimental conditions. Whether or not it affects fibrillogenesis, I don't know.

Lust: Does biglycan increase in osteoarthritic cartilage? Does cellular fibronectin bind as well as plasma fibronectin?

Rosenberg: Okay. Here we go. Lloyd Culp's studies used cellular fibronectin to which a mixture of biglycan and decorin is bound. These results are somewhat different from those reported by others, who prepared fragments from plasma fibronectin that did not contain the cell-binding domain, but did contain the carboxy terminal heparin-binding domain and the ED domain. Cells adhered to this fragment even though it did not contain the cell-binding domain. Therefore, their interpretation is more complex, suggesting that the core protein of these proteoglycans binds to more than just the cell-binding domain of fibronectin.

Kresse: I should say that it's even more complex. Decorin core protein binds to the heparin-binding domains near the N-terminus and also binds near the C-terminus of fibronectin, in addition to its interaction with the cell-binding domain.

Mason: The idea that these small dermatan sulfate proteoglycans inhibit tissue repair processes is very intriguing. How do you reconcile it with the fact that these proteoglycans are expressed in other tissues that readily undergo repair? Is it merely their concentration in cartilage that prevents repair, or is there some other factor involved?

Rosenberg: That is a wonderful question. A lesion restricted to cartilage which does not have access to macrophages and other cells which secrete proteolytic enzymes does not repair, and no cell migration occurs over its surface. If the lesion penetrates into subchondral bone, an entirely different set of events occurs. Proteoglycans decrease from the surface of the cartilage. Macrophages penetrate and probably degrade the dermatan sulfate proteoglycans from the surface. A fibrin clot can then form, and a full-blown reparative response is initiated which looks quite good after about 2 months. However, it then proceeds to fall apart. I think, then, that articular cartilage is walled off from a blood supply, and except under certain situations, like rheumatoid arthritis where there is an influx of inflammatory cells with their proteolytic enzymes, the dermatan sulfate proteoglycans are not degraded and thus shield the surface of collagen fibrils and prevent cell adhesion and migration. Ernst Hunziker has tested this hypothesis by removing proteoglycans from the surfaces of superficial defects that would be analogous to early human osteoarthritic lesions.

Hunziker: We created superficial defects in rabbit articular cartilage. The exposed surfaces were treated with chondroitinase to remove superficial proteoglycans. After 1 month, the surface is covered with mesenchymal-like cells that have migrated in and attached to the whole defect area. After about 6 months the cartilage matrix is refilled by intact, underlying chondrocytes that regenerate the depleted matrix.

Articular Cartilage and Osteoarthritis,
edited by K. Kuettner et al.
Raven Press, Ltd., New York © 1992.

Part II: Structural Components of Cartilage: Matrix Biology

Introduction

Marvin L. Tanzer

Department of Biostructure and Function, University of Connecticut Health Center, Farmington, Connecticut 06030

The study of cartilage matrix components is, in some ways, still in the descriptive stage. Various molecules have been identified, isolated, and characterized. The most abundant molecules, type II collagen and chondroitin sulfate proteoglycan, have well-defined roles in cartilage structure and function. Some of the less abundant molecules, decorin and fibromodulin, type IX and type XI collagens, are believed to play regulatory roles in collagen fibrillogenesis. They may act as nucleating substances (type XI collagen) for collagen fibril initiation, or as fibril-diameter limiting substances (type IX collagen, decorin, fibromodulin). Other molecules, biglycan, cartilage matrix protein, 36 kDa protein, COMP protein, and CH21 protein have less well-defined roles at present. In considering what these various substances might be doing in cartilage, we can suggest an analogy to the study of skeletal muscle. For many years, the major and minor protein constituents of muscle have been investigated and their interrelationships progressively deciphered. However, it is only recently that the dramatic progress provided by molecular genetics has not only discovered a new unsuspected protein, dystrophin, but has also pinpointed the importance of dystrophin in maintaining the normal integrity of skeletal muscle. Thus, not only may the previously mentioned minor components of cartilage be of great importance to the tissue, but there may be undiscovered substances which also play a critical role in the maintenance of tissue organization.

It is well established that some of the components of cartilage undergo time-dependent changes in their relative abundance, and their molecular composition in which the protein component may become shorter, and in which the post-translational modifications (primarily glycosylation) may be altered in their pattern of expression. The basis for these changes must ultimately be traced to the genome, which can regulate expression of the cartilage components in several ways. The relative abundance of a cartilage component is a reflection of its tissue half-life. This, in turn, is a balance of synthesis and degradation of the component.

Genetic regulation can modulate the balance, both in directly affecting production of the component and in affecting production of specific hydrolytic enzyme(s) and their inhibitor(s). The hydrolytic enzyme(s) would, in this case, be recognizing the particular cartilage component as a substrate. Regulation of genes can occur in two fundamental ways, via regulatory sequences within DNA itself, and via specific proteins which bind to DNA at regulatory sites. Both phenomena occur and may be important in regulating chondrocyte expression. Cytokines and growth factors act to signal cells, including chondrocytes, provoking a particular response. In this regard, it is important to note that cartilage, being relatively avascular tissue, may not receive signals from the circulation as rapidly as do vascular tissues. In fact, some of the low molecular weight factors appear to bind to the extracellular matrix which acts as a repository for them. Thus, chondrocytes may either be "protected" from their effects, or may be receiving a steady signal which is barely modulated. Given that there are a wide range of cytokines and growth factors, cells may respond to their collective stimuli by integration and summation of the signals. This type of response is reminiscent of neuronal cell responses to excitatory and inhibitory stimuli.

As in other tissues, the extracellular matrix molecules themselves may serve as stimuli for chondrocytes. Determining whether chondrocytes are equipped with the repertoire of cell surface receptors exhibited by other cells is certainly of interest. The territorial domain of chondrocytes differs substantially from the remainder of the matrix and may, in fact, serve as a source of signals to the circumscribed cells. Of interest here is the observation that some of the matrix components appear to be preferentially localized to the territorial zone. Whether integrins, cell surface lectins, selectins, or other types of cell surface receptors are operative for chondrocytes is an important point to investigate. Recent developments have implicated cell surface lectin-type receptors which recognize carbohydrate ligands of matrix molecules such as laminin, as well as recognize its peptide domains via the well-known integrin system of receptors. In fact, evidence suggests that laminin reciprocally serves as a lectin, recognizing the corresponding integrin. Given the carbohydrate-rich environment of cartilage cells, the incentive for seeking similar cell-matrix relationships and receptors on the surfaces of chondrocytes becomes even more compelling.

Molecular cloning of many of the cartilage matrix molecules now allows us to investigate structure/function relationships. Many of the matrix molecules exhibit discrete domains characterized by one or more types of posttranslational modification. It is most likely that the information for determining which substituents will be added is encoded by the core protein itself, but not uniquely in the domain which is to be modified. Other regions of the core protein may serve as routing addresses, enabling the core protein to arrive at the proper destination where posttranslational modification will occur. Current evidence indicates that chondrocytes have discrete intracellular distributions of type II collagen and the core protein of chondroitin sulfate proteoglycan. These matrix molecules, presumably en route to the cell surface for secretion, are modified in very different ways. Thus, it is not surprising that they may undergo selective intracellular routing as a means of achieving their mature forms.

Another mode of regulation found for molecules of the extracellular matrix is alternative splicing of the exons of various genes, e.g., those of fibronectin, some proteoglycans, and some collagens. In contrast, laminin expression relies on isoforms generated by a variety of genes. In the case of alternative splicing, the factors which determine the predominant mode of expression are not known. Conceivably, there may be transition states in which several molecular isoforms are present in the tissue, either in a territorial distribution or intermingled within the same areas. Alternative splicing thus provides yet another means for creating cellular and tissue diversity and flexibility. In essence, by using alternative splicing and the other regulatory mechanisms, the cell is manifesting a series of safety and control systems which protect its viability and allow alternative pathways of response. Perhaps in disease processes such regulatory systems go awry, losing their versatility and flexibility. The ability of adult human cartilage to repair itself properly is quite limited; a challenge for the future is to suppress inappropriate responses of the chondrocytes. Ideally, if we could induce them to return to an embryonic state at the cell physiology level, a more suitable tissue repair response might be generated. Such efforts have been partially successful in bone regeneration.

In summary, the powerful techniques of modern biology allow us to explore in great detail the behavior of chondrocytes in their normal environment of cartilage matrix. Comparison of normal behavior with response to injuries should provide new insights into the molecular bases for the regulation of chondrocytic gene expression.

Articular Cartilage and Osteoarthritis,
edited by K. Kuettner et al.
Raven Press, Ltd., New York © 1992.

5

Keratan Sulfate Substitution on Cartilage Matrix Molecules

Anna H. K. Plaas, Frank P. Barry, and Shirley Wong-Palms

Orthopaedic Research Lab, Shriners Hospital for Crippled Children, Tampa Unit, Tampa, Florida 33612, and Department of Biochemistry and Molecular Biology, University of South Florida Medical School, Tampa, Florida 33612

Keratan sulfate (KS) was first isolated from cornea by Meyer in 1953 (1) and was characterized as a sulfated glycosaminoglycan. The major repeat sequence of KS is the disaccharide *N*-acetyl-lactosamine (Gal β1,4 GlcNAc β1,3), which can be variably sulfated in the C6 position of both the galactose and *N*-acetyl-glucosamine moieties. In 1989 a book was published which contains an extensive review of research on the biochemistry of KS in a range of connective tissues, and the reader is referred to that text for general information on this subject (2).

In this chapter we present some studies comparing KS in epiphyseal and articular cartilages. In these cartilages, KS is present on two distinctly different proteoglycans, namely aggrecan and fibromodulin. Aggrecan is the major structural component of cartilage which is responsible for the tissue's ability to withstand compressive load. Fibromodulin is a recently described collagen-binding glycoprotein which is widely distributed in connective tissues.

A major distinguishing feature of the KS on these proteoglycans is the nature of the KS linkage to the core protein. On aggrecan, KS is attached to the terminal nonreducing galactose of an O-linked oligosaccharide structure, whereas on fibromodulin it is attached to the equivalent galactose on an N-linked oligosaccharide (Fig. 1). Results will be presented which indicate that the substitution of KS on these two proteoglycans is independently controlled, and the implications of this finding for an understanding of KS function in cartilage matrix are discussed.

SUBSTITUTION OF KS ON AGGRECAN

The current model for aggrecan, based on the human core sequence deduced from cDNA (3), is given in Fig. 2. The core protein consists of 2,316 amino acids and it is composed of N-terminal and C-terminal globular domains which

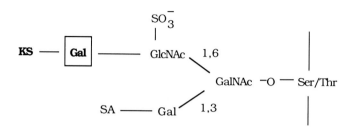

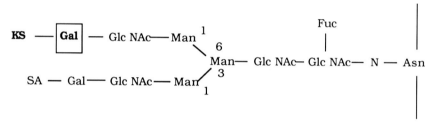

FIG. 1. The linkage region structures for O-linked keratan sulfate (12) and N-linked keratan sulfate (26).

are separated by an extended linear portion substituted with both chondroitin sulfate (CS) and KS. Between 100 and 150 CS chains are located in this region, and these are attached via xylose to serine residues in the sequence Ser-Gly (4). In addition to CS, aggrecan has been shown to contain a variable number of KS chains per molecule; the majority, if not all, of these KS chains are attached to serine or threonine (5) through the O-linked structure (6) shown in Fig. 1.

Heinegard and Axelsson (7) used enzymatic digestion and chemical methods to show that KS is distributed in a rather specific pattern on the aggrecan core protein. The majority (about 60%) was found to be located in a specific KS-rich domain, with another 20 to 30% in the chondroitin sulfate-rich region. There is also evidence to indicate KS substitution at sites in or near the G1 domain (8). This nonuniform distribution of KS on aggrecan must be related to the distribution of those specific serine and threonine residues which can serve as acceptors for O-linked oligosaccharide addition, and also the degree to which such individual O-linked oligosaccharides will further act as initiators of KS chain addition. Although there is presently no accepted consensus sequence for O-linked oligosaccharide initiation, it is interesting that in both the human (3) and bovine KS-rich (9) domains the sequence Pro-Ser is repeated about 20 times, and further, in both species these serine residues are often found within the sequence Pro-Phe-Pro-Ser. The Pro-Ser sequence is also repeated many times in the CS-rich

AGGRECAN

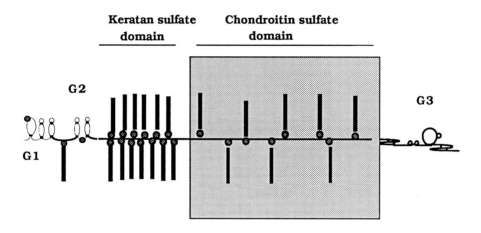

Keratan sulfate domain

Chondroitin sulfate domain

G2

G1

G3

FIBROMODULIN

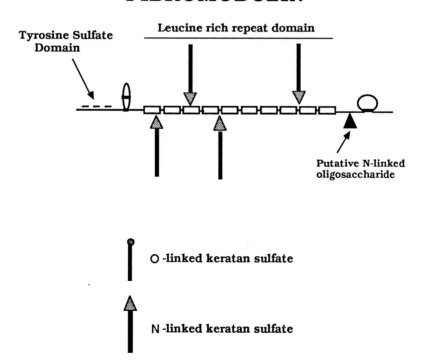

Tyrosine Sulfate Domain

Leucine rich repeat domain

Putative N-linked oligosaccharide

O -linked keratan sulfate

N -linked keratan sulfate

FIG. 2. Structural model of the keratan sulfate substituted proteoglycans in cartilage.

domains of human aggrecan; however, here it is almost always part of the consensus sequence for CS attachment, i.e., Pro-Ser-Gly. These serine residues are most likely substituted with CS rather than KS. On the other hand, the human CS domain contains many threonine residues within the repeating motif Thr-Thr-Ala-Pro or Thr-Ala-Ala-Pro, and many of these presumably carry O-linked oligosaccharide structures which may also serve as initiation sites for KS addition.

KS substitution sites on the N-terminal globular domains may also be predicted from these sequence considerations. Thus, the Pro-Ser sequence found repeated in the KS-rich domain is also found six times in the G1-G2 region and the Thr-Thr-Ala-Pro sequence commonly found in the CS-attachment region is also found once near the N-terminal of the G1 domain. It is not clear whether these serine and threonine residues can actually serve as acceptors for O-linked oligosaccharide addition in the Golgi compartment (12), since they might be masked by the globular conformation of this N-terminal domain of the aggrecan core.

The control of KS substitution on aggrecan cannot, however, simply reside in the primary sequence of the core protein. Thus, it has been shown that aggrecan in mature articular cartilage has a markedly higher KS content than that in young cartilage (10). This is apparently not due to the production of a "mature" form of the aggrecan core protein containing more KS attachment sites (9), but it appears to be due to an increased degree of substitution of the available O-linked oligosaccharides with KS (11).

The addition of KS to aggrecan is thought to occur in the Golgi compartment presumably in close temporal and spatial relationship to the addition of O-linked oligosaccharides (12). Therefore, to understand the mechanisms underlying the maturation-related increase in KS substitution, it will be necessary to establish what determines whether a particular O-linked oligosaccharide is further processed to KS. In this regard, it is possible that modification of the oligosaccharide structure may make it a preferential substrate for the action of the KS elongation enzymes. For example, the N-acetylglucosamine residue in the KS linkage region of bovine disc aggrecan (see Fig. 1) is sulfated, and this appears to distinguish it from other O-linked oligosaccharides on aggrecan (13). It is, of course, also possible that in mature chondrocytes, increased activities of the elongation and sulfation enzymes for KS result in rapid polymer addition to the terminal β-1,4 galactose before capping with sialic acid can occur.

STRUCTURE OF THE KS CHAINS ON AGGRECAN

In addition to variation in the abundance of KS on different aggrecan populations, it is now becoming increasingly clear that there is also a wide diversity in KS size and composition. For example, KS chains prepared by β-elimination from bovine nasal septum (14), bovine articular cartilage (15), and intervertebral disc (16) aggrecan have apparent molecular weights of about 4,500, 8,500, and 20,000, respectively.

Details of the range of possible substitutions on the polylactosamine backbone of KS are now becoming available through the pioneering high-field NMR studies of Nieduszynski and co-workers (15–17). For example, in an examination of KS chains from bovine nasal cartilage, a wide variation in the sulfation of polymer was noted (14), and this appeared to be due in large part to variation in the sulfation of galactose. Other studies from this group have shown that KS on articular cartilage aggrecan also contains a 1,3-linked fucose on the polylactosamine repeat sequence of the polymer (16) and this structure is apparently not present on aggrecan from nonweight-bearing cartilages, for example bovine tracheal and nasal septum cartilage.

KS SUBSTITUTION OF CARTILAGE FIBROMODULIN

In contrast to its linkage to aggrecan, KS is attached to fibromodulin through an Asn/N-acetylglucosamine linkage which is probably the same as that shown for corneal KS (Fig. 1). Thus tunicamycin, an inhibitor of N-linked oligosaccharide synthesis, inhibits the addition of KS to fibromodulin under conditions where KS addition to aggrecan is not affected (18).

The sequence of fibromodulin deduced from cDNA by Oldberg (19) shows five putative N-linked glycosylation sites (Asn-X-Thr/Ser). To identify which of these sites are indeed substituted with KS, we purified fibromodulin from bovine epiphyseal cartilage extracts by density gradient centrifugation, ion exchange chromatography, and gel permeation chromatography. Isolation of glycosylated peptides from tryptic digests of fibromodulin by ion exchange chromatography and reversed phase high-performance liquid chromatography revealed four separate hexosamine-rich species that were also immunoreactive with the KS monoclonal antibody 5D4. Sequence analysis of all of these glycopeptides gave blank cycles at the putative substitution sites, showing that all four Asn residues in the leucine-rich region of fibromodulin can serve as acceptor sites for KS addition (see Fig. 2).

During the course of these studies it became clear that only a portion of each of the glycosylation sites carried N-linked oligosaccharides substituted with KS. KS was defined in that case as a polymer composed of at least seven repeating disaccharides (Galβ1,4GlcNAcβ1,3) with a sufficient degree of sulfation to cause binding to a MonoQ anion exchange resin under the conditions described (17) (Fig. 3). In the same experiment, all four peptides containing the identified glycosylation sites were also isolated from the peptide pool which did not bind to the anion exchange resin. The glucosamine content of these species indicated that they were composed of polymer with no more than six repeating disaccharides with low levels of sulfation.

This finding of a significant population of peptides with N-linked oligosaccharides lacking KS was also suggested by a major difference in the glucosamine content of the purified fibromodulin preparation (37.6 mol/mol core protein),

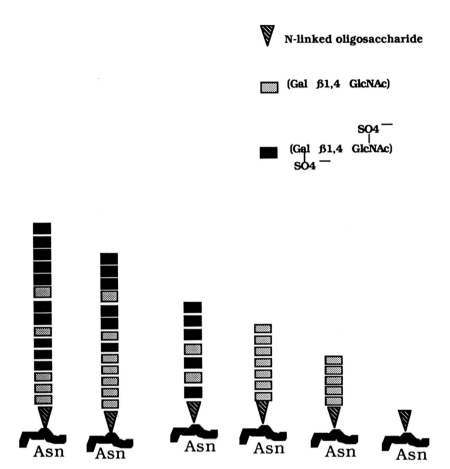

FIG. 3. Model of the modification of the N-linked oligosaccharides on bovine fibromodulin.

and that calculated by summation of the isolated KS-substituted peptides (103 mol/mol core protein). The exact proportion of each of these sites in fibromodulin which are substituted with the different types of polymer remains to be determined, however. Since individual sites in fibromodulin can be elongated to a variable extent (as shown in Fig. 3), it can be suggested that substitution of N-linked oligosaccharides with KS is probably regulated in a manner similar to that for KS addition to O-linkages; that is, by a specific processing of the linkage region and/or the prevailing activities of the glycosyltransferases and sulfation enzymes involved in the KS polymer synthesis.

In this regard it is interesting that the extent of KS substitution of cartilage fibromodulin varies markedly with development and maturation of the tissue. Western blots of guanidine HCl extracts of epiphyseal and mature articular cartilage (Fig. 4) have revealed a wide molecular weight range (60,000–100,000) for epiphyseal fibromodulin, indicating extensive glycosylation of the 40 kDa core

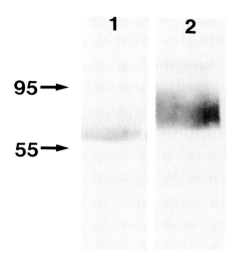

FIG. 4. SDS-PAGE of fibromodulin extracted from bovine epiphyseal and articular cartilage. Matrix components present in 4 M guanidine HCl extracts of epiphyseal (**Lane 2**) and articular cartilage (**Lane 1**) were electrophoresed on 10% SDS-PAGE gels and transferred to nitrocellulose. Fibromodulin was visualized by incubation of the nitrocellulose with a rabbit polyclonal antiserum to bovine fibromodulin as the primary antibody, followed by peroxidase conjugated goat anti-rabbit IgG and H_2O_2/4-chloro-1-napthol as substrate.

protein. In contrast, articular cartilage fibromodulin migrated as a relatively tight band between 50 kDa and 65 kDa. In addition, monosaccharide analyses of epiphyseal fibromodulin showed it to contain about 36 moles of glucosamine and 27 moles of galactose per mole of core protein. On the other hand, fibromodulin from mature articular cartilage contained only about 17 moles of glucosamine and 11 moles of galactose per mole of core protein.

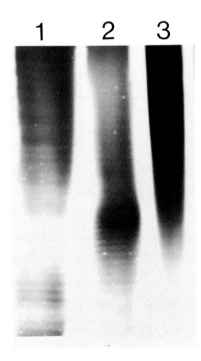

FIG. 5. Size distribution of keratan sulfate chains from bovine epiphyseal and articular cartilage fibromodulin. One hundred μg core protein equivalents of the different fibromodulin purified from epiphyseal and articular cartilage, using the method described in ref. 18, were digested with papain. Portions of papain digested epiphyseal fibromodulin, containing 9 μg glucosamine (**Lane 1**) and articular fibromodulin containing 1 μg glucosamine (**Lane 2**) were electrophoresed on a 24–30% polyacrylamide gradient gel with a 5% stacking gel. **Lane 3** shows the electrophoretic pattern of 10 μg of KS from bovine cornea (obtained from Seikagaku America, Inc., Rockville, MD). Electrophoresis conditions and visualization of the KS chains were by the method of Lyon and Gallagher (25).

Analysis of the size distribution of KS chains in papain digests of epiphyseal and mature fibromodulin (Fig. 5) has shown that at least part of the difference in carbohydrate content is due to a reduction in the size of the KS chains on fibromodulin during maturation. Moreover, these marked age differences in the extent of fibromodulin glycosylation appear to result from biosynthetic changes, since epiphyseal and mature chondrocytes in culture synthesize fibromodulin characteristic of the tissue source (A. Plaas and S. Wong-Palms, unpublished data).

CONCLUDING REMARKS

It is now clear that chondrocytes have the capacity to add KS to two abundant matrix macromolecules, namely aggrecan and fibromodulin, which are very different in both structure and proposed functions. A defined function for KS substitution on the two core proteins remains unclear. In aggrecan, KS will supplement the fixed charge density that is already provided by the CS chains, and which is clearly responsible for providing resistance to compressive loading. It has also been suggested that KS (or O- and N-linked oligosaccharide) substitution of matrix proteins may provide a degree of protection from proteolytic attack by enzymes involved in normal matrix turnover.

On the other hand, KS substitution might provide cartilage proteins with variable recognition structures which could react with carbohydrate-binding molecules within the extracellular matrix. This would be somewhat analogous to the role of polylactosamine (unsulfated KS) structures that are expressed on cell surface glycoproteins (20) and on other extracellular matrix macromolecules such as fibronectin (21) and bone sialoglycoprotein II (22). Moreover, in the systems studied, the expression of such polylactosamines changed in a predictable fashion during embryonic development and cell differentiation (23). Thus, elaboration of particular oligosaccharides on fibromodulin and aggrecan with N-acetyl-lactosamine sequences might have evolved as a mechanism by which the chondrocyte can modulate interactions of the major macromolecular structures (aggrecan aggregates and the collagen network) with other molecules involved in maintaining overall organization of the cartilage matrix.

The increased substitution of fibromodulin with KS in epiphyseal cartilage might be a reflection of the need for carbohydrate-rich domains on the collagen network in a growing and remodeling tissue. On the other hand, a more extensive substitution of aggrecan core protein with KS in mature articular cartilage might be an adaptation to increased need for interactions of aggrecan aggregates with other matrix components.

To ultimately understand the role of KS in cartilage matrix function, the similarities and differences in structural characteristics of the KS chains on both aggrecan and fibromodulin will have to be more clearly defined. Since KS substitution on both core proteins appears to vary with the developmental stage of the tissue, more work is needed to understand the biosynthetic mechanisms responsible for the variations. Thus, do the controlling steps occur during the addition or processing of the O- and N-linked oligosaccharide linkage regions? Is the amount of KS on a core protein simply dependent on the activities of the enzymes involved in KS elongation and sulfation? Since both N- and O-linked KS can be found in the same tissue, it also remains to be determined whether the same or different enzyme complexes are involved in the elaboration of KS on the two types of linkage structures, and if indeed both are products of the same chondrocyte.

It has been reported that in the repair attempt of the chondrocyte in an osteoarthritic lesion, the newly secreted aggrecan is substituted with CS that has structural characteristics of CS typically found on growth plate aggrecan (24). One might therefore speculate that such a repair response also involves an alteration in KS synthesis from the pattern of a mature chondrocyte to that more typical of a chondrocyte in growth cartilage. Thus, part of the inability of the articular chondrocytes to repair osteoarthritic lesions effectively might be because the "lightly substituted" fibromodulin and "heavily substituted" aggrecan which are required for a functional mature cartilage matrix are gradually replaced by molecules with a glycosylation pattern more suited to the requirements of a rapidly remodeling growth cartilage.

ACKNOWLEDGMENTS

The authors thank Dr. John Sandy for his critical review of the final version of the manuscript and our colleagues in the Research Laboratories of the Tampa Unit Shriners Hospital for their ongoing helpful discussion during the project. The work was supported by a grant from the Shriners of North America to Anna H. K. Plaas.

REFERENCES

1. Meyer K, Linker A, Davidson EA, Weissmann B. The mucopolysaccharides of bovine cornea. *J Biol Chem* 1953;205:611–616.
2. Greiling H, Scott JE. *Keratan sulphate, chemistry, biology, chemical pathology.* London: The Biochemical Society, 1989.
3. Doege K, Sasaki M, Kimura T, Yamada Y. Complete coding sequence and deduced primary structure of the human cartilage large aggregating proteoglycan, aggrecan. *J Biol Chem* 1991;266: 894–902.
4. Robinson HC, Hopwood JJ. The alkaline cleavage and borohydride reduction of cartilage proteoglycan. *Biochem J* 173;133:457–470.
5. Bray BA, Lieberman R, Meyer K. Structure of human skeletal keratosulfate. *J Biol Chem* 1967;242: 3373–3380.
6. Lohmander LS, De Luca S, Nilsson B, Hascall VC, Caputo CB, Kimura JH, Heinegard D. Oligosaccharides on proteoglycans from the Swarm rat chondrosarcoma. *J Biol Chem* 1980;255: 6084–6091.
7. Heinegard D, Axelsson I. Distribution of keratan sulfate in cartilage proteoglycans. *J Biol Chem* 1977;252:1971–1979.
8. Baker JR. Studies of keratan sulfates of aorta and cartilage utilizing MAb 6D2. In: Greiling H,

Scott JE., eds. *Keratan sulphate, chemistry, biology, chemical pathology.* London: The Biochemical Society, 1989:30–38.

9. Antonsson P, Heinegard D, Oldberg A. The keratan sulfate enriched region of bovine cartilage proteoglycan consists of a consecutively repeated hexapeptide motif. *J Biol Chem* 1989;264: 16170–16173.
10. Thonar EJMA, Kuettner K. Biochemical basis of age-related changes in proteoglycans. In: Wight TN, Mecham RP, eds. *Biology of proteoglycans.* New York: Academic Press, 1987;211–246.
11. Inerot S, Heinegard D. Bovine tracheal cartilage proteoglycans. Variations in structure and composition with age. *Coll Relat Res* 1983;3:245–262.
12. Lohmander LS, Hascall VC, Yanagashita M, Kuettner KE, Kimura JH. Posttranslational events in proteoglycan synthesis: kinetics of synthesis of chondroitin sulfate and oligosaccharides on the core protein. *Arch Biochem Biophys* 1986;250:211–227.
13. Dickenson JM, Huckerby TN, Nieduszynski IA. Two linkage region fragments isolated from skeletal keratan sulfate contain a sulfated N-acetylglucosamine residue. *Biochem J* 1990;269: 55–59.
14. Hascall VC, Riolo RL. Characteristics of the protein keratan sulfate core and of keratan sulfate prepared from bovine nasal cartilage proteoglycan. *J Biol Chem* 1972;247:4529–4538.
15. Thornton DJ, Morris HG, Cockin GH, Huckerby TN, Nieduszynski IA, Carlstedt I, Hardingham TE, Ratcliffe A. Structural and immunological studies of keratan sulfates from mature bovine articular cartilage. *Biochem J* 1989;260:277–282.
16. Dickenson JM, Morris HG, Nieduszynski IA, Huckerby TN. Skeletal keratan sulphate chain molecular weight calibration by HPGP-chromatography. *Anal Biochem* 1990;190:271–275.
17. Tai G-H, Brown GM, Morris HG, Huckerby TN, Nieduszynski IA. Fucose content of keratan sulfate from bovine articular cartilage. *Biochem J* 191;273:307–310.
18. Plaas AHK, Neame PJ, Nivens CM, Reiss L. Identification of the keratan sulfate attachment sites on bovine fibromodulin. *J Biol Chem* 1990;265:20634–20650.
19. Oldberg A, Antonsson P, Lindblom K, Heinegard D. A collagen-binding 59-kd protein (fibromodulin) is structurally related to the small interstitial proteoglycans PG-S1 and PG-S2. *EMBO J* 1989;8:2601–2604.
20. Fukuda M. Cell surface glycoconjugates as onco-differentiation markers in hematopoietic cells. *Biochim Biophys Acta* 1985;780:119–150.
21. Zhu BCR, Laine RA. Polylactosamine glycosylation of human fetal placental fibronectin weakens the binding affinity of fibronectin to gelatin. *J Biol Chem* 1985;260:4041–4045.
22. Kinne RW, Fisher LW. Keratan sulfate proteoglycan in rabbit compact bone is bone sialoprotein II. *J Biol Chem* 1987;262:10206–10211.
23. Feizi T. Demonstration by monoclonal antibodies that carbohydrate structures of glycoproteins and glycolipids are onco-developmental antigens. *Nature* 1985;314:53–57.
24. Caterson B, Blankenship-Paris T, Chandrasekhar S, Slater R. Biochemical characterization of guinea pig cartilage proteoglycans with the onset of spontaneous osteoarthritis. *Trans Orth Res Soc* 1991;16:251.
25. Lyon M, Gallagher JT. A general method for the detection and mapping of submicrogram quantities of glycosaminoglycan oligosaccharide on polyacrylamide gels by sequential staining with azure A and ammoniacal silver. *Anal Biochem* 1990;185:63–70.
26. Nilsson B, Nakazawa K, Hassell JR, Newsome DA, Hascall VC. Structure of oligosaccharides and the linkage region between KS and the core protein on proteoglycans from monkey cornea. *J Biol Chem* 1983;258:6056–6063.

DISCUSSION

Sandell: Are there molecules that change their N-linked substitution during development like you showed for fibromodulin?

Plaas: Yes, there are examples of extracellular matrix molecules such as fibronectin and laminin that are substituted with polylactosamine. Also intracellular molecules such as lysosomal membrane proteins can be variably substituted with polylactosamine.

Thonar: Your observation that the content of keratan sulfate on fibromodulin does not go up with aging is interesting. This appears to differ from keratan sulfate on aggrecan. Major changes in this parameter may occur early in life. Have you looked at this during cartilage development or in fetal cartilage?

Plaas: We have looked at fibromodulin in the growth plate of fetal calves. It appears to be identical to that in the newborn calf epiphysis with regard to glycosylation. So there doesn't appear to be much change between fetal and newborn. The major changes in glycolysation occur on maturation.

Hascall: Do you have any information on the half-life of fibromodulin in steer versus calf?

Plaas: When we looked at the fibromodulin content of calf explants before and after interleukin treatment, we found that the total tissue content remains unchanged. Our experiment did not address whether this is simply due to a resistance of fibromodulin to accelerated catabolic events in cartilage, or whether there has been removal of fibromodulin from the matrix which is replaced by newly synthesized molecules.

Peyron: Arthritic cartilage has very thick fibrils. Do you have any evidence of the state of fibromodulin in osteoarthritic cartilage?

Plaas: Our polyclonal antibody against bovine fibromodulin only shows weak cross-reactivity with human samples. We have now developed an antibody against human fibromodulin which should help us to address this question.

Bruckner: Have you studied immunolocalization of fibromodulin in association with collagen fibrils?

Plaas: No, but Dr. Heinegard can comment on that.

Heinegard: Our studies with Drs. Finn Reinholt and Olle Svensson show an extremely good correlation of fibromodulin with collagen distribution, such that in compartments where collagen is more abundant, fibromodulin is also more abundant. These studies were done at the electron microscopy-level using immunogold technology.

Plaas: In this regard we have maintained cells in the presence of ascorbate, where collagen is deposited primarily in the cell layer. Fibromodulin is almost exclusively associated with the cell layers and does not diffuse into the medium.

Caterson: Does the monoclonal antibody 5D4 interact with the keratan sulfate on fibromodulin and aggrecan differently? What proportion of the keratan sulfate in cartilage is on fibromodulin?

Plaas: We have not investigated the antigenicity of the keratan sulfate on fibromodulin to 5D4 in quantitative terms nor compared it to the KS on aggrecan. If the chemical and immunological properties of the keratan sulfate are the same, then about one-third of the total keratan sulfate in the growth plate would be fibromodulin.

Articular Cartilage and Osteoarthritis,
edited by K. Kuettner et al.
Raven Press, Ltd., New York © 1992.

6

Molecular Biology of Type II Collagen

New Information in the Gene

Linda J. Sandell,* Mary B. Goldring,† Oliver Zamparo,*
Jiangtao Wu,* and Rina Yamin†

*Departments of Orthopaedics and Biochemistry, University of Washington and
Veterans Administration Medical Center, Seattle, WA 98108; and †Massachusetts
General Hospital and Harvard University Medical School, Boston, MA 02129*

The predominant macromolecules of the cartilage extracellular matrix (ECM) are type II collagen and the proteoglycans aggrecan, fibromodulin, biglycan, and decorin. Chondrocytes resident in cartilage are responsible for the synthesis of proper ECM. Under pathological conditions, such as in rheumatoid arthritis and osteoarthritis, the functional characteristics of the chondrocyte are altered, resulting in changes in the composition of its products of ECM biosynthesis contributing to cartilage erosion and lack of tissue repair. For this reason, we have concentrated our studies on the mechanisms by which chondrocytes control synthesis of cartilage matrix molecules.

The isolation of complementary DNAs (cDNAs) encoding collagen and pro-teoglycan molecules has revealed the protein sequence and provided valuable probes for the study of biosynthesis. The recent isolation of genes encoding human type II procollagen and aggrecan allows the detailed investigation of the regulation of gene expression at the level at which biosynthesis is ultimately controlled. Unlike cDNAs, which are a direct copy of mature mRNA, genes contain both coding sequences (exons) and, importantly, regulatory sequences residing in the promotor domain and between exons (in the introns). In this chapter we will focus on new information regarding (a) transcriptional regulation of these molecules, using type II collagen as the prototypic chondrocyte gene, and (b) a second level of regulation involving the differential splicing of exons.

REGULATORY ELEMENTS IN NONCODING DOMAINS OF THE GENE: CONTROL AT TRANSCRIPTION

The spectrum of factors responsible for the altered function of the chondrocyte in conditions such as rheumatoid arthritis or osteoarthritis has not been fully defined. However, there is increasing evidence that the production of new cytokines or alterations in the amounts or temporal sequence of release of these soluble cell products may contribute to the abnormalities of connective tissue remodeling characteristic of these conditions. Various factors have been shown to be present in joint tissue normally, or in various stages of osteoarthritis. We know that the synthesis of type II collagen and the steady-state levels of collagen mRNA can be positively or negatively modulated *in vitro* by various cytokines and growth factors such as transforming growth factor-β (TGF-β) (1,2), insulin-like growth factor-I (IGF-I) (3), interleukin 1 (IL-1) (4,5), and γ-interferon (6). Many of these studies indicate transcriptional regulation of type II collagen synthesis. This knowledge has pinpointed our investigations of regulatory mechanisms to the gene level. A summary of growth factor and cytokine effects on steady-state mRNA levels for the major structural macromolecules is presented in Table 1.

Regulation of the gene involves two components: *cis*-acting sequences of the DNA itself and *trans*-acting protein factors that interact with the DNA sequences. In order to study transcriptional regulation, the DNA sequence is analyzed for potential sequence motifs implicated in the binding of regulatory factors, and then specific portions of the gene can be tested for activity in a functional assay. These functional assays are transient transfection experiments where the DNA of interest is coupled to a chloramphenicol acetyltransferase (CAT) reporter gene and transfected into cells. When the experiment is concluded, cell lysates are prepared and analyzed for enzyme activity. The activity of the CAT enzyme is proportional to the ability of the DNA construct to stimulate transcription. We initiated studies to determine which *cis* DNA sequences are involved in the transcription of the COLII gene. DNA segments 5′ from the start site of transcription and from the first intron of the gene were cloned into a pCAT vector.

TABLE 1. *Effect of cytokines on mRNA levels in chondrocytes*

	DNA synthesis	Collagen I	Collagen II	Proteoglycans
Catabolic factors				
IL-1	−	+	−	−
TNF-α[a]	+	−, +	−	−
IFN-γ	+	−	−	−
Anabolic factors				
TGF-β	0	+	+	+
IGF-1	+	n/d	+	+
PDGF[b]	0	n/d	0	+
FGF[c]	+	+	+	+

[a] Tumor necrosis factor (12).
[b] Platelet derived growth factor.
[c] Fibroblast growth factor.
n/d, not determined.

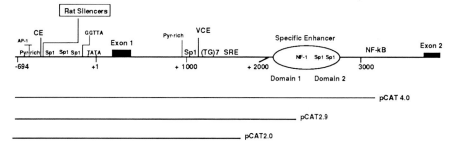

FIG. 1. Relative locations of the consensus sequence elements in the promoter and first intron of the human COLII gene. CE, cellular enhancer; VCE, viral core enhancer; pyr-rich, pyrimidine-rich stretch of nucleotides; other motifs are discussed in the text. Below the gene diagram are indicated the regions of the gene included in the chloramphenicol acetyltransferase (CAT) constructs used to transfect chondrocytes and fibroblasts.

The DNA constructs were transfected into human costal chondrocytes and human dermal fibroblasts. In addition, nucleotide sequences from the rat, mouse, and human COLII genes were compared to identify domains of high conservation.

Regulatory Sequences In the Promoter

The promoter domain (approximately 700 bp 5' to the start site of transcription) has a high G + C content, a high frequency of CpG dinucleotides, and various regions of very high conservation (shown in Fig. 1). Experiments with deletion constructs have shown that the human promoter itself contains very little ability to initiate transcription (Fig. 2). This was also true for the rat type II promoter (7). It is not clear at this time why there is so little activity attributable to the promoter when it contains elements that are stimulatory in other genes. Some

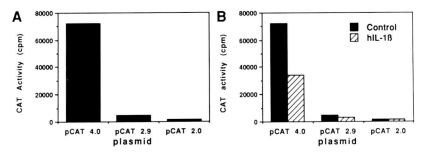

FIG. 2. Expression of human COLII gene regulatory sequences in human chondrocytes. Cells were transfected with 10 µg plasmid DNA/60 mm culture dish. Cells were harvested 48 hr after transfection. IL-1 was added to the cultures at 24 hr and CAT enzyme activity was monitored using radiolabeled acetyl coenzyme A. The pCAT constructs are shown in Fig. 1.

light has been shed on the role of the COLII promoter by transfecting dermal fibroblasts with the COLII constructs. When a human COLII construct conferring positive regulation in chondrocytes is transfected into fibroblasts, expression of the gene is inhibited (data not shown). Consistent with this result, Savagner et al., (8) have shown that the rat COLII promoter actually contains "silencer" elements that inhibit expression of the gene in fibroblasts. These negative regulatory elements are not used in chondrocytes, presumably due to the lack of the appropriate *trans*-acting protein factor. Consequently, evidence is beginning to accumulate indicating that the COLII promoter may play a slightly different role in the regulation of this gene compared to other genes. The negative control of transcription demonstrated by the COLII promoter may actually be an important aspect of tissue-specific gene expression, providing a mechanism by which COLII expression is repressed in most tissues.

A Functional Enhancer Is Located In the First Intron of the COLII Gene

Several members of the collagen gene family contain functional regulatory elements in the first intron (37), including the human (9,10), mouse $\alpha2(I)$ (11), mouse $\alpha1(IV)$ (12), and rat $\alpha1(II)$ (7) collagen genes. Like the promoter, the first 30% of intron 1 of the COLII gene has a high C + G content and a high frequency of CpG dinucleotides. Sequence analysis also reveals the presence of DNA sequences between +1068 and +2850 which are candidates for the binding of *trans*-acting factors (see Fig. 1) (13). The reverse complement of the hexanucleotide 5' GGGCGG 3' is located at +1068, +2821, and +2846. These regions may be able to bind Sp1, a factor that has been shown to activate transcription by RNA polymerase II from some promoters (14). At +1424 there is an inverted repeat similar to a serum responsive element (15) and at +2538 a recognition sequence for nuclear factor-1 (NF-1). Interestingly, in the mouse $\alpha2(I)$ collagen promoter, a similar NF-1 binding sequence is present and was shown to mediate the transcriptional effect of TGF-β (16). The same may be true for the COLII gene.

Three lines of evidence now indicate that the region of +2200 to +2850 contains a functional enhancer necessary for the expression of the COLII gene. (a) A construct (pCAT4.0) in Fig. 1 containing this domain was expressed at high levels when transiently transfected into human chondrocytes (Fig. 2). The activity could be greatly reduced by removing DNA sequences from +2300 to +3600 (pCAT2.9) and completely eliminated by reducing the construct to +1400 (pCAT2.0). (b) An intron domain of the rat COLII gene has been also shown to contain a functional enhancer (7). This is likely the same as the human enhancer because a fragment of the human intron from +2700 to +3400 hybridized to rat genomic DNA indicating an unusually high degree of homology in an intron. (c) Sequence comparison between the mouse intron sequence (E. Vuorio, personal communication) and the human COLII gene showed a striking degree of conservation. This high level of homology, 95% for 170 nts (domain 1 in Fig.

1) and 85% for an additional 320 nts (domain 2 in Fig. 1), is unique in our comparison of collagen DNA sequences and highly indicative of an important function. Obviously, an enhancer domain this large will be quite complex and probably contains multiple regulatory elements which may be functional under different conditions. The known regulatory elements, 2 Sp1 sites and a NF-1 site, are present in domain 2, where the majority of enhancer activity lies. Taken together, a picture is beginning to emerge defining the types of regulation and the important functional domains of this integral chondrocyte gene. Future experiments will be directed at the dissection of the enhancer domain and, in particular, the determination of sequences which specifically respond to agents known to effect COLII biosynthesis.

When IL-1 was added to cultures expressing the pCAT constructs, gene transcription was inhibited (Fig. 2). As found in analyses of mRNA levels after treatment with IL-1 (4), IL-1β was more effective than IL-1α (data not shown). Interestingly, IL-1β was also still able to inhibit this residual activity of the construct pCAT2.9 (Fig. 2). These preliminary results suggest that the negative regulatory element important for response to IL-1 is not contained in the DNA domain of +1400 to +3500, but is likely to be in the promoter or first part of intron 1.

DIFFERENTIAL SPLICING OF EXONS PRODUCES CUSTOMIZED PROTEINS: POSTTRANSCRIPTIONAL CONTROL

Splicing of pre-mRNA is the process by which noncoding DNA sequences (introns) are excised from the message, while the coding units (exons) are spliced together. Alternative splicing of pre-mRNA is now known to be of widespread importance for the generation of multiple transcripts from a single gene and, consequently, protein isoforms. By this mechanism functions ranging from intracellular and extracellular localization to enzyme activity can be modulated by expression of the appropriate protein domain. Alternative splicing is also used to quantitatively regulate gene expression by generating truncated open reading frames, or by regulating mRNA stability or translational efficiency via variability in the untranslated regions. Differential expression of specific domains within ECM proteins may be important in modulating interactions among components of the ECM and between the ECM and cell surface. In fibronectin, for example, alternative splicing provides a mechanism to generate functionally distinct forms of the protein during development (17), wound healing (18), and malignancy (18). There are other reports of alternative splicing in collagen genes. Both the type XIII (19) and $\alpha 2$ chain of type VI collagen (20) are alternatively spliced. The roles of these collagens and their splice variants are not known. In chondrocytes, two examples of alternative exon usage have been described which are relevant to the cartilage phenotype. First, type IX collagen, originally thought to be cartilage-specific, is expressed in developing cornea where a specific protein domain (NC4) is removed. Alternate usage of this exon is mediated by a second promoter within the intron immediately upstream of the alternatively spliced exon (21; see Olsen, this volume). Second, Bennett and Adams, (22) have shown that the $\alpha 2(I)$ chain of type I collagen is expressed in chondrocytes, but again, a different promoter is employed yielding a protein product that is shorter and, due to a shift in reading frame, not collagenous.

Alternative Splicing of Pre-mRNA Produces Two Isoforms of Type II Procollagen

Analysis of genomic clones for the COLII gene led to the identification of an exon (not known to be exon 2) encoding a 69-amino acid cysteine-rich domain in the NH_2-propeptide (13). This exon was not located in the corresponding cDNA clones for human (23) or rat (24) $\alpha 1(II)$ collagen mRNA. The apparent discrepancy between the genomic and cDNA clones was resolved by our findings that exon 2 can be alternatively spliced (Fig. 3) (25). Distinct oligonucleotide probes were designed to identify human $\alpha 1(II)$ collagen mRNA that spliced exon

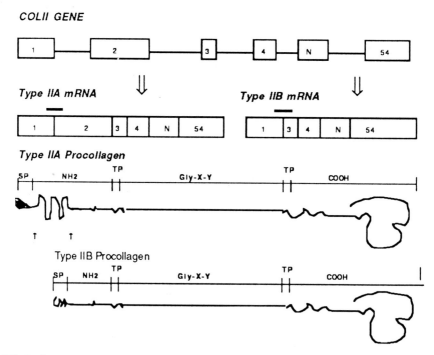

FIG. 3. Generation of type IIA and type IIB procollagen from the COLII gene. The *bars* above the mRNAs indicate the position of oligonucleotide probes used in the northern blots and *in situ* hybridizations. The alternative spliced domain is indicated by *arrows* in the procollagen chains. SP, signal peptide; TP, telopeptide.

1 to exon 2 (type IIA) or exon 1 to exon 3 (type IIB). Each probe was 24 nucleotides in length and used under conditions that would permit stable hybridization only across the exon boundaries. Figure 4 demonstrates that two populations of $\alpha 1(II)$ mRNA can be detected on a northern blot. Final proof for the existence of two mRNAs came from sequence analysis of the two mRNAs. Polymerase chain reaction technology was used to amplify cDNA synthesized from human chondrocyte RNA with primers flanking exon 2. The results of polymerase chain reactions show two amplified products, one with exon 1 spliced to exon 2 and one with exon 2 spliced to exon 3 (Fig. 5). As there is only one copy of the COLII gene, this evidence confirms that the 2 mRNAs are generated by alternate splicing of a single gene. We shown that both mRNAs can be translated and the proteins secreted into the extracellular environment (26). Importantly, the two procollagens were present in proportion to the amount of mRNA; consequently, analysis of mRNA levels is indicative of the presence of the protein.

Type IIB Procollagen mRNA is Expressed in Cartilage

Northern blot analyses of RNAs isolated from various cartilage sources clearly indicate that type IIB procollagen mRNA is the predominant type II message in chondrocytes (25). To avoid the problem of potentially heterogeneous cell populations in culture and in tissue, cartilage was examined directly using the same oligonucleotide probes (described above) used for hybridization *in situ*. Human and bovine cartilages were examined with the same result (an example

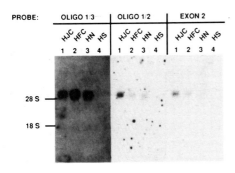

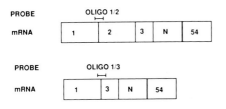

FIG. 4. Northern blot analysis show two distinct pro-$\alpha 1(II)$ transcripts. Oligonucleotide probes are indicated. The exon 2 probe was used to confirm the results of the oligo 1/2 probe and was isolated from a human genomic DNA clone. The following RNAs were used: **lane 1:** human juvenile chondrocyte (HJC); **lane 2:** human fetal chondrocyte (HFC); **lane 3:** human notochord (HN); **lane 4:** human bone marrow stromal RNA (HS). From ref. 27, with permission.

A

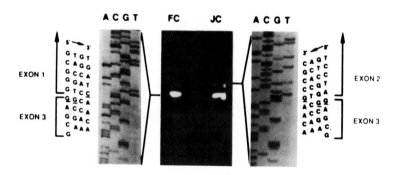

B

Exons 1, 2, and 3

EXON 1   EXON 2   EXON 3
ATGATT....GATGTCC AGGAG....GCCAGT<u>G</u> <u>G</u>GCAACCAGGACCAAAG
 M   I ... D   V   Q   E ...   A   S   <u>G</u>   Q   P   G   P   K

Exons 1 and 3

EXON 1   EXON 3
ATGATT   GATGTC<u>C</u> <u>G</u>GCAACCAGGACCAAAG
 M   I ... D   V   R   Q   P   G   P   K

FIG. 5. Agarose gel photograph of PCR products flanked by the autoradiogram of the sequencing gels. **A:** Primer-extended cDNA from fetal (FC) and juvenile (JC) chondrocyte was amplified and run on a 1% agarose gel: two bands are observed in the juvenile chondrocyte lane at 377 and 171 bp. The DNA sequence at the exon junctions is shown. **B:** The nucleotide and amino acid sequence show that splicing directly from exon 1 to exon 3 changes the first amino acid of exon 3 from glycine to arginine. Exon boundaries are indicated. The first amino acid residue of exon 3 and nucleotides of the split codon are underlined. From ref. 27, with permission.

is shown in Fig. 6); hybridization was observed only with the type IIB probe. Thus, posttranscriptional processing of the pre-mRNA qualitatively regulates the expression of the appropriate isoform.

Type II Procollagens Exist in Two Forms in Developing Tissue

After finding that type IIB was the major procollagen mRNA synthesized by chondrocytes, we asked whether differential expression of type II procollagen may be a marker for a distinct population of cells. Again, specific procollagen mRNAs were localized in tissue by *in situ* hybridization to oligonucleotide probes

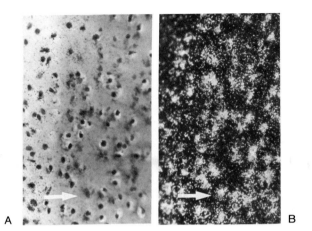

FIG. 6. Expression of type IIB by articular chondrocytes: a bright field photomicrograph is shown in *A* and the same field observed in dark field is shown in *B*. Magnification is 100×. Probes were labeled with [^{35}S]-ATP, hybridized and prepared for emulsion autoradiography. The oligonucleotide probe specific for type IIB procollagen mRNA hybridizes to all cells in the plane of the section while hybridization with the type IIA procollagen mRNA probe was not detectable.

spanning the exon junctions. Embryonic vertebral column was chosen as a source of tissue undergoing rapid chondrogenesis, allowing the examination of a variety of cell types related to cartilage. In this tissue, each procollagen mRNA had a distinct tissue distribution during chondrogenesis with type IIB expressed in chondrocytes and type IIA expressed in cells surrounding cartilage in prechondrocytes (Fig. 7). The morphology of the cells expressing the two collagen types was distinct: the cells expressing type IIA were narrow, elongated, and "fibroblastic" in character, while the cells expressing type IIB were large and round. The expression of type IIB appears to be correlated with abundant synthesis and accumulation of cartilagenous extracellular matrix. The expression of type IIB is spatially correlated with the high level expression of the cartilage proteoglycan, aggrecan, establishing type IIB procollagen and aggrecan as markers for the chondrocyte phenotype (Fig. 7). The cells surrounding the vertebral body that express type IIA are considered to serve as chondrogenic zones for the centra (27). Consequently, the alternative splicing of exon 2 may mark a new stage in chondrogenesis and may be relevant to cartilage repair.

Expression of type II procollagen has been observed in other tissues such as those in the vitreous (28), in embryonic tissues such as the developing epithelial-mesenchymal surface (29), and in basement membranes (30), in addition to "fibroblastic" cells adjacent to cartilage. These cells do not have morphological characteristics of chondrocytes and may actually synthesize the type IIA procollagen isoform. The removal of exon 2 may help to determine the developmental fate of the cell.

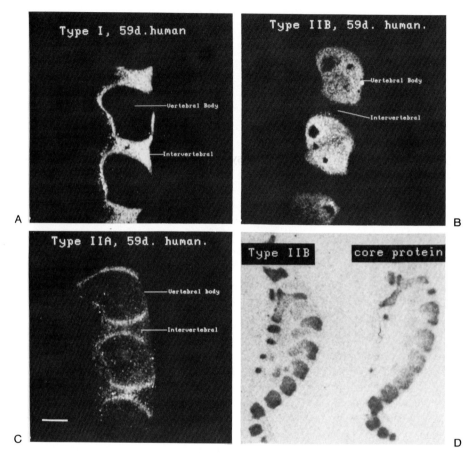

FIG. 7. Differential expression of types I, IIA, and IIB procollagen mRNA in vertebral column tissue. Type I (**a**) hybridizes to the cells of the intervertebral area while type IIB (**b**) hybridizes with the cartilagenous tissue (the apparent holes in the cartilage are due to artifacts of hybridization). The type IIA probe hybridizes only to the cells surrounding the vertebral body (**c**). After hybridization, sections were exposed to autoradiography film and visualized with an Image Analysis System. The same tissue was also hybridized with an oligonucleotide probe encoding the aggrecan core protein and shown in (**d**).

Function of the NH₂-Propeptide

The amino acid sequence deduced from the alternatively spliced exon 2 corresponds to the cysteine-rich portion of the NH$_2$-propeptide (see Fig. 1). The coding sequence of exon 2 is conserved across fibrillar collagens, and a homologous domain is also present in the extracellular matrix proteins thrombospondin and von Willebrand factor (25). Two major functions have been suggested for the NH$_2$-propeptide: (a) it plays a role in regulation of fibril diameter, and (b) it plays a role in feedback inhibition of collagen synthesis. Evidence has been presented to show that the diameter of type I collagen fibers was decreased from 35–40 nm to 20–30 nm by the presence of pN procollagen (31). The role of the NH_2-propeptide in feedback regulation of collagen synthesis has been suggested by studies on dermatosporactic sheep and the human disease Ehlers Danlos type IV. In both of these diseases, the NH_2-propeptide is retained in the mature collagen molecule and increased synthesis of both type I and type III collagens is observed. When isolated NH_2-propeptide was added directly to cultured fibroblasts, collagen synthesis was inhibited (32). Various *in vitro* studies now support the concept of feedback regulation of biosynthesis (33). The differential expression of this domain in developing cartilage is correlated with a change in the general characteristics of the ECM. It will be of interest to see whether a similar "feedback" occurs with collagen II gene expression.

Other cartilage proteins, link protein and aggrecan (34), also demonstrate diversity generated by alternative splicing of the pre-mRNA. In aggrecan, two domains are known to be alternatively spliced, an EGF-like domain (E domain) (35) and the complement regulatory domain (C domain) (36). Various mRNA transcripts are present in RNA preparations from different cartilages from different ages; however, it is not known whether all forms of the mRNA are represented proportionately at the protein level or if there is specific tissue or developmental expression. Tissue-specific expression and studies on the mechanisms of alternative splicing indicate that *cis*-acting sequences and *trans*-acting factors will be extremely important in the posttranscriptional regulation of mRNA splicing.

CONCLUSIONS

This chapter has considered basic mechanisms for the regulation of collagen II production by chondrocytes. The synthesis of cartilage proteoglycans will likely be controlled in a similar manner. Indeed, the gene for human aggrecan has been isolated (34); and there is even evidence for alternative splicing of exons. The differential expression of this cysteine-rich domain in developing cartilage is correlated with a change in the general characteristics of the ECM. When exon 2 is expressed, as it is in type I procollagen, the cells appear fibroblastic in character and do not deposit a cartilagenous matrix; however, when exon 2 is removed and the propeptide is not expressed, the cells appear rounded and deposit abundant ECM. It appears that the expression of this protein domain may be inhibitory to cartilage matrix accumulation. As our knowledge of control mechanisms increases, the possibility of controlling ECM production by chondrocytes and prechondrocytes becomes realistic. Regulation at the gene level is more complex than previously realized, but certain principles are beginning to emerge: both negative and positive regulatory elements are going to be important for the high level, tissue-specific expression of collagen (see ref. 37 for review). This is particularly important now that we know that type II collagen mRNA is expressed in mesenchymal cells or prechondrocytes (38) and in tissues other than cartilage (28), particularly during embryogenesis (29,30). The immediate challenge is to isolate and characterize the protein factors involved in initiation and fine-tuning of transcription.

An important second level of regulation of matrix production occurs after transcription of the initial pre-mRNA during removal of the introns and splicing together the mature mRNA. This event contributes to regulation in two ways: First, coding domains can be included or excluded, within the constraints of the gene sequence, and these domains may be important for interactions between molecules in the cartilage matrix. Second, for type II procollagen, a domain is included which may be actively involved in the regulation of biosynthesis by feedback inhibition. Future studies will be directed toward understanding the role played by type IIA procollagen during development and in processes related to cartilage pathology, such as inadequate repair and the formation of osteophyte.

REFERENCES

1. Rosen DM, Stempien SA, Thompson AY, Seyedin SM. Transforming growth factor-beta modulates the expression of osteoblast and chondroblast phenotypes *in vitro. J Cell Physiol* 1988;134: 337–346.
2. Sandell LJ, Dudek EJ, Bielaga B, Wight TN. Regulation of cartilage collagen and proteoglycan synthesis by transforming growth factor-beta. *Trans Orthopaedic Res Soc* 1989;14:280.
3. Sandell LJ, Dudek E. IGF-1 stimulates type II collagen gene expression in cultured chondrocytes. *Trans of the Orthopaedic Res Soc* 1988;13:300.
4. Goldring MB, Birkhead J, Sandell LJ et al. Interleukin-1 suppresses levels of procollagen mRNA and type II collagen synthesis in cultured human articular and costal chondrocytes. *J Clin Invest* 1988;82:2026–2037.
5. Chandrasekhar S, Harvey AK, Higginbotham JD, Horton WE. Interleukin-1-Induced Suppression of Type II Collagen Gene Transcription Involves DNA Regulatory Elements. *Exp Cell Res* 1990;191:105–114.
6. Goldring MB, Sandell LJ, Stephenson ML, Krane SM. Immune interferon suppresses levels of procollagen mRNA and type II collagen synthesis in cultured human articular and costal chondrocytes. *J Biol Chem* 1986;261:9049–9056.
7. Horton W, Miyashita T, Kohno K, et al. Identification of a phenotype-specific enhancer in the first intron of the rat collagen II gene. *Proc Natl Acad Sci USA* 1987;84:8864–8868.
8. Savagner P, Miyashita T, Yamada Y. Two silencers regulate the tissue-specific expression of the collagen II gene. *J Biol Chem* 1990;265:6669–6674.
9. Rossouw CMS, Vergeer WP, du Plooy SJ, et al. DNA sequences in the first intron of the human pro-α1(I) collagen gene enhance transcription. *J Biol Chem* 1987;262:151–157.
10. Bornstein P, McKay J, Morishima JK, et al. Regulatory elements in the first intron contribute to transcription control of the human α1(I) collagen gene. *Proc Natl Acad Sci USA* 1987;84: 8869–8873.
11. Rossi P, Karsenty G, Roberts AB, et al. A nuclear factor 1 site mediates transcription activation of a type I collagen promoter by transforming growth factor-beta. *Cell* 1988;52:405–414.
12. Killen PD, Burbela PD, Martin GR, Yamada Y. Characterization of the promoter for the α1(IV) collagen gene. *J Biol Chem* 1988;263:12310–12314.
13. Ryan MC, Sieraski M, Sandell LJ. The human type II procollagen gene: identification of an additional protein-coding domain and location of potential regulatory sequences in the promoter and first intron. *Genomics* 1990;8:41–48.

14. Kadonaga JT, Jones KA, Tjian R. Promoter-specific activation of RNA polymerase II transcription by Sp1. *Trends Biol Sci* 1986;11:20–23.
15. Treisman R. Identification of a protein-binding site that mediates transcriptional response of the c-fos gene to serum factors. *Cell* 1986;46:567–574.
16. Rossi P, de Crombrugghe B. Identification of a cell-specific transcription enhancer in the first intron of the mouse α2(type II) collagen gene. *Proc Natl Acad Sci USA* 1987;84:5590–5594.
17. french-Constant C, Van De Water L, Dvorak H, Hynes RO. Reappearance of an embryonic pattern of fibronectin splicing during wound healing in the adult rat. *J Cell Biol* 1989;109:903–914.
18. Oyama F, Hirohashi S, Shimosato Y, et al. Deregulation of alternative splicing of fibronectin pre-mRNA in malignant human liver tumors. *J Biol Chem* 1989;264:10331–10334.
19. Tikka L, Pihlajaniemi T, Henttu P, et al. Gene structure for the α1 chain of a human short-chain collagen (type XII) with alternatively spliced transcripts and translation termination codon at the 5′ end of the last exon. *Proc Natl Acad Sci* 1988;85:7491–7495.
20. Saitta B, Stokes DG, Vissing H, et al. Alternative splicing of the human α2(VI) collagen gene generates multiple mRNA transcripts which predict three protein variants with distinct carboxyl termini. *J Biol Chem* 1990;265:6473–6480.
21. Nishimura I, Muragaki Y, Olsen BR. Tissue-specific forms of type IX collagen-proteoglycan arise from the use of two widely separated promoters. *J Biol Chem* 1989;264:20033–20041.
22. Bennett VD, Adams SL. Identification of a cartilage-specific promoter within intron 2 of the chick α2(I) collagen gene. *J Biol Chem* 1990;265:2223–2230.
23. Baldwin CT, Reginato AM, Smith C, et al. Structure of cDNA clones coding for human type II procollagen. *Biochem J* 1989;262:521–528.
24. Kohno K, Martin GR, Yamada Y. Isolation and characterization of a cDNA clone for the amino-terminal portion of the pro-α1(II) chain of cartilage collagen. *J Biol Chem* 1984;259:13668–13673.
25. Ryan MC, Sandell LJ. Differential expression of a cysteine-rich domain in the NH$_2$-terminal propeptide of type II (cartilage) procollagen. *J Biol Chem* 1990;265:10334–10339.
26. Sandell LJ, Morris N, Robbins JR, Goldring MR. Alternatively spliced type II procollagen mRNAS define distinct populations of cells during vertebral development: differential expression of the amino-propeptide. *J Cell Biol* (in press).
27. O'Rahilly R, Gardner E. The initial appearance of ossification in staged human embryos. *Am J Anat* 1972;134:291–308.
28. Linsenmayer TF, Smith GN, Hay ED. Synthesis of two collagen types by embryonic chick corneal epithelium *in vitro*. *Proc Natl Acad Sci USA* 1977;74:39–43.
29. Thorogood P, Bee J, von der Mark K. Transient expression of collagen type II at epithelio-mesenchymal interfaces during morphogenesis of the cartilaginous neurocranium. *Dev Biol* 1986;116:497–509.
30. Kosher RA, Solursh M. Widespread distribution of type II collagen during embryonic chick development. *Dev Biol* 1989;131:558–566.
31. Fleischmajer R, Perlish JS, Timple R. Collagen fibrillogenesis in human skin. *Anal of the New York Academy of Sciences* 1985;460:246–257.
32. Wiestner M, Kreig T, Horlein D, et al. Inhibiting effect of procollagen peptides on collagen biosynthesis in fibroblast cultures. *J Biol Chem* 1979;254:7016–7023.
33. Wu CH, Walton CM, Wu GY. Propeptide-mediated regulation of procollagen synthesis in IMR-90 human lung fibroblast cell cultures. *J Biol Chem* 1991;266:2983–2987.
34. Doege K, Rhodes C, Sasaki M, et al. Molecular biology of cartilage proteoglycan (aggrecan) and link protein. In: Sandell LJ, Boyd CD, eds. *Extracellular Matrix Genes*, New York: Academic Press, 1990:137–155.
35. Baldwin CT, Reginato AM, Prockop DJ. A new epidermal growth factor-like domain in the human core protein for the large cartilage-specific proteoglycan. *J Biol Chem* 1989;264:15747–15750.
36. Doege KJ, Sasaki M, Kimura T, Yamada Y. Complete coding sequence and deduced primary structure of the human cartilage large aggregating proteoglycan, aggrecan. *J Biol Chem* 1991;266:894–902.
37. Sandell LJ, Boyd CD. Conserved and divergent sequence and functional elements within collagen genes. In: Sandell LJ, Boyd CD, eds. *Extracellular Matrix Genes*, New York: Academic Press, 1990;1–56.

38. Kravis D, Upholt WB. Quantitation of type II procollagen mRNA levels during chick limb cartilage differentiation. *Dev Biol* 1985;108:164–172.
39. Goldring MB, Birkhead J, Sandell LJ, Krane SM. Synergistic regulation of collagen gene expression in human chondrocytes by tumor necrosis factor-α and interleukin-1β. *Annals New York Acad Sci* 1990;580:536–9.

Kuettner: Do you know if the two different types of type II collagen appear or disappear in osteoarthritic lesions and osteophytes?

Sandell: We see type IIA procollagen in developing cartilage, but we do not see type IIA in growth plate cartilage. This suggests that expression of the two forms of type II collagen differs during differentiation of cartilage and growth. I don't know what happens in osteoarthritic cartilage, when matrix synthesis is stimulated, but we will find out.

Tanzer: Your results may help explain the mystery that during development, particularly in the chick embryo, immunostaining for type II collagen appeared in noncartilage regions such as basal lamina. Would you comment on that?

Sandell: Dr. Solursh as well as Drs. Kosher and Upholt have found that in model systems, mRNA for type II collagen appears before collagen protein and cartilage tissue are detected (17,18). This may be because cells which hybridize with probes to type IIA do not look cartilaginous and accumulate less matrix. The protein may not be easily detected. When cells switch to type IIB, they look like chondrocytes and synthesize significant amounts of matrix. We see type IIA expressed in notochord, spinal ganglia, and at facet joint interfaces, in cells that look fibroblastic.

von der Mark: You showed that transforming growth factor (TGF)-beta stimulates type II collagens. We do not see stimulation of type II collagen by TGF-beta, but do of type I collagen synthesis.

Sandell: I think there are a lot of reasons why investigators get different results with TGF-beta. One of them is cell density; another is serum concentration. TGF-beta acts more like a switch. If cells are not producing type II they may be switched on; if they are producing type II, they may be turned down. Our experiments are performed in low serum medium which lowers the concentration of type II mRNA greatly; thus, we can see a stimulation of type II with TGF-beta-1. If we culture cells in 10% serum where the expression is already very high, we do not see an increase. Long term effects are different from short-term effects and age and origin of the cells are also important.

Tanzer: Can you clarify your comments concerning the aminopropeptide of collagen?

Sandell: There is a large body of literature indicating that the aminopropeptide can regulate collagen levels by feedback inhibition of collagen synthesis. It has been shown that both the carboxy and the aminopropeptides can get into cells where they may show some transcriptional or translational regulation.

Heinegard: Why do cells switch from making type IIA to making type IIB collagen?

Sandell: Well, if one believes that aminopropeptide can regulate collagen synthesis by feedback inhibition, it fits very nicely. My current hypothesis is that cells making type IIA act more like fibroblastic cells and accumulate less matrix. When cells remove the exon and, consequently, the aminopropeptide, they may remove constraints to matrix production and can now produce an extensive collagen matrix typical for chondrocytes.

Articular Cartilage and Osteoarthritis,
edited by K. Kuettner et al.
Raven Press, Ltd., New York © 1992.

7

Cartilage Matrix Proteins

Dick K. Heinegård and Edson Rosa Pimentel

Department of Medical and Physiological Chemistry, S-221 00 Lund, Sweden

Cartilage is a composite tissue with a predominant intercellular matrix containing comparatively few cells. The various constituents in this matrix, however, are to a large extent produced by the cells, which also direct their assembly into an integrated functional matrix. An example of the low concentration of exogenous components in cartilage matrix is the observation that albumin is a very minor constituent in articular cartilage, in spite of its high concentration in surrounding synovial fluid.

Among the matrix proteins proper, collagen II represents one prominent constituent, where major processes of assembly occur in the matrix outside the cell. Thus the individual collagen molecules are secreted in proforms which are trimmed by propeptidases in a controlled way to form collagen molecules. These molecules then aggregate to form the collagen fibrils and fibril bundles. The cells appear to play a central role in this assembly by producing factors that are involved in its regulation as well as in the regulation of matrix formation.

Also, the other major matrix macromolecule, i.e., the large aggregating proteoglycan, aggrecan, is involved in major processes of self assembly outside the cell in the matrix. Thus the proteoglycan molecules are secreted in their monomeric form from the cell (1,2). Many proteoglycans then bind to a single hyaluronate molecule in the extracellular environment, thus forming the proteoglycan aggregate. The portion of the proteoglycan molecule located most closely to the hyaluronate represents one of several distinct protein domains (for refs. see 3) that lack major glycosaminoglycan substituents. As indicated in Fig. 1, this region is followed by the keratan sulfate-rich region carrying some 20 to 30 comparatively short keratan sulfate chains (for refs. see 3). The following chondroitin sulfate-rich region contains closely spaced and much longer chondroitin sulfate chains. At least a proportion of these aggregates appears to be formed with the hyaluronate still bound at the cell surface (4), as is schematically indicated in Fig. 1. Formation of such cell-bound aggregates has until now only been identified *in vitro* by using cell culture (5). Provided that they are present *in vivo* also, they should have important roles in sequestering and organizing the matrix constituents. In par-

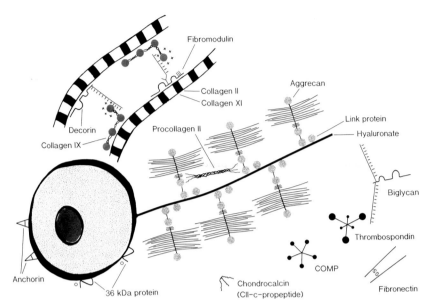

FIG. 1. Schematic illustration of cartilage matrix also indicating suggested interactions. The shorter side chains in aggrecan represent keratan sulfate, and the longer chains represent chondroitin sulfate.

ticular "channels" formed in the center of the aggregates, exemplified in Fig. 1, could have such important roles.

The major part of the matrix proteins in cartilage participate in interactions with other matrix molecules to form a network where most of the matrix molecules participate. These interactions are essential for the properties of the tissue. Thus an understanding of individual matrix constituents and their interactions with other matrix molecules is essential for understanding tissue properties.

MATRIX PROTEINS IN CARTILAGE

Studies of matrix proteins requires their extraction from the tissue, usually with chaotropic solvents, such as 4 M guanidine-HCl. A picture of the presence of matrix proteins can then be obtained by one or another fractionation scheme followed by analysis using SDS-polyacrylamide gel electrophoresis.

One approach, represented in Fig. 2, is to use initial gel chromatography on Superose 6 followed by electrophoresis on 4 to 16% SDS-polyacrylamide gradient gels with and without previous reduction to allow identification of oligomeric proteins. The two hyaline cartilages studied, i.e., tracheal and articular cartilage, show major differences. Thus, both cartilages contain oligomeric proteins present only in either articular or tracheal cartilage. These proteins are indicated by arrows in the figure. One of these proteins present only in tracheal cartilage is the cartilage matrix protein (CMP) (6).

Another approach for the fractionation of proteins extracted from a number of cartilage tissues, represented in Fig. 3, is to use chromatography on the anion exchanger Mono Q, eluted with a NaCl gradient in 7 M urea. Subsequent electrophoresis shows differences, indicated by arrows. Indeed, the structures of the intervertebral disc appear to contain proteins not present in articular and nasal cartilage.

It is thus clear that hyaline cartilages, although superficially similar, show clear differences in their patterns of matrix proteins. It should be stressed, however, that the basic pattern of proteins is similar and most of the proteins are present in all cartilages, e.g., collagen II, IX, and aggrecan.

It is likely that the fine tuning of the protein pattern reflects the different functional requirements encountered by a given cartilage. Knowledge of the structure and interactions of the proteins will provide important background for understanding their roles in the tissue. Therefore an account of some key cartilage noncollagenous proteins is provided below.

Cartilage Matrix Protein

Cartilage matrix protein, also called CMP or the 148 kDa protein, is made up of three apparently identical subunits with M_r of about 50,000 (6). The protein has been cloned and sequenced from chick chondrocytes. It contains two homologous repeat sequences of about 190 amino acids separated by a partial EGF-like domain. The total sequence contains 493 amino acids, including a 23 amino acid residue signal peptide. The single copy gene contains eight exons (7). Several other proteins contain sequences homologous to those of the repeat domains. These include the von Willebrand factor, complement factors B and C2, and the α-chains of the integrins LFA-1, Mac-1, and p150,95 (7). The protein has been identified in cartilage only and is even more restricted in its distribution in that it is not found in articular cartilage, while it is a major component in tracheal cartilage (8).

Cartilage matrix protein is a sensitive marker for aging. Its concentration in bovine tracheal cartilage is low during the fetal period and up to about 2 years of age. It then shows a rather linear increase up to some 10 years of age, where it constitutes more than 5% of the wet weight of the tissue. It is present in two pools, one that can be extracted with guanidine-HCl and one that requires additional trypsin digestion for solubilization (9).

The function of the protein is not clear. Early data indicated that the protein can bind to proteoglycans. It actually cochromatographed with aggrecan, also under denaturing conditions in several different fractionation procedures. Although providing indirect evidence, cochromatography of proteoglycan and CMP under dissociating and strongly denaturing conditions, with and without deter-

ARTICULAR +SH

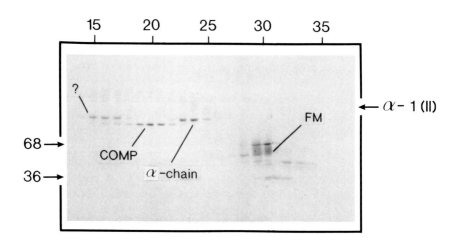

ARTICULAR −SH

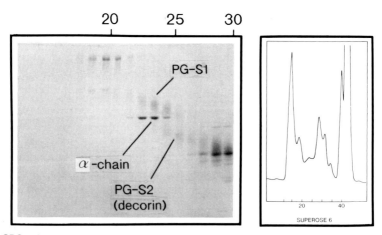

FIG. 2. SDS-polyacrylamide gel electrophoresis pattern of extracts from bovine tracheal and articular cartilages, respectively. The cartilage samples were extracted with 15 ml/g of 4 M guanidine-HCl, containing a number of proteinase inhibitors including N-ethylmaleimide to prevent disulfide exchange. The extract was then chromatographed on a column of Superose 6 (Pharmacia). Aliquots of the fractions were precipitated with ethanol and electrophoresed on 4–16% gradient SDS-polyacrylamide gels with (+SH) and without (−SH) previous reduction.

TRACHEAL +SH

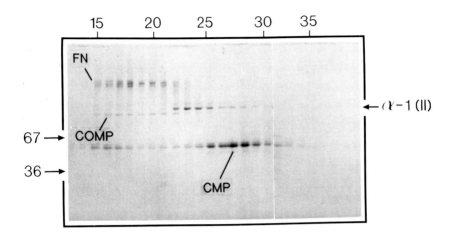

TRACHEAL −SH

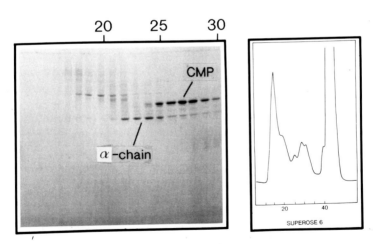

FIG. 2. *Continued.*

There are some major differences between the patterns. Thus fibronectin (FN) is much more prominent in tracheal cartilage and cartilage matrix protein is present in tracheal cartilage only. COMP is present in both types of cartilage, while other high M_r components are present in either tissue only. Also indicated are the low M_r proteoglycans fibromodulin (FM), decorin, and PG-S1 (biglycan).

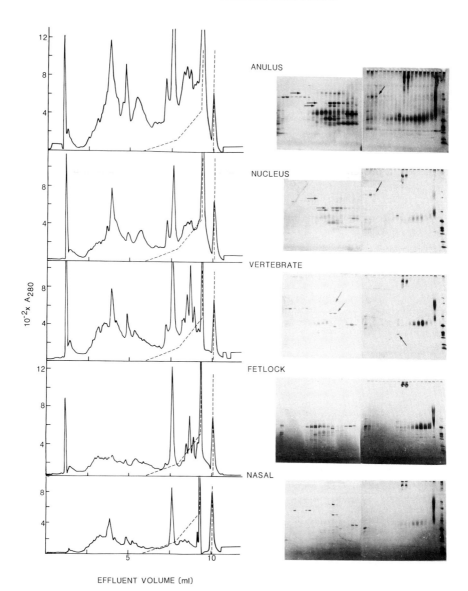

FIG. 3. Cartilaginous tissues were extracted with 4 M guanidine-HCl, transferred into 7 M urea, and chromatographed on a Mono Q column (Pharmacia Biotechnology) eluted with a 0–1 M NaCl gradient. Aliquots of the fractions were precipitated with ethanol and electrophoresed on 4–16% gradient SDS-polyacrylamide gels. Gels were stained with coomassie brilliant blue. Bovine tissues analyzed were from the intervertebral disc, i.e., anulus fibrosus, nucleus pulposus, the facet joints (vertebrate), articular cartilage from the fetlock joint, and nasal cartilage.

Several bands representing proteins not present in all of the tissues are indicated (*arrows*).

gent and also after chondroitinase digestion to remove the glycosaminoglycan side chains (Heinegård, unpublished), provides evidence that the protein is tightly bound.

Anchorin

Anchorin isolated from cartilage was originally identified as a protein mediating binding between collagen II and chondrocytes (for ref. see 10). It could therefore represent a protein that mediates interactions between cells and matrix, which are important for the regulation of cartilage matrix remodeling.

Anchorin has been cloned and sequenced (10,11). Its 329 amino acid long sequence does not contain any apparent signal peptide sequence. There is, however, a hydrophobic 25 amino acid sequence, that although interrupted by three polar residues, may represent a membrane-spanning domain. The protein contains four internal repeats of some 70 to 80 amino acids, each containing a highly conserved 17 amino acid residue domain. Interestingly, the protein shows some homology with calpactin, endonexin, protein II, and lipocortin, all primarily intracellular proteins. Anchorin CII appears to be at least partly located at the outside of the cell membrane (11).

Chondrocalcin or the C-terminal Propeptide of Collagen II

Cartilage contains an oligomeric protein made up of subunits, each migrating upon SDS-polyacrylamide gel electrophoresis with an apparent M_r of 35,000. This protein is present in all cartilages, most prominently in articular cartilage and in mineralized cartilage. The protein, first isolated from epiphyseal cartilage (12), binds to hydroxylapatite crystals and may have a role in the mineralization process. The protein can be extracted from cartilage using physiological strength salt solution (unpublished). This contrasts with most matrix proteins, which require denaturing solvents to release them from interactions with other matrix constituents. It therefore appears that in nonmineralized cartilage, the propeptide represents a pool of molecules released at the sites of collagen fiber formation and then cleared from the cartilage by diffusion out of the tissue.

PARP, Possibly Representing the Amino Terminal Domain of Collagen XI

This cationic low M_r protein with high contents of proline and arginine has been isolated from bovine articular and nasal cartilage and characterized (13). The protein, which is 218 amino acids long, shows 49% homology with the amino terminal domain of the α1-chain of human collagen XI. The protein is one of the minor components in the cartilage, and is present at less than 10% of the mass of the link protein (13). Its function is not known, but the protein is more abundant in nasal cartilage than in articular cartilage (13).

Cartilage Oligomeric Matrix Protein

The 100 kDa subunit protein, or the cartilage matrix oligomeric protein (COMP), was first identified in articular cartilage by Spitz-Fife et al. (14,15). Recent work in our laboratory has aimed at the structural and functional characterization of the protein. It contains subunits with an M_r of some 100,000 as determined by SDS-polyacrylamide gel electrophoresis, using 4 to 16% gradient gels. The intact protein appears to consist of four or five subunits apparently linked via disulfide bonds. The protein contains carbohydrate substituents, possibly including chondroitin sulfate (unpublished). COMP is present in cartilage only, as determined by enzyme-linked immunosorbent assay. Its concentration is somewhat higher in articular cartilage than in, e.g., nasal and tracheal cartilage (unpublished).

Functions of COMP are not known. Interestingly, release of the protein or fragments thereof is increased from articular cartilage when the tissue is apparently being repaired, e.g., when an inflammatory process has been shut off by intra-articular injection of glucocorticoids (Saxne and Heinegård, unpublished). This may indicate a role in the repair process and perhaps in the assembly of the matrix.

36 kDa Protein

A comparatively major component of cartilage, the 36 kDa protein, is somewhat basic and has a high content of leucine. The protein contains carbohydrate, but lacks sialic acid and hexosamines (Heinegård, unpublished). The protein has a restricted distribution and is found only in cartilage and bone. It is possible that its presence in bone is due to cartilage remnants.

Experiments with isolated chondrocytes show that the cells bind to plastic culture plates coated with the protein, indicating that it may represent one of several matrix molecules mediating interactions of cells with matrix (16). Such interactions could be essential for the ability of the cells to monitor alterations in matrix properties and thus for the regulation of tissue remodeling.

Interestingly, the 36 kDa protein is heterogeneous in some articular cartilage. Thus, fractionation of the articular cartilage proteins on CM-cellulose yields two components with somewhat different mobility by SDS-polyacrylamide gel electrophoresis (Fig. 4). The identity of both components as 36 kDa protein is clearly demonstrated by the reactivity with antibodies to the protein and the similar peptide patterns obtained after trypsin digestion (Fig. 4).

The nature of the difference between the two preparations is not clear. However, it is notable that the larger molecule is most cationic, i.e., it was more retarded on the column. This molecule appears to correspond to the single type of 36 kDa protein present in tracheal cartilage.

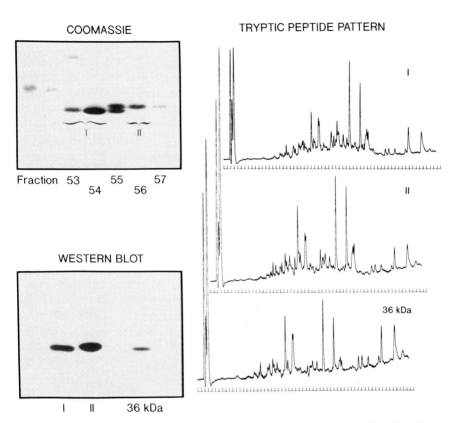

FIG. 4. Analysis of the 36 kDa protein from articular cartilage. An extract of bovine articular cartilage was fractionated by CsCl-4 M guanidine hydrochloride density gradient centrifugation as described (52). The top fraction was dialyzed into 7 M urea, 20 mM Tris, pH 8, and chromatographed on a DEAE-cellulose (DE-52) column (52). The flow-through fraction was adjusted to pH 4 and chromatographed on a CM-cellulose (CM-52) column eluted with a 0–0.5 M sodium chloride gradient in 7 M urea, 10 mM sodium acetate, pH 4. Aliquots of the fractions were analyzed by 4–16% SDS-polyacrylamide gradient gels. The coomassie stained gels showed two components with somewhat different mobilities, but with elution positions corresponding to the 36 kDa protein. Fractions were pooled and electrophoresed and transblotted onto nitrocellulose. Staining with an antibody to the 36 kDa protein isolated from tracheal cartilage show that both react with the antibody, as does the control (36 kDa).

The fractions containing the two components, respectively, were pooled and some larger sized components were removed by chromatography on Superose 12 (Pharmacia), data not shown. The pure proteins were digested with trypsin. They were further characterized by fractionation on a C-18 pep-RPC (Pharmacia Biotechnology) column eluted with a gradient of 0–70% acetonitrile in 0.1% trifluoroacetic acid.

The two components show almost identical peptide patterns, supporting that they are identical and also are identical to the 36 kDa protein isolated from tracheal cartilage analyzed for comparison.

Link Protein

This protein was originally isolated from cartilage as a component present in proteoglycan aggregates (17). When isolated from the tissue, several, usually two, isoforms are observed by SDS polyacrylamide gel electrophoresis (17). The protein is made up of three loops, showing extensive homology with the hyaluronate binding region in aggrecan (18–20). The most N-terminal of these folds shows homology with an immunoglobulin fold, while the other two folds have a different structure. It appears that hyaluronate binding depends on these two loop structures (18,19). Link protein is found in many connective tissues (15,17,21) and proteoglycans from several connective tissues can bind to hyaluronate and link protein in a manner typical for stabilized aggregates. The link protein stabilizes proteoglycan aggregates by binding both to the proteoglycan hyaluronate binding region and to the hyaluronate chain (22–24). Link protein has a similar specificity as the hyaluronate-binding region in aggrecan for a decasaccharide sequence (25).

One may speculate about the primary role of link protein. The stabilization of the strong association between the mature hyaluronate-binding region of the proteoglycan and hyaluronate, both present at high concentrations in the matrix, may seem superfluous. It is of interest that the newly secreted proteoglycan has lower affinity for hyaluronate, probably due to incomplete formation of disulfide bridges (26). The phenomenon has been referred to as delayed aggregation (27). However, it should be noted that the newly secreted proteoglycans also bind to hyaluronate when it is at high concentrations, as may exist in the tissue (1,5,28). With time in the matrix, reportedly over some 24 hr, the affinity increases and the proteoglycan attains full binding strength (26). In chondrocyte culture, the formation of link-stabilized aggregates occurs shortly after secretion from the cells (1,5). The newly secreted link protein, in contrast to the hyaluronate-binding region of the proteoglycan, was shown to have full capacity for binding both to the proteoglycan monomer and to the hyaluronate (Björnsson and Heinegård, unpublished; 28). Furthermore, other studies have indicated that the intermediate in aggregate formation may be a proteoglycan monomer-link protein complex (29). Thus, available data indicate that an important function of the link protein may be to mediate and provide some stability of early interactions between proteoglycans and hyaluronate by binding to the hyaluronate-binding region of the proteoglycan, thereby allowing the monomer to bind with some stability to hyaluronate. Still, such an arrangement may be important in conferring relatively stable binding of proteoglycans to hyaluronate. At the same time, it may permit some reshuffling of proteoglycans along the hyaluronate to modulate aggregate architecture to meet functional needs optimally.

Another hyaluronate-binding protein has been isolated from the Swarm rat chondrosarcoma and is referred to as HABP102. This glycoprotein of apparent M_r 102 kDa appears to be quite distinct from the hyaluronate binding region as demonstrated by peptide mapping. The specificity of its binding to hyaluronate is not known (30).

Thrombospondin

Thrombospondin is classically isolated from platelets. More recently, the protein has been identified in cartilage (31) also. It is apparently synthesized by cells in the tissue. It should be stressed that the protein is a minor product and its content in cartilage is low. The protein is made up of three very large subunits, each with an M_r of about 130,000. It contains many interesting substructures, including a cell-binding domain, apparently mediating cell attachment via an -RGD-sequence. It also contains a glycosaminoglycan-binding domain and substructures binding to the fibrillar elements in the tissues. Thrombospondin has been suggested to have major roles in repair of fibrous tissues. Whether it has functions in cartilage repair and remodeling is presently not known.

Tenascin

Tenascin is a very large oligomeric protein that contains three structurally related subunits: M_r 190 kDa, 200 kDa, and 230 kDa (32,33). The three subunits form a six-armed protein with an overall M_r in the order of 1,000,000. The protein has been cloned and sequenced and shows major homologies to other matrix molecules, e.g., fibronectin (32). Tenascin has not been identified in adult cartilage, but it is present during embryogenesis (for instance, surrounding budding limbs) (33). The protein appears to have major roles in embryogenesis. It is usually present in growing epithelium and functions in tissue/cell interactions.

Fibronectin

Fibronectin (for refs. see 34) is ubiquitous. It represents the first isolated and characterized cell-binding protein. Studies of the cell binding led to the first characterization of an integrin, i.e. a member of what later was found to represent a family of cell surface receptors particularly for matrix proteins. Fibronectin also binds to matrix macromolecules, e.g., the glycosaminoglycan chains of proteoglycans, where the far strongest binding is for heparan sulfate/heparin. This glycosaminoglycan is not a cartilage matrix constituent. Fibronectin, however, binds to other glycosaminoglycans, although with a lower affinity. Fibronectin has additional binding sites for collagens. This binding is most pronounced to denatured collagens, although native collagen III has been shown to interact. Clear binding has only been demonstrated to native collagen III, normally not present in tissues like bone and cartilage. It is possible that additional binding may be to some of the more recently described minor collagens. Fibronectin has major roles in tissue repair. Whether it has a role in repair processes in cartilage is not known. In this context it is of some interest that the articular cartilage content of the molecule increases as a result of increased synthesis in the degenerative process of osteoarthritis (35), indicative of attempted repair.

Ch21

This protein consists of 158 amino acid residues and has an M_r of 18 kDa (36). It belongs to a superfamily of proteins that appear to bind and transport small hydrophobic molecules, e.g., retinoids. The protein is expressed by hypertrophic chick chondrocytes and may have a role as a carrier for a hydrophobic molecule involved in the regulation of morphogenesis (36).

Low Molecular Weight Proteoglycans With Few Side Chains: Biglycan, Decorin, and Fibromodulin

Cartilage contains structurally very different proteoglycans of much smaller size, i.e., biglycan (PG-S1), decorin (PG-S2), and fibromodulin (37–41), schematically illustrated in Fig. 1. They represent a family of structurally related, but genetically distinct, molecules (38–42), with a wide tissue distribution. Their core proteins have M_r of about 40,000, and contain some 10 homologous repeats of about 25 amino acids (38,40–42). The cysteine residues are located in conserved locations, further corroborating the homology. In its N-terminal part, PG-S1 contains two closely spaced serine-glycine dipeptides, each containing a chondroitin sulfate or dermatan sulfate side chain, depending on the tissue (37–39,42,43). Decorin, on the other hand, contains only one glycosaminoglycan side chain in the corresponding domain (44,45). The chain may be either chondroitin sulfate or dermatan sulfate, depending on the tissue (39).

Fibromodulin is different in that there is no glycosaminoglycan chain in the N-terminal part. Instead, this domain contains several sulfated tyrosine residues (41; Antonsson, Oldberg, Heinegård, unpublished), such that this molecule is also strongly anionic in this region. Fibromodulin, interestingly, does not contain chondroitin/dermatan sulfate (41,46) but does contain keratan sulfate chains, linked via N-glycosidic linkage from N-acetylglucosamine to asparagine residues in the central domain of the molecule (41,46). This is similar to the keratan sulfate proteoglycans in cornea, which, however, appear distinct from fibromodulin (unpublished).

Functions of the Small Proteoglycans

Decorin and fibromodulin bind to fibril forming collagens *in vitro* and inhibit formation of collagen fibers (47–49). Both molecules are localized over the collagen fibers, as demonstrated by immunostaining at the ultrastructural level (Reinholt, Svensson, and Heinegård, unpublished).

Although PG-S1 has a very similar structure, it has so far not been possible to demonstrate that this proteoglycan can bind to any of the fibril-forming collagens. One of the important functions of these macromolecules that are bound along the collagen fibers may be to provide a coat that markedly alters the fibril surface properties. Also, other molecules bind along the collagen fibers. One example is collagen IX, having a cationic N-terminal globule of the α1 chain (for reference see Olsen). Thus, there are opportunities for ionic interactions between negatively charged decorin and fibromodulin and positively charged collagen IX on neighboring collagen fibrils. This may effectively make several shorter collagen fibers interact to mimic the properties of a very long collagen fiber. This hypothesis is schematically outlined in Fig. 1.

Another possibility is that the proteins/proteoglycans provide a space between collagen fibrils. It is likely that the coat prevents the collagen fibrils from growing either by including more collagen molecules or by fusion of neighboring fibrils.

One of the functions of the proteoglycans may be to immobilize growth factors. Recently it was shown that the small proteoglycans decorin and biglycan bind TGF-β via the protein core (50). The exact specificity of this binding has not yet been demonstrated. This aspect of proteoglycan function is particularly interesting in view of the potential role of the molecules in the regulation of tissue growth (51).

Interestingly, it has been shown that when the core protein of decorin is overexpressed in Chinese hamster ovary cells, this markedly affects cell shape and cell proliferation (51), perhaps as a result of binding of growth factors, e.g., TGF-β.

CONCLUDING REMARKS

Over recent years, several cartilage matrix macromolecules have been isolated and characterized. Studies of their structure and regulation have added insights into their roles. Key information on the functions of the proteins will be obtained in studies of their interactions. It is well documented that collagen molecules interact in a well-controlled manner such that they form fibrillar structures in the extracellular matrix. These interactions involve large parts of the molecules. Furthermore, collagens interact with other tissue molecules which may coat large parts of the collagen fibrillar surface, thereby not only preventing more collagen molecules from binding and thus limiting fiber growth, but also altering the surface properties and thus the interactions of the collagen fibers between themselves and with other matrix molecules. Other well-known interactions are those between proteoglycans and hyaluronate. These interactions serve important roles in maintaining proteoglycans fixed in the matrix.

In many disease processes early changes occur in the major matrix constituents. Thus, an early event in osteoarthritis appears to be fragmentation of proteoglycans and their release from the articular cartilage. This most likely aggravates the process by altering and impairing the mechanical properties such as resilience of the tissue. The cells may then become exposed to exceedingly high stress, impeding their possibilities to repair matrix.

ACKNOWLEDGMENTS

Grants were obtained from the Swedish MRC, Folksam's stiftelse, King Gustaf V:s 80-årsfond, Kock's stiftelse the medical faculty, Lund University, and Österlunds stiftelse. E. R. Pimentel was supported by a visiting scientist grant from CNP_q-conselho Nacional de Desenvolvimento Cientifico e Tecnológico.

REFERENCES

1. Björnsson S, Heinegård D. Assembly of proteoglycan aggregates in cultures of chondrocytes from bovine tracheal cartilage. *Biochem J* 1981;199:17–29.
2. Kimura JH, Hardingham TE, Hascall VC, Solursh M. Biosynthesis of proteoglycans and their assembly into aggregates in cultures of chondrocytes from the swarm rat chondrosarcoma. *J Biol Chem* 1979;254:2600–2609.
3. Heinegård D, Oldberg Å. Structure and biology of cartilage and bone noncollagenous macromolecules. *FASEB J* 1989;3:2042–2051.
4. Sommarin Y, Heinegård D. Four classes of cell associated proteoglycans in suspension cultures of articular cartilage chondrocytes. *Biochem J* 1986;233:715–724.
5. Sommarin Y, Heinegård D. Specific interaction between cartilage proteoglycans and hyaluronic acid at the chondrocyte cell surface. *Biochem J* 1983;214:777–784.
6. Paulsson M, Heinegård D. Purification and structural characterization of a cartilage matrix protein. *Biochem J* 1981;197:367–375.
7. Kiss I, Deák F, Holloway RG Jr, Delius H, Mebust KA, Frimberger E, Argraves WS, Tsonis PA, Winterbottom N, Goetinck PF. Structure of the gene for cartilage matrix protein, a modular protein of the extracellular matrix. *J Biol Chem* 1989;264:8126–8134.
8. Paulsson M, Heinegård D. Radioimmunoassay of the 148-kilodalton cartilage protein. Distribution of the protein among bovine tissues. *Biochem J* 1982;207:207–213.
9. Paulsson M, Inerot S, Heinegård D. Variation in quantity and extractability of the 148-kilodalton cartilage protein with age. *Biochem J* 1984;221:623–630.
10. Fernandez MP, Selmin O, Martin GR, Yamada Y, Pfäffle M, Deutzmann R, Mollenhauer J, von der Mark K. The structure of anchorin CII, a collagen binding protein isolated from chondrocyte membrane. *J Biol Chem* 1988;263:5921–5925.
11. Pfäffle M, Ruggiero F, Hoffmann H, Fernandez MP, Selmin O, Yamada Y, Garrone R, von der Mark K. Biosynthesis secretion and extracellular localization of anchorin CII, a collagen-binding protein of the calpactin family. *EMBO J* 1988;8:2335–2342.
12. Hinek A, Reiner A, Poole AR. The calcification of cartilage matrix in chondrocyte culture: studies of the C-terminal propeptide of type II collagen (chondrocalcin). *J Cell Biol* 1987;104:1435–1441.
13. Neame PJ, Young CN, Treep JT. Isolation and primary structure of PARP, a 24-kDa proline- and arginine-rich protein from bovine cartilage closely related to the NH_2-terminal domain in collagen α1(XI). *J Biol Chem* 1990;265:20401–20408.
14. Spitz-Fife R, Brandt KD. Identification of a high-molecular-weight (400,000) protein in hyaline cartilage. *Biochim Biophys Acta* 1984;802:506–514.
15. Spitz-Fife R. Identification of link proteins and a 116,000 dalton matrix protein in canine meniscus. *Arch Biochem Biophys* 1985;240:682–688.

16. Sommarin Y, Larsson T, Heinegård D. Chondrocyte-matrix interactions. Attachment to proteins isolated from cartilage. *Exp Cell Res* 1989;184:181–192.
17. Keiser HF, Schulman HJ, Sandson JL. Immunochemistry of cartilage proteoglycan. Immunodiffusion and gel-electrophoretic studies. *Biochem J* 1972;126:163–169.
18. Neame PJ, Christner JE, Baker JR. The primary structure of link protein from rat chondrosarcoma proteoglycan aggregate. *J Biol Chem* 1986;261:3519–3535.
19. Goetinck PF, Stirpe NS, Tsonis PA, Carlone D. The tandemly repeated sequences of cartilage link protein. *J Cell Biol* 1987;105:2403–2408.
20. Rhodes C, Doege K, Sasaki M, Yamada Y. Alternative splicing generates two different mRNA species for rat link protein. *J Biol Chem* 1988;263:6063–6067.
21. Gardell S, Baker J, Caterson B, Heinegård D, Rodén L. Link protein and a hyaluronic acid binding region as components of aorta proteoglycan. *Biochem Biophys Res Comm* 1980;95:1823–1831.
22. Heinegård D, Hascall VC. Aggregation of cartilage proteoglycans III. Characteristics of the proteins isolated from trypsin digests of aggregates. *J Biol Chem* 1974;249:4250–4256.
23. Hardingham TE. The role of link-protein in the structure of cartilage proteoglycan aggregates. *Biochem J* 1979;177:237–247.
24. Heinegård D, Hascall V. The effects of dansylation and acetylation on the interaction between hyaluronic acid and the hyaluronic acid binding region of cartilage proteoglycans. *J Biol Chem* 1979;254:927–934.
25. Tengblad A. A comparative study of the binding of cartilage link protein and the hyaluronate-binding region of the cartilage proteoglycan to hyaluronate-substituted Sepharose gel. *Biochem J* 1981;199:297–305.
26. Sandy JD, O'Neill JR, Ratzlaff LC. Acquisition of hyaluronate-binding affinity in vivo by newly synthesized cartilage proteoglycans. *Biochem J* 1989;258:875–880.
27. Oegema TR. Delayed formation of proteoglycan aggregate structures in human articular cartilage disease states. *Nature* 1980;288:583–585.
28. Björnsson S. Biosynthesis of cartilage proteoglycans in chondrocyte cell cultures (PhD thesis, Lund University, 1981).
29. Kimura JH, Hardingham T, Hascall VC. Assembly of newly synthesized proteoglycan and link protein into aggregates in cultures of chondrosarcoma chondrocytes. *J Biol Chem* 1980;255:7134–7143.
30. Crossman MV, Mason M. Purification and characterization of a hyaluronan-binding protein from rat chondrosarcoma. *Biochem J* 1990;266:399–406.
31. Miller R, McDevitt C. Thrombospondin is present in articular cartilage and is synthesized by articular cartilage. *Biochem Biophys Res Comm* 1988;153:708–714.
32. Vaughan L, Huber S, Chiquet M, Winterhalter KH. A major, six-armed glycoprotein from embryonic cartilage. *EMBO J* 1987;6:349–353.
33. Jones FS, Hofman S, Cunningham BA, Edelman GM. A detailed structural model of cytoactin: protein homologies, alternative RNA splicing and binding regions. *Proc Natl Acad Sci USA* 1989;86:1905–1909.
34. Ruoslahti E. Fibronectin and its receptors. *Ann Rev Biochem* 1988;57:375–413.
35. Wurster NB, Lust G. Synthesis of fibronectin in normal and osteoarthritic articular cartilage. *Biochim Biophys Acta* 1984;800:52–58.
36. Cancedda FD, Dozin B, Rossi F, Molina F, Cancedda R, Negri A, Ronchi S. The Ch21 protein, developmentally regulated in chick embryo, belongs to the superfamily of lipophilic molecule carrier proteins. *J Biol Chem* 1990;265:19060–19064.
37. Fisher LW, Hawkins GR, Tuross N, Termine JD. Purification and partial characterization of small proteoglycans I and II, bone sialoproteins I and II, and osteonectin from the mineral compartment of developing human bone. *J Biol Chem* 1987;262:9702–9708.
38. Fisher LW, Termine JD, Young MF. Deduced protein sequence of bone small proteoglycan I (biglycan) shows homology with proteoglycan II (decorin) and several nonconnective tissue proteins in a variety of species. *J Biol Chem* 1989;264:4571–4576.
39. Heinegård D, Björne-Persson A, Cöster L, Franzén A, Gardell S, Malmström A, Paulsson M, Sandfalk R, Vogel K. The core protein of large and small interstitial proteoglycans from various connective tissues form distinct subgroups. *Biochem J* 1985;230:181–194.

40. Krusius T, Ruoslahti E. Primary structure of an extracellular matrix proteoglycan core protein deduced from cloned cDNA. *Proc Natl Acad Sci USA* 1986;83:7683–7687.
41. Oldberg Å, Antonsson P, Lindblom K, Heinegård D. A collagen-binding 59-kd protein (fibromodulin) is structurally related to the small interstitial proteoglycans PG-S1 and PG-S2 (decorin). *EMBO J* 1989;8:2601–2604.
42. Neame PJ, Choi HU, Rosenberg LC. The primary structure of the core protein of the small, leucine-rich proteoglycan (PGI) from bovine articular cartilage. *J Biol Chem* 1989;264:8653–8661.
43. Heinegård D, Paulsson M, Inerot S, Carlström C. A novel low-molecular-weight chondroitin sulphate proteoglycan isolated from cartilage. *Biochem J* 1981;197:355–366.
44. Chopra RK, Pearson CH, Pringle GA, Fackre DS, Scott PG. Dermatan sulphate is located on ser-4 of bovine skin proteodermatan sulphate. *Biochem J* 1985;232:277–279.
45. Mann DM, Yamaguchi Y, Bourdon MA, Ruoslahti E. Analysis of glycosaminoglycan substitution in decorin by site-directed mutagenesis. *J Biol Chem* 1990;265:5317–5323.
46. Plaas AHK, Neame PJ, Nivens CM, Reiss L. Identification of the keratan sulfate attachment sites on bovine fibromodulin. *J Biol Chem* 1990;265:20634–20640.
47. Vogel KG, Paulsson M, Heinegård D. Specific inhibition of type I and type II collagen fibrillogenesis by the low-molecular-mass proteoglycan of tendon. *Biochem J* 1984;223:587–597.
48. Brown DC, Vogel KG. Characteristics of the *in vivo* interaction of a small proteoglycan (PGII) of bovine tendon with type I collagen. *Matrix* 1989;9:468–478.
49. Hedbom E, Heinegård D. Interaction of a 59-kDa connective tissue matrix protein with collagen I and collagen II. *J Biol Chem* 1989;264:6898–6905.
50. Yamaguchi Y, Mann DM, Ruoslahti E. Negative regulation of transforming growth factor-β by the proteoglycan decorin. *Nature* 1990;346:281–284.
51. Yamaguchi Y, Ruoslahti E. Expression of human proteoglycan in Chinese hamster ovary cells inhitis cell proliferation. *Nature* 1988;336:244–246.
52. Heinegård D, Larsson T, Sommarin Y, Franzén A, Paulsson M, Hedbom E. Two novel matrix proteins isolated from articular cartilage show wide distributions among connective tissues. *J Biol Chem* 1986;261:13866–13872.

DISCUSSION

Tanzer: I think there is something in this presentation for everybody in the audience.

Muir: Do proteoglycans influence fibrillogenesis of type II collagen?

Heinegård: Both decorin and fibromodulin bind to collagen types I and II and inhibit fibrillogenesis. However, these interactions require native collagen; denatured collagen will not bind.

Thonar: Does the keratan sulfate-rich fragment still bind to collagen after treatment with keratanase I?

Heinegård: Yes! Thus the interactions do not require the keratan sulfate chains.

Kuettner: You showed striking differences in pericellular distribution of fibromodulin. Was this from normal cartilage or was the section digested with chondroitinase?

Heinegård: The picture was from osteoarthritic cartilage. The pericellular area in osteoarthritic cartilage stained intensely with several antibodies to matrix molecules, including fibromodulin. Even though the cartilage appeared macroscopically normal, it was taken from a joint with advanced osteoarthritis. Therefore, most of the proteoglycans were already lost. In normal cartilage, digestion does not alter the appearance much. Fibromodulin at this level of resolution and staining is rather evenly distributed. The protein is more abundant in the superficial part of the articular cartilage.

Morales: Does fibromodulin bind to the surface of the fibril, or does it actually penetrate inside the fiber, possibly in the gap region?

Heinegård: I don't think fibromodulin binds at the gap region, judging from some preliminary data on binding specificity. John Scott has shown that decorin, on the other hand, is localized to the gap region. In his studies, he used staining for the side chains. The pictures nicely show that the proteoglycan binds at the outside of the collagen fibril. In order for the fibril to grow any further, the proteoglycans may have to be removed to allow an assembly of more collagen molecules onto the fibril surface.

Howell: Where does fibromodulin bind to individual collagen molecules?

Heinegård: Finn Reinhardt prepared rotary shadowed electron micrographs of fibromodulin bound to collagen. The fibromodulin appeared localized about one-fourth from one end of the collagen molecule, but this method could not resolve whether it is closest to the N- or the C-terminus.

Articular Cartilage and Osteoarthritis,
edited by K. Kuettner et al.
Raven Press, Ltd., New York © 1992.

8

General Discussion for Chapters 1–7

Pritzker: I have a question for Tim Hardingham and Dick Heinegård: Which matrix proteins or components of the proteoglycans resist proteolysis? These molecules may be present in osteoarthritic cartilages as memory molecules and provide information about the previous history of the events.

Hardingham: The G1-domain with its hyaluronic acid-binding region and the link proteins are protease-resistant to a large range of different proteinases. Under native conditions, they resist attack for quite some time. In denaturing conditions, they are more susceptible to degradation. In the aging process and in pathology, these molecules can be cleaved from proteoglycan aggregates, accumulate in the tissue, and can also be released into the synovial fluid. Further damage through other mechanisms, such as free radical attack, can produce smaller pieces. I don't know whether these will be useful molecules to follow during disease progression.

Heinegård: Tore Saxon has analyzed a number of matrix constituents released into the synovial fluid. The results were correlated with extent of cartilage destruction assessed by the Larsen system. At stage zero no cartilage destruction is observed, although the process is active, while at stage 5 there is extensive destruction. At stage zero the level of G1 is normal, although total proteoglycan epitope release is very high. Later, stage 4–5, release of G1 is much higher, while total proteoglycan epitope release is low. Thus early in the process of cartilage destruction, fragments from the CS-rich region are primarily released, and later the G1 is released into the synovial fluid.

Apparently the G1 is retained in the tissue bound to HA. Therefore, as the destruction of the cartilage progresses, different proportions of proteoglycan fragments can be detected. Incidentally, bone sialoprotein, which is bone-specific, increases in synovial fluid with disease progression, suggesting increased involvement or altered metabolism in the underlying bone.

Tyler: Many investigators have indicated that the small proteoglycans—biglycan, decorin, and fibromodulin—are fairly resistant to proteolysis. The total levels in various resorbing situations do not seem to change. Yet, if these molecules modify fibrillogenesis, they must go on and come off of the fibril during growth and during differentiation. Is this just a reversible ionic interaction in which these molecules are fairly stable, or does this process involve proteolysis followed by resynthesis during the course of cartilage life?

Heinegård: Kathy Vogel and Tom Koob have studied proteolytic fragmentation of decorin bound to collagen fibers. They found that only a fragment containing the side chain is released, while the major part of the molecule remains bound to collagen. It appears to be protected by this interaction with the collagen. It may be that measurements using antibodies do not detect the loss of the N-terminal part of the molecules where the side chains are.

Plaas: We have studied the fragmentation of decorin by stromelysin, and it can be cleaved in the leucine-rich repeated sequence. We are in the process of identifying cleavage sites for fibromodulin.

Rosenberg: In my chapter we suggest that in tissue during development, the cells first deposit a tissue with a particular matrix architecture, which is then coated with decorin or related molecules when the organization of the tissue is satisfactory. This stops further cell migration and major remodeling of the tissue until injury occurs and there is a need for repair.

Kresse: We find that normal rabbit and human cartilages contain significant amounts of core protein fragments of small proteoglycans which are generally devoid of glycos-aminoglycan chains. After treatment of rabbit knee joints with interleukin-1, the fragments disappeared with the same kinetics as the intact proteoglycans. Thus, there is limited proteolytic fragmentation, and the fragments remain for a long time. When an inflam-mation is induced, they disappear rapidly.

Cooke: I'm fascinated by the differential association of decorin with the surface layers of articular cartilage, while in fibrocartilage it seems to be permeated throughout the tissue. In our studies of experimental immune arthritis, the immune complexes, including fibrin, bind rapidly to the surface of articular cartilage, but are almost always bound throughout the meniscal fibrocartilage. The implication, if I understand Larry Rosenberg's hypothesis, in terms of decorin and its protective capacity, would be that the protective proteoglycans must be removed quickly for binding to occur.

Mason: Linda Sandell, do we know anything about the specific proteins which bind to the regulating sequences for transcription of the collagen II gene in chondrocytes? Do the same factors regulate transcription of the aggrecan gene?

Sandell: Thus far, only general factors are known. However, these proteins may be regulated by humoral factors known to affect type II collagen synthesis, for example, TGF-β or IGF-1. No chondrocyte-specific nuclear factors are known at present. With respect to co-expression of collagen and aggrecan, I think most of us who work with culture systems realize that expression of collagen, link protein, and aggrecan, major "cartilage-specific" molecules, can be quite easily uncoupled. However, there certainly may be as yet poorly understood common regulatory motifs. In the vertebral developmental system I described, aggrecan expression is actually coordinated with a change in the splice form of type II from A to B.

Kimura: While we know a vast amount about the structures of individual matrix com-ponents, we know very little about how these specific macromolecules interact with each other to provide a connective tissue which maintains appropriate mechanical properties during tissue differentiation and remodeling, such that the tissue continues to bear load. There must be orderly transitions of macromolecules in the extracellular matrix to maintain the mechanical properties during skeletal growth. Studies of these processes may help us understand the disorganized disassembly of the matrix that might occur during degenerative joint diseases, where mechanical properties of the matrix are impaired.

Articular Cartilage and Osteoarthritis,
edited by K. Kuettner et al.
Raven Press, Ltd., New York © 1992.

Part III: Structural Components of Cartilage: Collagens

Introduction

Michel van der Rest

Institute of Biology and Chemistry of Proteins (CNRS-UPR 412) and
École Normale Supérieure de Lyon, France

The biomechanical properties of cartilage are usually and very properly described as the result of the containment of the swelling pressure of highly charged proteoglycans by entrapment into a network of tension-resistant collagen fibrils. The definition of the biochemical nature of this network has rapidly progressed in the last few years. Three main collagenous constituents have been described: collagen types II, IX, and XI. Most of their primary structures has been elucidated through protein and cDNA sequencing and much information has been gained about their organization in an aggregated fibril. The available biochemical and immunochemical data clearly support the notion that the fibrils are heterotypic and are made of a mixture of these three collagen types in a very defined architecture. Type II collagen is, of course, the main building block of the fibril, while type XI collagen may serve as a core to the fibrils; type IX collagen appears to be an intermediate between the fibrils and the extrafibrillar space or between the fibrils themselves. Additional components, such as proteoglycans, are very likely involved in fibril assembly. The study of the crosslinking of the collagen molecules as presented by David Eyre and his colleagues reveals some of the three-dimensional relationships between the fibril constituents.

Important biochemical questions about the cartilage collagens remain unanswered however. At the levels of protein structure and of supramolecular aggregation, type XI collagen still poses several problems. Its tissue form has been shown to retain a globular domain whose structure and location within the molecule is still unknown, although it is likely to be at the N-terminus (1). Are thin type XI collagen fibrils assembled first and then reinforced by the accretion of type II collagen molecules? Such a scheme may explain some of the immunolocalization data which have initially suggested a limited pericellular localization for type XI collagen. The immunohistochemical masking of type XI collagen by type II collagen in the mature fibril has now been clearly established.

Type XI collagen presents a close homology to type V collagen which may likewise be a core to fibrils made of type I collagen. The distinction between collagen types V and XI is not clear-cut. Data from several laboratories indicate that some cells synthesize simultaneously $\alpha 1(XI)$ and type V chains in ratios that suggest the existence of hybrid molecules (2). Type V collagen chains have also been reported in some cartilages. The possibility that these chains participate in hybrid molecules with type XI chains should be considered. The $\alpha 3(XI)$ chain has a primary structure identical, as far as it could be established, with $\alpha 1(II)$. cDNA sequencing data indicate the existence of alternate splicing for the $\alpha 1(II)$ mRNA. This may be related to the assembly of type XI collagen molecules.

Type IX and possibly other fibril-associated collagens present new challenges in our understanding of cartilage matrix assembly. The existence of two alternate promoters for the $\alpha 1(IX)$ gene gives some clues about the functions of the various parts of the molecule (3). The triple helical domains, which are always expressed, would serve as a mean to anchor different functionalities to the fibril. The globular and basic NC4 domain, which is only expressed when the cartilage promoter is used, provides a means of interaction, probably between the aggregating proteoglycan network and the collagen fibril. In its absence, such as in the chicken vitreous humour, the most notable function of type IX collagen appears to be the direct attachment of a very large glycosaminoglycan chain to the fibrils (4). In the avian vitreous, this glycosaminoglycan chain is a substitute for the hyaluronic acid found in the mammalian tissue. The role of the glycosaminoglycan side chain of type IX collagen in cartilage remains unclear.

The biosynthesis of type IX collagen has not been much investigated yet. It must nevertheless differ from the well-described fibrillar collagen pathway in several aspects. For example, there is no globular domain similar in size or structure to the C-propeptide of fibrillar collagen, a region which is known to play a critical role in chain recognition and assembly of the molecule. The precise assembly in register of the three different polypeptide chains of type IX collagen must involve a recognition system for which the information must reside either in the chains themselves or in a complex with a molecular chaperone. The addition of the glycosaminoglycan side chain implies posttranslational steps which are not found in other collagen types.

The chondrocytes handle collagen fibril assembly in a very different way from other cells, tendon fibroblasts for example. While the fibroblast assembles fibril bundles in membrane invaginations and extrudes this bundle by moving itself away, the chondrocyte appears to be immobile and to throw away components that are assembled in a location remote from itself. The description of the mechanisms of fibril aggregation at the molecular level, as described by Eikenberry et al. (this volume), will certainly contribute to the understanding of the ways by which chondrocytes control cartilage matrix assembly.

The biochemical analysis of normal hyaline cartilage has failed to reveal the presence of any other collagenous constituent that would represent a substantial proportion of the matrix macromolecules (say over 1%). There is, however, a large body of evidence indicating that certain regions of the cartilage have different collagen compositions. For example, the surface of fetal human articular cartilage contains type I collagen and the calcified zone of adult articular cartilage contains type X collagen. Under pathological conditions and in aging, the collagen composition of cartilage also changes, and several additional collagen types can be found, such as collagen types I, III, V, and VI. Some of these collagens may actually be present at low levels in normal cartilage.

The growth plate cartilage constitutes a very different tissue with the abundant synthesis by hypertrophic cells of a molecule found only in calcifying cartilage, namely type X collagen. While the structure of the molecule is well established, its function as a collagen, i.e., as a structural element of the matrix, remains unclear. As discussed by Bjorn Olsen (this volume), its structure is remarkably homologous to that of type VIII collagen, which forms the hexagonal lattice of corneal Descemet's membrane. The supramolecular assembly of type X collagen has thus to be reassessed from this perspective.

While much work remains to be done by "classical" biochemical and histological approaches, it is becoming evident that these approaches fail to give us complete understanding of the detailed molecular events that lead to the formation of a functional cartilage matrix. The study of natural and induced mutations of structural molecules of the matrix will undoubtedly provide new insights into cartilage biology. Several mutations of type II collagen leading to some chondrodysplasias and familial osteoarthritis have now been characterized, as presented by Sergio Jimenez and his co-workers. The genetic linkage between the COL2A1 gene and some familial cases of osteoarthritis has also been established. This conforms with the view that the main function of type II collagen is to provide internal resistance to cartilage. Mutations of other, less abundant collagens may actually prove to produce more severe phenotypes as their functions are probably mainly at the level of matrix organization. Some studies will require the use of transgenic animals. However, the complexity of the development process and the central role played by cartilage in this process may actually limit the usefulness of this approach for the study of matrix assembly. The development of stable chondrocyte cultures, which lend themselves to transfection experiments, might prove to be the approach of choice for the study of the molecular events leading to the formation of the multimolecular aggregates that give cartilage its unique biomechanical and biochemical properties.

REFERENCES

1. Morris NP, Bächinger HP. Type XI collagen is a heterotrimer with a composition ($1\alpha,2\alpha,3\alpha$) retaining non-triple-helical domains. *J Biol Chem* 1987;262:11345–11350.
2. Niyibizi C, Eyre DR. Identification of the cartilage $\alpha1(XI)$ chain in type V collagen from bovine bone. *FEBS Lett* 1989;242:314–318.
3. Muragaki Y, Nishimura I, Henney A, Ninomiya Y, Olsen BR. The $\alpha1(IX)$ collagen gene gives rise to two different transcripts in both mouse embryonic and human fetal RNA. *Proc Natl Acad Sci USA* 1990;87:2400–2404.
4. Brewton RG, Wright DW, Mayne R. Structural and functional comparison of type IX collagen-proteoglycan from chicken cartilage and vitreous humor. *J Biol Chem* 1991;266:4752–4757.

Articular Cartilage and Osteoarthritis,
edited by K. Kuettner et al.
Raven Press, Ltd., New York © 1992.

9

Cartilage-Specific Collagens

Structural Studies

David R. Eyre, Jiann-Jiu Wu, and P. Woods

*Departments of Orthopaedics and Biochemistry, University of Washington,
Seattle, Washington 98195*

The different genetic types of collagen present in articular cartilage are listed in Table 1 (1). Type II collagen is the most abundant. Its fibrils form the basic framework of the tissue. Of the less abundant collagen species identified in cartilage, types IX and XI are notable in that they also are cartilage-specific and are found wherever type II collagen is found. Growing evidence points to hybrid polymerization and covalent interactions between collagens II, IX, and XI in forming the fibrillar matrix of cartilage.

TYPE II COLLAGEN

The type II collagen molecule is a homotrimer of $\alpha 1(II)$ chains, the product of a single gene, COL2A1. Its molecular dimensions and polymeric form, a 67 nm-repeat banded fibril by electron microscopy, resemble closely those of the other class I fibril-forming collagens, types I and III (Fig. 1).

The tensile strength of the collagen, and hence of cartilage, depends on intermolecular cross-linking. The principal cross-linking residues in the mature type II collagen fibril are hydroxylysyl pyridinoline residues (2). Each of these trivalent cross-links forms by a maturation reaction between two adjacent divalent keto-amines that are the initial products of lysyl oxidase-mediated cross-linking in the newly polymerized collagen fibrils (Fig. 2).

With development and maturation of cartilage tissue, the diameters of the collagen type II fibrils increase from less than 20 nm in fetal tissue to a range of 50 to 100 nm or more in adult human articular cartilage (3). The diameters remain thin in the uppermost (tangential) zone of the tissue where the fibrils lie primarily parallel to the plane of the articular surface. The collagen fibrillar

TABLE 1. *Collagen types present in adult articular cartilage*

Fibril-forming molecules	Molecular formula	% of total collagen	Distribution
Type II	$[\alpha 1(II)]_3$	95	Throughout
Type XI	$[\alpha 1(XI)\alpha 2(XI)\alpha 3(XI)]$	3	Throughout; $\alpha 1(V)$ partially replaces $\alpha 1(XI)$ in mature tissue
Short-helix molecules			
Type VI	$[\alpha 1(VI)\alpha 2(VI)\alpha 3(VI)]$	0–1	May be concentrated pericellularly
Type IX	$[\alpha 1(IX)\alpha 2(IX)\alpha 3(IX)]$	1	Throughout
Type X	$[\alpha 1(X)]_3$	1	Zone of calcified cartilage only

Based on analyses of bovine articular cartilage (Eyre et al., ref. 1.).

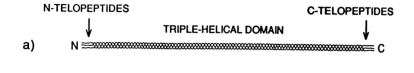

a)

N-TELOPEPTIDES   **C-TELOPEPTIDES**

TRIPLE-HELICAL DOMAIN

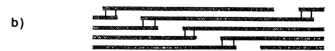

b)

FIG. 1. Structure of (**a**) the type II collagen molecule and (**b**) its cross-linked polymer, the 67 nm-periodic fibril. All class I collagens (types I, II, III, V, and XI) have this basic molecular and fibrillar form.

→

FIG. 2. Collagen cross-linking chemistry. **A:** Structures of the two forms of mature, pyridinoline cross-links. Hydroxylysyl pyridinoline (HP) is essentially the only form in articular cartilage. Lysyl pyridinoline (LP) appears, with HP, in significant amounts only in bone. **B:** Pyridinoline residues are believed to form essentially by an interaction between two keto-amine cross-links (in turn the products of interaction between an hydroxylysine aldehyde and an hydroxylysine). Collagen molecules are illustrated in cross-section here. **C:** The two molecular sites of intermolecular cross-linking in the type II collagen fibril. Two telopeptides containing a hydroxylysine aldehyde residue (derived by lysyl oxidase) react with a 4D-staggered triple-helical site in an adjacent molecule. The two telopeptides are probably in different collagen molecules, as shown here and in Fig. 2B. The amino acid sequences forming the pyridinoline (HP) cross-link sites in bovine $\alpha 1(II)$ are shown.

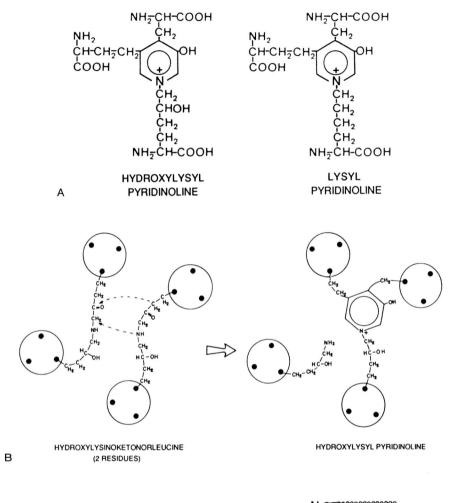

A HYDROXYLYSYL PYRIDINOLINE — LYSYL PYRIDINOLINE

B HYDROXYLYSINOKETONORLEUCINE (2 RESIDUES) — HYDROXYLYSYL PYRIDINOLINE

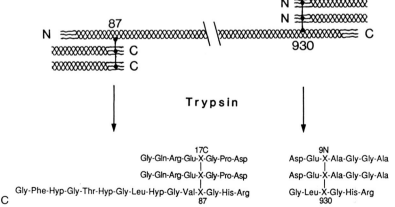

C

network provides a cohesive framework which entraps aggregating proteoglycans and to which the small proteoglycans (decorin and fibromodulin) bind (4).

It was shown recently that two forms of COL2A1 mRNA are expressed by variable splicing of the primary transcript. One contains and the other lacks the cysteine-rich exon 2 coding domain (5). These messages appear to be differentially expressed in different tissues during development. Differences in function of these splicing variants are not yet known.

There is growing evidence that type IX collagen and possibly type XI collagen contribute critically to the organization and mechanical stability of the collagen type II fibrillar network.

TYPE XI COLLAGEN

Type XI collagen was originally discovered in a salt-precipitated fraction (1.2 M NaCl) of pepsin-solubilized cartilage collagen (6). Three distinct α-chains were resolved: $\alpha1(XI)$ (initially called 1α), $\alpha2(XI)$ (2α), and $\alpha3(XI)$ (3α) in a 1: 1:1 ratio. The $\alpha3(XI)$ chain is indistinguishable in primary sequence from $\alpha1(II)$ (7). The $\alpha1(XI)$ chain shows close sequence homology to a $\alpha1(V)$ but is nevertheless a distinct gene product; $\alpha2(XI)$ is also a distinct gene product. The three chains probably form primarily a heterotrimeric native molecule of composition $[\alpha1(XI)\ \alpha2(XI)\ \alpha3(XI)]$, at least in young cartilage, although many chain combinations are theoretically possible (see below).

The functioning type XI collagen molecule in the extracellular matrix retains its N-propeptide extensions judging by SDS-PAGE of neutral salt and denaturant extracts of cartilage (8). As with the α-chains of the other class I collagens, the N-propeptide sequences of $\alpha1(XI)$ and $\alpha2(XI)$ include short segments of triple-helix $(GlyXY)_n$ and an amino terminal globular domain (Fig. 3). Retention of the N-propeptides may prevent the lateral growth of fibrils.

In tissues based on type II collagen, type XI collagen seems to be the molecule equivalent to type V collagen in tissues based on type I collagen. The situation is not quite so simple, however. During the maturation of articular cartilage, the type XI collagen fraction contains an increasing proportion of the $\alpha1(V)$ chain, apparently at the expense of $\alpha1(XI)$ (7). By contrast in bone, the type V collagen fraction contains an increasing proportion of $\alpha1(XI)$ at the expense of $\alpha1(V)$ going from fetal to adult tissue (9). The significance of these apparent developmental switches in gene expression from $\alpha1(XI)$ to $\alpha1(V)$, and vice versa is unknown. The stoichiometry in the yields of α-chains suggests that hybrid heterotrimeric molecules exist in which $\alpha1(V)$ and $\alpha1(XI)$ can substitute for each other. In adult articular cartilage, therefore, type XI collagen may consist of more than one molecular species assembled from different combinations of the type XI/V family of gene products.

Polymers of type XI collagen are cross-linked by the lysyl oxidase mechanism. However, even in mature tissue the cross-links seem to remain as the immature,

N-PROPEPTIDE

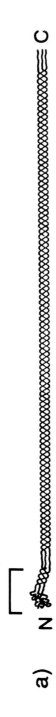

a)

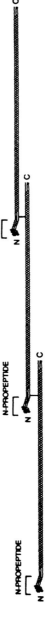

b)

FIG. 3. a: Structure of the type XI collagen molecule. **b:** Current extent of knowledge of its polymeric form based on cross-linking data. Unlike type I or II collagen molecules, the N-propeptide domain is retained in the functioning molecule in the extracellular matrix.

divalent keto-amines without a significant level of pyridinoline being formed (10). Analyses of cross-linked peptides from type XI collagen (35) indicated that the intermolecular links are between N-telopeptide and C-helix sites only (Fig. 3b).

TYPE IX COLLAGEN

Type IX collagen accounts for about 1% of the collagenous protein in adult mammalian articular cartilage but 10% or more in fetal cartilage, the amount decreasing with increasing cartilage maturity (11). The molecule is a proteoglycan and a collagen. In the chick, it has a single site of attachment for a chondroitin sulfate (CS) chain on the $\alpha 2(IX)$ chain in the NC3 domain, as shown by direct chemical analysis (12) and by predictions from the chick $\alpha 2(IX)$ cDNA sequence (13,14). It is possible that all molecules of type IX collagen do not bear CS chains, however. The molecule appears to be a heterotrimer of three distinct gene products $[\alpha 1(IX)\ \alpha 2(IX)\ \alpha 3(IX)]$. It consists of three triple-helical domains: COL 1, COL 2, and COL 3 (Fig. 4). The $\alpha 1(IX)$ chain is expressed in two different forms in different tissues as a result of variable mRNA splicing, one form having a large globular domain (NC4) at its amino-terminus, and the other lacking it (15).

Cross-linking sites have been identified in the COL 2 domain to which the telopeptides of type II collagen become covalently attached (16,17). One site is within a few amino acid residues of the N-terminus of COL 2. All three chains in this domain have at least one hydroxylysine residue to which the $\alpha 1(II)$ N-telopeptide cross-link site can attach (18). In addition, an $\alpha 1(II)$ C-telopeptide attachment site is located farther into the COL2 triple-helix, but only in $\alpha 3(IX)$ (16; unpublished results; Fig. 5). The distance of this site from the $\alpha 1(II)$ N-telopeptide attachment site is exactly 0.6 D, which is the length of the hole zone in a collagen fibril. This predicts an antiparallel relationship between the cross-linked type II and IX molecules (Fig. 4b), since this is the only relationship that would allow both $\alpha 1(II)$ N-telopeptide and $\alpha 1(II)$ C-telopeptide sites to be occupied in a single type IX collagen molecule. This has important implications when considering the physical mechanisms that cause type IX collagen molecules to associate with type II collagen fibrils.

The stoichiometric yield of cross-linked peptides predicts that essentially every type IX collagen molecule in fetal or adult bovine articular cartilage is covalently linked through at least one site to one or more molecules of type II collagen. The chemistry of the cross-linking is similar to that between type II collagen molecules, with keto-amines that can mature to hydroxypyridinium residues. Moreover, the aldehyde precursors were shown to originate in the type II collagen telopeptides, which must interact with the triple-helical sites in type IX collagen (18,36). Electron microscopy has shown that molecules of type IX collagen do indeed decorate the surface of type II collagen fibrils (19).

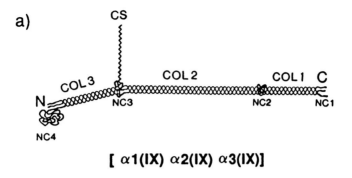

$$[\; \alpha1(\text{IX}) \; \alpha2(\text{IX}) \; \alpha3(\text{IX})]$$

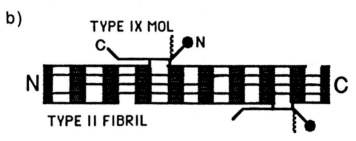

FIG. 4. Type IX collagen. **a:** Domain structure of the type IX collagen molecule showing the three collagenous domains and glycosaminoglycan attachment site in the NC3 domain of α2(IX). **b:** Most molecules function in the extracellular matrix in covalent linkage to the surface of type II collagen fibrils. The lateral interrelationship is antiparallel based on the spacing of α1(II) N-telopeptide and α1(II) C-telopeptide cross-linking sites in the COL2 domain.

α3(IX) COL2

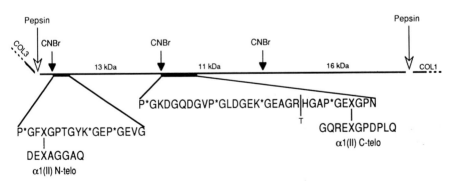

FIG. 5. Sites of cross-linking in the type IX collagen molecule: The sequences of interaction sites for the type II collagen N-telopeptide and C-telopeptide in the α3(IX)COL2 domain are shown. The α1(II) N-telopeptide can also cross-link to equivalent sites in α1(IX) and α2(IX) (18), but the α1(II) C-telopeptide apparently links only to the α3(IX) chain at the site shown. The distance between the N-telopeptide and C-telopeptide linkage sites is exactly 0.6D, predicting an antiparallel association between type IX collagen molecules and type II fibrils as illustrated in Fig. 4b.

The findings imply that type IX collagen provides a covalent interface between the surface of the type II collagen fibril and the interfibrillar proteoglycan domain. It has also been proposed (10,20) that type IX collagen is a source of covalent links between different type II collagen fibrils (i.e., interfibrillar links). This would enhance the mechanical stability of the fibril network and help resist the swelling pressure of the entrapped proteoglycans. If, in fact, type IX collagen molecules can also self-polymerize, then the suspected role of type IX collagen in interfibrillar cross-linking would have a clearer molecular mechanism. Preliminary data do indeed indicate that covalent cross-links are formed between different type IX collagen molecules (Eyre, Wu, and Woods, unpublished results).

TYPE X COLLAGEN

Collagen type X is another short-helix collagen. The molecule is a homotrimer, $[\alpha1(X)]_3$, which consists of a single triple-helical domain with a globular C-terminal extension and shorter nonhelical sequences at the N-terminus (21,22). It seems to be restricted in expression to the hypertrophic zone of the growth plates of growing animals and to the deep calcified layer of mature articular cartilages, although a recent report identifies type X collagen in the chicken eggshell membrane (34). Its polymeric form is as yet undefined, but the $\alpha1(X)$ protein sequence is closely homologous to that of type VIII collagen (23), which forms a distinctive hexagonal lattice in Descemet's membrane of the eye and in other endothelial basal laminae. Type X collagen appears to be cross-linked intermolecularly by bonds other than disulfides since pepsin digestion is needed to solubilize monomers.

TYPE VI COLLAGEN

Collagen type VI, another short-helix collagen molecule, is widely distributed in small amounts in most types of connective tissue (24). Small amounts of the protein can be extracted from articular cartilage. It forms a microfibril which can aggregate and present a distinctive 110 nm periodicity.

Type VI collagen molecules form disulfide-bonded tetramers, but do not appear to form the aldehydic cross-links that are characteristic of other collagen types. Most of the protein can be extracted from tissue by denaturing solvents (25). Three distinct chains—$\alpha1(VI)$, $\alpha2(VI)$, and $\alpha3(VI)$—have been characterized at the protein and gene levels. There is evidence for variable splicing of the $\alpha2(VI)$ and $\alpha3(VI)$ mRNAs (26), so tissue-specific forms of the molecule may exist. There are also several arginine-glycine-aspartic acid (RGD) sequences in each chain (27), implying that it has cell-attachment properties. Enrichment in the pericellular space around the chondrocytes of articular cartilage has been reported (28). Increased amounts of type VI collagen have also been found in articular cartilage in an experimental model of osteoarthrosis (29).

ACTION OF STROMELYSIN ON THE CARTILAGE COLLAGENS

The matrix metalloproteinase, stromelysin (MMP3), has a well-documented action in degrading proteoglycans, link protein, and probably other matrix proteins, but was generally believed to be ineffective in degrading collagen (30). However, recent studies showed that stromelysin can indeed cleave each of the cartilage-specific collagens, but only at highly specific sites in the molecules (31,32). This activity may be important for the remodeling of the extracellular matrix of cartilage to accommodate normal turnover and growth, and may also be a key, early event in the destruction of joints in osteoarthrosis.

Salt-extracted, intact molecules of type IX collagen are cleaved into two pieces by stromelysin (31,32). Recombinant human stromelysin-1 cleaves bovine type

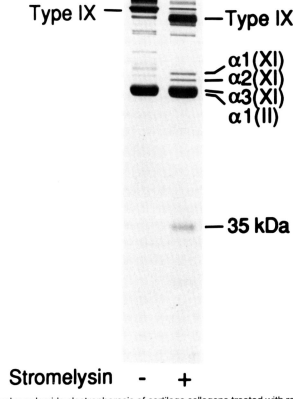

FIG. 6. SDS-polyacrylamide electrophoresis of cartilage collagens treated with recombinant human stromelysin-1. A mixture of intact collagen molecules II, IX, and XI, extracted by neutral salt from fetal bovine cartilage, was run on 7.5% polyacrylamide without disulfide cleavage, before and after stromelysin digestion. The 35 kDa fragment released by stromelysin is the disulfide-bonded COL1 trimer of type IX collagen.

IX collagen, primarily at sites in the NC2 domain in all three chains [$\alpha 1$(IX), $\alpha 2$(IX), and $\alpha 3$(IX)]. These sites were identified by microsequencing analysis of the COL1(IX) products of digestion (Fig. 6) (32). Stromelysin also cleaved salt-extracted native molecules of intact bovine type II collagen within their N-telopeptide cross-linking site. This action predicts that stromelysin can depolymerize polymeric type II collagen. Consistent with this prediction, incubation of cartilage matrix with stromelysin showed significant swelling and release of soluble type II monomers (32). It should be noted that such cleavage of type II collagen telopeptides would also provide a mechanism for the removal of covalently bound type IX collagen molecules from the surface of type II collagen fibrils. Growth in diameter of type II collagen fibrils coated by type IX molecules presumably would require such an activity.

In the same study (32), stromelysin cleavage sites were also found in the α-chain sequences of native type XI collagen (within the N-telopeptide cross-linking domain) and in the triple-helical domain of type X collagen.

RELEVANCE TO OSTEOARTHRITIS

Type IX collagen, through its ability to link covalently to type II collagen fibrils, is believed to contribute to the structural framework and tensile strength of the matrix and therefore to its resistance to proteoglycan swelling pressure. Stromelysin, which is known to be a product of chondrocytes and other connective tissue cells stimulated by interleukin-1, is predicted to cause, or at least contribute to, the collagen network swelling seen in articular cartilage as an early event in experimental animal osteoarthrosis (33). We suspect that the cleavage of type IX collagen molecules may be a critical mediator of this swelling.

The collagen network of cartilage is a hybrid polymer of different types of collagen which interact specifically at the molecular level. The importance of maintaining the integrity of the collagen network for the longevity of articular cartilage is clear. Learning the precise details of the molecular architecture, and of mechanisms of remodeling that can accommodate growth and participate in the cellular response to damage incurred during normal joint function, are crucial for understanding the pathological process of cartilage destruction in osteoarthorisis.

REFERENCES

1. Eyre D, Wu J-J, Apone S. A growing family of collagens in articular cartilage: identification of 5 genetically distinct types. *J Rheumatol* 1987;14:25–27.
2. Eyre DR, Oguchi H. The hydroxypyridinium crosslinks of skeletal collagens: their measurement, properties and proposed pathway of formation. *Biochem Biophys Res Commun* 1980;92:403–410.
3. Lane JM, Weiss C. Review of articular cartilage collagen research. *Arthritis Rheum* 1975;18:553–562.

4. Rosenberg LC, Choi HU, Poole AR, Lewandowska K, Culp LA. Biological roles of dermatan sulphate proteoglycans. In: *Functions of the proteoglycans.* New York: John Wiley and Sons, 1986;47–68.

5. Ryan MC, Sandell LJ. Differential expression of a cysteine-rich domain in the amino-terminal propeptide of type II (cartilage) procollagen by alternative splicing of mRNA. *J Biol Chem* 1990;265:10334–10339.

6. Burgeson RW, Hollister DW. Collagen heterogeneity in human cartilage: identification of several new collagen chains. *Biochem Biophys Res Commun* 1979;87:1124–1131.

7. Eyre DR, Wu J-J. Type IX or $1\alpha2\alpha3\alpha$ collagen. In: Mayne R, Burgeson RE, eds. *Structure and function of collagen.* Orlando, FL: Academic Press, 1987;261–281.

8. Morris NP, Bachinger HP. Type XI collagen is a heterotrimer with a composition (1α, 2α, 3α) retaining non-triple-helical domains. *J Biol Chem* 1987;262:11345–11350.

9. Niyibizi C, Eyre DR. Identification of the cartilage $\alpha1(XI)$ chain in type V collagen from bovine bone. *FEBS Lett* 1989;242:314–318.

10. Wu J-J, Eyre DR. Cartilage type IX collagen is cross-linked by hydroxypyridinium residues. *Biochem Biophys Res Commun* 1984;123:1033–1039.

11. Eyre DR, Wu J-J, Niyibizi C. The collagens of bone and cartilage: molecular diversity and supramolecular assembly. In: Cohn DV, Glorieux FH, Martin TJ, eds. *Calcium regulation and bone metabolism.* Elsevier, 1990;188–194.

12. Huber S, Winterhalter KH, Vaughn L. Isolation and sequence analysis of the glycosaminoglycan attachment site of type IX collagen. *J Biol Chem* 1988;263:752–756.

13. McCormick D, van der Rest M, Goodship J, Lozano G, Ninomiya Y, Olsen BR. Structure of the glycosaminoglycan domain in the type IX collagen-proteoglycan. *Proc Natl Acad Sci USA* 1987;84:4044–4048.

14. van der Rest M, Mayne R, Ninomiya Y, Seidah NG, Chretien M, Olsen BR. The structure of type IX collagen. *J Biol Chem* 1985;260:220–225.

15. Muragaki Y, Nishimura I, Henney A, Ninomiya Y, Olsen BR. The $\alpha1(IX)$ collagen gene gives rise to two different transcripts in both mouse embryonic and human fetal RNA. *Proc Natl Acad Sci USA* 1990;98:2400–2404.

16. Eyre DR, Apone S, Wu J-J, Ericksson LH, Walsh KA. Collagen type IX: evidence for covalent linkages to type II collagen in cartilage. *FEBS Lett* 1987;220:337–341.

17. van der Rest M, Mayne R. Type IX collagen proteoglycan from cartilage is covalently cross-linked to type II collagen. *J Biol Chem* 1988;263:1615–1618.

18. Wu J-J, Eyre DR. Covalent interactions of type IX collagen in cartilage. *Connect Tissue Res* 1989;20:241–245.

19. Vaughn L, Mendler M, Huber S, Bruckner P, Winterhalter KH, Irwin MI, Mayne R. D-Periodic distribution of collagen type IX along cartilage fibrils. *J Cell Biol* 1988;106:991–997.

20. Muller-Glauser W, Humbel B, Glatt M, Strauli P, Winterhalter KH, Bruckner P. On the role of type IX collagen in the extracellular matrix of cartilage. Type IX collagen is localized to inter-sections of collagen fibrils. *J Cell Biol* 1986;102:1931–1939.

21. Schmid TM, Conrad HE. A unique low molecular weight collagen secreted by cultured chick embryo chondrocytes. *J Biol Chem* 1982;257:12333–12340.

22. Ninomiya Y, Gordon M, van der Rest M, Schmid T, Linsenmayer T, Olsen BR. The developmentally regulated type X collagen gene contains a long open reading frame without introns. *J Biol Chem* 1986;261:5041–5050.

23. Yamaguchi N, Benya P, van der Rest M, Ninomiya Y. The cloning and sequencing of $\alpha1(VIII)$ collagen cDNAs demonstrate that type VIII collagen is a short chain collagen and contains triple helical and carboxy-terminal non-triple-helical domains similar to those of type X collagen. *J Biol Chem* 1989;264:16022–16029.

24. Timpl R, Engle J. Type VI collagen. In: Mayne R, Burgeson RE, eds. *Structure and function of collagen types.* Orlando, FL: Academic Press, 1987;105–143.

25. Wu J-J, Eyre DR, Slayter HS. Type VI collagen of the intervertebral disc. Biochemical and electron microscopic characterization of the native protein. *Biochem J* 1987;248:373–381.

26. Chu M-L, Zhang RZ, Pan T, et al. Mosaic structure of globular domains in the human type VI collagen $\alpha3$ chain. Similarity to von Willebrand factor fibronectin, actin, salivary proteins and aprotinin type protease inhibitors. *EMBO J* 1990;9:385–393.

27. Aumailley M, Mann K, von der Mark H, Timpl R. Cell attachment properties of collagen type VI and Arg-Gly-Asp dependent binding to its $\alpha2(VI)$ and A3(VI) chains. *Exp Cell Res* 1989;181:463–474.

28. Poole CA, Ayad S, Schofield JR. Chondrons from articular cartilage. 1. Immunolocalization of type VI collagen in the pericellular capsule of isolated canine tibial chondrons. *J Cell Sci* 1988;90: 635–643.
29. McDevitt CA, Pahl JA, Ayad S, Miller RR, Uratsuji M, Andrish JT. Experimental osteoarthritic articular cartilage is enriched in guanidine-soluble type VI collagen. *Biochem Biophys Res Commun* 1988;157:250.
30. Chin JR, Murphy G, Werb Z. Stromelysin, a connective tissue-degrading metalloendopeptidase secreted by stimulated rabbit synovial fibroblasts in parallel with collagenase. *J Biol Chem* 1985;260:12367–12376.
31. Okada Y, Honomi H, Yada T, Kumata K, Nagase H. Degradation of type IX collagen by matrix metalloproteinase 3 (stromelysin) from human rheumatoid synovial cells. *FEBS Lett* 1989;244: 473–476.
32. Wu J-J, Lark MW, Chun LE, Eyre DR. Molecular sites of stromelysin cleavage in collagen types II, IX, X and XI of cartilage. *J Biol Chem* 1991;226:5625–5628.
33. Eyre DR, Wu J-J, Woods PE. The cartilage collagens: structural and metabolic studies. *J Rheumatol* 1991;18(Suppl. 27):49–51.
34. Arias JL, Fernandez MS, Dennis JE, Caplan AI. Collagens of the chicken eggshell membrane. *Connect Tissue Res* 1991;26:37–45.
35. Wu J-J, Eyre DR. Covalent interactions of the cartilage collagens. *Trans Orthop Res Soc* 1991;27.
36. Eyre DR, Wu J, Niyibizi C, Chun L. The cartilage collagens: analysis of their cross-linking interactions and matrix organization. In: Maroudas A, Kuettner K, Bullough P, eds. *Methods in cartilage research.* Academic Press, 1990;28–33.

DISCUSSION

Kuettner: In your hypothesis for remodeling, type II has a slow turnover rate. When remodeling is necessary, removal and resynthesis of type IX, and maybe even type XI, has to occur. Is anything known about the half-lives of the minor collagens?

Eyre: Not a lot. In work with Jeff Friedmann and Linda Sandell, we used the rabbit meniscectomy model of osteoarthrosis to ask two questions: What are the relative rates of synthesis of types II, IX, and XI collagens in the normal joint cartilage, and second, is cartilage of the operated joint showing accelerated turnover of matrix after surgical meniscectomy? The results showed that the relative rates of synthesis of type II, IX, and type XI collagens were roughly in proportion to their relative amounts as proteins in the tissue. However, our data suggested that type IX collagen may turn over faster in the operated joint.

Muir: When preexisting functional tissue is remodeled, will newly formed collagen molecules be deposited on old fibrils? Second, if the collagen network is loosened, which occurs within a week in experimental canine osteoarthritis, the network never tightens up again, even after many months, and the hydration persists. How can this be reversed and the collagen network tightened up again?

Eyre: I don't know the answer to your second question. As to the first, I don't think there are any definitive data showing collagen molecules going from the cell and adding to fibrils that are old, meaning that they have been there for months or years. But intuitively, and from what is known about the increasing diameter of collagen fibrils in articular cartilage with increasing age, it's very clear that fibrils do grow considerably in diameter. They go from a mean diameter of about 200 angströms to as great as 4,000 angströms in adult cartilage. So I believe that the fibrils can indeed grow by accretion.

Muir: If preexisting collagen is modified in any way, will new molecules bind to it?

Eyre: That is the proposition. The chondrocytes don't have to keep sticking finger-like projections out to all the little sites in the matrix where remodeling has to occur.

Assembly occurs because of the inherent properties of the molecules themselves, which can self-assemble and disassemble, as a consequence of the effects of specific proteases that the cell can release in defined local domains.

Maroudas: Can two fibrils come together to form one thicker fibril, or alternatively, can one fibril dissociate and the molecules deposit on another fibril?

Eyre: I think there is reasonable evidence in the literature that thin fibrils can fuse together to form thicker fibrils. It doesn't have to be simply accretion of individual molecules on old fibrils. Both mechanisms probably occur. If you strip two adjacent collagen fibrils of coating molecules down to bare type II collagen, the very thing they want to do physicochemically is to fuse and interact in the way inherent to collagen.

Articular Cartilage and Osteoarthritis,
edited by K. Kuettner et al.
Raven Press, Ltd., New York © 1992.

10

Fibrillar Organization in Cartilage

Eric F. Eikenberry,* Markus Mendler,† Renate Bürgin,†
Kaspar H. Winterhalter,† and Peter Bruckner†

*Department of Pathology, Robert Wood Johnson Medical School, UMDNJ,
Piscataway, New Jersey 08854 and †Laboratorium für Biochemie I,
Eidgenössiche Technische Hochschule, 8092 Zurich, Switzerland*

Near the surface of normal adult articular cartilage, cells have very low metabolic activity and also divide infrequently. Disruption of the extracellular environment, such as in degenerative disease, leads to profound changes in cellular activity. Near fissures in delaminating articular cartilage, so-called brood capsules occur in which cell proliferation is markedly enhanced and biosynthetic activity is increased. These changes are presumed to be brought about by altered cell-matrix interactions (1). The sensitivity of cartilage cells to their stationary surroundings can also be demonstrated *in vitro*. Chondrocytes placed in monolayer culture under appropriate conditions modulate their phenotype and with time, increasingly resemble fibroblasts in both morphology and biosynthetic activity. These same cells when reintroduced into three-dimensional matrices resume the chondrocytic phenotype (2,3). These examples illustrate the importance of the extracellular matrix in the homeostasis of cartilage. Therefore, to better understand cell-matrix interactions, it is important to improve our knowledge of the structure and biogenesis of cartilage matrix.

The extracellular matrices of connective tissues generally contain fibrils that serve as tensile elements. Tissues vary widely with respect to fibril sizes and orientation according to biomechanical requirements. In hyaline cartilage, particularly in young animals, fibrils with seemingly random orientation serve to contain the osmotic pressure generated by water bound to molecules of the extrafibrillar matrix. In tendons, large bundles of parallel fibrils give the tissue its tensile strength, while in cornea and some skins, layered sheets of parallel fibrils resist stretching of the tissue. These examples underscore the importance of fibrillar organization to the function of connective tissues, in particular to overall biomechanical properties. Here we discuss the morphogenesis of cartilage fibrils, structural elements central to the biomechanical properties of cartilage.

The structures of connective tissue fibrils have been studied by electron microscopy and x-ray diffraction complemented by biochemical analyses. The structure of rat tail tendon has been elucidated in considerable detail because the collagen is in part organized into large crystalline domains, making this tissue particularly suitable for x-ray diffraction studies. The structure that emerged is considered a prototype of the packing of collagen molecules in fibrils. Collagen molecules are assembled laterally in a quasi-hexagonal pattern and are staggered longitudinally with a $D = 67$ nm periodicity as schematically represented in Fig. 1 (4). The axial periodicity of the gap-overlap structure shown in Fig. 1 (5) gives rise to the characteristic x-ray diffraction pattern of this tissue and is also readily apparent in electron micrographs. The basic quasi-hexagonal model of lateral packing also applies to fibrils of origins other than rat tail tendon, albeit with variable distortion of an ideal hexagonal lattice (6,7).

The composition of connective tissue fibrils is complex. Generally, such fibrils contain two or more distinct collagen types and therefore are called heterotypic. For example, the coexistence of collagens I and V within the same fibrils in chicken cornea has been documented (8). Similarly, tendons and skin have heterotypic fibrils containing collagens I and III (9,10). Another well-studied case is that of hyaline cartilage where collagens II, IX, and XI are coassembled (11). Fibril composition is rendered even more complex by the probable inclusion of noncollagenous proteins and/or proteoglycans. Glycosaminoglycans have been observed associated with specific bands in the D-period of native collagen fibrils, associations that vary in a tissue-specific manner (12,13). Decorin (14) and fibronectin also bind to collagen, though the latter binds more effectively to the denatured protein (15). This spectrum of potential interactions between matrix components may have an influence on fibril morphology.

A striking feature of many connective tissues is the uniformity of the diameters of the fibrils. In cornea, for example, such uniformity is required for transparency. But in other tissues, including some forms of hyaline cartilage, where the necessity

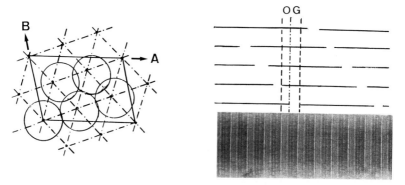

FIG. 1. Structure of collagen I. **Left:** Quasi-hexagonal lateral packing of collagen molecules in rat tail tendon. The dimensions of the unit cell are A, 4.0 nm; B, 2.6 nm; γ, 105°. **Right:** Schematic illustration of the staggered longitudinal arrangement of collagen molecules that gives rise to the D-periodic gap-overlap structure seen in negative stain electron microscopy. *G*, gap; *O*, overlap-region.

for uniform diameters is less obvious, fibrils also exhibit this property. Interestingly, the vitreous body (16), the primary corneal stroma (17), and the sheath of lamprey notochord (18), which contains collagens that are biochemically similar to those of cartilage, also contain thin fibrils with very narrow distributions of diameters.

Several mechanisms have been proposed for the control of lateral growth of fibrils. Cells themselves may provide this function. In electron micrographs of embryonic tendons, deep invaginations of cell membranes containing bundles of collagen of defined width are observed. This has been interpreted as representing fibril precursors in the process of being joined to an existing fibril in the extracellular space (19,20). Lateral growth can be controlled by the cells either by steric constraint in the limited space of the compartment, by a specific temporal sequence of assembly, or by the addition of components to block further accretion of collagen molecules after a given diameter has been reached.

An alternative mechanism that has been suggested for diameter control consists of the regulation of procollagen processing in the extracellular space during fibrillogenesis (21,22). In this model, fibril diameters are limited by selective removal of either the amino-terminal or the carboxyl-terminal propeptide from collagen molecules at the surface of the fibrils as they grow. The observation that antibodies to the amino-propeptides of collagens I and III preferentially label the smallest diameter fibrils seen in skin and tendon was interpreted as supporting this mechanism (23). Diameter control has also been investigated in fibrillogenesis *in vitro* of procollagen I treated with procollagen N- and C-proteinases (24). Asymmetric growth at the ends could be demonstrated, leading to fibrils of various widths. However, uniform populations were not observed. A drawback of this mechanism, however, is that it is difficult to predict how a constant and specific diameter can be achieved and maintained since collagen biosynthesis, including the conversion of procollagen into collagen, is a continuous process that could be expected to vary with the metabolic state of the tissue.

Another proposed mechanism is based on the propagation of strain in fibrils with helically arranged molecules. Filaments in a helical fibril are under tension at the periphery of the fibril and under compression at the center. As fibril diameter increases, elongation of protofilaments involved in assembly of the fibril eventually reaches a level at which addition of further molecules becomes energetically unfavorable (25). Helical collagen fibrils from skin, for example, have indeed been observed by electron microscopy, a finding that has been supported by x-ray diffraction results (26–29). While this mechanism may act to limit the diameter of the large fibrils of skin, it is difficult to reconcile with small diameter fibrils such as those in cartilage which appear not to have a significant helicity (30). Further, an implication of this mechanism is that fibrils containing only one collagen type should have uniform diameters. However, in the one tissue in which homotypic fibers seem to exist, namely mammalian tail tendon, diameter control is absent, indicating that this mechanism is less generally applicable in collagen fibrils than to other protein aggregates.

Fibril diameter could in principle be regulated by the kinetics of assembly in a nucleation-growth mechanism. In this model, fibril width would vary according to the relative rate of formation of nuclei and could be modulated by the presence of other components, such as chondroitin sulfate or other polyanions (31). However, the fibril diameter distributions predicted by this theory are considerably wider than those observed *in vivo,* and the distributions seen in experiments are wider still (32).

Finally, fibril width may be set by the thermodynamics of fibril assembly from a mixture of components. The mixtures may consist solely of collagens, or of collagens and other fibril-associated materials. In this concept, as fibril width increases, specific interaction sites are created for agents blocking further growth. Hence, diameter control is an intrinsic property of the materials involved, making the diameter inherently stable and invariant. Such a mechanism is attractive because of the implied stability of tissue architecture.

The validity of the latter mechanism can best be tested by reconstitution experiments. Most experiments on reconstitution of fibrils from purified collagens in solution have been carried out with single collagen types. The progression and the extent of fibril formation have been monitored by turbidity, and fibril morphology has been evaluated by electron microscopy and x-ray diffraction. The kinetics of reconstitution of both collagens I and II exhibited a critical concentration below which no fibrils were formed (33). This concentration was much higher for collagen II than for collagen I. The reconstituted fibrils were similar to natural ones in that they exhibited the same banding pattern by electron microscopy, and had comparable x-ray diffraction patterns. However, no control of fibril width was achieved. Further, fibrils formed by collagen II did not form long fibrils, but rather tactoids with lengths of several microns and symmetrically tapering ends. Their maximal width varied widely up to 2 μm.

Collagen V added to collagen I in varying proportions restricted the width of the resulting fibrils, albeit not to the extent seen in tissues from which the components were derived (34,35). This supported the hypothesis that the role of collagen V was to limit lateral growth of fibrils, but was not completely effective either because of the absence of further required components or because of damage done to the collagen during preparation. Partial control over fibrillogenesis *in vitro* for collagens I and II by the proteoglycans fibromodulin and decorin has also been observed (36).

The structure of cartilage fibrils has extensively been investigated. Cartilage contains tissue-specific collagens II, IX, and X, as well as collagen XI which is found in other tissues such as placenta (37) and bone (38) as well. Collagen X is unique to hypertrophic zones of cartilage undergoing endochondral ossification (39). All of these collagens are components of the same fibrils (11,40,41), with collagens II, IX, and XI being obligatory (11). Cartilage collagens are much more highly modified posttranslationally than those of tendon, with collagen XI especially containing large amounts of hydroxylysyl glycosides in the helical portions of the molecule (42). This could be expected to lead to a larger intermolecular distance between laterally adjacent triple-helices in fibrils, particularly in regions containing collagen XI. Such a larger intermolecular spacing has been observed in lamprey notochord sheath, a tissue with fibrils that are chemically and morphologically similar to those in cartilage, but which is amenable to structure analysis by x-ray diffraction. The unit cell describing the molecular packing is 42% larger than in rat tail tendon, indicating that the center-to-center spacing between molecules is larger. Further, there is a different angular geometry, indicating that the molecular contacts between the triple helices differ in the two structures. However, the axial periodicity of the collagen molecules is identical in the two tissues (30).

Biochemical and immunochemical methods have also been used to probe the organization of collagens in cartilage fibrils. Not only do collagens II, IX, and XI form heterotypic fibrils, but these collagens are incorporated into a specific topology. Collagen IX has been immunochemically localized to the surface of isolated fibril fragments where the globular and helical domains nearest the amino-terminal end protrude from the surface in a D-periodic pattern (43). The bulk of the fibril body is composed of collagen II, which is accessible to antibodies in intact fibrils. However, collagen XI was strongly masked toward immuno-chemical labeling in isolated fibrils, suggesting that this protein is buried within the fibrils (11). The presence of collagen XI could be demonstrated immuno-chemically only after extensive disruption of the fibrils by proteolytic digestion.

The question of how diameter is controlled, and the role played by each of the three individual cartilage collagens in fibril assembly, can be addressed by reconstitution experiments. This chapter provides evidence that typical cartilage fibrils can be assembled from the collagens alone, and that a simple mechanism applies to fibrillogenesis in cartilage.

METHODS

Preparation of Collagens

A mixture of cartilage collagens in 0.4 M NaCl, 0.1 M Tris-HCl, pH 7.4 at 25°C (buffer A) was prepared from cultures of chick embryo sternal chondrocytes embedded in agarose as described (44). The mixture was stored in liquid nitrogen until used.

Separation of Collagens

The crude mixture of collagens was dissolved in 100 ml of buffer A, dialyzed against 2 M urea, 0.2 M NaCl, 0.05 M Tris-HCl, pH 7.3 at 4°C, and passed over a column (15 × 60 mm) of DEAE-cellulose equilibrated with the same buffer. Breakthrough fractions contained collagens II and XI and part of collagen IX. After washing the column, pure collagen IX was eluted with 0.4 M NaCl.

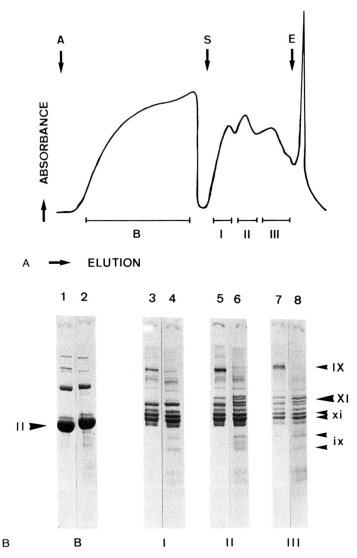

FIG. 2. A: Separation of collagens II and XI on DEAE-cellulose. The sample was applied at A. Elution of the gradient from 0.02 to 0.25 M NaCl was initiated at S. E denotes the end of the salt gradient and the beginning of the washing of the column with 1 M NaCl. Released proteins were monitored by absorbance at 225 nm. **B:** Electrophoresis on a 4.5–15% polyacrylamide gradient gel in SDS of purified collagens stained with coomassie blue. Proteins were run without (*lanes 1, 3, 5, 7*) or with (*lanes 2, 4, 6, 8*) reduction with 2% mercaptoethanol prior to electrophoresis. *II,* $\alpha1$(II)-chain (the faint band above the $\alpha1$(II) chain is pN-$\alpha1$(II)); *IX,* unreduced collagen IX; *XI,* several variants of the $\alpha1$(XI)-chain; *xi,* $\alpha2$(XI) and $\alpha3$(XI); *ix,* $\alpha1$(IX) and $\alpha3$(IX) of reduced collagen IX. *B, I, II,* and *III* refer to pooled fractions as shown in Fig. 2A.

The breakthrough fractions were dialyzed overnight against 9 volumes of 10% glycerol, 2 M urea, 0.05 M Tris-HCl, pH 8.0 at 4°C and passed over a DEAE cellulose column equilibrated in 10% glycerol, 2 M urea, 0.02 M NaCl, 0.05 M Tris-HCl, pH 8.0 at 4°C. After washing, the column was eluted by a gradient of 0.02 to 0.25 M NaCl. As shown in Fig. 2, collagen II eluted in the breakthrough fractions, whereas collagen XI was recovered from gradient fractions. Separated collagens were dialyzed against buffer A, precipitated with 176 g/l $(NH_4)_2SO_4$, recovered by centrifugation at 17,500 × g for 30 min, dissolved in a minimal amount of buffer A, and dialyzed against buffer A. For some experiments, collagens II and IX were prepared from organ cultures of 17 d chick embryo sterna as described (33,44,45).

Fibril Reconstitution

Solutions of collagen II in 0.02 M acetic acid were diluted with an equal volume of 0.28 M NaCl, 0.06 M sodium phosphate, pH 7.4 at 37°C containing collagen IX at a ten-fold lower concentration than that of collagen II. Fibrils were reconstituted from collagen II alone by omitting collagen IX from the phosphate buffer.

To induce fibril formation in all other cases, collagen solutions in buffer A were mixed appropriately, diluted with an equal volume of distilled water, and warmed to 37°C. After incubating for various lengths of time, fibrils were separated from soluble components by centrifugation at room temperature. Collagens in the fibrils were analyzed by SDS polyacrylamide gradient (4.5–15%) gel electrophoresis (SDS-PAGE) (46). Quantitation of protein on gels was carried out by stain extraction (47).

Electron Microscopy

Samples were taken from fibril reconstitution experiments before centrifugation and were adsorbed to carbon coated collodion film grids for 3 min. After washing three times with distilled water, grids were negatively stained with saturated aqueous uranyl acetate and were observed in a Philips 300 or a Hitachi H-600 electron microscope. Fibril widths were estimated on negatives taken at instrumental magnifications greater than 50,000-fold using an 8-fold magnifier with a measuring reticle. For immunolabeling, reconstituted fibril samples were diluted 100-fold with 0.15 M NaCl, 0.02 M sodium phosphate, pH 7.4, adsorbed onto grids, and floated on a solution of 0.15 M NaCl, 0.04 M $MgCl_2$, 0.2% Tween 20, and 0.01 M Tris-HCl, pH 7.4 (25°C) containing 5% normal goat serum (blocking buffer) for 10 min. Reactions with antibodies specific for collagens II, IX, or XI were carried out for 75 min at appropriate dilutions in blocking buffer (11). After washing six times with blocking buffer, samples were reacted with gold particles coated with protein A, rinsed six times with blocking buffer and three times with water, and were negatively stained as above.

RESULTS

Chick embryo chondrocyte cultures in agarose gels at low density in the presence of fetal bovine serum were established as described (48). After 14 days, collagens were extracted from the homogenized cultures by neutral saline and dissolved in storage buffer. SDS-PAGE revealed that this preparation contained collagens II, IX, and XI, and was essentially free of other proteins (not shown). This preparation was used as the native collagen mixture in some of the reconstitution experiments described below.

Individual collagens were purified from this mixture (Fig. 2A) and were characterized by SDS-PAGE (Fig. 2B). Collagen II contained some pN-collagen chains, whereas collagen XI exhibited several variants of the $\alpha 1(XI)$ chain as described (49). Collagen IX contained some residual collagen II, perhaps covalently cross-linked (50) (see chapter by Eyre et al.). Efforts to remove these contaminants under conditions which preserved native conformation and competence to form fibrils were unsuccessful because of the insolubility of the native protein in low ionic strength buffers.

Collagen II purified from 17 d chick embryo sternal cartilage without proteolytic treatment was reconstituted into fibrils following the protocol of Vogel et al. (14), which differed from the procedure of Lee and Piez (33) in that phosphate was substituted for N-Tris(hydroxymethyl)methyl-2-aminoethanesulfonic acid (TES) as the buffer. Electron microscopy showed large, banded tactoids with long tapering ends similar to those reported (33), demonstrating the lack of diameter control when fibrils were reconstituted from collagen II alone (Fig. 3A). Therefore, we turned to mixtures of collagen II with the minor cartilage collagens.

Mixtures of collagen II and IX in a 10:1 ratio were prepared as described "Methods," and fibrillogenesis was induced by adjusting the pH to 7.4 with NaOH and by warming. After incubation at 36°C for 2 hr, or up to 12 hr, tactoids were again observed with closely similar banding patterns. However, in this case the ends of the tactoids were more sharply tapered and were frequently split (Fig. 3B).

Collagen XI was soluble in high ionic strength neutral buffer. No discernible supramolecular aggregates could be detected by negative stain electron microscopy in these solutions prior to initiation of fibril formation. Fibril formation was induced by mixing the collagen solution with an equal volume of water and warming to 37°C for 2 hr. The preparation of collagen XI produced thin, flexible filaments immediately upon reduction of the buffer ionic strength, even at 4°C (Fig. 4A). When the solutions were incubated at 37°C for 2 hr, they formed

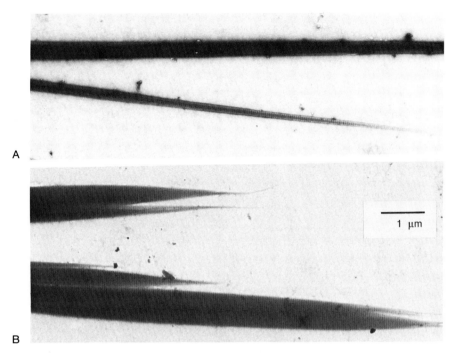

FIG. 3. Electron micrograph of tactoids reconstituted from collagen II (**A**) or from a mixture of collagens II and IX (87:13) (**B**).

uniformly thin fibrils similar to those seen with the native mixture (not shown). Addition of collagen II at nine-fold excess over collagen XI resulted in an abundant formation of tactoidal aggregates mixed with thin, uniform fibrils (Fig. 4B). Even with as little as 1% of type XI collagen in this binary mixture, frequent formation of tactoids were observed. By contrast, collagen II alone reconstituted under similar conditions, i.e., by diluting with water solutions of the protein in Tris (buffer A), formed few if any aggregates. As mentioned above, however, collagen II exclusively produced tactoidal aggregates under the conditions used by Vogel et al. (14) or Lee and Piez (33).

Mixtures of collagens II, IX, and XI were obtained by extraction of chondrocyte cultures with high ionic strength neutral buffer. Fibril formation in this ternary system was induced by lowering the ionic strength as described above. Electron microscopy revealed thin fibrils with a manifestly uniform width (Fig. 4C). In common with cartilage fibrils, and fine fibrils from many other sources, the reconstituted material showed only a faint D-periodic banding. The width, measured in a number of micrographs, was 19.7 ± 4.7 nm (N = 74), although in any single micrograph the fibril diameters were always similar. This width is comparable to the diameter of fibrils *in vivo*. The fibrils contained each of the

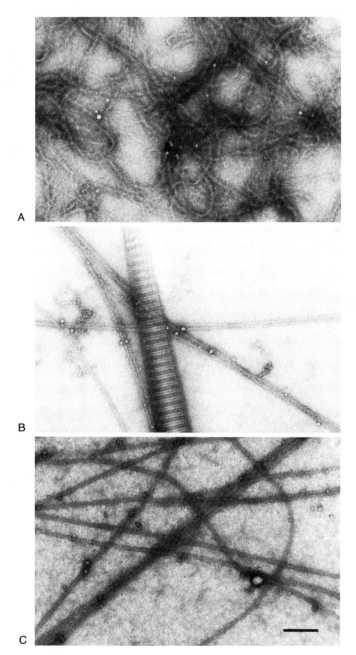

FIG. 4. A: Electron micrograph of filaments formed by collagen XI at 4°C immediately after adjustment to 0.2 M NaCl. **B:** Electron micrograph of tactoids and fibrils formed by a mixture of collagens II and XI (8:1) after 2 hr at 37°C. **C:** Electron micrograph of fibrils formed by a mixture of collagens II, IX, and XI (8:1:1) after 2 hr at 37°C. Bar: 300 nm.

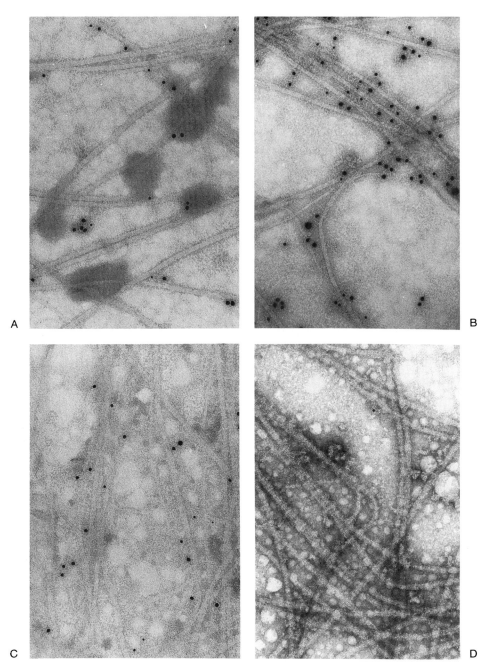

FIG. 5. Immunoelectron micrographs of fibrils as shown in Fig. 4C. Fibrils were treated with specific antisera to **A,** collagen II; **B,** collagen IX; and **C,** collagen XI. Fibrils in **D** were treated with nonimmune serum. Bound antibodies were visualized with protein A-gold. Magnification: ×60,000.

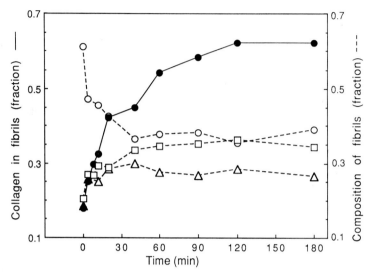

FIG. 6. Kinetics of fibril reconstitution from a mixture of collagens II, IX, and XI. *Closed symbols:* Fraction of collagens in the mixture that is pelletable as a function of time. *Open symbols:* (O--O) collagen II as a fraction of pelletable collagens; (△--△) collagen IX; (□--□) collagen XI.

three collagen types since it was possible to stain the fibrils with indirect immunogold labeling using antibodies against collagens II, IX, and XI, respectively (Fig. 5).

Figure 6 shows the kinetics of fibrillogenesis in a ternary mixture of collagens II, IX, and XI. The reaction was initiated as described above, and protein incorporated into fibrils was quantified by centrifugation followed by SDS-PAGE of the pellets. Relative amounts of collagen were determined by extracting the coomassie blue from the stained bands (47). Fibrillogenesis started immediately upon adjustment of the ionic strength, with no lag phase (filled symbols). A comparable result has also been obtained by turbidity measurements (data not shown). These results differ from those obtained with collagen I or II alone, both of which showed a lag of at least several minutes before typical lateral growth of fibrils occurred (33,51). Figure 6 also shows the composition of the fibrils as a function of time (open symbols). The pelletable material was initially rich in collagen XI but its proportion declined, whereas that of collagen II increased. The contribution of collagen IX appeared to be constant throughout the experiment within the limits of error, but may have increased near the beginning.

CONCLUDING REMARKS

A prerequisite for the fibrillogenesis *in vitro* of collagens II, IX, and XI was the development of solvent conditions which permitted initial solubilization of all three collagen types. The conditions adopted represent a compromise between fibril-formation efficiency, which is favored by lower ionic strength and certain ions such as phosphate, and solubilization, which requires higher ionic strength or the presence of polyols (Tris) in the buffer. Though no protein was pelleted from this preparation under our protocol, the presence of small aggregates of collagen molecules is not excluded. Only the ternary mixture of collagens gave fibrils resembling those found in chick embryo sterna in that they had uniform small diameters and were composed of collagens II, IX, and XI. As in native fibrils, collagens IX and XI were quantitatively minor.

This system represents an opportunity to study *in vitro* the self-limited assembly of a biological suprastructure with the inherent capability of infinite growth. We propose the following model. Collagen XI first forms a core filament, the lateral organization of which may be based on either a quasi-hexagonal or microfibrillar structure. The core then grows by the epitaxial deposition of collagen II. This concept is consistent with the kinetics of fibrillogenesis, and the early stages could be expected to give rise to thin, flexible filaments such as those shown in Fig. 4A, which contain as much as 45% collagen XI. Because of the high degree of glycosylation of collagen XI, the packing of the molecules is distorted with respect to the packing of collagen II alone. These distortions cause lattice dislocations which are propagated and enlarged as collagen II is added to the growing fibril. When the diameter reaches about 17 nm, the dislocations are of such size and configuration as to become optional binding sites for collagen IX. When collagen IX is absent or scarce, continued growth of the fibrils is permitted. When collagen IX is present in sufficient quantities, however, attachment of the protein inhibits further growth. This process results in relatively stiff, diameter-controlled mature fibrils, as shown in Fig. 4C. The model is shown schematically in Fig. 7. It is interesting to note that electron micrographs of cross-sections of lamprey notochord consistently showed a small staining discontinuity at the center of most fibrils (6).

In our fibril model, the surface is largely coated by collagen IX which provides or modulates most of the interaction sites with extrafibrillar material. A particular function of collagen IX could be to join fibrils into a three-dimensional network that can resist deformation. This may be accomplished by collagen IX being incorporated into the structure of more than one fibril by means of its multiple helical domains connected by flexible regions. This model predicts that fibril intersections would not be randomly distributed along the fibrils, but rather would be related to the underlying D-periodicity. Our preliminary observations showed that distances between adjacent intersections were indeed not random.

Other considerations follow from our model of collagen structure in cartilage fibrils. Collagen IX with its glycosaminoglycan and its cationic domain (NC4) protruding from the surface renders fibrils highly charged. Electrostatic and other hydrophilic interactions with other matrix macromolecules are likely to make an important contribution to the stability of cartilage matrix because the extra-fibrillar matrix itself is composed largely of highly polyanionic macromolecules.

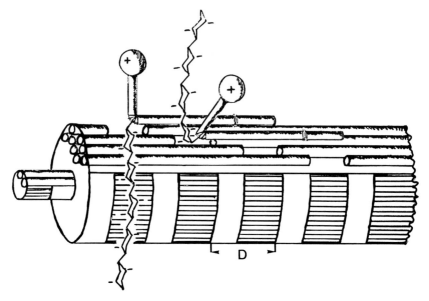

FIG. 7. Schematic representation of the collagen arrangement in cartilage fibrils. The core filament is formed by collagen XI and is surrounded by collagen II. Collagen IX with its chondroitin sulfate chain is at the surface. The cationic nature of the N-terminal globular domain (NC4) is symbolized by a (+); the negative charges on chondroitin sulfate by (−).

Proteoglycans other than collagen IX, such as decorin and fibromodulin, both of which have been shown to interact with collagens, may also play an important role in tethering the extrafibrillar matrix to the fibrils. These components, however, do not appear important to the regulation of the collagen structure within fibrils.

It will be interesting to learn how the interaction between chondrocytes and fibril surfaces is mediated. Based on our model for fibril structure, it would be logical to look for interactions with fibril surface components other than just those with collagen II.

REFERENCES

1. Sokoloff L. Pathology and pathogenesis of osteoarthritis. In: McCarthy DJ, ed. *Arthritis and allied conditions.* Philadelphia: Lea and Ferbiger, 1979;1135–1153.
2. Benya PD, Shaffer JD. Dedifferentiated chondrocytes re-express the differentiated collagen phenotype when cultured in agarose gels. *Cell* 1982;30:215–224.
3. Gibson GJ, Schor SL, Grant ME. Effects of matrix macromolecules on chondrocyte gene expression: synthesis of a low molecular weight collagen species by cells cultured within collagen gels. *J Cell Biol* 1982;93:767–774.
4. Hulmes DJS, Miller A. Quasi-hexagonal molecular packing in collagen fibrils. *Nature* 1979;282:878–880.
5. Hodge AJ, Petruska JA. Recent studies with the electron microscope on ordered aggregates of

the tropocollagen molecule. In: Ramachandran GN, ed. *Aspects of protein structure.* New York: Academic Press, 1963;289–300.

6. Brodsky B, Eikenberry EF. Supramolecular collagen assemblies. *Ann NY Acad Sci* 1985;460:73–84.

7. Brodsky B, Eikenberry EF, Cassidy Belbruno K, Sterling K. Variations in collagen fibril structure in tendons. *Biopolymers* 1982;21:935–951.

8. Birk DE, Fitch JM, Babiarz JP, Linsenmayer TF. Collagen type I and type V are present in the same fibrils in the avian corneal stroma. *J Cell Biol* 1988;106:999–1008.

9. Keene DR, Sakai LY, Burgeson RE, Bächinger HP. Type III collagen can be present on banded collagen fibrils regardless of fibril diameter. *J Cell Biol* 1987;105:2393–2402.

10. Fleischmajer R, Perlish JS, Burgeson RE, Shaikh-Bahai F, Timpl R. Type I and type III collagen interactions during fibrillogenesis. *Ann NY Acad Sci* 1990;580:161–175.

11. Mendler M, Eich-Bender SG, Vaughan L, Winterhalter KH, Bruckner P. Cartilage contains mixed fibrils of collagen types II, IX and XI. *J Cell Biol* 1989;108:191–197.

12. Scott JE, Haigh M. Proteoglycan-collagen interactions in intervertebral disc. A chondroitin sulphate proteoglycan associates with collagen fibrils in rabbit annulus fibrosus at the d-e band. *Biosci Rep* 1986;6:879–888.

13. Scott JE. Proteoglycan—collagen interactions and subfibrillar structure in collagen fibrils. Implications in the development and ageing of connective tissues. *J Anat* 1990;169:23–35.

14. Vogel KG, Paulsson M, Heinegård D. Specific inhibition of type I and type II collagen fibrillogenesis by the small proteoglycan of tendon. *Biochem J* 1984;223:587–597.

15. Ruoslahti E, Hayman EG, Pierschbacher M, Engvall E. Fibronectin: purification, immunochemical properties, and biological activities. *Methods Enzymol* 1982;82:803–831.

16. Wright DW, Mayne R. Vitreous humor of chicken contains two fibrillar systems: an analysis of their structure. *J Ultrastruct Mol Struct Res* 1988;100:224–234.

17. von der Mark K, von der Mark H, Timpl R, Trelstad R. Immunofluorescent localization of collagen types I, II, and III in the embryonic chick eye. *Dev Biol* 1977;59:75–85.

18. Sheren SB, Eikenberry EF, Broek DL, van der Rest M, Doering T, Kelly J, Hardt T, Brodsky B. Type II collagen of lamprey. *Comp Biochem Physiol* 1986;85B:5–14.

19. Trelstad RL. Multistep assembly of type I collagen fibrils. *Cell* 1982;28:197–198.

20. Birk DE, Zycband EI, Winkelmann DA, Trelstad RL. Collagen fibrillogenesis *in situ.* Discontinuous segmental assembly in extracellular compartments. *Ann NY Acad Sci* 1989;580:176–194.

21. Hulmes DJS, Mould AP, Kadler KE, Chapman JA, Prockop DJ. Procollagen processing control of type I collagen fibril assembly. In: Aebi U, Engel J, eds. *Structure, assembly, and interactions of cytoskeletal and extracellular matrix proteins.* New York: Springer, 1989;292–301.

22. Chapman JA. The regulation of size and form in the assembly of collagen fibrils *in vivo.* *Biopolymers* 1989;28:1367–1382, 2201–2205.

23. Fleischmajer R, Timpl R, Tuderman L, Raisher L, Wiestner M, Perlish JS, Graves PN. Ultrastructural identification of extension amino propeptides of type I and type III collagens in human skin. *Proc Natl Acad Sci USA* 1981;78:7360–7364.

24. Kadler KE, Hojima Y, Prockop DJ. Collagen fibrils *in vitro* grow from pointed tips in the C-terminal to N-terminal direction. *Biochem J* 1990;268:339–343.

25. Makowski L, Magdoff-Fairchild B. Polymorphism of sickle cell hemoglobin aggregates: structural basis for limited radial growth. *Science* 1986;234:1228–1231.

26. Lillie JH, McCallum DK, Scaletta LJ, Occhino JC. Collagen structure: evidence for helical organization of the collagen fibril. *J Ultrastruct Res* 1977;58:134–143.

27. Ruggeri A, Benazzo F, Reale E. Collagen fibrils with straight and helicoidal microfibrils: a freeze-fracture and thin-section study. *J Ultrastruct Res* 1979;68:101–108.

28. Stinson RH, Sweeny PR. Skin collagen has an unusual d-spacing. *Biochim Biophys Acta* 1980;621:158–161.

29. Brodsky B, Eikenberry EF, Cassidy K. An unusual collagen periodicity in skin. *Biochim Biophys Acta* 1980;621:162–166.

30. Eikenberry EF, Childs B, Sheren SB, Parry DAD, Craig AS, Brodsky B. Crystalline fibril structure of type II collagen in lamprey notochord sheath. *J Mol Biol* 1984;176:261–277.

31. Wood GC, Keech MK. The formation of fibrils from collagen solutions. 1. The effect of experimental conditions: kinetics and electron-microscope studies. *Biochem J* 1960;75:588–598.

32. Wood GC. The formation of fibrils from collagen solutions. 3. The effect of chondroitin sulfate

and some other naturally occurring polyanions on the rate of formation. *Biochem J* 1960;75: 605–612.

33. Lee SL, Piez KA. Type II collagen from lathyritic rat chondrosarcoma: preparation and in vitro fibril formation. *Coll Relat Res* 1983;3:89–103.

34. Adachi E, Hayashi T. In vitro formation of hybrid fibrils of type V collagen and type I collagen. Limited growth of type I collagen into thick fibrils by type V collagen. *Cell Tissue Res* 1986;14: 257–266.

35. Birk DE, Fitch JM, Babiarz JP, Doane KJ, Linsenmayer TF. Collagen fibrillogenesis *in vitro*— interaction of type I and type V collagen regulates fibril diameter. *J Cell Sci* 1990;95:649–657.

36. Hedbom E, Heinegård D. Interaction of a 59-kDa connective tissue matrix protein with collagen I and collagen II. *J Biol Chem* 1989;264:6898–6905.

37. Bernard M, Yoshioka H, Rodriguez E, van der Rest M, Kimura T, Ninomiya Y, Olsen BR, Ramirez F. Cloning and sequencing of pro-α1(XI) collagen cDNA demonstrates that type XI belongs to the fibrillar class of collagens and reveals that the expression of the gene is not restricted to cartilagenous tissue. *J Biol Chem* 1988;263:17159–17166.

38. Niyibizi C, Eyre DR. Identification of the cartilage α1(XI) chain in type V collagen from bovine bone. *FEBS Lett* 1989;242:314–318.

39. Schmid TM, Linsenmayer TF. Type X collagen. In: Mayne R, Burgeson RE, eds. *Structure and function of collagen types.* New York: Academic Press, 1987;223–259.

40. Poole AR, Pidoux I. Immunoelectron microscopic studies of type X collagen in endochondral ossification. *J Cell Biol* 1989;109:2547–2554.

41. Schmid TM, Linsenmayer TF. Immunoelectron microscopy of type X collagen: supramolecular forms within embryonic chick cartilage. *Dev Biol* 1990;138:53–62.

42. Eyre D, Wu J-JW. Type XI or 1α2α3α collagen. In: Mayne R, Burgeson RE, eds. *Structure and function of collagen types.* New York: Academic Press, 1987;261–281.

43. Vaughan L, Mendler M, Huber S, Bruckner P, Winterhalter KH, Irwin MI, Mayne R. D-periodic distribution of collagen IX along cartilage fibrils. *J Cell Biol* 1988;106:991–997.

44. Mayne R, van der Rest M, Bruckner P, Schmid T. Approaches for isolating and characterizing the collagens of cartilage (Types II, IX, X and XI) and the type IX-related collagens of other tissues. In: Haralson MA, Hassell JR, eds. *Extracellular matrix molecules. A practical approach.* Oxford, Washington, DC: IRL Press, (*in press*).

45. Huber S, van der Rest M, Bruckner P, Rodriguez E, Winterhalter KH, Vaughan L. Identification of type IX collagen polypeptide chains; the α2(IX) polypeptide carries the chondroitin sulfate chain(s). *J Biol Chem* 1986;261:5965–5968.

46. King J, Laemmli UK. Polypeptides of the tail fibres of bacteriophage T4. *J Mol Biol* 1971;62: 465–477.

47. Ball EH. Quantitation of proteins by elution of coomassie brilliant blue R from stained bands after sodium dodecyl sulfate-polyacrylamide gel electrophoresis. *Anal Biochem* 1986;155:23–27.

48. Bruckner P, Hörler I, Mendler M, Houze Y, Winterhalter KH, Eich-Bender SG, Spycher MA. Induction and prevention of chondrocyte hypertrophy in culture. *J Cell Biol* 1989;109:2537–2545.

49. Morris NP, Bächinger HP. Type XI collagen is a heterotrimer with the composition (1α, 2α, 3α) retaining non-triple helical domains. *J Biol Chem* 1987;262:11345–11350.

50. van der Rest M, Mayne R. Type IX collagen-proteoglycan from cartilage is covalently linked to type II collagen. *J Biol Chem* 1988;263:1615–1618.

51. Gelman RA, Williams BR, Piez KA. Collagen fibril formation. Evidence for a multistep process. *J Biol Chem* 1979;254:180–186.

DISCUSSION

Sandell: The proportions of different collagen types change in development. Can you predict any differences in fibrils observed in development, for instance, when the ratio of type XI to type II increases?

Bruckner: Collagen type IX appears to decrease with age, as do the wider fibrils. Collagen type XI is more complicated. Type V collagen appears to occur in cartilage as well and may substitute for collagen type XI, which also appears to decrease with age. So the answer is less clear in that case.

Sandell: Can type IX collagen be replaced by proteoglycans in reconstitution experiments?

Bruckner: I haven't tried that.

Oegema: Your model predicts that at a certain concentration, type IX collagen will saturate the fibrils. Is there evidence for this? Do you have any idea about what regulates the length of the fibrils?

Bruckner: If collagen type IX is underrepresented, both tactoids and thin fibrils are formed. That is why we believe this regulation is thermodynamic. The tactoids that formed when either type IX or XI or both are missing have a limited length, but the ternary fibrils are very long, as long as you can realistically observe in the electron microscope. For all practical purposes, they have an infinite length when reconstituted.

Muir: What happens if type XI is added last?

Bruckner: Tactoids form as if there were no collagen XI at all. Formation of tactoids is irreversible. You cannot convert them back into fibrils.

Oegema: There is almost 10% of type IX collagen in the young cartilage, but only 1 to 2% in older cartilage. Is a couple of percent enough to control fibril diameter?

Bruckner: We don't know how much type IX is needed to cover the surface of a fibril or whether you need to cover the surface entirely to get the effect.

Werb: Do the type XI microfilaments really get incorporated in these fibrils? Each component appears to be able to aggregate into fibrils by itself. If type XI fibrils are preformed and then type II is added followed by type IX, is the same final structure obtained?

Bruckner: We haven't done that. However, the aggregated evidence supports our model. Type XI is not accessible to antibodies, which suggests that it may be buried inside the fibril. Further type XI filaments precipitate first, and finally nascent fibrils contain a high proportion of type XI, which decreases during fibril maturation. The arguments are indirect, since it is beyond the reach of ultrastructural immunochemistry to show directly that type XI is inside the fibril.

Werb: Type XI seemed to be more accessible in the reconstituted fibrils than in the real ones, however.

Bruckner: That is true. The reconstituted fibrils are also less densely packed than the native ones, but I suspect that after formation and cross-links, this accessibility would be lost.

Articular Cartilage and Osteoarthritis,
edited by K. Kuettner et al.
Raven Press, Ltd., New York © 1992.

11

Molecular Biology of Cartilage Collagens

Bjorn R. Olsen

*Department of Anatomy and Cellular Biology, Harvard Medical School,
Boston, Massachusetts 02115*

During chondrogenesis, chondrocytes secrete and assemble a highly complex extracellular matrix in which the fibrillar collagen framework and proteoglycans interact to create a tissue of unique biological properties. A molecular understanding of the structure of the fibrils, the proteoglycans, and their interactions is essential for understanding the biogenesis of this complex tissue and the disease processes (rheumatoid arthritis, osteoarthritis, chondrodysplasias) associated with it. The assembly of the collagenous framework requires the participation of a large number of components. Several of the genes that encode these components have been identified and characterized. Many are undoubtedly not yet discovered.

In this chapter, what is known about the genes encoding proteins with collagenous sequences in cartilage will be briefly discussed. Cartilage collagen fibrils are composed of quarter-staggered arrays of the fibrillar collagen molecules types II and XI, encoded by the $\alpha1(II)$, $\alpha1(XI)$, and $\alpha2(XI)$ genes. The three human genes have been cloned and localized on chromosomes 12q13, 1p21, and 6p21, respectively. Their exon structures have been studied extensively, and they clearly belong to the same homology subclass of collagen genes. Since several recent reviews deal with the structure and expression of the fibrillar collagen genes (3), they will not be discussed further here.

A third collagenous component of cartilage fibrils, type IX collagen, is encoded by three genes that do not belong in the fibrillar collagen subclass. In fact, extensive studies of type IX and the partially homologous collagens XII and XIV have demonstrated that the $\alpha1(IX)$, $\alpha2(IX)$, and $\alpha3(IX)$, as well as the $\alpha1(XII)$ and $\alpha1(XIV)$ genes, are members of a unique subclass of collagen genes called FACIT (fibril associated collagens with interrupted triple-helices) collagens (1–3).

Type IX collagen molecules are associated with the surface of collagen fibrils in hyaline cartilage (4). It is not known at what point in the fibril assembly process this association takes place, or what the precise roles of type IX molecules are, once they occupy the fibril surface. However, the structure and location of the molecules suggest a bridging function, and it has been suggested that type IX molecules may interact with proteoglycans (2,5).

During maturation of cartilage and chondrocyte hypertrophy, chondrocytes express a unique short-chain collagen, type X, which is incorporated into the matrix in areas of endochondral ossification (6). Type X molecules are homotrimers, encoded by the $\alpha1(X)$ gene. Molecular cloning studies have shown that this gene belongs to a unique class of collagen genes, called short-chain collagens (7,8). Noncartilaginous members of this class currently include $\alpha1(VIII)$ and $\alpha2(VIII)$, in addition to $\alpha1(X)$ in cartilage. The three short-chain collagen genes have a similar exon structure, with one large exon encoding the entire triple-helical and carboxyl non–triple-helical domain of the protein products (7,9,10). This lack of introns within the region that codes for triple-helical sequences is a hallmark of the short-chain genes and distinguishes the subclass from all other collagen genes.

Immunoelectron microscopical studies suggest that type X collagen in hypertrophic cartilage is associated, at least in part, with collagen fibrils (11,12). Thus, in hypertrophic cartilage several different kinds of collagenous molecules, fibrillar, FACIT, and short-chain collagens are colocalized in the perifibrillar region. What are the biological consequences of this colocalization? What are the precise molecular interactions involved? How are these interactions regulated? The answers to these questions are essential for a molecular understanding of cartilage function. We do not yet know the precise answers, but the structural analysis of the components involved and an examination of the expression of their genes are providing ideas and hypotheses that can be experimentally tested.

TYPE IX COLLAGEN GENES

Type IX collagen-proteoglycan (collagen IX) is a multidomain molecule associated with collagen fibrils in cartilage and noncartilage tissues such as the vitreous and embryonic cornea (13). Extensive studies have demonstrated that the molecule contains three different polypeptide subunits and that one of these, the $\alpha2(IX)$ chain, contains a glycosaminoglycan chain attached to a seryl residue within the sequence -glu-gly-ser-ala- (14,15). A second subunit, the $\alpha1(IX)$ chain, is synthesized in two different forms (Fig. 1).

One form of the $\alpha1(IX)$ chain is the major form in cartilage and contains a globular domain of about 250 amino acid residues-long at the amino terminus (5), while a second form, predominant in the embryonic chick cornea (16,17), contains instead a short alternative sequence. This form is probably also present in the vitreous of both birds (18) and mammals (19,20). The different sequences of the two forms have been determined for $\alpha1(IX)$ chains in the chicken, mouse, and human, and analysis of the $\alpha1(IX)$ gene [located in the 6q13 region of the human chromosome 6 (21)] in all three species has shown that the two forms are generated by the alternative use of two transcription start sites and RNA splice patterns (17,22). The long form is the product of transcripts generated from an upstream start site, with the amino-terminal globular domain encoded

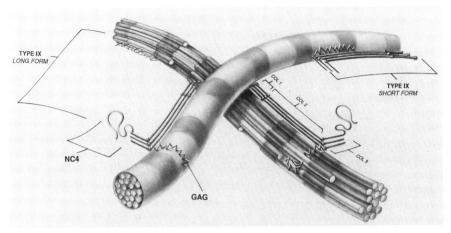

FIG. 1. Diagram showing type II collagen-containing fibrils with type IX molecules on the surface. Two forms of type IX molecules are illustrated; a long form containing a large globular domain (NC4) at the amino end of the $\alpha1$(IX) chain, and a short form lacking the NC4 domain. Both forms are shown with a glycosaminoglycan side chain (GAG) attached to the non–triple-helical region that separates the triple-helical domains COL2 and COL3 in the $\alpha2$(IX) chain. The precise spatial positioning of the GAG chain is not known; it is therefore shown in three different configurations. (From Jacenko et al., ref. 3, with permission.)

by exons 1–7 (counted from the 5' end of the gene). The short form is the product of a transcript generated from a downstream start site located in the intron between exons 6 and 7, and the amino-terminal region of this form is encoded by an alternative exon located within that intron (Fig. 2).

The tissue-specific expression of two distinct forms of $\alpha1$(IX) chains leads to the synthesis of type IX collagen molecules, with large differences in their amino-terminal non–triple-helical domains. Since these domains are located in the perifibrillar space along type II-containing collagen fibrils, it seems reasonable to conclude that this variation represents a molecular mechanism by which fibrils in different tissues can have different interaction properties. This conclusion is based on the assumption that the amino-terminal domain of collagen IX molecules in cartilage interacts with ligands in the perifibrillar matrix. The nature of these ligands is not known. However, the glycosaminoglycan chains of proteoglycans are good candidates, since the calculated pI for the long form globular domain is about 10 for the chicken, mouse, and human $\alpha1$(IX) chains. Type IX collagen in cartilage may therefore be considered a molecular bridge between major matrix components. We believe that the triple-helical domains COL1 and COL2 link collagen IX molecules to collagen fibrils, while the COL3 domain provides the physical linkage between the fibril-associated domains and the amino-terminal globular domain (Fig. 1).

The glycosaminoglycan side chain, attached to the non–triple-helical region of the $\alpha2$(IX) chain between the COL3 and COL2 domains, may serve to provide additional stability to the type IX-collagen fibril association. Also contributing

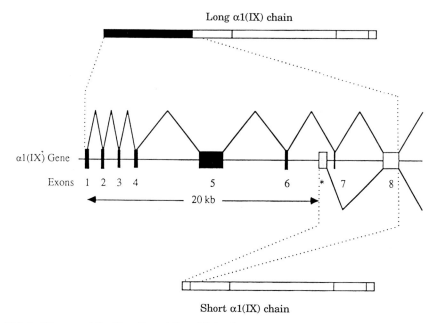

FIG. 2. Diagram of the 5′ portion of the $\alpha 1$(IX) collagen gene with exons 1–8. An exon utilized to generate a short transcript is located within the intron between exons 6 and 7. The long $\alpha 1$(IX) transcripts code for a chain with a large amino-terminal globular domain encoded by exons 1–7, whereas the short transcripts encode only a short peptide [encoded by exon (*asterisk*)] connected to the sequence of exon 8. (Modified from Nishimura et al., ref. 17.)

to that stability are the covalent cross-links that form between lysyl residues in the $\alpha 2$(IX) and $\alpha 3$(IX) chains and the amino and carboxyl telopeptides of type II collagen molecules within fibrils (23–25).

TYPE IX COLLAGEN AS A MEMBER OF THE FACIT COLLAGEN SUBCLASS

Type XII and XIV collagens (26–29) show partial homology with type IX, in that all three collagens contain a similar carboxyl-terminal triple-helical domain COL1 with several conserved structural features. In addition, both $\alpha 1$(XII) and $\alpha 1$(XIV) chains contain a globular domain that is homologous to the amino-terminal globular domain of the cartilage form of $\alpha 1$(IX). We hypothesize that the similar triple-helical domain COL1 represents a region that binds to specific sites along fibril surfaces—a fibril "docking" domain (Fig. 3). The initial interactions with fibrils through this domain in type IX collagen are then further stabilized by covalent cross-links involving residues in the COL2 domain and by the interaction of the glycosaminoglycan side chain with the fibril. Since type XII and XIV collagens do not contain glycosaminoglycan chains or domains

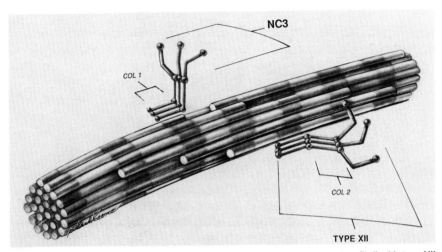

FIG. 3. Diagram showing the staggered array of type I collagen molecules in a fibril with type XII collagen molecules on the surface. Type XII molecules contain two triple-helical domains (COL1 and COL2) separated by a non–triple-helical sequence. The COL2 domain is attached to a globular region from which three non–triple-helical finger-like regions (NC3) extend. It is hypothesized that the molecules interact with fibrillar surfaces through their COL1 domains. (From Jacenko et al., ref. 3, with permission.)

that are homologous to the COL2 domain in type IX, one prediction of this model is that the fibril associations for types XII and XIV collagen are based on noncovalent interactions. The model also predicts that matrix molecules which contain a triple-helical domain of COL1 homology belong to the FACIT class of collagens. A component recently identified by sequencing of cDNA from a human fibroblast library (M.-L. Chu and R. Timpl, personal communication) probably represents such a new member of the FACIT class.

Molecules of the FACIT class are expressed in a tissue-specific manner, but not in a mutually exclusive fashion. For example, type IX, XII, and XIV collagen mRNAs are all present in cartilage. Immunostaining of embryonic chick tissues with monoclonal antibodies against type IX and XII collagens show that while type IX is abundant in the cartilage matrix, type XII is found in the perichondrium (13,30). However, in the subperichondrial region of cartilage, a positive reaction is seen with both antibodies. An antibody against chicken type XIV collagen is not yet available, so the distribution of type XIV protein is not known, but the mRNA is widely distributed and clearly present in cartilage. Also, it is likely that the protein called TL-B, recently isolated from fetal bovine skin (31), is identical or closely related to type XIV, and antibodies against TL-B do stain cartilage (31). We suspect, therefore, that type XIV collagen is coexpressed with type IX collagen in cartilage matrix.

What are the consequences of coexpression of different FACIT molecules in cartilage? It seems reasonable to assume that type IX and XIV collagens, by having homologous COL1 domains, would compete for the same binding sites along collagen fibrils. Therefore, the relative abundance of the two types may regulate the surface properties of the fibrils, since the amino-terminal portions of the molecules are so different (see Figs. 1 and 2). As discussed above, the major cartilage form of type IX contains a globular amino-terminal domain. In contrast, type XIV molecules (like type XII) contain very large (>1,500 amino acid residues) non–triple-helical regions organized as three fingers projecting from a central globule (27,29,31). The finger-regions contain domains that are homologous to the repeat domains of cartilage matrix protein as well as several type III fibronectin repeats (32).

THE TYPE X COLLAGEN GENE: A MEMBER OF A DISTINCT CLASS WITHIN THE SUPERFAMILY OF COLLAGEN GENES

Collagen types X and VIII belong to the same subclass within the collagen gene superfamily. We have given this subclass the designation short-chain collagen because of the relatively small size (<750 amino acid residues) of the protein products as compared with the proα-chains of fibrillar collagens (2,8). The initial cloning and characterization of the chicken $\alpha1(X)$ collagen gene demonstrated that it had a unique exon structure, totally different from that of fibrillar and basement membrane collagen genes (7,33). The gene was not only small (<10 kb in size) and contained only three exons, but one of the exons was large (2137 bp) and encoded the entire triple-helical (460 amino acid residues) and carboxyl non–triple-helical (162 amino acid residues) domains of the $\alpha1(X)$ collagen chain (Fig. 4). Subsequent isolation and characterization of the rabbit, mouse, and human $\alpha1(VIII)$ and $\alpha2(VIII)$ collagen genes have further shown that the genes encoding the two collagen VIII polypeptides have a similar exon structure with a large 3′ exon (2278 bp for the rabbit $\alpha1(VIII)$ gene) (8–10).

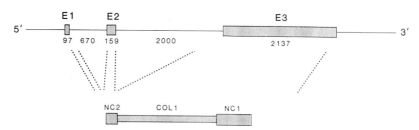

FIG. 4. Diagram showing the exon structure of the chicken type X collagen gene and the locations of exon-intron splice junctions relative to the translation product (*bottom*). The exons are numbered from the 5′ to the 3′ end of the gene. The sizes (in nucleotides) of the exons are indicated below each exon, together with the sizes of the introns. Below the gene are indicated the three domains (NC1, COL1, NC2) of the $\alpha1(X)$ translation product. (Modified from Ninomiya et al., ref. 41, with permission.)

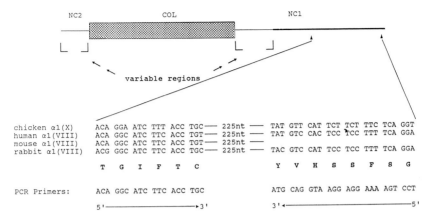

FIG. 5. Diagram showing the domain structure of short-chain collagen chains. Non–triple-helical domains (NC1 and NC2) are indicated (*lines*); the triple-helical region (COL) is also represented (*boxed-in area*). The sequence of the carboxyl three-quarters of the NC1 domain (*heavy line*) is highly conserved between $\alpha1(X)$ and $\alpha1(VIII)$ collagen chains, whereas the amino-terminal one-quarter of NC1 and the NC2 domain (*thin lines*) are more variable in sequence. Below the diagram, the nucleotide sequence of two selected regions within the conserved portion of NC1 is shown, together with the amino acid sequences, for chicken $\alpha1(X)$ and $\alpha1(VIII)$ chains from three mammalian species. Based on these sequences, two primers were synthesized for PCR and used to isolate human and mouse $\alpha2(VIII)$ and human $\alpha1(X)$ genes. (Modified from Muragaki et al., ref. 10.)

A comparison of the $\alpha1(X)$, $\alpha1(VIII)$, and $\alpha2(VIII)$ genes shows also a high degree of sequence similarity in their coding regions. This similarity is especially striking within the sequences of the large exons that encode the carboxyl-terminal non–triple-helical domains (Fig. 5). In fact, the conservation of sequences within this region at both the nucleotide and amino acid levels has provided the basis for molecular cloning of the human and mouse $\alpha2(VIII)$ gene and the human $\alpha1(X)$ gene (10,34). Using genomic DNA as a template and oligonucleotides from within the highly conserved regions as primers, the three genes have been cloned through a PCR-approach. The same approach can undoubtedly be used to clone additional members of the short-chain family. The availability of clones encoding the human $\alpha1(VIII)$, $\alpha2(VIII)$, and $\alpha1(X)$ collagen chains has permitted the chromosomal assignment of their genes. By *in situ* hybridization on chromosome spreads, the $\alpha1(VIII)$ gene has been located on chromosome 3 (3q12-3q13.1), the $\alpha2(VIII)$ gene on chromosome 1 (1p32.3-1p34.3), and the $\alpha1(X)$ gene on chromosome 6 (6q21-6q22) (9,10,34).

DEVELOPMENTAL REGULATION
OF THE $\alpha1(X)$ COLLAGEN GENE

The onset of type X collagen expression in cartilage is accompanied by a large increase in the levels of $\alpha1(X)$ collagen mRNA (Fig. 6). To find out whether this

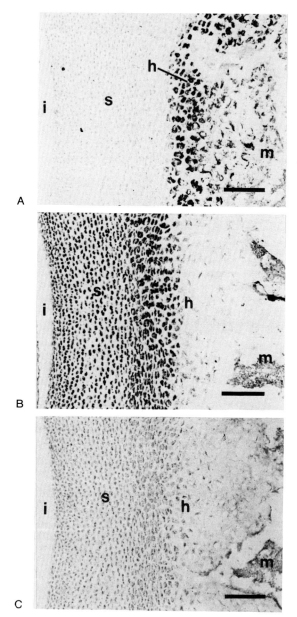

FIG. 6. Consecutive longitudinal sections of vertebrae of a stage 45 chick embryo processed for *in situ* hybridization with probes for $\alpha1(X)$ (**A**) $\alpha1(II)$, (**B**) and $\alpha1(IX)$, (**C**) collagen. Grains representing $\alpha1(X)$ collagen mRNA are noted over hypertrophic chondrocytes (*h*), while there are virtually no grains over small chondrocytes (*S*). Numerous grains for $\alpha1(II)$ collagen mRNA are seen over small chondrocytes (*S*). *i*, intervertebral joint space; *m*, marrow cavity. Bar = 100 μm. (From Iyama et al., ref. 39, with permission.)

is due to transcriptional regulation, we have performed run-off transcription assays with chondrocyte nuclei isolated from the cephalic, calcified portion of 18-day-old sternal cartilage of chick embryos (which expresses type X), from the caudal, permanently cartilaginous portion of sternal cartilage (which does not express type X collagen), and from fibroblasts (no expression of type X). We have also examined nuclei from different stages, such as days 15–18. The results demonstrate that nuclei from cells that express type X collagen have a very high rate of transcription of the $\alpha 1(X)$ gene, whereas nuclei from cells that do not express type X collagen transcribe the gene at a low background rate. Also, analysis of nuclei of different developmental stages shows that the rate of transcription of the $\alpha 1(X)$ gene increases rapidly with the appearance of type X protein, as detected with a monoclonal antibody. We conclude, therefore, that the developmental and tissue-specific expression of type X collagen *in vivo* is primarily regulated by a transcriptional mechanism (35).

What is the nature of this transcriptional mechanism? The definition of the complete exon structure of the chicken $\alpha 1(X)$ gene and isolation of >2,000 nucleotides of sequence in the 5' upstream region of the gene have permitted cloning of several type X promoter-CAT expression constructs for transient assays in cultured cells. Constructs containing various portions of the $\alpha 1(X)$ 5' region, exon 1 (all untranslated), and intron 1 have been transfected into chick embryo fibroblasts, sternal and tibial chondrocytes, and the rat chondrocyte line RCJ-3.1C5.25, using Lipofectin and $CaPO_4$ transfection protocols. All transfections include as an internal control a construct, pCH110, encoding β-galactosidase regulated by the SV40 early promoter. All CAT activities can thus be expressed relative to β-galactosidase activities (36).

The results from these transient transfection assays show that a 640 bp region immediately upstream of the transcription start acts as a powerful promoter in chicken fibroblasts and chondrocytes as well as in rat chondrocytes. In fact, it is a stronger promoter in fibroblasts than the herpes virus thymidine kinase promoter. When sequences further upstream are added to the 640 bp piece, the expression of CAT is suppressed 15- to 20-fold in fibroblasts and small chondrocytes, suggesting that factors in these cells recognize this upstream region and suppress transcription. In hypertrophic chondrocytes, CAT constructs containing the 640 bp piece and constructs with more extensive 5' sequences are expressed equally well, suggesting an absence of such suppression in these cells.

FUNCTIONAL ROLE OF TYPE X AND OTHER SHORT-CHAIN COLLAGENS

Except for the hen oviduct and the eggshell membrane (37), expression of type X collagen *in vivo* is restricted to cartilage tissues that undergo endochondral ossification (6). The association between chondrocyte hypertrophy during endochondral ossification and type X collagen expression has prompted several suggestions for the role of the molecule in hypertrophic cartilage. One suggested function is that of facilitating the removal of hypertrophic cartilage. Since chicken type X molecules have been found to contain two cleavage sites for vertebrate collagenase, it has been concluded that type X collagen is more rapidly degraded by vertebrate collagenase than is type II collagen (38). However, the two cleavage sites are located toward the two ends of the triple-helical 45 kDa domain and cleavage at the sites releases a fragment of 32 kDa with a Tm of 43°C. Collagenase cleavage of type X is therefore more a processing than a degradation process.

It has also been suggested that type X collagen plays a role in mineralization of cartilage (6,12). However, while calcification occurs in a matrix that contains type X collagen, there is a considerable delay between the deposition of type X collagen and the onset of calcification (39).

A role in vascular invasion has also been considered for type X collagen. Interestingly, the deposition of type X collagen precedes the invasion of blood vessels from the perichondrium into hypertrophic cartilage, and although there is no reason to believe that type X collagen has angiogenic activity, it is possible

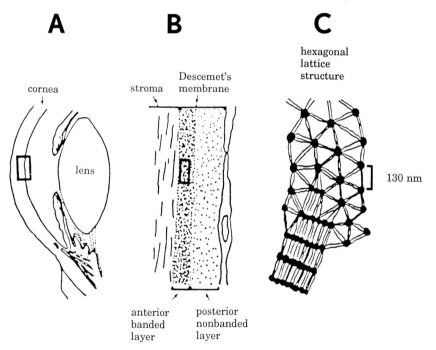

FIG. 7. A: A sagittal section through the anterior region of the eye. **B:** The posterior portion of the cornea [rectangular area in (A)] contains the Descemet's membrane. The anterior banded layer of Descemet's membrane [rectangular area in (B)] contains a hexagonal lattice structure **(C)** with nodes spaced about 130 nm apart, connected by thin strands. The internodal distance corresponds to the length of type VIII collagen molecules. (Courtesy of Dr. Y. Ninomiya.)

that the type X-rich hypertrophic matrix may promote vascularization (39). The role of type X collagen within this matrix may be essentially structural in nature. In fact, the strong homology between $\alpha1(X)$, $\alpha1(VIII)$, and $\alpha2(VIII)$ collagen chains suggests that type X and VIII molecules may form similar supramolecular structures *in vivo.*

Clues about the precise nature of such supramolecular structures come from recent studies of Descemet's membrane. Within this membrane, an hexagonal lattice with nodes interconnected by rods contains type VIII collagen molecules as major constituents. The internodal distance corresponds to the length of type VIII collagen molecules, and Sawada et al. (40) have demonstrated that the nodes and rods are recognized by monoclonal antibodies against the $\alpha1(VIII)$ triple-helical domain. Type VIII molecules must therefore participate in the formation of a network by end-to-end interactions involving both amino- and carboxyl-terminal non–triple-helical domains (Fig. 7).

Given the structural homology between type X and VIII collagens, it seems reasonable to suggest that type X molecules may form similar structures in hypertrophic cartilage (2). Using gold-labeled antibodies against type X collagen, Schmid and Linsenmayer (11) have reported the presence of collagen X in pericellular fine networks in hypertrophic cartilage, and these may somehow be structurally related to the hexagonal lattices formed with type VIII molecules. Lattices of a similar nature may also form along type II-containing fibrils in hypertrophic cartilage, since gold-labeled anti-type X antibodies also show fibrillar labeling (11,12). The role of these lattices may be to provide a temporary scaffold around cells and fibrils as the fibrils and proteoglycans are degraded by stromelysin/collagenase.

HOW DOES THE NEW INFORMATION ON THE MOLECULAR BIOLOGY OF NONFIBRILLAR CARTILAGE COLLAGENS HELP OUR UNDERSTANDING OF OSTEOARTHRITIS?

The new data on nonfibrillar collagens have significantly increased our knowledge of cartilage matrix structure. The isolation and sequencing of DNAs is obviously an effective approach to obtaining precise structural information. The large amount of sequence data now available for nonfibrillar collagens could not have been collected by protein chemical methods alone. However, the use of molecular cloning techniques has not only provided structural information about known components but molecules such as type XII were discovered by isolation and sequencing of cDNA, and the complex, multidomain structure of type IX became apparent only by analysis of cDNA sequences. The continued use of cloning methods will undoubtedly lead to the discovery of a large number of additional cartilage components. The identification of such components will continue to provide a general basis for understanding disease processes involving cartilage. In addition, the availability of DNA probes, sequences, and sequence-specific antibodies makes it possible to consider the development of novel assays to measure degradation of cartilage. For example, the degradation of collagen fibrils may produce peptide fragments derived from collagen types IX and XIV, and possibly type X, that could be detected in synovial fluid or serum. Finally, as we learn more about the mechanisms which control the expression of non-fibrillar collagens in chondrocytes and how these mechanisms are tied to the genetic controls of chondrocyte differentiation and maturation, we may learn how to alter these control mechanisms and stimulate the formation/regeneration of cartilage. It will clearly also be possible to use cloned cartilage-specific promoters, such as the upstream promoter of the $\alpha 1(IX)$ gene or the $\alpha 1(X)$ promoter, to drive the expression of cartilage-degrading enzymes, such as stromelysin, or cytokines, such as interleukin-1 in the cartilage of transgenic animals. Such animals may provide useful models of both osteoarthritis and rheumatoid arthritis.

REFERENCES

1. Olsen BR. The next frontier: molecular biology of extracellular matrix. *Connect Tiss Res* 1989;23: 115–121.
2. Gordon MK, Olsen BR. The contribution of collagenous proteins to tissue-specific matrix assemblies. *Curr Opinion Cell Biol* 1990;2:833–838.
3. Jacenko O, Olsen BR, LuValle P. Organization and regulation of collagen genes. *Crit Rev Eukaryot Gene Express* 1991;1:327–353.
4. Vaughan L, Mendler M, Huber S, Bruckner P, Winterhalter KH, Irwin MH, Mayne R. D-Periodic distribution of collagen type IX along cartilage fibrils. *J Cell Biol* 1988;106:991–997.
5. Vasios G, Nishimura I, Konomi H, van der Rest M, Ninomiya Y, Olsen BR. Cartilage type IX collagen proteoglycan contains a large amino-terminal globular domain encoded by multiple exons. *J Biol Chem* 1988;263:2324–2329.
6. Schmid TM, Linsenmayer TF. Type X collagen. In: Mayne R, Burgeson RE, eds. *Biology of extracellular matrix: structure and function of collagen types.* New York: Academic Press, 1987;223–259.
7. LuValle P, Ninomiya Y, Rosenblum ND, Olsen BR. The type X collagen gene: intron sequences split the 5' untranslated region and separate the coding regions for the non-collagenous amino-terminal and triple-helical domains. *J Biol Chem* 1988;263:18378–18385.
8. Yamaguchi N, Mayne R, Ninomiya Y. The $\alpha 1(VIII)$ collagen gene is homologous to the $\alpha 1(X)$ collagen gene and contains a large exon encoding the entire triple-helical and carboxyl-terminal non–triple-helical domains of the $\alpha 1(VIII)$ polypeptide. *J Biol Chem* 266:4508–4513.
9. Muragaki Y, Mattei M-G, Yamaguchi N, Olsen BR, Ninomiya Y. The complete primary structure of the human $\alpha 1(VIII)$ chain and assignment of its gene (COL8A1) to chromosome 3. *Eur J Biol* 1991;197:615–622.
10. Muragaki Y, Jacenko O, Apte S, Mattei M-G, Ninomiya Y, Olsen BR. The $\alpha 2(VIII)$ collagen gene—a novel member of the short-chain collagen family located on the human chromosome 1. *J Biol Chem* 1991;266:7721–7727.
11. Schmid TM, Linsenmayer TF. Immunoelectron microscopy of type X collagen: supramolecular forms within embryonic chick cartilage. *Dev Biol* 1990;138:53–62.
12. Poole AR, Pidoux I. Immunoelectron microscopic studies of type X collagen in endochondral ossification. *J Cell Biol* 1989;109:2547–2554.
13. van der Rest M, Mayne R. Type IX collagen. In: Mayne R, Burgeson RE, eds. *Biology of extracellular matrix: structure and function of collagen types.* New York: Academic Press, 1987;195–221.

14. Huber S, Winterhalter R, Vaughan L. Isolation and sequence analysis of the glycosaminoglycan attachment site of type IX collagen. *J Biol Chem* 1988;263:752–756.
15. McCormick D, van der Rest M, Goodship J, Lozano G, Ninomiya Y, Olsen BR. Structure of the glycosaminoglycan domain in the type IX collagen-proteoglycan. *Proc Natl Acad Sci USA* 1987;84:4044–4048.
16. Svoboda KK, Nishimura I, Sugrue SP, Ninomiya Y, Olsen BR. Embryonic chicken cornea and cartilage synthesize type IX collagen molecules with different amino-terminal domains. *Proc Natl Acad Sci USA* 1988;85:7496–7500.
17. Nishimura I, Muragaki Y, Olsen BR. Tissue-specific forms of type IX collagen-proteoglycan arise from the use of two widely separated promoters. *J Biol Chem* 1989;264:20033–20041.
18. Yada T, Suzuki S, Kobayashi K, Kobayashi M, Hoshino T, Horie K, Kimata K. Occurrence in chick embryo vitreous humor of a type IX collagen proteoglycan with an extraordinary large chondroitin sulfate chain and short $\alpha1$ polypeptide. *J Biol Chem* 1990;265:6992–6999.
19. Wright DW, Mayne R. Vitreous humor of chicken contains two fibrillar systems: an analysis of their structure. *J Ultrastruct Molec Struct Res* 1988;100:224–234.
20. Seery CM, Warman ML, Olsen BR, Davison PF. $\alpha1(IX)$ collagen chain of mammalian vitreous (submitted).
21. Kimura T, Mattei M-G, Stevens JW, Goldring MB, Ninomiya Y, Olsen BR. Molecular cloning of rat and human type IX collagen cDNA and localization of the $\alpha1(IX)$ gene on the human chromosome 6. *Eur J Biochem* 1989;79:71–78.
22. Muragaki Y, Nishimura I, Henney A, Ninomiya Y, Olsen BR. The $\alpha1(IX)$ collagen gene (COL9A1) gives rise to two different transcripts in mouse embryonic and human fetal RNA. *Proc Natl Acad Sci USA* 1990;87:2400–2404.
23. van der Rest M, Mayne R. Type IX collagen proteoglycan from cartilage is covalently cross-linked to type II collagen. *J Biol Chem* 1988;263:1615–1618.
24. Eyre DR, Apon S, Wu J-J, Erickson LH, Walsh KA. Collagen type IX: evidence for covalent linkage to type II collagen in cartilage. *FEBS Lett* 1987;220:337–341.
25. Eyre D, Wu J-J, Woods P. The cartilage-specific collagens: structural studies (this volume).
26. Gordon MK, Gerecke DR, Dublet B, van der Rest M, Olsen BR. Type XII collagen: a large multidomain molecule with partial homology to type IX collagen. *J Biol Chem* 1989;264:19772–19778.
27. Dublet B, van der Rest M. Type XIV collagen, a new homotrimeric molecule extracted from fetal bovine skin and tendon, with a triple helical disulfide-bonded domain homologous to type IX and type XII collagens. *J Biol Chem* 1991;266:6853–6858.
28. Gordon MK, Castagnola P, Dublet B, Linsenmayer TF, van der Rest M, Olsen BR. Cloning of a cDNA for a new member of the FACIT class of collagenous proteins. *Eur J Biochem* (in press).
29. Castagnola P, Gerecke DR, Gordon MK, Olsen BR. Type XIV collagen: a multidomain matrix component encoded by a widely expressed mRNA (submitted for publication).
30. Sugrue SP, Gordon MK, Seyer J, Dublet B, van der Rest M, Olsen BR. Immunoidentification of type XII collagen in embryonic tissues. *J Cell Biol* 1989;109:939–945.
31. Keene DR, Lunstrum GP, Morris NP, Stoddard DW, Burgeson RE. Two type XII-like collagens localize to the surface of banded collagen fibrils. *J Cell Biol* 1991;113:971–978.
32. Gerecke D, *et al.* (in preparation).
33. Ninomiya Y, Gordon M, van der Rest M, Schmid T, Linsenmayer T, Olsen BR. The developmentally regulated type X collagen gene contains a long open reading frame without introns. *J Biol Chem* 1986;261:5041–5050.
34. Apte S, Mattei M-G, Olsen BR. Cloning of human $\alpha1(X)$ collagen DNA and localization of the COL10A1 gene to the q21-q22 region of human chromosome 6. *FEBS Lett* 1991;282:393–396.
35. LuValle P, Hayashi M, Olsen BR. Transcriptional regulation of type X collagen during chondrocyte maturation. *Dev Biol* 1989;133:613–616.
36. LuValle P, *et al.* (in preparation).
37. Arias JL, Fernandez MS, Dennis JE, Caplan AI. The fabrication and collagenous substructure of the eggshell membrane in the isthmus of the hen oviduct. *Matrix* 1991 (in press).
38. Schmid TM, Mayne R, Jeffrey JJ, Linsenmayer TF. Type X collagen contains two cleavage sites for a vertebrate collagenase. *J Biol Chem* 1986;261:4184–4189.
39. Iyama K-I, Ninomiya Y, Olsen BR, Linsenmayer TF, Trelstad RL, Hayashi M. Spatio-temporal pattern of type X collagen gene expression and collagen deposition in embryonic chick vertebrae undergoing endochondral ossification. *Anat Rec* 1991;229:462–472.

40. Sawada H, Konomi H, Hirosawa K. Characterization of the collagen in the hexagonal lattice of Descemet's membrane: its relation to type VIII collagen. *J Cell Biol* 1990;110:219–227.
41. Ninomiya Y, Castagnola P, Gerecke D, Gordon M, Jacenko O, LuValle P, McCarthy M, Muragaki Y, Nishimura I, Oh S, Rosenblum N, Sato N, Sugrue S, Taylor R, Vasios G, Yamaguchi N, Olsen BR. The molecular biology of collagens with short triple-helical domains. In: Sandell LJ, Boyd CD, eds. *Extracellular matrix genes.* New York: Academic Press, 1990;79–114.

DISCUSSION

Sandell: Your *in situ* hybridization studies on growth plate appeared to show that type X was expressed differently from type II. Is that correct?

Olsen: Yes. But if you expose those slides longer, you do see type II hybridization also in the hypertrophic region. The same is true for type IX. Analyses of total tissue mRNA by Northerns shows some type IX, but it is decreased in the hypertrophic zone. If one looks at the two forms of alpha 1 (IX), the long and short forms, depending on which one of the two transcription start sites are used, the major form in cartilage by PCR and Northern analysis is the long form. In hypertrophic cartilage, the short form becomes dominant. I don't think there is an up-regulation of the short form in hypertrophic cartilage, but rather, there is a relative shift in the ratio of the two messages. This is mainly because the long form mRNA disappears while there is always some background transcription from the downstream start site for the short form in the alpha 1 (IX) gene.

Bruckner: Can you comment on the observations by Tom Schmid and Robin Poole on the immunolocalization of collagen type X on fibrils in cartilage?

Olsen: Schmid and Linsenmayer found type X epitopes in two locations. One is in pericellular mats or networks that may correspond to the polymeric structures I proposed for type X collagen. A careful analysis of their microscopic images reveals networks within these mats. The second location is fibrillar in nature and was also seen by Robin Poole. The same types of networks could form around fibrils and not necessarily only around the cells. It would be very difficult to see such networks in cartilage, much more difficult than in Descemet's membrane.

Eyre: Can you rule out heterotrimer molecules between type XII and XIV chains simply because their triple helical domains are of different lengths?

Olsen: The sequences of the type XII and XIV collagenous domains are highly homologous, but have different lengths. In the middle of the COL 1 domain there is an insertion of a Gly-X-Y triplet in XIV compared to XII. The COL 1 domain is therefore longer in XIV than in XII. Similarly, two triplets are inserted in the COL 2 domain of type XIV, making it six residues longer than COL 2 in type XII. These differences make it unlikely that the two chains form heterotrimers. In Robert Burgeson's group the two homotrimers have been isolated and purified as two distinct molecules from fetal calf tissues.

van der Rest: We have isolated homotrimers of types XII and XIV also from the same tissue, making it very unlikely that they form heterotrimers.

Howell: Chondrocytes in the growth plate remodel their matrix. Antibodies to interstitial collagenase localize in the vertical septa and rims around the cells in the hypertrophic zone. Micropuncture of these regions reveals latent collagenase. Can factors such as the small proteoglycans regulate the access of collagenase to collagen substrates during remodeling?

Olsen: Tom Linsenmayer showed that vertebrate collagenase cuts chicken type X in two places, and this has been taken as evidence of rapid degradation. I suggest that this is not degradation but processing. The Tm of intact type X is very high, close to 50°. After cleavage with collagenase, the noncollagenous regions and a very small portion of the triple helix are removed. Most of the triple helix is intact and the Tm of the fragment is as high as that of an intact type I triple helix. Perhaps type X forms a polymer that would remain stable even in the presence of high levels of collagenase. If type X is a structural component that reinforces the matrix around hypertrophic chondrocytes, it may help prevent collapse of the local matrix around the cells.

Articular Cartilage a
edited by K. Kuettner
Raven Press, Ltd., New

12

Type II Collagen Gene Mutations in Familial Osteoarthritis

Sergio A. Jimenez,*† Leena Ala-Kokko,† Nina Ahmad,†
Clinton Baldwin,† Rita Dharmavaram,* Anthony Reginato,*
Robert Knowlton,† and Darwin J. Prockop*†

*Departments of Medicine, and Biochemistry and Molecular Biology and
†Jefferson Institute of Molecular Medicine, Jefferson Medical College,
Thomas Jefferson University, Philadelphia, Pennsylvania 19107*

INHERITED FORMS OF OSTEOARTHRITIS (OA)

Human osteoarthritis (OA) is a heterogeneous and multifactorial disease characterized by the progressive degeneration of the hyaline cartilage of diarthrodial joints. Multiple pathogenetic mechanisms have been implicated in its development and progression (for review see ref. 1). In many instances, OA is an acquired process secondary to various metabolic, mechanical, or inflammatory-immunologic events. However, epidemiological and large population studies have provided compelling evidence that several distinct forms of OA are inherited as dominant traits with a Mendelian pattern (2,3). The most common form of inherited OA is primary generalized OA (PGOA) in which the development of Heberden's and Bouchard's nodes and the premature degeneration of multiple joints are prominent. A characteristic feature of PGOA is the symmetric and concentric, or uniform loss of articular cartilage, particularly apparent in the hip and knee joints (2–4). A second type of inherited OA is that associated with familial chondrocalcinosis due to the deposition of calcium pyrophosphate dihydrate (CPPD) crystals in fibrous and hyaline cartilages (5). Because occasionally the degenerative arthritis precedes or is not associated with demonstrable deposition of CPPD crystals (6), it has been suggested that structural abnormalities in articular cartilage matrix may be a primary common event leading to cartilage degeneration and/or to CPPD crystal deposition. A third familial form of OA is the Stickler syndrome, or hereditary progressive arthro-ophthalmopathy (7). This syndrome is characterized by progressive vitreo-retinal degeneration, severe myopia and premature degenerative joint disease. Other heritable disorders accompanied by premature OA include hydroxyapatite deposition disease (8) and certain forms of multiple epiphyseal dysplasias (reviewed in ref. 9).

The Mendelian pattern of inheritance of these diseases suggests that defects in one or more of the genes encoding for the structural components of articular cartilage may be responsible for the premature and generalized degenerative changes in the tissue. Identification of mutations in the multiplicity of genes that may be affected would represent a monumental task because of the enormous effort required to determine the sequence of all the possible genes, and the incomplete knowledge of their structure and organization.

COLLAGEN, THE STRUCTURAL COMPONENT OF ARTICULAR CARTILAGE MOST LIKELY TO BE DEFECTIVE IN FAMILIAL OA

There are several reasons to support the hypothesis that failure of the collagenous components of articular cartilage may be responsible for the degeneration of this tissue in familial OA. The collagens are predominant components of the organic matrix of articular cartilage, and play a crucial role in the maintenance of its biomechanical properties (10). Although early studies suggested that articular cartilage collagen consisted almost exclusively of type II collagen, current evidence indicates that at least five different collagen types (types II, V, VI, IX, and XI) are present in this tissue (reviewed in ref. 11). In addition, collagen type X, which is a specific biosynthetic product of hypertrophic chondrocytes, may also be a component of articular cartilage. The demonstration that type IX collagen contains a glycosaminoglycan molecule covalently attached to one of its α-chains suggests that it may be intimately involved in the interaction of the collagen network with the surrounding proteoglycans in the tissue matrix. It has recently been suggested that type IX and type XI collagen molecules may play a role in the formation of type II collagen fibrils (reviewed in ref. 11). The complexity of the collagenous components in articular cartilage and the important roles that these molecules play in the maintenance of the normal architecture of the tissue indicate that alterations in their structure may have profound effects on the normal function of articular cartilage. Furthermore, the normal supramolecular assembly of the collagens in cartilage serves as a mechanical constraint to prevent the expansion of proteoglycans into the large hydrodynamic domains characteristic of proteoglycans in free solution (12). A failure of this collagenous network would result in swelling of the proteoglycans, increased tissue water content, softening of the matrix, and eventual cartilage degeneration.

RESTRICTION FRAGMENT LENGTH POLYMORPHISM ANALYSIS IN FAMILIAL OA

The development of recombinant probes that allow the detection of polymorphic sites in human DNA by restriction fragment length polymorphism

(RFLP) analysis has made available a vast resource of genetic markers to follow the inheritance of specific DNA sequences in families (13). These polymorphic sites occur frequently in the flanking regions of most genes as well as in randomly selected genomic DNA. Molecular probes that detect these polymorphisms can now be used to identify abnormal alleles of many genes and to trace their familial pattern of cosegregation with a given disease phenotype. Recently, several polymorphisms in the type II procollagen gene (COL2A1) and surrounding DNA sequences have been identified (14–16). The identification of these polymorphisms has permitted the application of RFLP analysis to test the possibility that mutations in COL2A1 may be responsible for familial OA. Francomano et al. (17) and Knowlton et al. (18) recently examined the coinheritance of type II

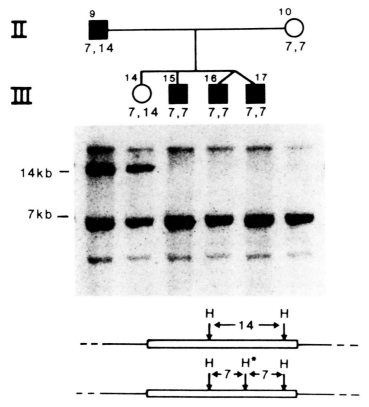

FIG. 1. Inheritance of COL2A1 RFLP alleles in members from the second and third generations of a large family with premature OA and mild chondrodystrophy. The diagram at the bottom shows the allelic variants of the COL2A1 gene that arise from the presence or absence of a polymorphic *Hind* III site (H*) halfway between two invariable *Hind* III sites (H) that are separated by 14 kb. *Hind* III digestion yields a 14 kb band from the nonpolymorphic allele and two comigrating 7 kb bands from the allele containing the H* polymorphism. The mother is homozygous for the 7 kb allele, and the father is heterozygous. The healthy daughter inherited the normal paternal 14 kb allele, whereas the three affected sons (including two twins) inherited his abnormal 7 kb allele. From ref. 19, with permission.

procollagen gene polymorphisms with the expression of the Stickler syndrome. The study of Knowlton et al. (18) analyzed three large families for coinheritance of the genetic defect with the *Hind* III restriction enzyme and the variable number tandem repeat (VNTR) polymorphisms in COL2A1. Genetic linkage between the disease phenotype and COL2A1 was demonstrated in the largest family. The results from the second family also supported linkage to COL2A1. The studies of Francomano et al. (17) also showed coinheritance of the disease with COL2A1 in two families with Stickler syndrome. These observations are consistent with the conclusion that mutations in the COL2A1 gene are responsible for the disease in these families.

More recently, Knowlton et al. (19) examined the coinheritance of a phenotype of premature OA and a mild chondrodysplasia with the type II procollagen gene in a large family. In this study, the genotypes of 18 family members were determined with the *Hind* III RFLP. This analysis showed that in every informative meiosis in two generations, the joint disease segregated with the abnormal COL2A1 allele transmitted from an affected male. There was no evidence for recombination between the phenotype and COL2A1. Figure 1 shows the inheritance of the *Hind* III RFLP in the COL2A1 alleles in selected members of the family. These studies provided statistically significant evidence that the defective gene was in close genetic linkage with COL2A1. A similar study of a large family from Finland with a phenotype of severe PGOA also found coinheritance of the disease with polymorphisms in COL2A1 (20).

IDENTIFICATION OF COL2A1 MUTATIONS IN AFFECTED INDIVIDUALS WITH FAMILIAL OA

The development of methods for cloning and sequencing complementary and genomic DNA has resulted in substantial advances in our understanding of the structure of normal articular cartilage matrix. The recent cloning and sequencing of a full-length cDNA for human type II procollagen (21) and the determination of the entire sequence of the gene (22) have allowed the search for mutations in COL2A1 in affected members from families with OA. Ala-Kokko et al. (23) obtained genomic DNA from cultured skin fibroblasts from one affected member of the family in which cosegregation of the phenotype of PGOA and mild chondrodysplasia with COL2A1 was previously demonstrated by Knowlton et al. (19). The genomic DNA was partially digested, and following gel fractionation and electroelution, it was cloned into a cosmid vector engineered to receive the appropriate restriction fragments of 25–35 kb. One clone containing the abnormal allele, as identified by *Hind* III RFLP, was plaque-purified, subcloned, and used for double-stranded DNA sequencing. A total of >20 kb, including all of the nucleotides for exons 2B to 52 from the allele, were sequenced. A single base mutation that changes the codon for arginine into a codon for cysteine at position 519 of the type II procollagen triple helix was found. To confirm that this mutation was coinherited with the disease, Ala-Kokko et al. (23) examined DNA samples from affected and unaffected members of the family by allele-specific hybridization of polymerase chain reaction-amplified genomic DNA. All nine affected members of the family had the mutation, whereas ten unaffected members and 57 controls did not.

In a more recent study, Ahmad et al. (24) identified a mutation that results in the introduction of a stop codon in the coding region of COL2A1 in affected individuals from a family with the Stickler syndrome. Thus, it is clear that mutations in COL2A1 are responsible for the OA phenotype in these two families.

IDENTIFICATION OF MUTATED TYPE II COLLAGEN MOLECULES IN ARTICULAR CARTILAGE FROM AFFECTED MEMBERS OF A FAMILY WITH PGOA

Intact, native type II collagen was extracted from articular cartilage from two affected individuals from the family with PGOA and mild chondrodysplasia in

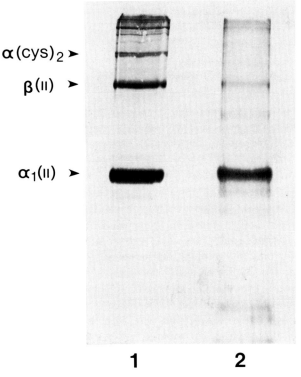

FIG. 2. Western blot analysis under nonreducing conditions of type II collagen extracted from articular cartilage of one affected individual from the family with premature OA and mild chondrodystrophy before and following NTCBA cleavage. **Lane 1:** Before cleavage. Note $\alpha(Cys)_2$ type II collagen dimers migrating above normal β chains. **Lane 2:** After cleavage. Note the disappearance of the $\alpha(Cys)_2$ chains following specific cleavage of intrahelical cysteine residues.

which the arginine to cysteine mutation at position 519 of the triple helix was identified (23). The extracted collagen was characterized by immunoelectrophoresis under reducing and nonreducing conditions employing human type II procollagen-specific polyclonal antibodies. The results showed that articular cartilage from the two affected individuals contained type II collagen α chains that assembled into disulfide-bonded dimers [$\alpha(Cys)_2$ in Fig. 2]. The disulfide-bonded dimers displayed a slower electrophoretic mobility than did normal β chains of type II procollagen, but under reducing conditions their individual chains comigrated with the normal type II collagen α chains. The presence of cysteine within the triple helical domain of the mutated type II collagen was demonstrated by treatment of the samples with 2-nitro-5-thiocyanobenzoic acid (NTCBA), a reagent that causes a specific cleavage at cysteine residues. The results (Fig. 2) showed the selective cleavage of the $\alpha(Cys)_2$ chains, indicating that the mutation resulted in the change of one of the residues within the triple helical domain of the α chains for a cysteine residue and that these chains accumulated as disulfide-bonded dimers in the cartilage matrix. Because cysteine residues are not normally present within the triple helical domain of type II collagen, it is likely that this mutation causes structural alterations in articular cartilage matrix that may lead to the premature failure and degeneration of the tissue. A study by Eyre et al. (25) also showed the presence of abnormal type II procollagen molecules containing cysteine at the amino acid location expected from the mutation in the gene in articular cartilage from one affected member of the same family.

NEW APPROACHES TO IDENTIFY TYPE II COLLAGEN GENE MUTATIONS WHEN ARTICULAR CARTILAGE TISSUE IS NOT AVAILABLE

Confirmation that a mutation identified at the DNA level is responsible for a given disease phenotype is the finding of the corresponding mutated protein in the affected tissues and the demonstration that it displays an abnormal function or has an altered structure. The demonstration of abnormalities in the function of the macromolecular components of articular cartilage in OA has been severely hampered by the difficulty of obtaining sufficient amounts of intact, native molecules from the tissues. Extraction of collagens from cartilage usually involves the use of denaturing agents such as guanidine hydrochloride, lithium salts, etc., and/or limited proteolysis with pepsin or chymotrypsin. Identification of structural defects at the mRNA level has also been limited by the availability of sufficient amounts of type II procollagen mRNA from tissues or chondrocyte cultures from affected individuals. Therefore, recent interest has been placed on the identification of type II collagen gene mutations when cartilage or chondrocytes are not available. To this end, Ala-Kokko et al. (26) examined the possibility of obtaining expression of the human type II procollagen gene in cultured NIH 3T3 cells, starting with genomic DNA obtained from human peripheral blood mononuclear cells or cultured fibroblasts. A chimeric gene construct was designed to test the hypothesis that the promoter of the proα1(I) collagen gene would drive expression of human type II procollagen in NIH 3T3 cells that normally express type I procollagen but do not synthesize any cartilage-specific proteins such as type II procollagen. The chimeric gene was inserted into the cosmid vector pJB8. The resulting modified vector contained (a) the promoter region, the first exon, and part of the first intron of the proα1(I) collagen gene (COL1A1); (b) two fragments of 14 kb and 12 kb isolated from a cosmid clone of the human type II procollagen gene (the two fragments contained exons 2B to 52 of the gene); (c) a 3.5 kb fragment from the 3′ end of the normal human type II pro-collagen gene containing the proper signals for termination of transcription; and (d) a 7 kb stuffer fragment (Fig. 3). The cosmid vector containing the chimeric type I/type II procollagen gene was used for cotransfection with a neomycin-resistant gene into NIH 3T3 cells by calcium phosphate precipitation. Clones of NIH 3T3 cells resistant to the neomycin analog G418 were isolated and the levels of type II procollagen mRNA as assayed by slot-blot and Northern blot hybridization with a human cDNA for COL2A1 (21) were examined. Several stable clones that expressed high levels of type II procollagen mRNA were selected and expanded. The production of human type II collagen in the permanently transfected NIH 3T3 cells was demonstrated employing type II collagen-specific antibodies to detect the protein by immunoelectrophoresis (Fig. 4).

The system will make it possible to obtain mRNA for human type II procol-lagen and the corresponding protein in mouse cells from cosmid clones prepared with genomic DNA from patients with familial OA. In addition to obtaining type II procollagen mRNA, large-scale production of the recombinant human

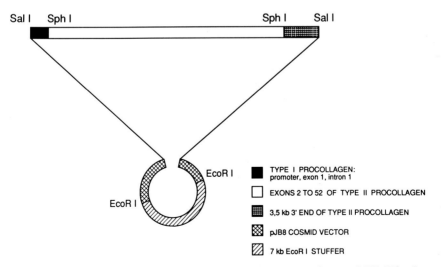

FIG. 3. The chimeric gene construct employed for permanent transfection of NIH 3T3 cells.

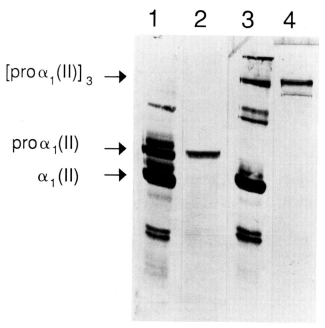

FIG. 4. Western blot analysis of proteins from NIH 3T3 cells transfected with a chimeric gene construct containing the human type I procollagen gene promoter ligated to exons 2B to 52 of the human type II procollagen gene. **Lane 1:** Standard; **lane 2:** media plus cell extract; **lanes 3,4:** same as lanes 1 and 2, nonreduced.

type II procollagen in native and pure form appears feasible. The availability of quantitative amounts of the protein will permit, for the first time, the performance of extensive structural and functional studies. For example, it will be possible to determine the thermal stability of the intact procollagen, the kinetics of procollagen cleavage and collagen fibril formation, the assembly of supramolecular aggregates with proteoglycans, and the role of the minor collagens (types VI, IX, and XI collagens) in regulating type II collagen fibril size and structure, etc.

IDENTIFICATION OF MUTATIONS IN GENES FOR OTHER CARTILAGE COLLAGENS

In addition to the benefits of RFLP genetic linkage analysis to identify the genes that may be at fault in heritable OA, RFLP analysis can give valuable negative information, because the absence of cosegregation (i.e., recombination) with the disease phenotype can exclude a candidate gene in a given family. Knowlton et al. showed the presence of recombination between the disease phenotype and the type II procollagen gene in one of the families with Stickler syndrome they studied (18). This observation conclusively excluded a mutation in COL2A1 as the cause of the disease phenotype in this family. Similar analyses of another family with Stickler syndrome and a large family with severe premature OA associated with CPPD deposition failed to show cosegregation of COL2A1 polymorphisms with the disease phenotype (Knowlton et al., unpublished observations). These results suggest that mutations in genes other than COL2A1 may be responsible for the disease phenotype in certain subsets of heritable OA. It is apparent, therefore, that a careful search for mutations in other genes expressed in articular cartilage matrix should be carried out in families with OA. In the past, attempts to identify such mutations would have been nearly impossible with the small amounts of articular cartilage available to extract mRNA. The recent introduction of the polymerase chain reaction (PCR) and the explosive developments in PCR technology have rendered these tasks feasible even when only minute amounts of tissue are available. For example, we have recently been able to obtain cDNAs encompassing the entire coding region of the type II procollagen gene from human chondrocytes isolated from OA cartilage employing the PCR (unpublished data). Even the small amounts of articular cartilage obtained from arthroplasty or from arthroscopic surgery can be successfully utilized to prepare cDNAs for the various collagens present in articular cartilage employing appropriate oligonucleotide primers. The PCR products can be sequenced directly or can be cloned into bacterial vectors for standard sequencing procedures. Given the advances in DNA sequencing, as many as 350 bp can now be read from a single sequencing reaction. Thus, to sequence the entire coding region of the mutant genes is feasible. Single base mutations or small insertions/deletions in coding or regulatory sequences can be identified. Mutations in sequences important for splicing can also be detected utilizing oligonucleotide primers specific for intron sequences at the intron-exon boundaries when the structure of the respective genes is known. Thus, PCR amplification will allow the rapid and efficient identification of mutations not only in the genes for type II procollagen, but also in the genes for other structural components of articular cartilage from minute amounts of tissue.

CONCLUSION

The studies reviewed above have clearly confirmed the hypothesis that certain inherited forms of OA are caused by mutations in genes expressed in cartilage and specifically in the gene for the cartilage-specific type II procollagen. Further study of other forms of familial OA with the innovative techniques of molecular biology currently available or being developed will allow investigators to define the exact molecular causes of these diseases and to establish whether or not they are single entities at the molecular level. Eventually these studies may lead to the development of simple DNA tests that will permit the definitive diagnosis of the molecular defects in individual patients in whom it may be possible to initiate preventive forms of therapy before the disease becomes clinically apparent.

ACKNOWLEDGMENTS

This work was supported by Program Project Grant #AR 39740-01 from the National Institutes of Health. The expert assistance of Meredith Billman in the preparation of this manuscript is thankfully acknowledged.

REFERENCES

1. Moskowitz RW. Clinical and laboratory findings in osteoarthritis. In: McCarty DJ, ed. *Arthritis and allied conditions,* 11th ed. Philadelphia: Lea & Febiger, 1989;1605–1630.
2. Stecher RM, Hersh AH, Hauser H. Heberden's nodes: the family history and radiographic appearance of large family. *Am J Hum Genet* 1953;5:46–60.
3. Kellgren JH, Lawrence JS, Bier F. Genetic factors in generalized osteo-arthrosis. *Ann Rheum Dis* 1963;22:237–255.
4. Marks JS, Stewart IM, Hardinge K. Primary osteoarthrosis of the hip and Heberden's nodes. *Ann Rheumat Dis* 1979;38:107–111.
5. Reginato AJ. Articular chondrocalcinosis in the Chiloe islanders. *Arthritis Rheum* 1976;19:395–404.
6. Bjelle A. Cartilage matrix in hereditary pyrophosphate arthropathy. *J Rheumatol* 1981;8:959–964.
7. Stickler GB, Belau PG, Farrell FJ, Jones JD, Pugh DG, Steinberg AG, Ward LE. Hereditary progressive arthro-ophthalmopathy. *Mayo Clin Proc* 1965;40:433–455.
8. Marcos JC, DeBenyacar MA, Garcia-Morteo O, Maldonado-Cocco JA, Morales VH, Laguena RP. Idiopathic familial chondrocalcinosis due to apatite crystal deposition. *Am J Med* 1981;71: 557–564.
9. Spranger J. The epiphyseal dysplasias. *Clin Orthop Rel Res* 1975;114:46–59.
10. Kempson GE, Muir H, Pollard C, Tuke M. The tensile properties of the cartilage of human femoral condyles related to the content of collagen and glycosaminoglycans. *Biochem Biophys Acta* 1973;297:456–472.
11. Mayne R. Cartilage collagens. *Arthritis Rheum* 1989;32:241–246.
12. Comper WD, Laurent TC. Physiological function of connective tissue polysaccharides. *Physiol Rev* 1978;58:255–315.
13. Lander ES, Botstein D. Strategies for studying heterogeneous genetic traits in humans by using a linkage map of restriction fragment length polymorphisms. *Proc Natl Acad Sci USA* 1986;83: 7353–7357.
14. Sangiorgi FO, Benson-Chanda V, de Wet WJ, Sobel ME, Tsipouras R, Ramirez F. Isolation and partial characterization of the entire human proα1(I) collagen gene. *Nucleic Acids Res* 1984;13: 1025–1038.
15. Nunez AM, Francomano C, Young MF, Martin GR, Yamada Y. Isolation and partial characterization of genomic clones coding for a human proα1(II) collagen chain and demonstration of restriction fragment length polymorphism at the 3′ end of the gene. *Biochemistry* 1985;24:6343–6348.
16. Weaver EJ, Knowlton RG. A PvuII polymorphism near the 5′ end of the type procollagen gene (COL2A1). *Nucleic Acids Res* 1989;17:6429.
17. Francomano CA, Liberfarb RM, Hirose T, Maumenee IH, Streeten EA, Meyers DA, Pyeritz RE. The Stickler syndrome: evidence for close linkage to the structural gene for type II collagen. *Genomics* 1987;1:293–296.
18. Knowlton RG, Weaver EJ, Struyk AF, Knobloch WH, King RA, Norris K, Shambam A, Uitto J, Jimenez SA, Prockop DJ. Genetic linkage analysis of hereditary arthro-ophthalmopathy (Stickler syndrome) and the type II procollagen gene. *Am J Hum Genet* 1989;45:681–688.
19. Knowlton RG, Katzenstein PL, Moskowitz RW, Weaver EJ, Malemud Ch J, Pathria MN, Jimenez SA, Prockop DJ. Demonstration of genetic linkage of the type II procollagen gene (COL2A1) to primary osteoarthritis associated with a mild chondrodysplasia. *N Engl J Med* 1990;322:526–530.

20. Palotie A, Vaisanen P, Ott J, Ryhanen L, Elima K, Vikkula M, Cheah K, Vuorio E, Peltonen L. Predisposition to familial osteoarthrosis linked to type II collagen gene. *Lancet* 1989;1:924–927.
21. Baldwin CT, Reginato A, Smith C, Jimenez SA, Prockop DJ. Structure of a cDNA clone coding for human type II procollagen. The $\alpha 1(II)$ chain is more similar to the $\alpha 1(I)$ chain than two other α chains of fibrillar collagens. *Biochem J* 1989;162:521–528.
22. Ala-Kokko L, Prockop DJ. Completion of the intron-exon structure of the gene for human type II procollagen (COL2A1): variations in the nucleotide sequences of the alleles from three chromosomes. *Genomics* 1990;9:454–460.
23. Ala-Kokko L, Baldwin CT, Moskowitz RW, Prockop DJ. Single base mutation in the type II procollagen gene (COL2A1) as a cause of primary osteoarthritis associated with a mild chondrodysplasia. *Proc Natl Acad Sci USA* 1990;87:6565–6568.
24. Ahmad NN, Ala-Kokko L, Knowlton RG, Jimenez SA, Weaver EJ, Maguire JI, Tasman W, Prockop DJ. Stop codon in the procollagen II gene (COL2A1) in a family with the stickler syndrome (arthro-ophthalmopathy). 1991;88:6624–6627.
25. Eyre DR, Weis MA, Moskowitz RW. Cartilage expression of a type II collagen mutation in an inherited form of osteoarthritis associated with a mild chondrodysplasia. *J Clin Invest* 1991;87:357–361.
26. Ala-Kokko L, Hyland J, Smith C, Kivirikko K, Jimenez SA, Prockop DJ. Expression of a human cartilage procollagen gene (COL2A1) in mouse 3T3 cells. *J Biol Chem* 1991;226:14175–14178.

DISCUSSION

von der Mark: If these patients have a defect in the type II collagen gene, do they also have growth abnormalities during development?

Jimenez: Yes, these patients have a mild form of epiphyseal dysplasia. However, the presence of mild growth plate abnormalities is not unexpected because type II collagen is also expressed in the growth plate. The affected individuals have flattening of multiple ephiphyses and most are 4 to 5 inches shorter in stature than nonaffected siblings.

Peyron: Is this novel method for transfecting cells with a defective gene going to be practical on as large a scale as is needed to scrutinize the osteoarthritic population?

Jimenez: The length of time required to sequence large regions of DNA has been shortened dramatically by the recent developments in PCR technology, cloning, and other strategies. The construction of the chimeric genes and their transfection have also been advanced by development of new cosmic vectors that accept very large fragments of DNA. Therefore these techniques are becoming more feasible. Once the cells are transfected, they can be grown in large amounts and produce large quantities of protein.

van der Rest: Do the transfected cells lay down any cartilage-like matrix?

Jimenez: We were interested in examining whether or not the transfected cells would accumulate a cartilaginous matrix. However, the NIH 3T3 cells assemble very little matrix and most of the collagens synthesized are secreted into the medium.

Hascall: Did the patient that had the termination codon accumulate any mutant chains in the tissue?

Jimenez: Unfortunately, we did not have cartilage available from that patient for biochemical analyses. The limitation imposed by the difficulty in obtaining articular cartilage from affected individuals is one of the problems that we hope to overcome by the approach I described of inducing noncartilaginous cells to express the cartilage-specific proteins of interest.

Pritzker: In molecular terms, why is osteoarthritis so common while the hereditable forms are so rare?

Jimenez: We have been very surprised by the relatively large number of families with osteoarthritis in several generations that we have identified. It is possible that in the past we were not examining patients with osteoarthritis with the idea of its being genetically determined. Now we are obtaining more detailed family histories and are evaluating several members of each family. It is also possible that mutations that cause milder defects in the protein may become apparent much later in life and may, therefore, be considered sporadic rather than familial. Furthermore, milder mutations may be a predisposing factor that causes accelerated degeneration of cartilage in response to environmental or mechanical injuries. In these cases, the disease would be erroneously considered to be secondary.

Benya: Has anyone looked at the morphology of the cartilage and collagen fibrils in the patient with the cysteine mutation?

Jimenez: We unfortunately have not. The cartilage we had available was processed for biochemical studies before the mutation was identified. However, David Eyre and ourselves have shown that abnormal type II collagen molecules are present in the cartilage from affected individuals.

Eyre: In a preliminary examination with transmission electron microscopy, fibrils appeared to fuse into abnormally thick structures.

Articular Cartilage and Osteoarthritis,
edited by K. Kuettner et al.
Raven Press, Ltd., New York © 1992.

Part IV: Structural Components of Cartilage: Morphological Aspects

Introduction

T. Derek V. Cooke

Surgery Arthritis Laboratory, Department of Surgery, Queen's University, Kingston, Ontario K7L2VF, Canada

In this section are chapters by Hunziker, Poole, and von der Mark et al. Each group has contributed unique data to our expanding yet incomplete knowledge of cartilage and of its form development, maintenance, and response in disease.

This inert-appearing tissue exemplifies a highly specific, unique organization of matrix molecules to provide an extraordinary functional role of load transmission and motion between limb segments. Without disease, it functions without wear in the lifetime of the individual. The matrix, in which generally sparse cell elements are located, provides for the physical work of motion and load transmission without any direct and immediate interaction of cells. Yet the cells—often widely separated and devoid of vascular or neural connections—work under major fluctuations of physical stress to maintain and regulate the matrix.

Much of past data on cartilage were suppositions based on imperfect technology for tissue preparation, inspection, and extraction. Major advances, which included light and electron microscopy and a variety of biochemical and cellular extraction techniques, have allowed much better understanding of the tissues and cells. These are well described in chapters elsewhere in the volume as well as in this section.

We may better define structure and cell makeup as an anisotropic organization from surface to depth and in transverse planes (see chapter by Hunziker). For example, the surface tissue is rich in collagen, has a tightly bound complement of smaller molecular weight proteoglycan (PG) (decorin, etc.), but much less aggregating PG and a fiber collagen mesh-oriented parallel to the surface (see chapters by Aydelotte et al., Rosenberg, Eyre, and ref. 1). Scattered flattened cells within this zone exist without extensive capsular basketry around them (3). This surface zone, lacking the capacity to retain water, is readily deformable (see discussion in chapter by Grodzinsky); it has a cell population with important functional and possible protective role(s) (see chapter by Aydelotte et al.).

In contrast, the deep zones feature marked variations in matrix organization in the horizontal plane. Cells clustered in columns are located within dense collagenous capsules, chondrons, that contain type II, VI, IX, and XI collagens. The pericellular zone contains varying concentrations of proteoglycans. Between chondrons, the interstitial regions contain a complex, three-dimensional organization of collagen fibers weaving toward the surface. Their base seems firmly fixed within the calcified deepest zone. This interstitial basketry is subjected to tension by the high concentration of PG aggrecan, retains water strongly, and thereby transmits loads and strongly resists deformation. The turnover of matrix elements is usually slow, especially that of collagen. Thus, *in situ* hybridization for type II collagen production by chondrocytes in normal tissue shows no mRNA activity (see chapter by von der Mark et al.). But proteoglycans may be degraded rapidly from the immobilized joint and are readily restored by reactivation of chondrocytes after reintroducing load. How these processes occur and what controls them is less clear. The basal layers of cartilage cells, visualized by usual LM techniques, appear necrotic; in fact, cells are alive, intact, and actively synthesizing substrate and restraining invasion of bone (see chapter by Hunziker).

The redefinition of a functional cell unit in cartilage, the chondrone, has been revived by Poole. The concept has considerable attraction in enabling one to assess the support provided by the cell for "zones" in the cartilage. It is also attractive to consider that the capsule around the cell may provide protection or stability to resist sudden deformation or pressure change. But why do we not see these capsular structures in young cartilages or in the surface of mature tissue? How do they come to be? How do they change with disease? Poole argues that in osteoarthritis, local digestion of pericellular matrix opens the capsule which he has shown to be disorganized and have an ultrastructure. He feels the weakening may allow (i.e., promote) clonal proliferation.

Interestingly, on the question of its origin, the chondrone shows striking similarity to the strong structural organization of capsule and cells in the growth plate (see chapter by Hunziker). Shown by SEM, the interior capsular organization is amazingly similar to that of the extracted chondrone (see chapter by Poole). Both Hunziker and Poole agree (informal discussion) that prehypertrophic growth plate cells most near the surface are likely "the chondrones" in their infancy. Further histochemical and time-based extraction studies on developing cartilage will likely answer this question.

In osteoarthritis (OA), marked perturbations occur. The cartilage surface is eroded and often grossly disrupted by splits and craters that enter the basal areas. *In situ* hybridization using cDNA probes in conjunction with immunohistochemistry documents activation of cells to synthesize type II collagen at all levels in the damaged tissue (see chapter by von der Mark et al). Some limited dedifferentiation of cell type (production types I and III collagen) occurs. But an increase in type X collagen synthesis is remarkable, deposited mainly around the cells representing the most marked alteration of collagen synthesis, which are those of the mid-zone between cell clusters. Yet, mRNA message was seen only in basal layer cells! These features were taken as evidence of hypertrophy reactions by chondrocytes. This activation of type X collagen production was also evident in forming tissue of osteophytes. Thus, the "OA cell" may revert to a "hypertrophic" cell in a phase of precalcification. Corroborating evidence on similar lines has also been shown for enzyme activity using the immunohistochemical studies (see chapters by von der Mark et al. and Poole).

The cells, examined by the newly developed chondron extractions taken from normal and osteoarthritic cartilage, reveal capsular disorganization, progressive cloning, and cell replication in disease. Strong evidence now exists for significant matrix enzyme activation in conjunction with increased synthesis (see chapter by Poole). Collectively, these features support long-held beliefs that the cartilage tissue *does* have repair capacity. Evidently this capacity is far less than the rate of the degradative processes involved in its breakdown (see also final discussion).

We also now know that the turnover of matrix PG occurs within days of injury and well before any overt or microscopic signs of change occurs (see chapter by Lohmander). Thus, the data on OA described in this section likely represent advanced stages of destruction.

Should we wish to test the hypothesis that cartilage may repair itself, we must define the nature of the mechanical lesion (injury) extremely early, counter or limit the destructive pathway, and then promote repair mechanisms which these observations clearly define to be available responses of all cells at even the advanced stages of damage.

REFERENCES

1. Clark JM. The organization of collagen in cryofractured rabbit articular cartilage: a scanning electron microscopic study. *J Orthop Res* 1985;3:17–29.
2. McClure J, Bates GP, Rowston H, Grant ME. A comparison of the morphological, histochemical and biochemical features of embryonic chick sternal chondrocytes in vivo with chondrocytes cultured in three-dimensional collagen gels. *Bone Min* 1988;3:235–247.
3. Poole AR, Pidoux I, Reiner A, Rosenberg L. An immunoelectron microscope study of the organization of proteoglycan monomer, link protein, and collagen in the matrix of articular cartilage. *J Cell Biol* 1982;93:921–937.

Articular Cartilage and Osteoarthritis,
edited by K. Kuettner et al.
Raven Press, Ltd., New York © 1992.

13

Articular Cartilage Structure in Humans and Experimental Animals

Ernst B. Hunziker

M. E. Müller Institute for Biomechanics, University of Bern, 3010 Bern, Switzerland

The synovial joint ensures load transmission within skeletal structures and provides the basis for their movement towards one another. It is organized to provide almost frictionless movement, thereby preventing wear of tissue, and to act as an effective shock absorber during periods of active loading. Because these various functions are achieved simultaneously and performed in a coordinated manner, it is not surprising that joints are made up of a variety of tissues between which a close structural and functional relationship exists. The three tissue types which function in this capacity are as follows: (i) the articular cartilage tissue itself, (ii) the synovial membrane along the joint capsule together with its secretory product, the synovial fluid, and (iii) the subchondral bone plate, bone trabeculae, and associated marrow space. The coordination which exists between these tissues and various external (capsular ligaments, muscles, tendons, etc.) and internal (cruciate ligaments, menisci, etc.) components represents a finely tuned equilibrium state for optimizing functional activity combined with nutritional and structural maintenance. Under pathological conditions, each of the various joint tissues may contribute to (and be affected by) the disease process and determine the healing potential.

The structure of the joint is similar in all mammals, although significant organizational differences do exist. It is the purpose of this chapter to briefly review the basic structure, development, and function of articular cartilage tissue and to highlight certain differences existing between humans and experimental animals.

IMMATURE AND MATURE ARTICULAR CARTILAGE TISSUE

In synovial joints, the layer of hyaline articular cartilage tissue faces the joint cavity (i.e., the synovial fluid space) on one side and is linked to the subchondral bone plate via a narrow layer of calcified cartilage tissue on the other. In the mature state, its structural organization is characterized by a high degree of

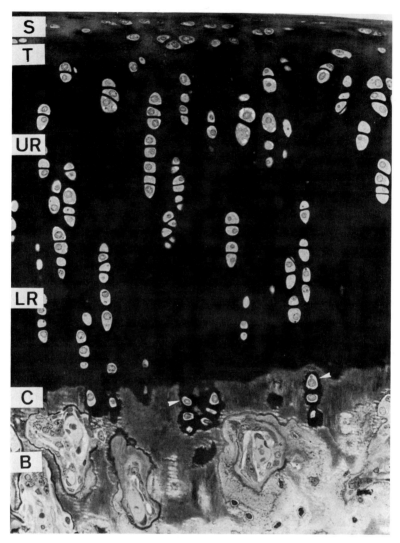

FIG. 1. Light micrograph of mature rabbit articular cartilage (femoral condyle; NZW rabbit). S, tangential zone; T, transitional zone; UR, upper radial zone; LR, lower radial zone; C, calcified cartilage; B, subchondral bone plate; *arrowheads,* chondrocytes in calcified cartilage. One-micron-thick section, stained with toluidine blue O. ×300.

anisotropy, with the cells and matrix being arranged into clearly defined zones (1,2) (Figs. 1–3). In the immature state, the layer of articular cartilage tissue is generally much thicker and unstratified, with chondrocytes being distributed in a more random, isotropic pattern. A gradient in cell size, from the superficial zone to the calcifying zone, does, however, exist with chondrocytes near the

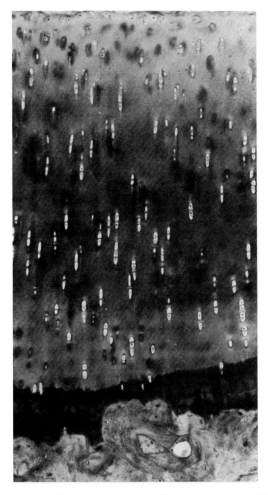

FIG. 2. Light micrograph of adult human articular cartilage (femoral condyle). Note the oblate spheroid shape of chondrocytes in the tangential zone, and the relative thinness of the calcified cartilage zone. Chemical fixation in the presence of ruthenium hexaamine trichloride. ×120.

latter region being much larger (hypertrophic). This feature reflects the growth function which the cartilage tissue additionally fulfills during postnatal development (2–4). Thus it is not surprising that during the prepubertal growth spurt, a tissue reorganization process takes place whereby articular cartilage develops a close structural resemblance to the growth plate (5). This process is, however, not achieved by a process of tissue transformation (i.e., remodeling per se) but rather by the addition of new tissue which is characterized by an increased structural anisotropy (*unpublished data*). It coincides with the increase in bio-

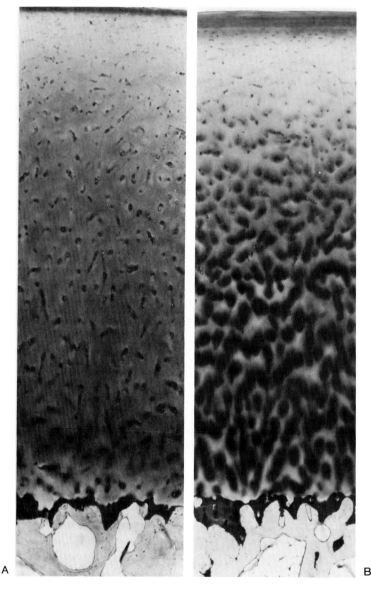

FIG. 3. Light micrographs of adult human articular cartilage (femoral condyle), chemically fixed in the presence of alcian blue (**A**) or ruthenium red (**B**). Note the difference in staining profile. ×45.

mechanical competence of mature articular cartilage tissue—that is, a dramatic improvement in its stiffness and resistance to shearing and compressive forces (6).

The differences in biomechanical properties between immature and mature articular cartilage tissue are reminiscent of those found between immature (woven) and mature (lamellar) bone forms (i.e., isotropic versus parallel organization of osteocytes and collagen fibrils within bone matrix). However, the improved mechanical competence of mature bone is achieved by a process of remodeling (i.e., tissue transformation).

HYALINE ARTICULAR CARTILAGE STRUCTURE IN HUMANS AND EXPERIMENTAL ANIMALS

A comparative analysis of hyaline articular cartilage structure in humans and experimental animals reveals significant differences with respect, for example, to anisotropic organization, zone height, cell size, and matrix mass per cell. These differences, which extend also to the neighboring tissue layers, such as calcified cartilage and subchondral bone, appear to represent species-specific adaptations.

In the medial femoral condyle, for instance, the layer of hyaline articular cartilage is 10 times thicker in humans ($\sim$2–3 mm) than in the mature rabbit ($\sim$200–300 μm) (Figs. 1 and 2). Individual zones also occupy different proportions of this layer in the two species. In humans, the tangential zone constitutes about 2–3% of the total hyaline articular cartilage height, whereas in the mature rabbit it occupies about 10% of the total thickness. In the transitional and radial zones, these differences are 5% (human) versus 10% (rabbit) and 92% (human) versus 80% (rabbit), respectively (*unpublished data*). Differences also exist in the comparative thicknesses of the underlying calcified cartilage zone and subchondral bone plate. These constitute 1–2% (human) versus 20% (rabbit) and 7–10% (human) versus 100% (rabbit), respectively, of the total height occupied by the layer of hyaline articular cartilage.

Another experimental animal also frequently used in our laboratory is the Yucatan minipig. In this animal, zonal thickness proportions within the layer of hyaline articular cartilage are closer to those in humans. Values for the tangential, transitional, and radial zones are 5% (human: 2–3%), 5% (human: 5%), and 90% (human: 92%), respectively. The total hyaline articular cartilage thickness is, however, much smaller (i.e., 800 μm as compared to 2–3 mm). The underlying calcified cartilage zone and subchondral bone plate occupy 15% (human: 1–2%) and 35% (human: 7–10%), respectively, of the thickness taken up by the layer of hyaline articular cartilage. These structural differences between the species suggest that the various layers fulfill diverse biomechanical functions according to the different postural and locomotive habits of the animal (7).

With respect to the structure of individual chondrocytes within the various zones of hyaline articular cartilage, differences between mature humans and rabbits are much smaller (Figs. 2 and 4). The superficial zone generally consists of flat, spindle-like, or elipsoidal-like chondrocytes (Fig. 4A), surrounded by a network of fine collagen fibrils (8–13). This region is less rich in proteoglycans [as indicated by staining density in the light microscope and by numerical density of matrix granules (precipitated proteoglycans) in the electron microscope] than are the deeper zones. Human chondrocytes here tend to have a more elipsoidal-

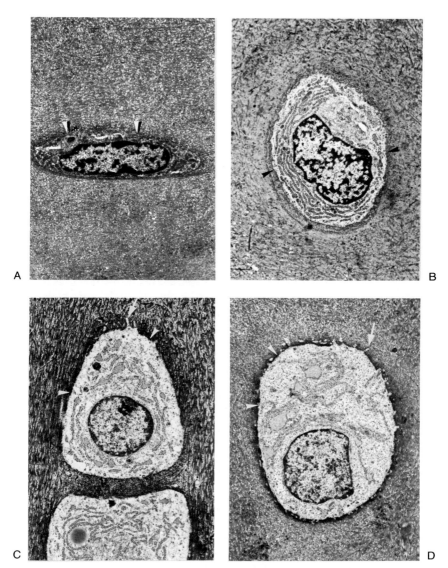

FIG. 4. Electron micrographs of chondrocytes originating from the different zones of mature articular cartilage (femoral condyle; NZW rabbit). **A:** Tangential zone chondrocyte; oblate spheroid or spindle-like in shape. ×3550. **B:** Transitional zone chondrocyte; spheroid in shape. ×3550. **C, D:** Upper (**C**) and lower (**D**) radial zone chondrocytes, frequently prolate spheroid ("super-egg-like") in shape. ×3550. *Arrowheads,* pericellular matrix compartment; *arrows,* cell processes.

like (oblate spheroid) profile, whereas rabbit chondrocytes are generally flatter or even spindle-like.

In the transitional zones (Fig. 4B) of both species, the cells are more spherical. The collagen fibrillar architecture in the interterritorial matrix compartment is relatively disorganized (8,9). This impression most likely reflects the arcade-like organization in various directions of space, as originally described by Benninghoff (14). The vertical orientation of this framework begins at the calcified cartilage–bone interface (cement line) and continues through the region of calcified cartilage and the radial zone of hyaline articular cartilage. The fibrils start to curve within the transitional zone, and they assume a tangential orientation with respect to the articular cartilage surface in the interterritorial matrix compartment of the tangential zone. In both the superficial and transitional zones, chondrocytes usually exist as single entities within their territorial matrix compartment. Chondrocytes of the radial zone (Figs. 3, 4C, and 4D) are the largest in size (15–19). In the upper portion they are frequently present as single cells, whereas in the middle and lower portions they usually occur in groups (Fig. 5) of three to four (also called *chondrones*). In general, they exhibit a prolate spheroid (super-egg-like) profile. All cells within this zone are both structurally and functionally integral. In the upper and lower regions, they are rich in cytoplasmic organelles (such as endoplasmic reticulum and the Golgi apparatus). In the middle portion, they frequently contain large numbers of intermediate filaments, which are often in the form of whirls. The typical organization of these chondrocytes into vertical

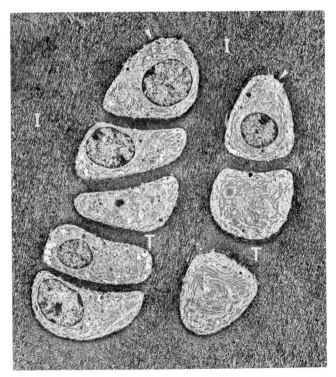

FIG. 5. Electron micrograph of two chondrocyte groups (chondrones) in the radial zone of mature articular cartilage (femoral condyle; NZW rabbit). The pericellular (*arrowheads*) and inner territorial (T) matrix compartments are included within the definition of a chondrone. The interterritorial (I) matrix compartments and the outer part of the territorial compartments together comprise the largest proportion of the mature articular cartilage matrix. ×2200.

columns and cell groups most likely reflects the previous double function which articular cartilage tissue played during postnatal growth—namely, as hyaline articular cartilage and as a superficial growth plate. In this latter capacity, stem cells were produced, passed through a proliferative phase in the transitional and upper radial zones, and then underwent hypertrophic changes in the middle and lower radial zone. On the basis of this analogy to growth-plate structure and function, the mechanism by which chondrones are formed may be readily understood.

MATRIX COMPARTMENTALIZATION

The staining profile observed in microscopic sections of cartilage tissue originally served as the basis for delineating its various matrix compartments (20). It was soon realized, however, that their appearance varied considerably according to the fixation (21) and staining (20) protocol adopted. This phenomenon is illustrated with adult human articular cartilage that is (a) fixed in the presence of either alcian blue, ruthenium red, or ruthenium hexaamine trichloride and (b) surface-stained using McNeil tetrachrome and toluidine blue O (Figs. 2, 3, and 6). Clearly, matrix compartmentalization had to be based on more reliable criteria, and this was provided by the organization of the collagen fibrillar network (10,12,13,20) (Figs. 5 and 7). The pericellular (or lacunar) matrix compartment, which immediately surrounds the chondrocyte plasmalemma, is characterized by the absence of cross-banded fibrillar collagen and a richness in proteoglycans (Fig. 7). Adjacent to this lies the territorial (or capsular) matrix compartment, which is characterized by a fine network of fibrillar (cross-banded) collagen ex-

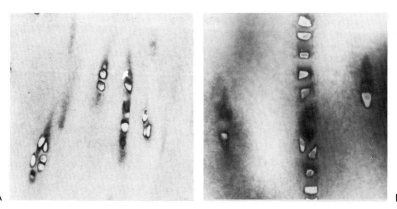

A   B

FIG. 6. Light micrograph of chondrocyte groups (chondrones) in the radial zone of human adult articular cartilage (femoral condyle). Chemical fixation was carried out in the presence of either ruthenium hexaamine trichloride (**A**) or ruthenium red (**B**). Note the difference in chondrone staining profile. ×250.

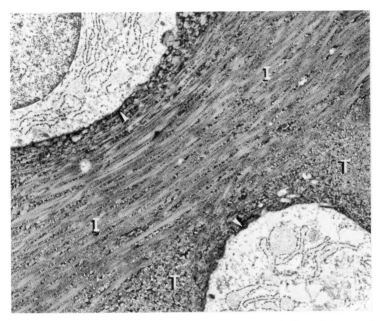

FIG. 7. High-power electron micrograph of matrix compartments in the radial zone of mature articular cartilage (femoral condyle; NZW rabbit). *Arrowheads,* pericellular matrix; T, territorial matrix; I, interterritorial matrix. ×8700.

tending around individual chondrocytes and, in its outer extremities, around groups of chondrocytes [i.e., chondrones (13)]. This compartment exhibits a high mechanical resistance during homogenization procedures (13). Chondrocytes establish contact with collagen fibrils of the territorial matrix via the protrusion of fine cytoplasmic processes (4,16,22) which contain abundant microfilaments; the plasma membrane of their outer extremities is rich in anchorin (23). The structural coherence of these cell processes within the collagen fibril network of the territorial matrix is well illustrated in tissue fixed according to routine chemical methods in the absence of a cationic dye. Under these conditions, the pericellular matrix compartment becomes completely depleted of proteoglycans, and the cell collapses and retracts [giving rise to the so-called lacuna (2,24)]. A few of its cytoplasmic processes do, however, usually withstand the retraction forces and remain lodged in the territorial network. This phenomenon gives rise to the star-like appearance of chondrocytes preserved by such means (2,24).

The interterritorial and outermost matrix compartment constitutes the largest domain in most hyaline cartilages. It is characterized by cross-banded collagen fibrils or fibers running in parallel (Fig. 7). The concentration of proteoglycans in the interfibrillar space varies according to the zone within which the chondrocytes are functioning.

CHONDROCYTE METABOLIC DOMAIN

The basic organization of the matrix into pericellular, territorial, and interterritorial compartments (10,12,13) remains the same in all zones of hyaline articular cartilage tissue. However, the size of the whole matrix coat surrounding each chondrocyte, as well as the relative thicknesses of individual compartments, may vary considerably.

The size of the matrix domain under metabolic control by an individual chondrocyte [defined as the ratio of matrix mass (per unit volume of tissue) to the number of cells (per unit volume of tissue)] also shows species-specific variation (Figs. 1 and 2). For example, in immature articular cartilage of the rabbit—in which the matrix has not yet been compartmentalized, but exists as an isotropic homogenous mass around the cells—the mean metabolic domain of a single chondrocyte is about 4000 μm^3. The corresponding volume for a mid-radial zone cell in the mature rabbit is 30,000 μm^3, and that for the adult human is 180,000 μm^3. Differences are also apparent with respect to other parameters. For example, the volume densities of chondrocytes within the mid-radial zone for mature rabbit and adult human articular cartilage are approximately 15% (15,16) and 4.7% (17–19), respectively, and the corresponding numbers of chondrocytes per cubic millimeter of zone tissue for these two species are 55,000 and 1800, respectively.

The idea of isolating chondrones (13,25,26) rather than chondrocytes from cartilage tissue has recently gained a new foothold for studies carried out *in vitro* (see chapter by Poole, also see refs. 25 and 26). In this case, the innermost part of the matrix coat surrounding a cell or cell group is isolated together with its encased chondrocyte(s). In the superficial, tangential, and upper radial zones, single-cell chondrones normally exist, whereas in the mid- and lower radial zones, multiple-cell chondrones are present (Fig. 5), and it is usually the latter which are analyzed *in vitro*. It is important to remember that only about 5% of the original "metabolic" matrix coat of the chondrone remains adherent after the isolation procedure. In the case of mature rabbit articular cartilage, the total matrix volume per chondrone in the mid-radial zone is approximately 80,000 μm^3; after isolation of the chondrone and destruction of the interterritorial and outer territorial matrix compartments, the "metabolic" domain controlled by these cells will be reduced to about 5000 μm^3. In the case of mature human articular cartilage, the corresponding reduction is from 550,000 μm^3 to 25,000 μm^3. As such, the isolated chondrone represents a very artificial unit, and great caution must be exercised in interpreting data from these studies and in extrapolating to the physiological situation.

CALCIFIED CARTILAGE

This generally narrow layer is interposed between the hyaline articular cartilage tissue and the subchondral bone plate (Figs. 8–10). The interposition is char-

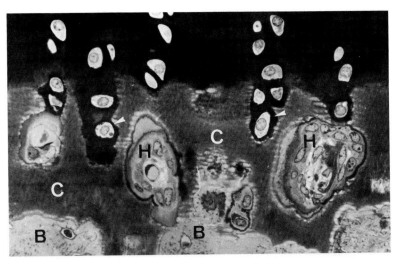

FIG. 8. Light micrograph of the calcified cartilage zone of mature rabbit articular cartilage (femoral condyle; NZW rabbit). *Arrowheads,* calcified zone chondrocytes, exhibiting structural integrity; C, calcified cartilage; H, Haversian remodeling; B, subchondral bone tissue. ×390.

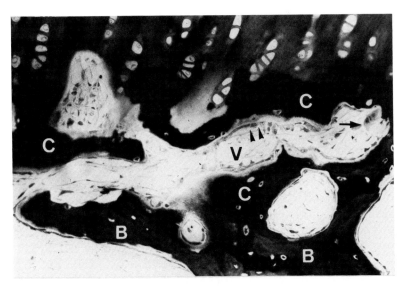

FIG. 9. Light micrograph of calcified cartilage zone penetrated by a Haversian canal, longitudinally sectioned (femoral condyle; NZW rabbit). The canal contains a blood vessel (V) and is lined laterally by osteoblasts (*arrowheads*) and apically by osteoclasts (*arrow*). C, calcified cartilage; B, subchondral bone tissue. ×200.

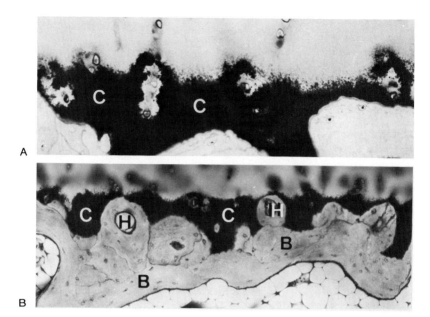

FIG. 10. Light micrograph of calcified cartilage zones (C) in human adult articular cartilage (femoral condyle). **A:** Structurally intact chondrocytes control matrix metabolism within this zone. ×150. **B:** Haversian remodeling processes (H) govern the progressive transformation of calcified cartilage tissue (C) into bone (B). ×75.

acterized by extensive interdigitation, which most likely serves for structural and mechanical integration. When routine chemical fixation procedures are adopted, as is frequently the case in pathology laboratories, chondrocytes within this tissue layer usually appear collapsed or disintegrated or may even be completely dissolved away [27,28 (review)]. For these reasons, numerous investigators believe that the chondrocytes here are necrotic or dead. However, when appropriate chemical fixation (including a cationic dye) and embedding procedures are adopted, chondrocytes within this layer exhibit a normal structure (Figs. 8 and 10–12), a precondition for which is (of course) that they are functioning normally (28). We have recently tested this capacity in mature rabbit calcified cartilage and, indeed, found that these chondrocytes take up [^{35}S]sulfate and incorporate it into their pericellular and territorial matrix compartments (light-microscopic autoradiography, *unpublished data*).

The borderline—or, rather, the interface plane—between hyaline articular cartilage and the zone of calcified cartilage is called the *tidemark* (29–31). This represents none other than a normal mineralization front (Fig. 13A). During postnatal growth, this front advances and the matrix compartment becomes actively mineralized (Fig. 13B), whereas in the adult the reverse mechanism is operative: Mineralization in this region must be continuously suppressed in order to prevent its progression and potential destruction of the hyaline articular car-

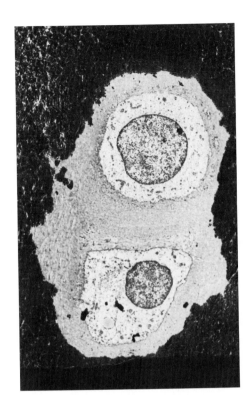

FIG. 11. Electron micrograph of chondrocytes in mature rabbit articular cartilage (femoral condyle; NZW rabbit). The pericellular and inner territorial matrix compartments remain uncalcified, and the cells remain structurally intact. ×2750.

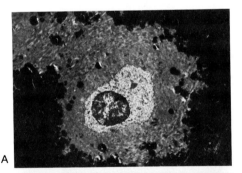

A

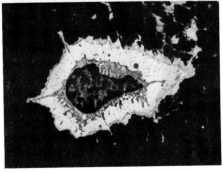

B

FIG. 12. A: Electron micrograph of a chondrocyte in the calcified cartilage zone of human adult articular cartilage (femoral condyle). The pericellular and inner territorial matrix compartments remain unmineralized. ×2100. **B:** Osteocyte and its surrounding lacuna in the subchondral bone tissue of adult human articular cartilage (femoral condyle). Note the radiating canaliculi containing fine cell processes. ×2100.

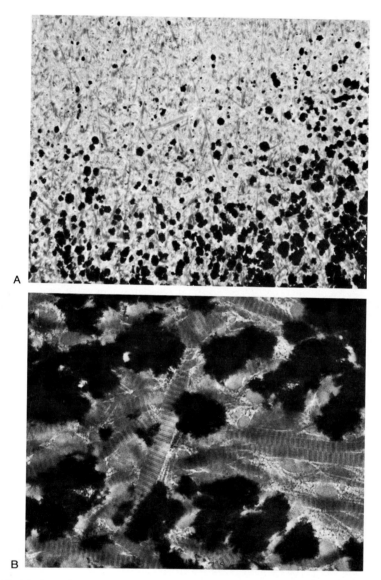

FIG. 13. Electron micrographs of the tidemark (**A**) and mineralized material (**B**) in the calcified cartilage zone of adult human articular cartilage (femoral condyle). Note that the tidemark does not appear as a discrete line, but rather as a "fuzzy" zone of increasing mineral density which represents a mineralization front. As seen in **B**, collagen fibers become completely embedded within the mineralized mass. **A:** ×4900. **B:** ×33,000.

tilage tissue. We thus hypothesize that the cells near the tidemark, (i.e., predominantly those of the lower radial zone) exert a continuous and active suppression of the mineralization processes in this area. This view conflicts with that most frequently presented in the literature (see chapter by Oegama and Thompson). It is generally believed that cell activity and mineralization in this region is low or even completely absent, and that only after traumatic insults or during the early phases of osteoarthritis do chondrocytes near the tidemark become activated and induce mineralization for a period of time. As a consequence of this, the mineralization front advances for a limited spatial interval. We believe the reverse situation to be the case—namely, that following trauma (or during the early active phase of osteoarthritis) the metabolic activity of chondrocytes in this region becomes transiently impaired, thereby allowing mineralization to become possible once again. However, this hypothetical interpretation of data still requires experimental confirmation.

In physiologically calcified tissues, such as woven and lamellar bone, the incorporated cells (osteocytes) (Fig. 12B) cannot undertake a complete remodeling of the matrix, particularly not the mineralized component. The same applies for the zone of calcified cartilage with its incorporated chondrocytes [which are always surrounded by an unmineralized pericellular and interterritorial matrix (Fig. 11)]. The only means by which compact calcified tissue layers (such as cortical bone) may be transformed in mammalian organisms is via the process of Haversian remodeling. This mechanism is also operative in the calcified cartilage zone (Figs. 8, 9, and 10B) and is the reason why this layer becomes progressively narrower with increasing age (32,33). In this context, it is interesting to note that osteoclasts, which are responsible for the resorption phase in Haversian remodeling processes, apparently cannot distinguish between calcified cartilage matrix and calcified bone matrix nor indeed between enclosed chondrocytes and enclosed osteocytes; remodeling of these two tissue types is thus achieved by the same mechanism.

ACKNOWLEDGMENTS

The author is indebted to Ceri England for her English correction of the manuscript, to Eva Kapfinger for her technical assistance and help with the artwork, and to Verena Rickli for her secretarial assistance. This work was supported by the AO/ASIF Foundation (Switzerland) and by the Swiss National Science Foundation, grant no. 31-25723.88.

REFERENCES

1. Buckwalter J, Hunziker E, Rosenberg L, Coutts R, Adams M, Eyre D. Articular cartilage: composition and structure. In: Woo SLY, Buckwalter JA, eds. *Injury and repair of the musculoskeletal soft tissues.* Park Ridge, IL: American Academy of Orthopaedic Surgeons, 1987;405–425.

2. Hunziker EB, Herrmann W. Ultrastructure of cartilage. In: Bonucci E, Motta PM, eds. *Ultrastructure of skeletal tissues.* Boston: Kluwer Academic Publishers, 1990;79–109.

3. Hunziker EB. Struktur und Funktion des Gelenkknorpels. In: Glinz W, Kieser C, Munzinger U, eds. *Arthroskopie bei Knorpelschäden und bei Arthrose.* Stuttgart: Ferdinand Enke Verlag, 1990;1–7.

4. Schenk RK, Eggli PS, Hunziker EB. Articular cartilage morphology. In: Kuettner KE, Schleyerbach R, Hascall VC, eds. *Articular cartilage biochemistry.* New York: Raven Press, 1986;3–22.

5. Hunziker EB, Schenk RK, Cruz-Orive LM. Quantitation of chondrocyte performance in growth-plate cartilage during longitudinal bone growth. *J Bone Joint Surg* 1987;69A(2):162–173.

6. Mow V, Rosenwasser MP. Articular cartilage: biomechanics. In: Woo SLY, Buckwalter JA, eds. *Injury and repair of the musculoskeletal soft tissues.* Park Ridge, IL: American Academy of Orthopaedic Surgeons, 1987;427–463.

7. Athanasiou KA, Rosenwasser MP, Buckwalter JA, Malinin TI, Mow VC. Interspecies comparisons of in situ intrinsic mechanical properties of distal femoral cartilage. *J Orthop Res* 1991;9:330–340.

8. Clark JM. The organisation of collagen fibrils in the superficial zones of articular cartilage. *J Anat* 1990;171:117–130.

9. Clark JM. Variation of collagen fiber alignment in a joint surface: a scanning electron microscope study of the tibial plateau in dog, rabbit and man. *J Orthop Res* 1991;9:246–257.

10. Eggli PS, Herrmann W, Hunziker EB, Schenk RK. Matrix compartments in the growth plate of the proximal tibia of rats. *Anat Rec* 1985;211:246–257.

11. Ghadially FN. *Fine structure of synovial joints: a text and atlas of the ultrastructure of normal and pathological articular tissues.* London: Butterworths, 1983.

12. Poole CA, Flint MH, Beaumont BW. Morphological and functional interrelationships of articular cartilage matrices. *J Anat* 1984;138(1):113–138.

13. Szirmai JA. Structure of cartilage. In: Engel A, Larsson T, eds. *Aging of connective and skeletal tissue. Thule international symposia.* Stockholm: Norkiska Bokhandelns Förlag, 1969;163–200.

14. Benninghoff A. Ueber den funktionellen Bau des Knorpels. *Anat Anz* 1922;55:250–267.

15. Brighton CT, Kitajima T, Hunt RM. Zonal analysis of cytoplasmic components of articular cartilage chondrocytes. *Arthritis Rheum* 1984;27(11):1290–1297.

16. Eggli PS, Hunziker EB, Schenk RK. Quantitation of structural features characterizing weight- and less-weight-bearing regions in articular cartilage: a stereological analysis of medial femoral condyles in young adult rabbits. *Anat Rec* 1988;222:217–227.

17. Gilmore RStC, Palfrey AJ. Chondrocyte distribution in the articular cartilage of human femoral condyles. *J Anat* 1988;157:23–31.

18. Stockwell RA. Cell density, cell size and cartilage thickness in adult mammalian articular cartilage. *J Anat* 1971;108:584–593.

19. Vignon E, Arlot M, Patricot LM, Vignon G. The cell density of human femoral head cartilage. *Clin Orthop* 1976;121:303–308.

20. Szirmai JA. Quantitative approaches in the histochemistry of mucopolysaccharides. *J Histochem Cytochem* 1963;11:24–34.

21. Hunziker EB, Ludi A, Herrmann W. Preservation of cartilage matrix proteoglycans using cationic dyes chemically related to ruthenium hexaammine trichloride. *Histoch. Cytoch.* 1992 (in press).

22. Hunziker EB, Herrmann W, Schenk RK. Improved cartilage fixation by ruthenium hexammine trichloride (RHT): a prerequisite for morphometry in growth cartilage. *J Ultrastruct Res* 1982;81:1–12.

23. Fernandez MP, Selmin O, Martin GR, et al. The structure of anchorin CII, a collagen binding protein isolated from chondrocyte membrane. *J Biol Chem* 1988;263(12):5921–5925.

24. Hunziker EB, Herrmann W, Schenk RK. Ruthenium hexaamine trichloride (RHT)-mediated interaction between plasmalemmal components and pericellular matrix proteoglycans is responsible for the preservation of chondrocytic plasma membranes *in situ* during cartilage fixation. *J Histochem Cytochem* 1983;31(6):717–727.

25. Poole CA, Flint MH, Beaumont BW. Chondrons in cartilage: ultrastructural analysis of the pericellular microenvironment in adult human articular cartilages. *J Orthop Res* 1987;5:509–522.

26. Poole CA, Matsuoka A, Schofield JR. Chondrons from articular cartilage. III. Morphologic changes in the cellular microenvironment of chondrons isolated from osteoarthritic cartilage. *Arthritis Rheum* 1991;34(1):22–35.

27. Green WT, Martin GN, Eanes ED, Sokoloff L. Microradiographic study of the calcified layer of articular cartilage. *Arch Pathol* 1970;90:151–158.
28. Stockwell RA. *Biology of cartilage cells.* Cambridge, England: Cambridge University Press, 1979.
29. Havelka S, Horn V. Joint cartilage tidemark and periosteum: two components of one envelope. *Acta Univ Carol [Med] (Praha)* 1986;32(5/6):311–318.
30. Havelka S, Horn V, Spohrová D, Valouch P. The calcified–noncalcified cartilage interface: the tidemark. *Acta Biol Hung* 1984;35(2–4):271–279.
31. Redler I, Mow VC, Zimny ML, Mansell J. The ultrastructure and biomechanical significance of the tidemark of articular cartilage. *Clin Orthop* 1975;112:357–362.
32. Holmdahl DE, Ingelmark BE. Der Bau des Gelenkknorpels unter verschiedenen funktionellen Verhältnissen: experimentelle Untersuchung an wachsenden Kaninchen. *Acta Anat* 1948;6(4): 310–375.
33. Müller-Gerbl M, Schulte E, Putz R. The thickness of the calcified layer of articular cartilage: a function of the load supported? *J Anat* 1987;154:103–111.

DISCUSSION

Howell: Have you examined the matrix next to the tidemark with the same techniques you use to see matrix vesicles in the growth plate?

Hunziker: We have looked at about six or seven samples of human articular cartilage from young adults between 20 and 40 years of age. They all showed matrix vesicles in the interterritorial matrix compartment of the lower radial zone and near the tidemark. Mature rabbit articular cartilage also shows their presence. Exactly what role they play there is not clear.

Campion: To what extent are the differences you showed between rabbit and human cartilage species-specific, and to what extent do they reflect different joint sites with different loading? After all, there is very different loading across the human hip compared with that across a rabbit joint.

Hunziker: It is very hard to assess what is species-specific and what is dependent on mechanical load forces transmitted by the joint. In the joints of the various species we examined, namely pig, rabbit, rat, mouse, and human, the zonal organization varies considerably. We have not tried to correlate this variation with load or load transmission. This would require a comparison of the same types of joint and calculation of their average force transmissions, etc. The outcome most likely won't be a clear correlation. I suspect that the differences are predominantly genetically determined rather than mechanically.

Caterson: How often do you see cell divisions in human cartilage? How does this vary between, for example, a 20-year-old and an 80-year-old individual?

Hunziker: In tissue from human adults, I have not seen cells dividing. Mitosis can be seen, but very rarely in the mature rabbit articular cartilage.

Articular Cartilage and Osteoarthritis,
edited by K. Kuettner et al.
Raven Press, Ltd., New York © 1992.

14

Chondrons

The Chondrocyte and Its Pericellular Microenvironment

C. Anthony Poole

Department of Anatomy, University of Auckland School of Medicine, Private Bag, Auckland, New Zealand

EVOLUTION OF THE CHONDRON CONCEPT

Since the earliest studies of hyaline cartilage structure it has been recognized that the chondrocyte is surrounded by a specialized matrix distinctly different from the bulk of the intercellular matrix which makes up more than 90% of the tissue volume (1). In the 1920s, Benninghoff studied hyaline cartilages with polarized light microscopy and showed that the chondrocyte was surrounded by a specialized matrix to form a unit he named the *chondron* (discussed in ref. 1). He showed that each chondron consists of a chondrocyte, its "lacunar space," and a "perilacunar rim," and he suggested that they represent the primary functional and metabolic unit responsible for cartilage matrix homoeostasis (1). However, Benninghoff's new observations were not in accord with the established histochemical interpretations of the period, and relatively few authors over the ensuing decades have embraced his concept of the chondron as a compression-resistant, water-filled bladder which protects chondrocyte function during mechanical loading.

The expansion of research in the 1960s and 70s led to the emergence of new histochemical concepts, improvements in ultrastructural techniques, refinement of biochemical technology, and, ultimately, to new interpretations of articular cartilage structure, composition, and function. Each of these disciplines has been consistent in showing (a) a progressive increase in the concentration of chondroitin sulfate and keratan sulfate from the superficial to the deep layers of the cartilage matrix and (b) a clear subdivision of the middle and deep layers into pericellular, territorial, and interterritorial matrices (2). Alcian blue histochemistry has also shown that keratan sulfate is concentrated in the interterritorial matrix and increases with aging, whereas chondroitin sulfate is concentrated in the territorial matrix and decreases with aging. The pericellular matrix contains chondroitin sulfate and a significant proportion of the total matrix hyaluronic acid (2). Ultrastructural studies using cationic, electron-dense stains confirmed the high proteoglycan concentrations in the pericellular microenvironment, whereas conventional electron microscopy revealed large numbers of fine collagen fibers and other filamentous material forming a woven enclosure in the vicinity of the chondrocyte (2).

Yet despite the mounting evidence in support of a specialized microenvironment around the chondrocyte, Szirmai (1) was one of the few authors to support Benninghoff's original concept of the chondron. Using contemporary histochemical interpretations in conjunction with microchemical analyses, he argued that the heterogeneous distribution of proteoglycans and collagen in the matrix of horse nasal cartilage was consistent with the chondron concept. He also demonstrated that chondrons were mechanically robust structures, citing as evidence the presence of intact chondrons in the sediment resulting from high-speed homogenization of horse nasal septum and in the cartilage–bone fracture plane of an accident victim. These results prompted Szirmai to describe the chondron as a separate anatomical, mechanical, and physiological unit of cartilage, but again, little attention has been given to the subject since his retirement in the early 1970s (*personal communication*).

The introduction and application of immunohistochemical techniques at the light- and electron-microscopic levels have significantly advanced our understanding of the complex heterogeneity of the articular cartilage matrix. Numerous studies have now reported the distribution of collagens (3), glycoproteins (3), and proteoglycans (4) in the matrix of articular cartilages and are consistent in showing high pericellular concentrations of many of these components. Given the continued accumulation of data indicating a specialized microenvironment around the chondrocyte, it is surprising that the original concept of the chondron has continued to be ignored for so many years.

In an attempt to address this conundrum, we decided to repeat Szirmai's original homogenization experiments with samples of adult canine and human tibial cartilage using lower homogenization speeds. The discovery of intact chondrons in the homogenate convincingly proved that chondrons could be extracted and isolated from adult articular cartilage and therefore represent a separate microanatomical unit unique to hyaline cartilage.

ISOLATED CHONDRON MODEL

The details of chondron extraction methods have now been published (5,6). Briefly, 1-g samples of diced cartilage were homogenized at slow speeds for short periods and the larger cartilage chips allowed to settle. The flocculent suspension was collected, the sediment washed, and the suspensions pooled. This process was repeated until the sample was exhausted. Pooled suspensions were filtered through a series of nylon filters, and the final filtered suspension was collected by centrifugation. This filtered homogenate contains a heterogeneous mixture of intact chondrons, ruptured capsular ghosts lacking a chondrocyte, small cartilage chips, and collagenous debris.

Homogenization, however, is a mechanically destructive process, and yields of viable chondrons are significantly lower than those achieved by traditional enzymatic extraction of the chondrocytes. Nevertheless, the routine use of 5,6-carboxyfluorescein diacetate as a viability marker will produce yields ranging from 0.2 to 1.0×10^6 viable chondrons per gram of tissue (6). Understandably, these techniques are very much in their infancy, and further improvements in the yield of viable chondrons will be critical in the future expansion of the isolated chondron model.

Studies to date have focused on developing a variety of techniques to exploit the isolated chondron as a model of cell–matrix interactions in a natural microanatomical unit of adult articular cartilage. Our first priority has been to identify the components which constitute a normal chondron, because an understanding of composition, organization, and function is fundamental to the interpretation of degenerative changes which occur in the cellular microenvironment during osteoarthritis.

CHONDRONS: THE CHONDROCYTE AND PERICELLULAR MICROENVIRONMENT

In initial studies, wet mount preparations were viewed by phase contrast and differential interference contrast microscopy to determine chondron morphology. Single chondrons consist of a chondrocyte and a birefringent pericellular matrix enclosed within a moderately dense pericellular capsule which often extends from the basal pole to form a thick "tail." In double and multiple chondrons, each chondrocyte–pericellular matrix complex was separated from its adjacent neighbor by a dense capsular sheath continuous along the length of the linearly arranged chondron column. These morphologies are consistent with previous studies of capsular structure and its columnar organization in the middle and deep layers of vertebrate articular cartilages.

Scanning electron microscopy of chondrons collected onto millipore filters confirmed the felt-like texture of the pericellular capsule surrounding each chondrocyte (5). However, preliminary ultrastructural studies of randomly sectioned chondron pellets proved unproductive, and new correlative light- and electron-microscopic techniques have now been developed.

Histochemical methods have proved important for the routine assessment of the chondron homogenate (7). For these studies, we adapted cytological methods and collected chondrons onto cellulose acetate filters which could be cleared after staining to allow detailed light-microscopic examination of proteoglycan and protein distribution in the chondron. Preliminary results using a battery of conventional histochemical stains in conjunction with selective hyaluronidase, chondroitinase, keratanase, and collagenase extraction show that the chondron is rich in hyaluronate and chondroitin sulfate, with lesser amounts of keratan sulfate. Further studies of chondrons extracted with 4 M guanidine hydrochloride showed that the small fraction of proteoglycans traditionally resistant to extraction could be histochemically localized in the cellular microenvironment. Biochemical analyses of this resistant fraction have shown that elevated levels of hyaluronate, but reduced levels of chondroitin sulfate, are retained within the chondron, possibly by chemical or physical interactions with the pericellular collagens (7). Indeed recent studies now indicate a chondroitin sulfate chain is covalently linked to type IX collagen, demonstrating a potential link between the collagen and proteoglycan components of the pericellular matrix (for review see ref. 8).

Studies with suspensions of isolated porcine chondrons and rat chondrosarcoma chondrons reacted with monoclonal antibodies to type IX and type II collagens indicate that type IX collagen is preferentially distributed in the chondron and colocalizes with type II collagen (9). These results are consistent with recent evidence indicating that type IX collagens are cross-linked to type II collagen fibrils and project from the fibril surface in a "bottle-brush" array (8). The function of this interaction is not yet clear, although it could serve to control lateral growth of type II collagen fibrils in areas rich in type IX collagen (8).

In further studies, canine chondron suspensions reacted positively to an anti-type VI collagen antibody, with intense staining in the pericellular matrix immediately adjacent to the chondrocyte and a less intense, but quite distinct, boundary staining at the outer margins of the pericellular capsule, in the tail and in the interconnecting segments between columnated chondrons (10). Type VI collagen has only recently been identified in articular cartilage, and although its function in the chondron is not known, it has been implicated in cell-matrix adhesion and proteoglycan interaction and recently, as an anchoring network involved in stabilization of the dominant collagen network (8).

Type XI ($1\alpha,2\alpha,3\alpha$) collagen has also been immunolocalized in articular cartilage (3) and identified in the pericellular microenvironment surrounding suspension cultured chondrocytes (11). The function of this collagen also remains unclear (11), although recent results from this rapidly developing field indicate that embryonic chick cartilage contains mixed fibrils of types II, IX, and XI collagens (12). Current evidence suggests that type XI collagen may form an internal component of the type II collagen fibril (see chapter by Eikenberry et al.), further complicating our interpretation of the functional interdependency of the major and minor collagen components in the cellular microenvironment.

Preliminary experiments using antibodies to a variety of other extracellular matrix components suggest that fibronectin is also present in isolated chondrons (6). Detailed examination of the distribution and role of cell-matrix adhesion proteins, fibronectin, and glycoproteins (such as cartilage matrix glycoprotein, chondronectin, and thrombospondin) is planned in future experiments.

However, a major problem with many of these techniques is the use of chondron suspensions which require repeated centrifugation during the numerous washing procedures necessitated by these methods. In an effort to overcome these potentially damaging steps, we have been experimenting with a variety of techniques which allow us to immobilize isolated chondrons and better maintain the natural relationship between the chondrocyte and its pericellular microenvironment. These techniques have been adapted from a variety of disciplines and include collection onto filters, filter imprinting onto glass, and, most significantly, suspension of chondrons in thin layers of low-melting-point agarose gel for *in vitro* maintenance culture. Correlative light- and electron-microscopic, immunohistochemical, and preliminary autoradiographic studies of normal and osteoarthritic chondrons show that they undergo dramatic structural remodeling during degenerative osteoarthritis.

CHONDRON ULTRASTRUCTURE

Chondron Pellets

Initial studies of chondron ultrastructure utilized small samples of homogenate spun into a pellet at the bottom of an Eppendorf tube. Experience with this method indicates that the pellet must be well-compacted to survive the rigors of electron-microscopic processing. However, the centrifugation required to produce such a compact pellet exceeds that used for packing viable cells; consequently, most chondrons in the pellet were deformed to some degree. Additional problems with this method relate to the random orientation of chondrons within the block and the large amount of sectioning required. Nevertheless, many chondrons and capsular ghosts were examined and revealed a dense fibrous capsule surrounding the chondrocyte (Fig. 1A). The introduction of distortive artifacts and the laborious nature of random sectioning have prompted us to explore alternative methods of chondron preparation for transmission electron microscopy (TEM).

Filter Handling Methods

We have now developed filter collection techniques for TEM. Six filters are set in a Teflon block, and 10–20 μl of fresh homogenate was drawn onto the filter and washed with 20 ml of phosphate-buffered saline. For conventional fixation the filter was fixed *in situ* for 15 min and then transferred to fresh fixative for a further 45 min. These filters were then post-fixed in osmium, dehydrated, and processed into resin. A critical component of this technique was to render the filter transparent during the final mounting step by matching the refractile indices of the filter and the resin as closely as possible. Several filters and resin types have now been tested, and in our laboratory we have found that cellulose acetate or nucleopore filters in either Epon or LR White's resin perform satis-

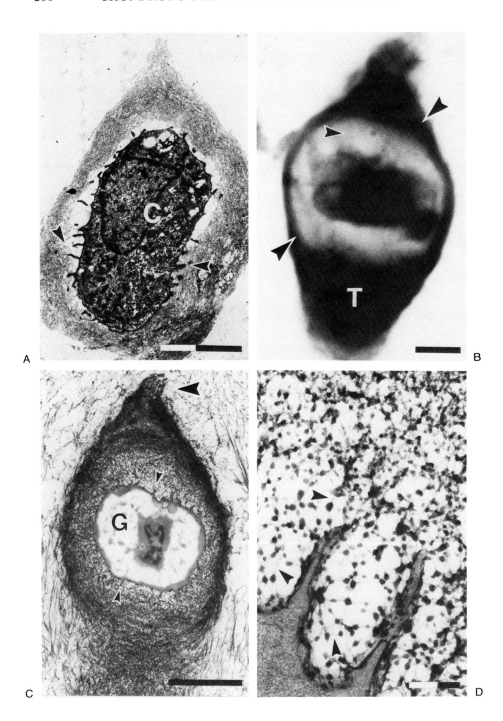

factorily. To embed the filter, it was laid sample side down on a drop of fresh resin on a slide or coverslip, with thin acetate spacers at the margins; a second drop of resin was added to the filter, and, finally, a second coverslip was placed on top which settled onto the spacers during curing. Once cured, the glass was removed from both sides of the resin with hydrofluoric acid to produce a thin, chondron-filter wafer which could be mounted on a glass slide and examined by light microscopy.

Unfortunately, conventionally prepared chondrons have little contrast, making selection difficult. This led to the introduction of the cationic proteoglycan dyes ruthenium red and ruthenium hexamine trichloride to provide contrast. Fresh filter-collected chondrons were floated, chondron side down, onto a dish of ruthenium fixative prepared according to standard protocols. Following osmium–ruthenium post-fixation, the filter was prepared according to the methods described above. The densely stained chondrons in these preparations were contrasted against the poorly stained filter and thereby facilitated the introduction of correlative light- and electron-microscopic techniques. By this method we can now examine large numbers of chondrons by light microscopy and select specific chondrons for detailed study by inscribing their position with a diamond-tipped objective. Selected chondrons were cut from the resin wafer, mounted on blocks, trimmed, and sectioned at 0.1–1.0 μm for electron microscopy. Initial studies were completed using the high-voltage electron microscope (HVEM) facility at the Wadsworth Center for Laboratories and Research, Albany, New York, and sections up to 300 nm thick were examined at a range of magnifications and goniometer tilts.

Figure 1B shows a chondron photographed in the block and subsequently examined by HVEM (Fig. 1C). Ruthenium-stained proteoglycans dominate the chondron and show a gradation in size and packing density from the cell surface to the abrupt outer margin of the capsule. Staining of the tail was consistently less intense and compacted than was the pericellular capsule surrounding the

---

FIG. 1. Chondron ultrastructure. **A:** A single chondron prepared in a pellet by conventional TEM techniques. The chondrocyte (C) has multiple cell processes, many of which remain in contact with the fine fibrous material of the pericellular capsule (*arrowheads*). Bar represents 5 μm. **B:** A single filter-collected chondron stained with ruthenium red and photographed in a resin wafer. Staining in the pericellular matrix (*small arrowhead*) is markedly less intense than that in the pericellular capsule (*large arrowheads*) and tail (T). Bar represents 5 μm. **C:** The chondron from **B** sectioned at 250 nm and viewed by using a high-voltage electron microscope. This section through the margins of the chondron shows large glycogen deposits (G) within the chondrocyte and exhibits cell processes extending into the pericellular matrix (*small arrowheads*). The density of ruthenium deposits is minimal at the cell surface and maximal at the outer boundary of the chondron. A pericellular channel (*large arrowhead*) (5) is seen at the articular pole, and the tail stains intensely. Bar represents 5 μm. **D:** Detail from a section adjacent to **C**. Note the fine filamentous connections (*arrowheads*) between ruthenium-dense proteoglycan granules attached to cell processes and the plasma membrane, and also note large granules in the adjacent pericellular matrix. The size of these granules decreases as one moves outward from the chondrocyte, but their packing density increases. Bar represents 0.5 μm.

chondrocyte. Stereoscopic examination of the interaction between the cell membrane and the pericellular matrix reveals large proteoglycan granules adhering to the plasma membrane and cell processes, which are connected three-dimensionally by fine filamentous threads to large, widely spaced granules in the immediate pericellular matrix (Fig. 1D). The average size of these granules progressively decreases towards the outer margin of the capsule. However, their packing density increases dramatically and obscures all but the dominant fibrillar structure of the chondron.

We have recently attempted a variation on filter collection termed *filter imprinting*. By this method, fresh filter-collected chondrons were firmly pressed onto a cooled glass slide and the filter peeled away, leaving an imprint of the chondrons adhering to the slide. This imprint was immediately flooded with cationic fixatives and processed into resin as described above. The resin wafers produced are virtually identical to those described above, with the added advantage that the absence of the filter creates a thinner resin wafer with increased optical clarity. These methods have only recently been used for immunohistochemistry, and preliminary results have confirmed the distribution of type VI collagen in imprinted chondrons.

CHONDRONS *IN VITRO*

Radiolabeling in Suspension

A critical component of our research is to develop culture conditions to maintain isolated chondrons *in vitro*. In initial studies, chondrons were labeled in suspension with [^{35}S]sulfate and [^{3}H]glucosamine over a 12- to 24-hr period. Labeled chondrons were collected and washed by centrifugation and prepared in one of two ways: (i) A small aliquot of labeled chondrons was mixed with agarose gel, spread thinly on a glass slide, air dried, dipped in nuclear tack emulsion, and exposed for 5–15 days. These whole-mount preparations gave strong indications of sulfate and glucosamine incorporation into viable chondrons, with the intense and discrete pericellular labeling contrasting markedly with the absence of label in adjacent nonviable chondrons (Fig. 2A and 2B). This method, however, has proved of limited value at the present time, and alternative techniques have been developed. (ii) Labeled chondrons were collected onto cellulose acetate filters, fixed in Karnovsky's fixative with and without cetylpyridinium chloride, stained with alcian blue to visualize the chondrons, and embedded in resin as described above. Chondrons considered viable by morphological criteria could then be selected by light microscopy, sectioned at 1 μm, mounted on glass slides, dipped in emulsion, and exposed for 7–21 days. The increased resolution afforded by these techniques allows clear identification of chondron compartments and confirms that synthesized material is preferentially localized in the pericellular matrix around the chondrocyte, with significantly less label penetrating the tail or interconnecting segments between adjacent chondrons (Fig.

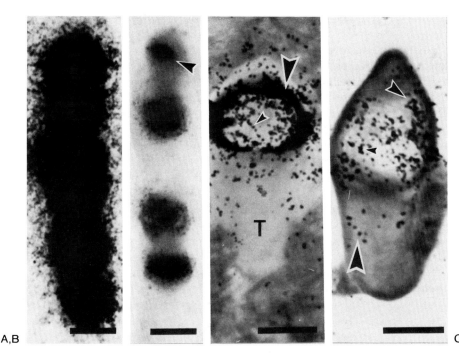

A,B   C,D

FIG. 2. Radiolabeling of chondrons in suspension. **A:** Whole-mount preparation of a chondron column continuously labeled with [^{35}S]sulfate for 24 hr. Intense labeling is seen over all five chondrocytes within the column, indicating sequestration and retention of synthesized material within the chondron. Bar represents 20 μm. **B:** Whole-mount preparation labeled with [^{3}H]glucosamine over a 24-hr period. Dense silver granules can be seen around three of the chondrocytes in the column, indicating synthesis and retention of glycosaminoglycans within the pericellular matrix. One nonviable cell showed a complete absence of label (*arrowhead*). Bar represents 20 μm. **C:** Single chondron labeled with [^{35}S]sulfate for 24 hr, embedded in resin and sectioned at 1 μm prior to autoradiography. The increased resolution afforded by this technique shows intracellular processing of label (*small arrowhead*) and intense sequestration of secreted material in the pericellular matrix around the chondrocyte (*large arrowhead*). Smaller quantities of label have diffused radially from the chondron, but there is no evidence of a preferential accumulation of newly synthesized material within the tail (T). Bar represents 10 μm. **D:** Single chondron labeled with [^{3}H]glucosamine and processed as described for **C.** Although incorporation of this label is significantly less than that for [^{35}S]sulfate, intracellular processing (*small arrowhead*) and pericellular sequestration are clearly evident (*medium arrowhead*). There seems little evidence of diffusion, and some material has entered the tail region (*large arrowhead*). Bar represents 10 μm.

2C and 2D). Although these studies indicate a discrete pericellular sequestration of synthesized proteoglycans within the chondron, material passing outside the confinement of the chondron was lost in this type of analysis. Recent studies have now shown that chondrocytes cultured in agarose gel retain synthesized material and form a pericellular matrix (13) which may resemble that found in isolated chondrons. We have recently introduced agarose gel culture to maintain the isolated chondron phenotype *in vitro*.

Chondron–Agarose Gels

No attempts have yet been made to preferentially select viable chondrons from a cartilage homogenate. Instead, the entire sample was mixed with low-melting-point agarose gel according to previously published methods (13). One-milliliter aliquots of the chondron–agarose gel were spread on a basal layer of agarose, allowed to gel, flooded with medium, and incubated at 37°C. Initial studies used a combination of alcian blue histochemistry and 5,6-carboxyflu-orescein diacetate as viability markers and showed that differentiated chondron structures can be successfully maintained *in vitro* for periods up to 4 weeks. Metabolic studies with this system are planned, and autoradiography of pulse-chased cultures are currently in progress. When the basal acellular layer is omitted, viable chondrocytes within chondrons and small cartilage chips dedifferentiate on the plastic culture dish and proliferate over the entire surface beneath the gel during 4 weeks of culture. Accordingly, this system was only used for short-term culture of 1–3 days.

An interesting feature of agarose gel culture methods is the accessibility of histochemical and immunohistochemical probes to the structures immobilized within. In a recent study (Poole and Aydelotte, *unpublished observations*), we have shown that chondrocytes isolated from bovine cartilage and cultured in agarose produce a highly differentiated pericellular matrix which contains, among other things, type VI collagen as visualized by immunohistochemistry (Fig. 3A). In addition to identifying the production of a "chondron-like" structure in long-

⟶

FIG. 3. Distribution of anti-type VI collagen antibody. **A:** Fixed whole-mount preparation of a bovine chondrocyte cultured for 15 weeks in agarose gel, digested with testicular hyaluronidase, reacted with antibody, and visualized with peroxidase-DAB without counterstaining. The pericellular calyx (*arrowheads*) surrounding the chondrocyte stains intensely for type VI collagen, suggesting the formation of "chondron-like" structures in long-term culture of isolated chondrocytes. Bar represents 10 μm. **B:** Whole mount of an isolated chondron immunolabeled in suspension and visualized using FITC. Labeling was most intense in the capsule surrounding the chondrocyte (*small arrowheads*), but persists as a patchy array in the tail (*large arrowhead*). Bar represents 10 μm. **C:** Two single chondrons immunolabeled in agarose gel with peroxidase-DAB-OsO$_4$ and photographed in the resin wafer prior to selection and sectioning. A pericellular channel is seen at the articular pole (*small arrowhead*), whereas the characteristic gap between the tail of one chondron and the capsule of its subjacent neighbor seen with type VI collagen antibody is clearly evident (*large arrowhead*). Bar represents 20 μm. **D:** Detail from a 1-μm section of the chondrons shown in **C.** Dense antibody labeling is evident around the chondrocyte (*small arrowhead*) and, in the tail, has a defined but clumpy distribution (*medium arrowhead*). The gap between the tail and capsule contains no label (*large arrowhead*), but chondron continuity was maintained by other fine fibers which do not react with this antibody. Similarly, type II collagen fibers adhering to the chondron are not stained (*double-headed arrow*). Bar represents 10 μm. **E:** Detailed electron micrograph from a section adjacent to that shown in **D.** Antibody label appears as a dense granular precipitate which was concentrated and clumped in the pericellular capsule (*large arrowheads*), and it was totally absent from type II collagen fibers adjacent to the chondron (*medium arrowheads*). Granular reaction product was also evident over the surface of cell processes and the plasma membrane, and it forms a filamentous continuum (*small arrowheads*) with the densely labeled capsule. The section was counterstained with uranyl acetate and lead citrate. Bar represents 0.5 μm.

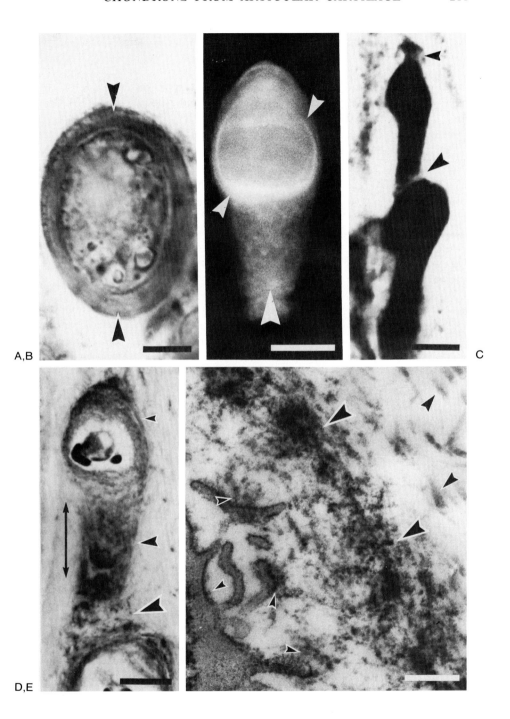

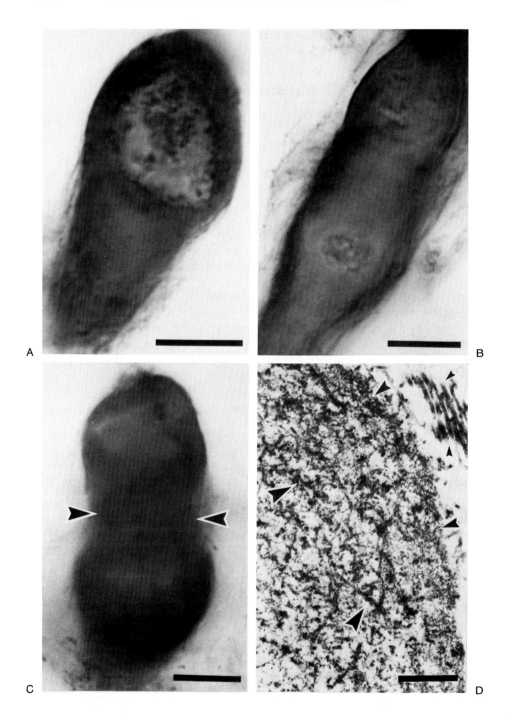

term agarose gel culture, these studies highlight the potential to immobilize chondrons for immunohistochemistry.

Immunohistochemistry

For these studies, we omit the basal agarose layer to produce a thinner, more optically transparent gel. After 12–48 hr of culture, the samples were fixed *in situ* for 1 hr and were washed extensively with PBS; plugs 5 mm in diameter were then cored from the center of the culture dish. These plugs are quite robust and can be stored in PBS for several weeks at 4°C (14).

A variety of fixatives have been qualitatively tested for structural preservation and epitope retention (14). Acid alcohol (99% of 95% ethanol, 1% glacial acetic acid) gave the best epitope retention, but chondrocyte structure was poorly preserved. Conversely, 2% glutaraldehyde gave the best structural preservation, but retention of epitope activity was reduced compared with acid alcohol or formaldehyde. We finally compromised on a combination of 2% formaldehyde–1% glutaraldehyde which gave reasonable ultrastructural preservation and sufficient epitope retention to allow visualization by electron microscopy (14).

For immunohistochemical experiments, individual plugs are transferred to PBS in a multiwell plate and preparative enzyme pretreatment is completed under appropriate conditions. Type VI collagen antibody has been used to validate this system because it has previously been shown to stain isolated chondrons in suspension (Fig. 3B) (10). Using fluorescent and peroxidase-DAB probes, we identified a type VI collagen distribution in chondron–agarose gels which was almost identical with that found in chondron suspensions (Fig. 3C). More im-

←————————————————————————————————————

FIG. 4. Immunolocalization of proteoglycan–GAG epitopes in chondron–agarose gels. **A:** A single chondron, fixed in glutaraldehyde–formaldehyde, digested with chondroitinase ABC, and reacted with antibody MK-302 which recognizes chondroitin-6-sulfate stubs attached to the core protein through linkage tetrasaccharides. The intense and uniform reaction throughout the capsule and tail indicates that high levels of chondroitin-6-sulfate-rich proteoglycans are retained within the chondron. Bar represents 10 μm. **B:** A fresh untreated double chondron reacted with antibody BCD-4 which recognizes keratan sulfate attached to core protein peptides of the proteoglycan monomer. Staining intensity with this antibody was consistently less than that seen with MK-302, but its distribution remained fairly uniform throughout the capsule. Bar represents 10 μm. **C:** Fresh untreated double chondron reacted with antibody αHABR which recognizes the hyaluronic acid (hyaluronate) binding region of the proteoglycan core protein. Again, a strong reaction persists throughout the pericellular capsule and was particularly intense in the tail and interconnecting segment between adjacent chondrons (*arrowheads*). Bar represents 10 μm. **D:** Detailed electron micrograph of a chondron labeled prior to resin embedding with antibody 2B6 which recognizes chondroitin-4-sulfate attached to the core protein through linkage tetrasaccharides. Chondroitinase ABC pre-digestion is required to expose the epitope. The antibody distribution was visualized using peroxidase-DAB-OsO$_4$, which appears as dense granules distributed throughout the capsule. Granules decorate most of the fine fibers within the capsule (*large arrowheads*) and are densely packed at the abrupt margin of the chondron (*medium arrowheads*). A small bundle of adherent type II collagen fibers shows a complete absence of antibody reaction (*small arrowheads*). Bar represents 1.0 μm.

portantly perhaps, we successfully post-fixed peroxidase-DAB-labeled chondrons in osmium and processed chondron–agarose gels into resin for correlative light and electron microscopy (Fig. 3C, 3D, and 3E). Ultrastructural examination shows the label as dense granular deposits concentrated and clumped in the pericellular capsule, but forming filamentous connections with the cell processes and the plasma membrane (Fig. 3E). Granular deposits could be identified in close association with fine capsular fibrils, but type II collagen-fibers adhering to the chondron showed no evidence of antibody reaction. These results suggest that type VI collagen may interact with both the cell membrane and other collagen species within the chondron and could conceivably act to stabilize the interaction between the chondrocyte and its pericellular microenvironment. The use of type VI collagen antibodies as a chondron marker has validated the use of the chondron–agarose gel system for immunohistochemistry, and it has now been used to study the localization of proteoglycan–glycosaminoglycan (GAG) epitopes in the isolated chondron.

A wide range of monoclonal antibodies to a variety of proteoglycan–GAG epitopes have now been tested on chondron–agarose plugs (14). Initial studies concentrated on the light-microscopic distribution of the epitopes (Fig. 4A, 4B, and 4C), but more recently they have been expanded to include electron-microscopic examination of peroxidase-DAB-osmium labeled chondrons (Fig. 4D). Using comparable antibodies from alternative sources, we have shown that chondrons are rich in chondroitin-4-sulfate, chondroitin-6-sulfate, keratan sulfate, and hyaluronic acid binding region epitopes, that these components are differentially organized within the chondron, and that staining can be eliminated by treatment with enzymes disruptive to these epitopes (14). Electron-microscopic studies to date confirm the high density of proteoglycan epitopes in the fibrous capsule and tail of the chondron (Fig. 4D). Gold-particle labeling methods are currently being developed to clarify the structural interaction between the proteoglycan and collagen components of the chondron.

OSTEOARTHRITIC CHONDRONS

A critical component of our studies has been to examine the role and fate of the chondron during osteoarthritic degeneration, because recent studies have shown this to be a key area in the initiation of degradative matrix changes. In the course of our studies, occasional samples of osteoarthritic canine tibial cartilage were identified. They showed significant changes in the morphology of the chondron during the transition from a normal to an osteoarthritic form, ultimately characterized as a "clonal" cluster of chondrocytes (15). The expansion of this study to include samples of osteoarthritic human cartilage removed during arthroplasty of the knee shows structural changes identical to those seen in spontaneous canine osteoarthritis.

Morphology

A diverse range of chondron morphologies were observed in the osteoarthritic cartilage homogenates, but the preparation contained relatively few chondrons typical of normal cartilage (Fig. 5) (15). More frequently, isolated osteoarthritic chondrons appeared swollen and distended, particularly in the tail region and in the interconnecting segments between adjacent chondrons (Fig. 5A and 5B). This was accompanied by a decrease in the refractile properties of the capsule (15) and proliferation of the chondrocytes within the chondron. Following the initial cell division, the chondrocytes seem to move apart and continue to divide as the pericellular microenvironment progressively expands to maintain the overall integrity of the developing cluster (Fig. 5C). Ultimately this progressive proliferation and expansion forms a discrete cluster of densely packed chondrocytes (Fig. 5D), many of which can be isolated intact and which, in fresh samples, often contain many viable chondrocytes (15).

Histochemistry

Histochemical studies of osteoarthritic chondrons collected onto filters confirmed the general morphological changes described above. In addition, they show dramatic changes in the distribution and organization of chondron components. The first identifiable histochemical changes appeared in the immediate vicinity of the chondrocyte, where the optically uniform texture of the capsule gave way to fibrous condensations easily observed by light microscopy (15). Pericellular proteoglycan staining persisted in isolated osteoarthritic chondrons but was consistently weaker and more patchy than that in normal chondrons. Staining with hematoxylin and eosin and van Gieson's stain confirmed the proliferation and migration of chondrocytes within the swollen microenvironment, but the traditionally dense hematoxylin reaction seen in normal chondrons was lost while the pericellular capsule and tail stained with the eosin counterstain (Fig. 5A). Chondrocyte clusters showed the greatest variation in staining, with chondrocytes located at the margins of a large pool of mildly metachromatic material representing the remnants of the pericellular microenvironment (Fig. 5C). In their final stages of development, large clusters of densely packed chondrocytes showed a total absence of pericellular metachromasia (Fig. 5D) and were thought to represent the massive clusters typically identified at the eroding surface or margins of deep fissures in osteoarthritic cartilage.

Although the mechanisms controlling chondrocyte cluster formation are unclear, previous studies have shown that the normally dormant chondrocyte can proliferate under degenerative conditions. This is consistent with the formation of isolated chondrocyte clusters reported here (15). However, it has yet to be established if all the chondrocytes within these clusters derive from the one

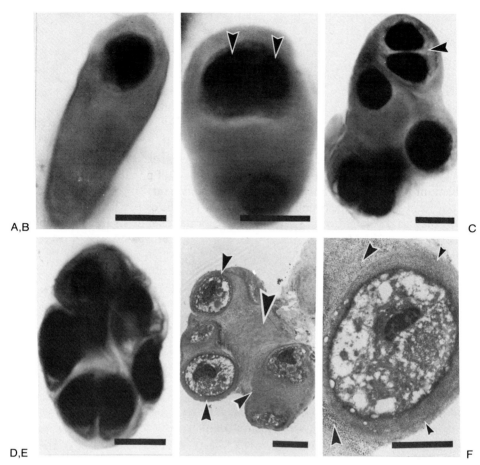

A,B

C

D,E

F

FIG. 5. Chondrons isolated from osteoarthritic cartilage. **A:** A single chondron extracted from human tibial plateau, collected onto a filter, and stained with hematoxylin and eosin. Note the swollen, amorphous appearance of the pericellular capsule and tail, and also note the absence of a typical hematoxylin reaction. Bar represents 10 μm. **B:** Double osteoarthritic chondron from human patella stained with van Gieson's stain. The pericellular capsule and interconnecting segment appears swollen and lacks the defined substructure typical of normal double chondrons. The upper chondrocyte is binucleated (*arrowheads*). Bar represents 10 μm. **C:** Developing osteoarthritic chondrocyte cluster extracted from human tibial cartilage and stained with van Gieson's stain. The pericellular microenvironment continues to expand, and staining becomes patchy. Two of the chondrocytes share a common pericellular matrix (*arrowhead*) and suggest that a recent cell division may have occurred. Bar represents 10 μm. **D:** A small, tightly packed osteoarthritic chondrocyte cluster extracted from human femoral cartilage and stained with van Gieson's stain. The expanded pericellular microenvironment has been replaced by the proliferation of chondrocytes which occupy most of the cluster's volume. Bar represents 10 μm. **E:** Osteoarthritic chondrocyte cluster extracted from canine tibial cartilage, stained with ruthenium hexamine trichloride, and processed for TEM. This low-power scan shows that chondrocytes at the margins of the cluster are surrounded by a moderately dense calyx (*small arrowheads*) which interfaces with the central mass of the cluster where ruthenium-dense proteoglycan granules vary in size and density (*large arrowhead*). Bar represents 10 μm. **F:** Detailed micrograph of a chondrocyte and its pericellular calyx at the margin of the cluster shown in **E**. The calyx totally encloses the chondrocyte and consists of small ruthenium-dense granules embedded in a moderately dense amorphous material (*small arrowheads*). The outer portion of the calyx provides a barrier between the chondrocyte and the extracellular material, whereas the inner portion is continuous with the larger proteoglycan granules in the central mass of the cluster (*large arrowheads*). Bar represents 5 μm.

original chondrocyte within a chondron to form a true "clone." Studies in this area are currently in progress.

Ultrastructure

A number of osteoarthritic chondrons have now been examined by correlative light and electron microscopy after cationic staining of proteoglycans with ruthenium (Fig. 5E and 5F). The results were consistent with those illustrated above and show that the overall staining intensity of the osteoarthritic chondron was markedly reduced compared to that of normal chondrons in comparable preparations (15). The tail region and interconnecting segments were most obviously affected, with randomly sized proteoglycan granules spread throughout the distended microenvironment. The fibrillar substructure of the capsule, partially evident in normal ruthenium-treated chondrons, was absent from osteoarthritic chondrons (Fig. 5E and 5F), suggesting a breakdown in the fine collagenous components of the chondron during osteoarthritic degeneration.

Within the clusters, each chondrocyte was surrounded by a distinct pericellular calyx containing small proteoglycan granules and a mildly dense amorphous material (Fig. 5F). Chondrocytes were often located at the margins of the cluster, with one portion of the pericellular calyx forming a thin interface with the adjacent matrix, whereas the remaining portion retains continuity with the central mass of the cluster (Fig. 5E and 5F). In this regard, the ultrastructure of clustered chondrocytes and their pericellular calyx is similar to the pericellular coat described around rat chondrosarcoma chondrocytes (9) and observed in agarose-cultured chondrocytes (Fig. 3A). The formation and function of this pericellular calyx is unknown.

The sum of these results indicates that the chondrocyte can remodel the pericellular microenvironment in response to changing environmental factors, but the initiation and regulation of these events are poorly understood. Degradation of pericellular collagens has recently been shown to be a primary event in the onset of osteoarthritis (15). It is tempting to speculate that this disorganization of the capsular collagens allows increased hydration of the pericellular proteoglycans and permits the chondron to swell during the initial phases of degenerative osteoarthritis. This enzymatically induced remodeling of the constrictive microenvironment around the chondrocyte could then remove the mechanical and physicochemical restraints imposed on the chondrocyte by the structure of the pericellular capsule, and could ultimately facilitate the proliferation of the chondrocytes to form the massive clusters typical of articular cartilage pathology. The presence of a pericellular calyx around each chondrocyte in these clusters may represent the final abortive attempt by the cell to construct a protective "chondron" prior to their demise as the fibrillation progressively erodes toward the tidemark. Investigation of the mechanisms responsible for the remodeling of the chondron and the proliferation of chondrocytes to form osteoarthritic clusters represents a new phase in our studies of the isolated chondron model and the role played by the pericellular microenvironment in degenerative joint disease.

SUMMARY AND CONCLUSIONS

A multiplicity of etiological factors have been implicated in the onset of osteoarthritis, but despite significant advances in cartilage research over recent decades we do not yet have a clear indication as to the mechanisms operating in the etiopathogenesis of this disease. What is clear, however, is that once skeletal maturity has been achieved, the chondrocyte is solely responsible for the production and maintenance of the extracellular matrix which surrounds it. It is this matrix which must physically transmit the applied load to the underlying bone, and ultimately the health of the cartilage matrix must depend on the health of the chondrocytes and the quality of the matrix it produces.

Ultrastructural studies of adult canine and human articular cartilages have now defined a specialized microenvironment around each chondrocyte, and we have previously suggested that this microanatomical structure represents the chondron originally described by Benninghoff (discussed in ref. 1). We subsequently developed methods to extract and isolate chondrons from low-speed homogenates of adult articular cartilage and have shown that they are sufficiently robust to enable extraction of chondrons which contain viable chondrocytes. Several techniques have now been introduced to advance our understanding of the structure, composition, and function of this important physiological unit of adult articular cartilage. Moreover, recent studies of chondrons extracted from human and canine osteoarthritic cartilage show dramatic remodeling of the pericellular microenvironment which suggests a role for the chondron in the genesis of osteoarthritis.

Three key areas need to be considered if we are to expand the chondron concept and the potential offered by this model to study the role and fate of the chondrocyte and its pericellular microenvironment in articular cartilage biology and pathology.

First, improvements in homogenization techniques and technology are required to achieve improved yields of viable chondrons. Work in this area is critical for the development of reliable and quantifiable techniques for *in vitro* culture.

Second, little is known of chondron function *in vivo*. Historical and contemporary arguments suggest that the chondron acts as a fluid-filled, compression-resistant bladder which serves to protect chondrocyte function by dampening the mechanical, physicochemical, and osmotic changes induced in the matrix by dynamic loading. The isolated chondron model now offers the potential to study dynamic chondron function independently of the bulk extracellular matrix, and development of techniques in this area is vital for understanding articular cartilage function.

Finally, the role of the chondron in osteoarthritis is an intriguing problem which can only be answered by improvements in the areas identified above. Nevertheless, the isolation of viable osteoarthritic chondron clusters and developments in agarose gel techniques offer the potential to answer the question, What mechanisms control chondron remodeling and chondrocyte proliferation during osteoarthritic degeneration?

ACKNOWLEDGMENTS

This work was funded by the Health Research Council of New Zealand. Studies with the New York State high-voltage electron microscope were assisted by PHS grant number RR01219 as a National Biotechnology Resource, awarded by the Division of Research Resources, DHHS. Antibodies supplied by Drs. S. Ayad, B. Caterson, and T. Glant are gratefully acknowledged.

REFERENCES

1. Szirmai JA. Structure of cartilage. In: Engel A, Larrson T, eds. *Aging of connective and skeletal tissue.* Stockholm: Nordiska Bokhandelns, 1969;163–184.
2. Meachim G, Stockwell RA. The matrix. In: Freeman MAR, ed. *Adult articular cartilage,* 2nd ed. Tunbridge Wells: Pitman Medical, 1979;1–68.
3. Evans HB, Ayad S, Abedin MZ, Hopkins S, Morgan K, Walton KW, Weiss JB, Holt PJL. Localisation of collagen types and fibronectin in cartilage by immunofluorescence. *Ann Rheum Dis* 1983;42:575–581.
4. Ratcliffe A, Fryer PR, Hardingham TE. Distribution of aggregating proteoglycans in articular cartilage: comparison of quantitative immunoelectron microscopy with radioimmunoassay and biochemical analysis. *J Histochem Cytochem* 1984;32:193–201.
5. Poole CA, Flint MH, Beaumont BW. Chondrons extracted from canine tibial cartilage: preliminary report on their isolation and structure. *J Orthopaed Res* 1988;6:408–419.
6. Poole CA. Chondrons extracted from articular cartilage: methods and applications. In: Maroudas A, Kuettner KE, eds. *Methods in cartilage research.* London: Academic Press, 1990;78–83.
7. Poole CA, Honda T, Skinner SJM, Schofield JR, Hyde KF, Shinkai H. Chondrons from articular cartilage. II. Analysis of the glycosaminoglycans in the cellular micro-environment of isolated canine chondrons. *Connect Tissue Res* 1990;24:1–12.
8. Mayne R. Cartilage collagens. What is their function, and are they involved in articular disease? *Arthritis Rheum* 1989;32:241–246.
9. Poole CA, Wotton SF, Duance VC. Localisation of type IX collagen in chondrons isolated from porcine articular cartilage and rat chondrosarcoma. *Histochem J* 1988;20:567–574.
10. Poole CA, Ayad S, Schofield JR. Chondrons from articular cartilage. 1. Immunolocalisation of type VI collagen in the pericellular capsule of isolated canine chondrons. *J Cell Sci* 1988;90: 635–645.
11. Smith GN, Hasty KA, Brandt KD. Type XI collagen is associated with the chondrocyte surface in suspension culture. *Matrix* 1989;9:186–192.
12. Mendler M, Eich-Bender SG, Vaughan L, Winterhalter KH, Bruckner P. Cartilage contains mixed fibrils of collagen types II, IX, and XI. *J Cell Biol* 1989;108:191–197.
13. Aydelotte MB, Kuettner KE. Differences between sub-populations of cultured bovine articular chondrocytes. I. Morphology and cartilage matrix production. *Connect Tissue Res* 1988;18:205–222.
14. Poole CA, Glant TT, Schofield JR. Chondrons from articular cartilage. IV. Immunolocalization of proteoglycan epitopes in isolated canine tibial chondrons. *J Histochem Cytochem* 1991;39: 1175–1187.

15. Poole CA, Matsuoka A, Schofield JR. Chondrons from articular cartilage. III. Morphologic changes in the cellular microenvironment of chondrons isolated from osteoarthritic cartilage. *Arthritis Rheum* 1991;34:22–35.

DISCUSSION

Pritzker: How do you know that the isolated chondrons (from which the chondrocytes have disappeared) and the fragmented chondrons are artifacts of the extraction procedure and not part of the natural history of chondrons? If the chondrocytes die, their capsules may remain intact, and if cartilage matrix is remodeled some of the chondrons may be disrupted. In transplanted cartilage, for example, one sees spaces with chondrons which are devoid of chondrocytes that presumably died and were resorbed.

Poole: Well, it's very difficult to tell. Examination of older cartilage does show some spaces where cells have died, and these are often filled with very massive collagen fibrils. However, we do not see these structures in our isolated chondrons. Usually, we do comparative samples, and we feel confident that the capsular ghosts that we see have in fact been produced more by disruption. We often see capsules that are torn open, with tear marks on them as if they were pulled out.

Muir: Do you find chondrons in cartilages other than articular cartilage—for example, trachea or nasal septum?

Poole: We have had little success in extracting chondrons from a number of different hyaline cartilages even though they are present by structural criteria.

Muir: If a specific protein like type VI collagen localizes in the chondron, can antibodies against that protein be used to identify chondrons in nonarticular cartilage, even though they are difficult to isolate from non-weight-bearing cartilages?

Poole: I am sure that you could. In fact, we think type VI is such a chondron-specific marker. In long-term chondrocyte agarose culture work with Margaret Aydelotte, after a couple of months the cells form beautiful chondron-like structures that stain for type VI collagen. This may provide a potential model to look at chondron development *in vitro.*

Benya: Have you done any metabolic studies to determine whether proteoglycan maturation (i.e., aggregation) occurs inside or outside the chondron domain?

Poole: When sulfate and glucosamine were used as metabolic precursors, after 24 hours we found virtually all the synthesized material trapped within the confines of the chondron microenvironment.

von der Mark: You put the chondrons of normal cartilage and the chondrocyte clusters of osteoarthritic cartilage in the same category. Is the pericellular matrix in osteoarthritic chondrocyte clusters really the same structure as that in chondrons of normal cartilage?

Poole: My view is that the normal chondron microenvironment is there, but the osteoarthritic cells start to remodel it. We think they first break down the collagen network which allows expansion due to the proteoglycans in the microenvironment. We are now starting a study with type VI, IX, and II collagen antibodies to probe osteoarthritic chondrons to see if they are resynthesizing a whole new chondron matrix or whether they are using parts of the old one and merely breaking it down.

Articular Cartilage and Osteoarthritis,
edited by K. Kuettner et al.
Raven Press, Ltd., New York © 1992.

15

The Fate of Chondrocytes in Osteoarthritic Cartilage

Regeneration, Dedifferentiation, or Hypertrophy?

K. von der Mark,* T. Kirsch,* T. Aigner,* E. Reichenberger,*
A. Nerlich,† G. Weseloh,‡ and H. Stöß¶

*Max Planck Society, Clinical Research Groups for Rheumatology, Medical Clinic III,
University of Erlangen-Nürnberg, 8520 Erlangen, Federal Republic of Germany;
†Institute of Pathology, University of Munich, Munich, Federal Republic of Germany;
and ‡Orthopedic Clinic and ¶Institute of Pathology, University of Erlangen-Nürnberg,
8520 Erlangen, Federal Republic of Germany*

Biochemical and immunohistological studies have provided some insight with regard to the degradation and turnover of the cartilage matrix in osteoarthritic joints (for review see ref. 1). In contrast, relatively little is known about the cellular responses and phenotypic changes of the articular chondrocytes in the various stages and forms of osteoarthritic cartilage degeneration.

The collagen types synthesized by chondrocytes can be used as specific markers to define various differentiation states of this cell type (Fig. 1): (a) Chondrocyte precursors as well as dedifferentiated chondrocytes synthesize types I and III collagen (2; for overview see refs. 3 and 4). (b) Functionally active chondrocytes of hyaline cartilage, such as articular chondrocytes, synthesize types II, IX, XI, and VI collagen (5–7). (c) Hypertrophic chondrocytes can be unequivocally identified on basis of their type X collagen synthesis (for review see ref. 8).

Several studies on collagen and proteoglycan synthesis in experimentally induced osteoarthritis in dogs (9,10) and on samples of human arthritic cartilage (11,12) have demonstrated enhanced matrix synthesis when compared to that of normal articular cartilage. The major collagen type which is synthesized by the articular chondrocytes 3 weeks after induction of osteoarthritis is type II collagen (10), indicating a stable cellular phenotype in the early phases of the disease. This finding is consistent with the biochemical analysis of osteoarthritic cartilage, which revealed type II collagen as the major collagenous component (5,7,13) besides the other cartilage collagen types, namely VI, IX, and XI. Type I collagen was found in significant amounts only in fibrocartilage (13). Immu-

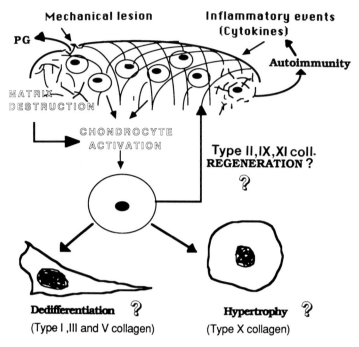

FIG. 1. Hypothetical pathways of phenotypic alterations of articular chondrocytes in osteoarthritis. PG, prostaglandin; coll., collagen.

nohistological studies with collagen-type-specific antibodies, however, detected clusters of chondrocytes synthesizing type I collagen in arthritic cartilage (14,15), suggesting focal "dedifferentiation" or modulation of arthritic chondrocytes to fibroblastic cells.

The appearance of chondrocyte clusters in osteoarthritic cartilage and of "hypertrophic" cells (16) suggested that continued stimulation of chondrocytes in osteoarthritis might eventually lead to chondrocyte hypertrophy, and thus to enhanced type X collagen synthesis. Type X collagen, a short, non-fibril-forming collagen with a triple-helical portion half the length of type II collagen (17,18), is found exclusively in the zone of hypertrophic and calcifying cartilage (5,6,8) and is thus a specific marker for hypertrophic chondrocytes.

In this chapter we present evidence using immunohistological, biochemical, and *in situ* hybridization methods to demonstrate that in various stages and sites of osteoarthritic cartilage, chondrocytes occur in all three differentiation stages: (i) differentiated, type II collagen producing chondrocytes in all phases of the disease; (ii) chondrocytes producing types I and III collagen (i.e., probably "dedifferentiated" or degenerating chondrocytes); and (iii) significant amounts of type X collagen producing chondrocytes, indicating chondrocyte hypertrophy. Type X collagen was located around chondrocyte clusters and single hypertrophic cells in the upper, middle, and deep zones, and it probably marks areas of severe osteoarthritic cellular hypertrophy.

CARTILAGE DEGRADATION AND REGENERATION

For examination of collagen type expression, deposition, and degradation, 34 samples of osteoarthritic condylar and femoral head cartilage obtained during endoprothesis operations or from autopsied femoral heads were graded morphologically and histologically according to Mankin et al. (19). Secondary repair cartilage and osteophytes were analyzed separately. For immunohistological analysis and *in situ* hybridization, full-thickness samples of 0.5 × 0.5 cm area were excised, fixed in 3% paraformaldehyde, and embedded in paraffin. Some samples were also quick-frozen for cryostat sections. Fourteen control cartilage samples were obtained from age-matched donors, either from amputated knees or from femoral heads after autopsy. Only white, solid cartilage showing a smooth, hard, and intact surface was used as control cartilage.

The immunohistological analysis of osteoarthritic cartilage samples with monoclonal antibodies to type II collagen showed two typical patterns of collagen distribution: In earlier stages of osteoarthritic degradation, before onset of intense surface fibrillation, type II collagen disappeared from the interterritorial matrix, in particular in the upper zone (Fig. 2c), whereas pericellular, type II collagen-positive halos suggested new synthesis of type II collagen and thus a stable chondrocyte phenotype. In areas of chondrocyte clusters, however, the contrary pattern was also found (Fig. 2e): Type II collagen-negative halos were observed around chondrocyte clusters, whereas the interterritorial matrix contained immunologically intact type II collagen.

This pattern suggests (a) the secretion of proteases by the chondrocytes within the clusters and (b) the suppression of type II collagen synthesis. Interestingly, *in situ* hybridization analysis of a parallel section with a ^{35}S-labeled, human α1(II) antisense RNA probe (20) demonstrated active type II collagen expression in such chondrocyte clusters (Fig. 2d), in contrast to normal, adult articular human cartilage which does not show any type II collagen expression (Fig. 2a). In 20 out of 25 investigated samples of osteoarthritic cartilage, areas of type II collagen-expressing chondrocytes were identified, predominantly in the middle zone (Fig. 2b). The extent of α1(II)-mRNA-positive cells varied considerably between samples; a correlation to clinical parameters could not yet be established. α1(II) mRNA was also detected in biopsies of osteoarthritic condylar cartilage obtained during arthroscopy (not shown).

The most intense signals were seen with the α1(II) probe in osteophytes, in particular in deep zones where the subchondral bone was opened to the bone marrow as well as in regenerated cartilage (Fig. 2h). Chondrocytes of hyaline which were fibrocartilage-like but which were also of hypertrophic appearance showed α1(II) signals, but the distribution was heterogeneous, and not all cells of chondrocytic morphology in metachromatic staining areas were positive. Of-

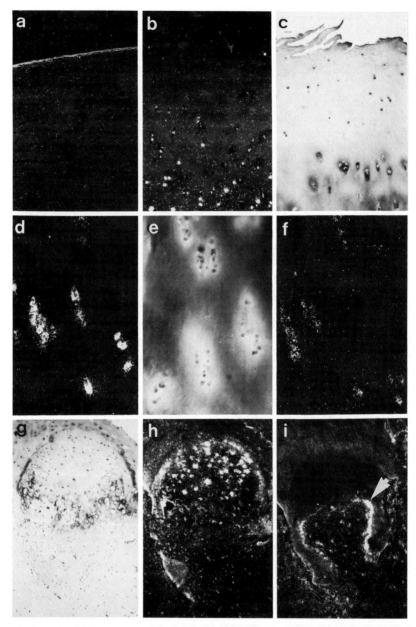

FIG. 2. Analysis of collagen expression in normal (**a**) and osteoarthritic articular cartilage (**b–i**) by *in situ* hybridization and immunostaining. **a,b:** *In situ* hybridization with a human $\alpha1$(II)-specific RNA probe reveals type II collagen expression in the middle zone of osteoarthritic articular cartilage (**b**), but not in normal adult articular cartilage (**a**). **a:** Amputated knee of a 28-year-old male. **b,c:** Varusgonarthrosis in a 68-year-old female. **c:** A similar section as in **b,** stained with a monoclonal antibody to type II collagen, followed by AP second antibody, shows extensive loss of type II collagen from the upper zone of osteoarthritic articular cartilage. **d,e,f:** Chondrocytes in the su-

ten, but not generally, there was a codistribution of $\alpha 1$(II)-mRNA-positive cells and extracellular staining with monoclonal antibodies to type II collagen. In other areas staining strongly with anti-type II collagen, however, no type II collagen-expressing cells were seen. This demonstrates the supplementary character of both techniques when used on parallel sections; antibody staining reveals extracellular deposits of collagen, whereas the *in situ* hybridization identifies cells actively transcribing collagen genes.

DEDIFFERENTIATION OF CHONDROCYTES

Most samples of osteoarthritic articular cartilage showed a slightly thickened type I collagen-positive layer at the surface. Occasionally, herds of chondrocytes in the upper zone stained intracellularly for type I collagen, confirming earlier observations (14,15). In adult control articular cartilage a slight staining for type I collagen was seen only in the superficial zone, about one cell layer thick (not shown). Using the *in situ* hybridization technique, however, no $\alpha 1$(I)-collagen-expressing cells were found in osteoarthritic cartilage, except in bone and fibrous cartilage that were regenerated (Fig. 2i). In several samples of osteoarthritic cartilage, however, areas of $\alpha 1$(III)-expressing cells were identified by *in situ* hybridization (Fig. 2f); immunohistological staining with an antibody to the pN peptide of type III procollagen confirmed a rather unexpected wide distribution of type III collagen at the articular surface and in chondrocytes of the upper and middle zone, as well as in osteophytes. Whether such chondrocytes that apparently showed coordinate expression of type II and III collagen (see Fig. 2d and 2f) are related to the type I and III collagen producing "dedifferentiated" chondrocytes remains to be determined. On the basis of the extent of $\alpha 1$(I) and/or $\alpha 1$(III) staining and RNA hybridization, the chance of "dedifferentiation" occurring in arthritic cartilage appears to be far less than the extent of cells showing type II collagen synthesis, confirming the strong tendency of osteoarthritic articular chondrocytes to repair eroded cartilage matrix with type II collagen.

CHONDROCYTE HYPERTROPHY

Hypertrophic differentiation of functional hyaline chondrocytes seems to be an inevitable event in the fetal growth plate as well as *in vitro,* when type II collagen producing fetal chondrocytes are allowed to divide for 8–10 passages

---

←

perficial zone of fibrillated osteoarthritic articular cartilage express $\alpha 1$(II) (**d**) and $\alpha 1$(III) (**f**) mRNA, whereas the antibody staining with a monoclonal anti-type II collagen (**e**) reveals extensive pericellular loss of type II collagen (79-year-old female, osteoarthritic femoral head). **g,h,i:** Cartilaginous cyst growing out of an eburnated osteoarthritic femoral head and undergoing endochondral ossification. Chondrocytes actively express $\alpha 1$(II) (**h**), whereas osteoblasts express $\alpha 1$(I) (**i**, *arrowhead*) (78-year-old female, femoral head. Magnification: **a,b,c,g,h,i:** $\times$ 64. **d,e,f:** $\times$150.

(21–23). Hypertrophy *in vitro* can be prevented only in the absence of serum at high cell density (24). The appearance of chondrocyte clusters resulting from a strong proliferation stimulus in osteoarthritic articular cartilage led to the analysis of osteoarthritic articular cartilage for the synthesis of type X collagen as a marker of chondrocyte hypertrophy (8,21).

Available antibodies to chick type X collagen did not cross-react with human type X collagen, nor was there cross-hybridization of the chick $\alpha 1(X)$ cDNA probe (17,18) with human or bovine type X collagen. Thus, type X collagen was extracted from human fetal cartilage and purified to homogeneity using DEAE anion-exchange chromatography and gel filtration on FPLC-superose (25,26). A rabbit antibody was prepared by immunization with the purified type X collagen coupled to hemocyanin and emulsified in poly A/poly U.

The specificity of the antibody for type X collagen was tested by enzyme-linked immunosorbent assay (ELISA) with human collagen types I, II, V, VII, IX, X, and XI, as well as with fibronectin. The antibody reacted only with human type X collagen, but not with the other collagens (26). In the immunoblot, the antibody stained only the band of human type X collagen (molecular weight: 66,000) (26). In frozen sections of human fetal cartilage (22 weeks' gestational age) derived from the femoral condyles, the antibody stained specifically the narrow zone of hypertrophic chondrocytes immediately adjacent to the chondro-osseous junction (26) (Fig. 3a). Immunofluorescence double staining with monoclonal antibodies to type II collagen revealed partial overlap of type II and X collagen-positive cells in the zone of proliferating chondrocytes, but absence from resting cartilage and from bone matrix (Fig. 3a and 3b), confirming the specificity of the antibody.

Examination of osteoarthritic cartilage samples with the anti-type X collagen antibody revealed pronounced extracellular staining, in particular around chondrocyte clusters, both in the middle zone (Fig. 3c and 3e) and in the deep zone (Fig. 3d). The most intense staining was seen in samples with a deeply fibrillated surface (Fig. 3f). This layer probably corresponds to the original middle zone of articular cartilage which has become the surface after extensive erosion. Although the distribution of type X collagen varied considerably between different samples, type X collagen was identified in 10 out of 14 investigated samples. It was absent from normal control cartilage and from samples of early stages of osteoarthritic degeneration. Extensive deposits of type X collagen were also seen in osteophytes and in nodules of regenerated cartilage, particularly in and around hypertrophic chondrocytes. The finding of type X collagen in the interterritorial matrix is consistent with a tendency to diffuse easily within the cartilage matrix (26).

The synthesis of type X collagen by osteoarthritic chondrocytes was confirmed biochemically by metabolic labeling of osteoarthritic articular chondrocytes, sodium dodecyl sulfate (SDS) gel electrophoresis of the newly synthesized proteins, and immunoprecipitation. For these experiments, only osteoarthritic cartilage obtained freshly during endoprothesis operations was used. Fourteen condyles showing homogeneously affected areas of yellow, fibrillated, soft primary articular

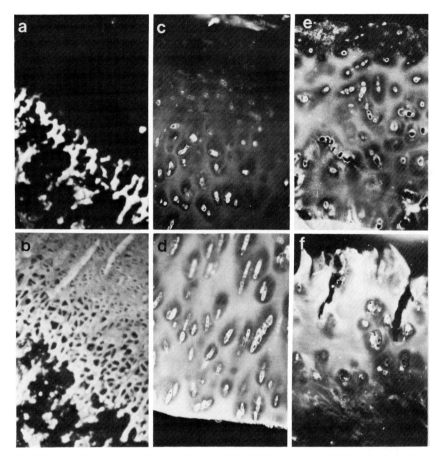

FIG. 3. Immunofluorescence staining of human fetal (**a,b**) and osteoarthritic (**c–f**) cartilage. **a,b:** Tibia epiphysis of a 22-week fetus; double staining with (**a**) rabbit anti-human type X collagen, followed by Texas-red conjugated goat anti-rabbit IgG, and (**b**) monoclonal anti-type II collagen, followed by FITC-labeled sheep anti-mouse. **c–f:** Anti-type X collagen staining. **c,d:** Varusgon-arthrosis, 77-year-old female. Anti-type X collagen reveals intracellular and interterritorial staining in the upper middle region (**c**) and deep zone (**d**). **e:** Gonarthrosis (lateral femoral condyle), 67-year-old female. Type X is seen mostly in the upper middle zone. **f:** Osteoarthritic femoral head, 63-year-old female. Type X collagen is most intense in the fibrillated surface layer around chondrocyte clusters. Magnification: ×64.

cartilage larger than 3 cm^2 were chosen. As controls, we used the following: (a) articular cartilage from amputated knees of one 28-year-old and one 16-year-old male and (b) two femoral heads obtained after autopsy of a 58-year-old and an 85-year-old male. All control joints were morphologically intact, were white, and had a smooth and hard surface. Full-thickness slices of cartilage were removed with a sharp blade under sterile conditions, and 5- × 5-mm slices were excised from the middle for histological examination. The rest was finely minced and digested with pronase for 30 min, followed by clostridial collagenase (1 mg/ml in F12 medium) for 6–12 hr. Between 2 and 8 million chondrocytes were obtained from 2 g of osteoarthritic cartilage. For immunofluorescence analysis, 0.5×10^6 cells were plated into 60-mm tissue culture dishes in Ham's F12 medium containing 10% fetal calf serum. For metabolic labeling, $3–5 \times 10^6$ cells were labeled for 18 hr in suspension with 200 μCi [^{3}H]proline in Dulbecco's modified Eagle's medium containing 25 mM HEPES, sodium ascorbate (50 μg/ml), sodium pyruvate, and 1% fetal calf serum. Half of the newly synthesized collagens from cells and culture medium was digested with pepsin at 4°C for 24 hr to remove procollagen peptides and noncollagenous proteins. The other half was dialyzed against NET medium (0.1 M NaCl, 0.05 M EDTA, 0.05 M Tris HCl, pH 7.2) containing protease inhibitors and used for immunoprecipitation.

SDS gel electrophoresis of the pepsin-digested [^{3}H]proline-labeled material synthesized by osteoarthritic articular chondrocytes revealed a major band (molecular weight: ~58,000) corresponding to the pepsin-resistant part of human type X collagen (26), but revealed little or no type II collagen (28). In contrast, the major collagen synthesized by control chondrocytes from normal adult articular cartilage was $\alpha 1(II)$, besides a minor fraction of the 58-kD protein.

The collagenous nature of the 58-kD molecule was confirmed by digestion with purified collagenase which almost completely digested the molecule (28). Furthermore, type X collagen synthesis by osteoarthritic articular chondrocytes

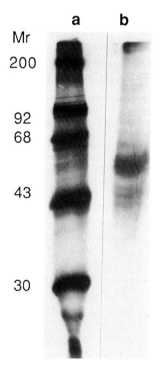

FIG. 4. Immunoprecipitation and SDS-gel electrophoresis of [^{3}H]proline-labeled type X collagen, synthesized by osteoarthritic chondrocytes from a femoral condyle. Chondrocytes were released by pronase collagenase 1 hr after operation, and then they were labeled in suspension with [^{3}H]proline for 18 hr. The collagens from medium and cell extract were precipitated with rabbit anti-type X collagen IgG, followed by protein A sepharose. **a:** Molecular-weight marker proteins. **b:** Immunoprecipitate showing a dominant band at Mr 58 kD, corresponding to $\alpha 1(X)$ (reduced).

was confirmed by immunoprecipitation of the [³H]proline-labeled material with rabbit anti-type X collagen antibodies, followed by protein A sepharose (Fig. 4b).

Out of 14 osteoarthritic articular cartilage samples analyzed, nine contained enough cells and incorporated sufficient amounts of [³H]proline to allow analysis of the synthesized collagen. The amount of radioactivity incorporated per cell, however, varied considerably between samples, not only in osteoarthritic but also in "normal" cartilage samples. This is consistent with a study by Lipiello et al. (11) which describes enhanced, but variable, collagen synthesis by human osteoarthritic cartilage and which reflects the circumstance that osteoarthritic degeneration of cartilage has a focal character and varies considerably with the progress of the disease, the site of the examined cartilage specimen, and the age of the patient.

IN SITU HYBRIDIZATION ANALYSIS OF TYPE X COLLAGEN EXPRESSION

To confirm the synthesis of type X collagen by osteoarthritic chondrocytes seen after metabolic labeling of isolated cells *in vitro,* attempts were made for *in situ* hybridization analysis of type X collagen mRNA expression in sections of osteoarthritic articular cartilage. A human $\alpha 1(X)$ DNA fragment was cloned by the polymerase chain reaction, using a set of 18-mer oligonucleotide primers designed after published chick $\alpha 1(X)$ cDNA sequences (18) and bovine $\alpha 1(X)$ protein sequences (29). The 329-base-pair cDNA clone covered most of the non-triple-helical domain at the 3' end and hybridized to a 2.9- to 3.0-kb mRNA in Northern blots, as expected for type X collagen (30). The fragment was cloned into the pGEM 42 vector (Promega) and transcribed into sense and antisense RNA probes using ³⁵S-UTP and T7 or SP6 polymerase, respectively (20).

In situ hybridization analysis of human fetal epiphyseal cartilage with the antisense $\alpha 1(X)$ probe revealed strong expression of type X collagen in the zone of hypertrophic chondrocytes above the chondro-osseous junction (Fig. 5a and 5b). The zones of proliferating and resting cartilage were negative for type X, but showed strong signals with an $\alpha 1(II)$-specific RNA probe (30). Hybridization experiments with sections of arthritic cartilage, however, showed only a few $\alpha 1(X)$-expressing chondrocytes, mostly in the deep zone of osteophytes and re-generated cartilage (Fig. 5c and 5d). Chondrocyte clusters in the fibrillated upper zone which showed extensive extracellular type X collagen antibody staining (Fig. 3f) were mostly negative in the *in situ* hybridization experiment. This apparent conflict underlines the different and supplementary character of the two methods: Whereas the immunohistological analysis revealed the presence of ex-tracellular type X collagen around chondrocyte clusters, the *in situ* hybridization results indicate that the chondrocytes in clusters close to the fibrillated surface have become silent by the time of operation in terms of type X collagen expression.

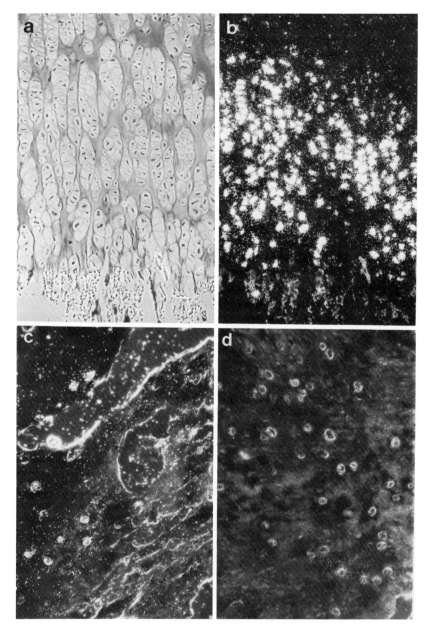

FIG. 5. *In situ* hybridization analysis of type X collagen expression in human fetal epiphyseal cartilage (**a,b**) and osteoarthritic articular cartilage (**c,d**). Paraformaldehyde-fixed specimens were embedded in paraffin, sectioned, and hybridized to the human-α1(X)-specific clone pERX (30) transcribed into ^{35}S-antisense RNA using the pGEM42 vector. **a,b:** Type X collagen is expressed by a sharply defined zone of hypertrophic chondrocytes in the growth plate. **c,d:** In osteoarthritic articular cartilage, areas of type X collagen-expressing chondrocytes are seen occasionally in the deep zone, but never in the upper, fibrillated area such as shown in Fig. 3f). Magnification: ×110.

The significant amounts of type X collagen synthesized by osteoarthritic articular chondrocytes after enzymatic release from cartilage also seem not in accordance with the *in situ* hybridization results. It is likely, however, that the enzymatic digestion of extracellular matrix reactivates collagen synthesis of arthritic chondrocytes that have become silent *in vivo*. Similarly, significant amounts of type II collagen are synthesized by chondrocytes freshly released from normal, adult articular cartilage (see ref. 7), whereas the *in situ* hybridization analysis with $\alpha1(II)$-specific probes can hardly detect any type II collagen expression in intact cartilage (Fig. 2a).

SUMMARY AND CONCLUSION

Using a combination of immunohistological, biochemical, and *in situ* hybridization methods of collagen type analysis, we demonstrated that osteoarthritic cartilage chondrocytes can be found in at least three different phenotypes: (i) functionally stable chondrocytes actively expressing type II collagen, (ii) "dedifferentiated" or modulated chondrocytes synthesizing types I and III collagen, and (iii) hypertrophic chondrocytes synthesizing type X collagen. Because of the focal character of osteoarthritic lesions, the distribution of these cell types varies considerably between samples. In general, early stages of osteoarthritic cartilage degeneration are marked by enhanced type II collagen expression—particularly in the middle zone of osteoarthritic articular cartilage, and most prominently in secondary osteophytic and regenerated cartilage. Relatively little type I collagen deposits were seen, whereas *in situ* hybridization occasionally revealed herds of $\alpha1(III)$-expressing chondrocytes in the upper zone. Type X collagen was identified in most osteoarthritic articular cartilage samples but not in normal adult articular cartilage. It was located predominantly in the extracellular matrix of chondrocyte clusters, as well as in osteophytes. By *in situ* hybridization criteria, cells in clusters did not actively express type X collagen, but enzymatic release of chondrocytes from osteoarthritic articular cartilage samples reactivated type X collagen synthesis, which was identified by immunoprecipitation.

The finding of type X collagen in osteoarthritic cartilage indicates that in certain areas and stages of the disease, chondrocytes become hypertrophic and lose their capability to synthesize a functional cartilage matrix, which contains type II collagen as its major collagenous constituent. Although the function of type X collagen is not clear yet, its occurrence in calcifying hypertrophic cartilage and the observation that it binds calcium (31) suggest that it is involved in the process of cartilage calcification.

ACKNOWLEDGMENTS

We gratefully acknowledge the technical assistance of Ms. Marion van Menxel and Ms. Barbara Brändlein. This work was supported by the German Ministry for Research and Technology (BMFT 01VM 8702/0).

REFERENCES

1. Poole AR. Changes in the collagen and proteoglycan of articular cartilage. In: Kühn K, Krieg T, eds. *Connective tissue: biological and clinical aspects. Rheumatology, an annual review.* Basel: Karger, 1986;316–371.
2. Benya PD, Padilla SR, Nimni ME. Independent regulation of collagen types by chondrocytes during the loss of differentiated function in culture. *Cell* 1978;15:1313–1321.
3. Mayne R, von der Mark K. Collagens of cartilage. In: Hall BK, ed. *The biochemistry of cartilage.* New York: Academic Press, 1983;181–214.
4. von der Mark K. Differentiation, modulation and dedifferentiation of chondrocytes. In: Kühn K, Krieg T, eds. *Rheumatology,* vol 10. Basel: Karger, 1986;272–315.
5. Eyre DR, Wu J-J, Apone S. A growing family of collagens in articular cartilage: identification of 5 genetically distinct types. *J Rheumatol* 1987;14:25–27.
6. Mayne R. Cartilage collagens: What is their function, and are they involved in articular disease? *Arthritis Rheum* 1989;32:241–246.
7. Ronziere M-C, Ricard-Blum S, Tiollier J, Hartmann DJ, Garrone R, Herbage D. Comparative analysis of collagens solubilized from human foetal, normal and osteoarthritic adult articular cartilage, with emphasis on type VI collagen. *Biochim Biophys Acta* 1990;1038:222–230.
8. Schmid TM, Linsenmayer TF. Type X collagen. In: Mayne R, Burgeson RE, eds. *Structure and function of collagen types.* New York: Academic Press, 1987;223–259.
9. McDevitt CA, Gilbertson EJJ, Muir H. An experimental model of osteoarthritis: early morphological and biochemical changes. *J Bone Joint Surg* 1977;59B:24–35.
10. Eyre DR, McDevitt CA, Billingham MEJ, Muir H. Biosynthesis of collagen and other matrix proteins by articular cartilage in experimental arthrosis. *Biochem J* 1980;188:823–837.
11. Lipiello L, Hall D, Mankin HJ. Collagen synthesis in normal and osteoarthritic human cartilage. *J Clin Invest* 1977;59:593–600.
12. Sandy JD, Adams ME, Billingham MEJ, Plaas A, Muir H. *In vivo* and *in vitro* stimulation of chondrocyte biosynthetic activity in early experimental osteoarthritis. *Arthritis Rheum* 1984;27: 388–397.
13. Goldwasser M, Astley T, van der Rest M, Glorieux FH. Analysis of the type of collagen present in osteoarthritic human cartilage. *Clin Orthop* 1982;167:296–302.
14. Gay S, Müller DK, Lemmen C, Remberger K, Matzen K, Kühn K. Immunohistological study on collagen in cartilage–bone metamorphosis and degenerative osteoarthritis. *Klin Wochenschr* 1976;54:969–976.
15. Adam M, Deyl Z. Altered expression of collagen phenotype in osteoarthrosis. *Clin Chim Acta* 1983;133:25–32.
16. Vignon E, Arlot M, Hartmann D, Moyen B, Ville G. Hypertrophic repair of articular cartilage in experimental osteoarthrosis. *Ann Rheum Dis* 1983;42:82–88.
17. Ninomiya Y, Gordon M, van der Rest M, Schmid T, Linsenmayer T, Olsen BR. The developmentally regulated type X collagen gene contains a long open reading frame without introns. *J Biol Chem* 1986;261:5041–5050.
18. LuValle P, Ninomiya Y, Rosenblum ND, Olsen BR. The type X collagen gene. *J Biol Chem* 263:18378–18385.
19. Mankin HJ, Dorfman H, Lippiello L, Zarins A. Biochemical and metabolic abnormalities in articular cartilage from osteo-arthritic human hips. II. Correlation of morphology with biochemical and metabolic data. *J Bone Joint Surg Am* 1971;53:523–537.
20. Aigner T, von der Mark K. 1991;in preparation.
21. Schmid TM, Linsenmayer TF. A short chain (pro)collagen from aged endochondral chondrocytes. *J Biol Chem* 1983;258:9504–9509.
22. Capasso O, Quarto N, Descalci-Cancedda F, Cancedda R. The low molecular weight collagen synthesized by chick tibial chondrocytes is deposited in the matrix both in culture and *in vivo.* *EMBO J* 1984;3:823–827.
23. Castagnola P, Dozin B, Moro G, Cancedda R. Changes in the expression of collagen genes show two stages in chondrocyte differentiation *in vitro. J Cell Biol* 1988;106:461–467.
24. Bruckner P, Hörler J, Mendler M, Honze Y, Winterhaller KH, Eich-Bender SG, Spycher MA. Induction and prevention of chondrocyte hypertrophy in culture. *J Cell Biol* 1989;109:2537–2545.

25. Kirsch T, von der Mark K. Isolation of bovine type X collagen and immunolocalization in growth-plate cartilage. *Biochem J* 1990;265:453–459.
26. Kirsch T, von der Mark K. Isolation of human type X collagen and immunolocalization in fetal human cartilage. *Eur J Biochem* 1991;196:575–580.
27. Chen Q, Gibney E, Fitch JM, et al. Long range movement and fibril association of type X collagen within embryonic cartilage matrix. *Proc. Natl. Acad. Sci. USA* 1990;87:8046–8050.
28. von der Mark K, Kirsch T, Nerlich A, et al. Type X collagen synthesis in human osteoarthritic cartilage: Indication of chondrocyte hypertrophy. 1991, submitted.
29. Thomas JT, Kwan APL, Grant ME, Boot-Handford RP. Analysis of the complete cDNA sequence encoding bovine type X collagen. Evidence for the conservation of a condensed gene structure across species. Presented at the Third International Conference on the Molecular Biology and Pathology of Matrix, Jefferson Institute of Molecular Medicine, Philadelphia; 1990.
30. Reichenberger E, Aigner T, von der Mark K, et al. In situ hybridization studies on the expression of type X collagen in fetal human cartilage. *Develop. Biol.* 1991; in press.
31. Kirsch T, von der Mark K. Manuscript in preparation, 1991.

DISCUSSION

Caterson: We have some monoclonal antibodies that recognize very subtle structures that are expressed in osteoarthritic proteoglycans but are not in normal articular cartilage proteoglycans. The only other tissue that they stain is the hypertrophic zone in fetal cartilage. This matches very closely the distributions you observed for type X collagen.

Howell: Yousuf Ali showed that the surface layer of articular cartilage in human osteoarthritis contains mineral crystals frequently. Would you speculate that the presence of these crystals might correlate with the presence of type X collagen?

von der Mark: We have also seen this in cases of chondrocalcinosis. The cartilage surfaces were covered with type X collagen in such samples as well. However the amounts of type X were similar in noncalcified osteoarthritic cartilage. So I really do not know whether there is any correlation.

Howell: Have you done morphometric analyses to see if the hypertrophic cells with type X collagen actually enlarge?

von der Mark: What is the definition of hypertrophic chondrocyte, and what marks the border to proliferating chondrocytes? You are right, not all cells which synthesize type X collagen or which have type X collagen around them seem to be very large. There may not be a tight correlation between morphological hypertrophy and type X collagen synthesis. How would Dr. Hunziker define a hypertrophic chondrocyte?

Hunziker: It is hard to define. In the growth plate, there is a vertical organization of the cells. First the cells proliferate, then they cease dividing, begin to mature, and finally become very hypertrophic. There is no clear-cut morphological borderline where hypertrophy starts and proliferation ends. In our morphometric studies we delineate the borders functionally. The cells still dividing are assigned to the proliferating pool, and those that have stopped dividing are assigned to the hypertrophic cells. Within the hypertrophic cell pool defined in this way, the early hypertrophic cells can structurally not be distinguished from late proliferating cells. The term "hypertrophic" cell should be reserved for the growth-plate chondrocytes. In this tissue the "proliferating pool" is the dividing pool. The rest of the cells underneath as far as the zone of vascular invasion are called the "hypertrophic pool." Type X collagen is found with cells in a certain phase within the hypertrophic pool (before they become eliminated). This phase, in the proximal tibial rat growth plate, lasts only about 3–5 hr, just before their matrix starts to mineralize. This is the final phase before the cells become eliminated. Following the development phase of articular cartilage, this tissue appears in the adult form like an "arrested growth plate." Based on this view you could call the lower radial zone cells also "hypertrophic chondrocytes." The term, however, should be reserved for the particular cell population within growth-plate cartilage and secondary centers for ossification.

Pritzker: The term "hypertrophic" should be reserved for chondrocytes that are truely enlarged. In adult articular cartilage, chondrocytes that express type X and/or type III collagens should be called "metaplastic chondrocytes," as they have altered their environment. I think this is a much more precise approach.

Sandell: Our *in situ* hybridization studies with type X in the growth-plate cartilage show exactly what Klaus von der Mark has found. Surprisingly, type X expression becomes very active in what is defined as a maturation zone, apparently after all division ceases. Maybe we should consider defining hypertrophic chondrocytes as those cells that begin to synthesize type X collagen.

Olsen: We have studied this in developing chicken vertebral cartilage in collaboration with Masando Hayashi. We used a combination of *in situ* hybridization and immuno-histochemistry. Type X mRNA levels increase transiently. Following the increase, the mRNA levels decrease even though the cells continue to synthesize type X protein. If one only took *in situ* hybridization data as a basis for defining hypertrophic chondrocytes, some cells that are hypertrophic would not be included—that is, those that have gone through a stage of high levels of type X mRNA and continue some type X synthesis after the levels of mRNA have become undetectable. Expression of type X mRNA, then, is really a wave. The gene is turned on, and then turned off again.

von der Mark: I think the same situation applies to osteoarthritic cartilage, where we see the extracellular matrix of chondrocyte clusters staining for type X but do not see the mRNA anymore.

Muir: How long do isolated chondrocytes synthesize type X collagen?

von der Mark: Usually we label cells immediately following dissociation to avoid culture artifacts. In some cultures that were kept 8 days, about 25% of the cells were stained for type X collagen.

Articular Cartilage and Osteoarthritis,
edited by K. Kuettner et al.
Raven Press, Ltd., New York © 1992.

Part V: Chondrocyte Metabolism

Introduction

Paul D. Benya

*Department of Orthopaedics, University of Southern California,
Orthopaedic Hospital, Los Angeles, California 90007*

The normal role of the differentiated aspect of chondrocyte metabolism is the elaboration of the proper spectrum of matrix molecules, integration of these into a functioning matrix, controlled degradation (normal turnover), and response to normal variation in stress with appropriate repair. This requires control (homeostasis) of multiple interacting systems. Chondrocytes must exhibit stable expression of a required pattern of genes for (a) structural molecules, (b) enzymes required for synthesis and turnover, (c) hormone/growth factor receptors, and (d) matrix receptors. The level of synthesis of both matrix molecules and receptors is regulated by the profile and concentration of extracellular growth factors. Endocrine, paracrine, and autocrine production of growth factors will establish the immediate extracellular milleu in concert with activation of latent forms, formation of matrix depots, and the presence of specific inhibitors. Secondary control is expected through the feedback of information concerning the integrity of the extracellular matrix transduced by cell-surface matrix receptors (integrins). Finally, the effects of most signaling molecules are mediated in the common arena of potentially interacting second messengers produced at the interior face of the plasma membrane and propagated through the cytoplasm. Each of these systems provides a challenge for our research and affords the opportunity to manipulate chondrocyte metabolism to influence the progression of degenerative cartilage disease.

In this section the autocrine production of transforming growth factor β (TGF-β) and insulin-like growth factor 1 (IGF-1) are discussed by Morales and Tyler et al., respectively. Both growth factors have been previously identified as exogenous stimulators of proteoglycan synthesis which are also able to interfere with normal and cytokine-induced degradation. The biosynthesis of these molecules by chondrocytes at levels sufficient to support the proteoglycan content *in vivo* (TGF-β) is in conflict with the observation that the such synthesis is not effective. Latent TGF-β and depot binding to biglycan and decorin may be responsible and functionally analogous to the production of IGF-1-binding proteins in preventing receptor binding and signaling. What are the circumstances required for liberation of active factor? Does this occur during normal turnover, and to what degree? Does the total production of factor vary with pathology? The answers to such questions may provide insight into feedback coupling of matrix synthesis and degradation and may describe an appropriate interface for the intervention of cytokines and their induced matrix proteases.

Aydelotte et al. discuss the metabolism of articular chondrocyte subpopulations with respect to the critical issues of stability and modulation of observed differences. Can exogenous growth factors elevate matrix synthesis in the superficial zone? Are the lower levels of synthesis due to lack of receptors or due to less autocrine production of growth factors? Insight into reversal of the metabolic state of surface cells, perhaps by limited proliferation in a factor-enriched monolayer environment, may facilitate repair *in vivo*. Van Kampen et al. discuss the existence of a metabolically stable pool of proteoglycans. It is important to distinguish between stability derived from increased presence or affinity in proteoglycan–hyaluronic acid (HA)–link-protein complexes and stability due to specific protective interactions with collagenous and/or noncollagenous matrix components. Is such a pool altered by interleukin-1 (IL-1) or altered in the presence of osteoarthrosis, or is it merely obscured by more rapid general degradation? The significance of such kinetic diversity might be enhanced if chondrocyte subpopulations produced different proportions of fast and slow pools— that is, if extracellular turnover were under cellular control. It is still not clear whether proteoglycan function is more effectively served by slower or faster turnover of proteoglycan.

Articular Cartilage and Osteoarthritis,
edited by K. Kuettner et al.
Raven Press, Ltd., New York © 1992.

16

Heterogeneity of Articular Chondrocytes

Margaret B. Aydelotte,* Barbara L. Schumacher,*
and Klaus E. Kuettner*†

*Departments of Biochemistry and †Orthopedic Surgery, Rush Medical College
at Rush–Presbyterian–St. Luke's Medical Center, Chicago, Illinois 60612*

The structure of articular cartilage has been described in detail in earlier chapters of this book (see chapters by Hunziker and by Poole); further elaboration is not necessary here except in relation to the zonal variation in depth, which provides the most striking heterogeneity in articular cartilage and is the focus of the present discussion. Four layers are generally recognized from the articular surface to the subchondral bone, namely the superficial (tangential), middle (transitional), deep (radial), and calcified zones (I–IV, respectively). These subdivisions are based on well-recognized morphological differences in (a) cell density and orientation, (b) nature, content, and distribution of proteoglycans, and (c) organization of the collagenous fibrillar network, which all vary with distance from the articular surface (for a recent review see ref. 1). The material properties of the cartilage at different depths also change because they are determined by the biochemical nature, content, and organization of the matrix macromolecules.

Because the living chondrocytes elaborate and maintain this complex matrix in which they reside, the zonal variations in the extracellular matrix must result from metabolic differences among the cells. However, it is not known to what degree the metabolism of articular chondrocytes varies because of intrinsic cellular specializations that arise during growth and differentiation, or because of modulation in response to the cells' environment within the tissue. Several investigators have recently addressed this question by examining the morphology and metabolism of subpopulations of cultured articular chondrocytes following their isolation from different depths of the cartilage (2–7). Results show striking differences between chondrocytes derived from the superficial and the deep slices of cartilage in terms of their morphology, metabolism, phenotypic stability, and responsiveness to interleukin-1α (IL-1). Zonal differences in metabolism have also been demonstrated in cartilage explant cultures when chondrocytes are left undisturbed within their original matrix (8,9). Such studies may provide one way to understand better how these diverse cell populations contribute to the long-term maintenance of healthy articular cartilage.

MORPHOLOGY OF CULTURED CHONDROCYTES

Current methods of dissecting articular cartilage to separate groups of cells have not yielded pure preparations of different types of chondrocytes, because the slices do not correspond precisely with the different zones of the tissue. Furthermore, changes in the tissue with depth are gradual, not abrupt, and even within one zone there may be considerable cellular heterogeneity. These considerations must be kept in mind when studies of chondrocytes derived from superficial, middle, and deep regions of cartilage (i.e., cells from zones I, II, and III) are described. Nevertheless, the cell populations from these individual zones are certainly more homogeneous than are preparations isolated from the entire thickness of the tissue, and they show marked morphological and metabolic differences in culture. There is generally good agreement in results with these populations of chondrocytes from bovine, porcine, and human articular cartilage (4,6,7). The middle slices of cartilage which are harvested include some residual tangential tissue, most of the transitional zone, and the upper part of the radial zone; these slices yield a heterogeneous population of chondrocytes which always gives results that are similar to those of the full population and that are intermediate between populations from superficial and deep slices. In intact tissue, this region has the highest concentration of proteoglycans, and it is frequently the source of cells which proliferate to form cell nests in damaged osteoarthritic cartilage.

Chondrocytic metabolism is readily modulated by alterations in cell shape (10) or by changes in the organization of cytoskeletal microfilaments (11). Thus, the results of experiments with isolated cells depend to some extent on the environmental conditions provided by the particular culture method. For example, differences exhibited initially between the populations of cells derived from superficial and deep zones of cartilage diminished with time in monolayer culture at low density under conditions in which the chondrocytic phenotype is labile (6,7). However, in high-density monolayers, and especially in suspension culture either within an agarose gel or in liquid medium over agarose, some phenotypic differences between chondrocytes from zones I and III were retained for extended periods (4,6,7). Chondrocytes from zone I, cultured in agarose gel, became irregular in shape, with numerous processes (3,4), and in liquid medium they formed clusters covered by flattened cells resembling a perichondrium (7). Some of the cells from zone I produced very little extracellular matrix, whereas others became surrounded by a highly fibrillar matrix poor in proteoglycans (4,7). In contrast, chondrocytes from the deep zone retained a rounded shape and morphological features typical for chondrocytes. These cells, cultured within an agarose gel, accumulated an extensive extracellular matrix rich in proteoglycans and containing collagen fibrils (4,7). Similarly, in liquid medium the clusters of rounded chondrocytes from the deep zone produced large quantities of matrix that contained proteoglycan granules and fine collagen fibrils, and they lacked a covering of flattened cells (7). The matrix which is formed in these agarose cultures is denser and more highly organized than that formed in liquid medium, presumably because the agarose is more effective in trapping the matrix macromolecules close to the cells.

CELL PROLIFERATION IN CULTURE

Although there is little, if any, cell division in healthy adult articular cartilage, chondrocytes cultured in medium containing fetal bovine serum proliferated in response to serum growth factors. The doubling time for bovine chondrocytes

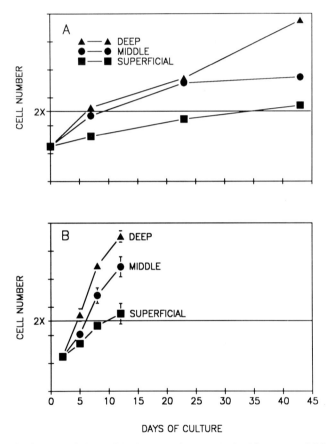

FIG. 1. Growth of subpopulations of bovine chondrocytes derived from superficial, middle, and deep regions of articular cartilage after different times of incubation within an agarose gel. **A:** At high density, mean cell numbers were calculated from measurements of DNA in duplicate samples using the fluorescent Hoechst dye 33258. **B:** Cells cultured at very low density (1/32 that for **A**) were counted under the microscope in defined areas on days indicated (vertical bars, visible only where larger than symbols, show standard deviations of the mean of three or four determinations). Note that proliferation was more rapid in low-density than in high-density cultures, but that under both conditions, chondrocytes from the deep zone of cartilage divided more rapidly than those from the middle region, and cells from the superficial zone showed the least proliferation. Horizontal lines at 2X mark doubling of the populations.

varied both with the cell density and with the source of cells within the articular cartilage (Fig. 1). Proliferation was more rapid in low-density than in high-density cultures, in agreement with results for porcine chondrocytes (6); however, at both high and low densities in agarose gels, chondrocytes from zone III divided more rapidly than did those from zone I. The doubling times for zone III chondrocytes at low and high density were approximately 5 days and 7 days, respectively, compared with 9 days and 32 days for the zone I cells. At high density, porcine chondrocytes from deep layers of cartilage reached greater numbers at confluence than did cells from superficial layers; this difference can be explained partly by the more flattened shape of cells from the upper zone (6). Subpopulations of human articular chondrocytes maintained in medium containing adult human serum, which has lower concentrations of growth factors than does fetal serum, showed little change in cell number during the culture period, and no difference in proliferation was reported between cells from the superficial and deep zones (12).

PROTEOGLYCAN SYNTHESIS

Chondrocytes derived from the proteoglycan-rich matrix of zone III consistently synthesized more proteoglycans than did cells from zone I, which normally reside in a matrix with a relatively low concentration of proteoglycans (4–7). Chondrocytes from both the superficial and deep zones of articular cartilage synthesized predominantly the proteoglycan, aggrecan, but zone I bovine and porcine cells produced relatively more of the small, nonaggregating proteoglycans than did zone III cells (5,6). In suspension cultures of human chondrocytes from both the superficial and deep regions of cartilage, aggrecan accounted for approximately 85% of the total ^{35}S incorporated into proteoglycans, although in the early stages of culture most cells were shown by immunohistochemistry to be positive for the dermatan sulfate proteoglycan, decorin (12). When grown as monolayers, in addition to aggrecan, human chondrocytes from both zones I and III also synthesized significant amounts of smaller, nonaggregating proteoglycans at later stages of culture (7). The quantitative differences in metabolism of proteoglycans observed in isolated chondrocytes cultured in suspension were retained throughout the culture period, and are in keeping with variations in the biochemical composition of matrix which surrounds these cells *in vivo.*

Keratan sulfate was synthesized during early stages of culture by most of the chondrocytes derived from zone III, but by only a few of those from the superficial zone, whether they were grown as monolayers or in suspension (2,6,7,13). Furthermore, keratan sulfate accounted for a higher percentage of ^{35}S in proteoglycans synthesized by zone III than by zone I chondrocytes (6,13). This metabolic difference coincides with the higher content of keratan sulfate in proteoglycans deep within the tissue than in those near the articular surface. With extended time *in vitro,* most of the zone I cells from porcine and human cartilage also began to synthesize keratan sulfate, but the reason for this modulation is not clear (2,7).

COLLAGEN SYNTHESIS

Collagen production by subpopulations of bovine articular chondrocytes has been examined in collaboration with Dr. Thomas Schmid, for periods of up to 6 weeks using [^{3}H]proline as a precursor (14). Type II collagen was the predominant form synthesized by all populations, and at all stages; no type I collagen was detectable after 1 week, although small quantities were synthesized at later stages of culture after cells had formed a monolayer underneath or on the surface of the agarose. Chondrocytes of zone III were the most active in collagen production; after 1 week, the proportions of collagen synthesized by chondrocytes from superficial, middle, and deep zones were approximately 1:2:3, respectively. These marked quantitative differences in collagen synthesis remained essentially unchanged after 3 and 6 weeks, although the net synthetic rate declined steadily with time in culture (14). Interestingly, small quantities of type X collagen were detected after 6 weeks in cultured bovine chondrocytes from zone III (T. Schmid, *personal communication*), but human chondrocytes from all zones initiated synthesis of type X collagen in liquid suspension culture (15).

Results of immunohistochemical staining with antibodies directed against collagens were in keeping with the more active synthesis of collagen by chondrocytes from zone III than by those from zone I. The percentage of cells with matrix binding an antibody for type II collagen (anti-chick type II collagen from Dr. T. Linsenmeyer) was much higher (and the staining was more intense) in the subpopulation from the deep zone than in that from the superficial zone. Extracellular matrix rich in proteoglycans which stained with alcian blue also stained for type II collagen. After 3 weeks in liquid suspension culture, over 90% of the chondrocytes from superficial and deep zones of human cartilage produced type II collagen detectable by immunofluorescence (7). Collagen of types IX and XI were also synthesized by bovine chondrocytes (detected by immunohistochemistry, using antibodies against bovine collagens, kindly provided by Dr. D. Hartmann), and their distribution was essentially similar to that of type II collagen.

RESPONSE TO INTERLEUKIN-1

Another important metabolic difference between chondrocytes derived from superficial and deep zones of the cartilage lies in their responsiveness to IL-1. Studies of cultured cartilage slices or the entire population of chondrocytes have demonstrated that this cytokine has a dual action. It inhibits synthesis of proteoglycans and also stimulates production of chondrocytic proteases (such as stromelysin, collagenase, and gelatinase), which results in enhanced catabolism of matrix—that is, chondrocytic chondrolysis (e.g., see refs. 16–19; also see chapter by Tyler et al.). Human articular chondrocytes cultured in either agarose gel or alginate beads also responded to IL-1 with diminished proteoglycan synthesis, but little catabolic response was observed (see chapter by Häuselmann et al., *this volume*). It is well accepted that IL-1 plays an important role in the pathology of inflammatory joint diseases, such as rheumatoid arthritis, but it may also contribute to cartilage damage during inflammatory episodes in osteoarthritis by stimulating matrix degradation and inhibiting repair. Therefore, it is important to understand how this cytokine influences chondrocytes and their surrounding matrix.

Bovine chondrocytes derived from zone I have consistently shown a greater sensitivity to IL-1α than have chondrocytes from the deep zone, based upon both their catabolic and anabolic responses (20). In control medium, chondrocytes from the superficial zone degraded their newly synthesized proteoglycans more rapidly than did zone III chondrocytes, but catabolism was greatly enhanced in the presence of IL-1 (Fig. 2). Zone III chondrocytes, on the other hand, showed only slightly accelerated catabolism at the same concentration of IL-1 (Fig. 2).

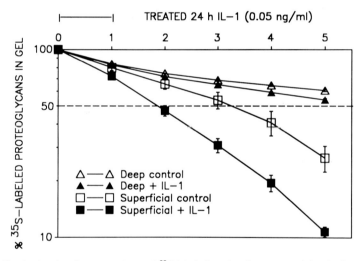

FIG. 2. Graph showing the percentage of ^{35}S-labeled proteoglycans remaining in the agarose-gel–cell layer on different days for control cultures (*open symbols*) and cultures treated for 24 hr with IL-1 (0.05 ng/ml) (*closed symbols*). After 4 days in control medium, cultures were labeled for 16 hr with [^{35}S]sulfate, then rinsed repeatedly to remove remaining free isotope, and the medium was changed and harvested daily for the remainder of the experiment. IL-1 was added to one group of cultures of superficial- and deep-zone chondrocytes for 24 hr. At the end of the experiment, the macromolecular radioactivity in harvested media and in the agarose-gel–cell layer was measured by liquid scintillation spectroscopy. Note that control cultures of chondrocytes derived from deep cartilage (*triangles*) retained a much greater percentage of proteoglycans than did cultures of cells from superficial cartilage (*squares*). In addition, IL-1 elicited a greater catabolic response in the population of superficial-zone chondrocytes, resulting in an additional loss of 16% ^{35}S-labeled proteoglycans, compared with only 7% for the deep-zone chondrocytes.

In terms of long-term damage to cartilage matrix by IL-1, the inhibition of proteoglycan synthesis may play a more important role than does the stimulation of matrix catabolism. In this context, it is interesting that the concentration of IL-1 required for 50% inhibition of proteoglycan synthesis for chondrocytes from zone III was approximately 25-fold that which elicited a similar response from cells of zone I. Further studies are needed to understand the basis for this cellular difference. The number of cellular receptors for IL-1 on the chondrocytes derived from superficial and deep cartilage may differ, the distribution of IL-1 in the vicinity of the cells may be affected by differences in the nature of their surrounding extracellular matrix, and subpopulations of chondrocytes may differ in their capacity for synthesis of endogenous IL-1 (21). However, these results with IL-1 on cultured subpopulations suggest that in intact articular cartilage, the chondrocytes which would be the most responsive to IL-1 *in vitro* are those which are close to the surface of the tissue, and most likely to be exposed to IL-1 in synovial fluid.

LONG-TERM CULTURES IN AGAROSE GEL

The different capacities of chondrocytes from zones I and III to accumulate an extracellular matrix when grown under similar conditions in agarose gel were obvious at early stages of culture, but became progressively more marked with time. The higher rates of synthesis of proteoglycans and collagens contribute to these differences, as does the greater retention of these macromolecules in the vicinity of zone III chondrocytes (4,5). Although some zone I cells produced a fibrillar matrix poor in proteoglycans, others retained very little morphologically distinct matrix. Even in a mixed population of chondrocytes from zone II, after an initial accumulation of compact matrix around some of the cells, this matrix was gradually lost at later stages of culture, coincident with an overgrowth of irregularly shaped cells which lacked matrix (Fig. 3A). Conversely, during a period of 2–6 weeks, chondrocytes from zone III surrounded themselves with a highly organized extracellular matrix and formed chondron-like structures (Fig. 3B). Such matrix consisted of both a proteoglycan-rich pericellular zone and a more peripheral layer resembling a territorial matrix, with collagen fibers oriented primarily parallel to the cell surface (Fig. 4). This matrix showed strong bire-fringence when examined by polarizing microscopy, as a result of the circular orientation of the collagen fibers (Fig. 5) (22). Chondrocytes from deep layers of cartilage which elaborated this kind of matrix were stable in culture for long periods and could be maintained for over 6 months with little change except for growing cell-clusters near the periphery of the culture. In our experience, zone I chondrocytes have not assembled a similar cartilaginous matrix nor formed stable populations when cultured within agarose.

Many chondrocytes from deep layers of cartilage, but not those from other zones, enlarged and became hypertrophic after several weeks. Changes charac-

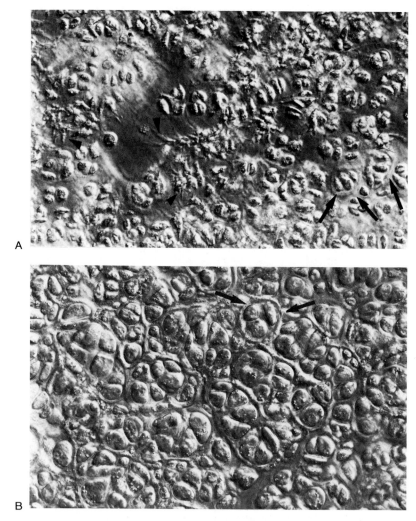

FIG. 3. Bovine articular chondrocytes cultured for 6 weeks in an agarose gel (Hoffman modulation contrast, ×225). **A:** Mixed population derived from middle-depth slices of cartilage; some chondrocytes are rounded and enclosed in matrix (*arrows*), whereas others lack visible matrix but have long cell processes (*arrowheads*). **B:** Chondrocytes isolated from deep slices of cartilage are more homogeneous; note the preponderence of groups of large, rounded hypertrophic cells encircled by dense matrix (*arrows*).

teristic of chondrocyte hypertrophy (e.g., synthesis of alkaline phosphatase) were also observed in porcine chondrocytes derived from deep cartilage and cultured as a monolayer (6). Human chondrocytes in liquid suspension also initiated synthesis of alkaline phosphatase, but cells from both the superficial and deep regions of the cartilage showed similar biochemical changes characteristic of maturation, although apparently without accompanying morphological changes

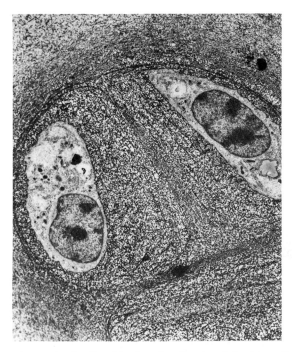

FIG. 4. Electron micrograph of cultured bovine chondrocytes derived from the radial zone of articular cartilage (×3160). These cells were cultured for 9 weeks in an agarose gel, and then they were fixed in the presence of ruthenium hexamine trichloride to stain proteoglycans. Note the extensive, well-organized matrix produced *in vitro,* with a pericellular region rich in proteoglycans; also note the collagen fibrils in the territorial matrix oriented predominantly parallel to the cell surface. (Electron microscopy courtesy of J. R. Kuszak.)

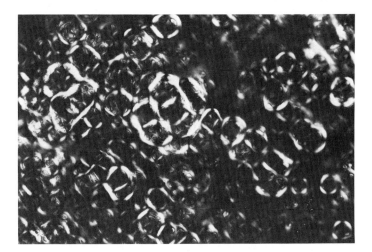

FIG. 5. Bovine articular chondrocytes derived from the entire thickness of cartilage. These cells were cultured for 11 weeks within agarose, and then they were viewed by polarizing microscopy (×75). Note the strong birefringence of the matrix partitions surrounding groups of cells.

(15). The calcium content of the medium was low, and the matrix did not become mineralized in these cultures (15).

CARTILAGE ORGAN CULTURES

The metabolism of different groups of chondrocytes has also been studied in organ cultures with the cells retained in their original matrix (8,9). When initially placed in culture, or after maintenance in medium lacking serum or other growth factors, the superficial zone showed the lowest rate of proteoglycan synthesis based upon the wet weight of the tissue, even though this region was the most cellular (8,9). However, proteoglycan synthesis was stimulated by serum growth factors, and interestingly, in organ cultures, the chondrocytes of the superficial zone showed the greatest response (8). It seems unlikely that the rate of diffusion of growth factors through the tissue was a limiting factor, because the results were similar whether the cartilage was (a) cultured as full-depth plugs and sub-divided later for analysis or (b) cultured as thin slices separated according to distance from the articular surface (8). By contrast with serum, insulin (which can readily permeate cartilage matrix) stimulated proteoglycan synthesis to a similar degree in all zones of the tissue (8). The variation in response of chon-drocytes to serum may have resulted from a differential partition of high-molecular-weight growth factors, which could readily penetrate the superficial zone but would have only limited access to cells in the middle and deep zones of cartilage which lie within a matrix rich in proteoglycans (8).

CONCLUSIONS AND FURTHER CHALLENGES

Subpopulations of chondrocytes isolated from their native matrix in superficial and deep regions of articular cartilage and cultured either as suspensions or as high-density monolayers show both morphological and quantitative metabolic differences which persist over a period of many weeks. These results are consistent with the retention and continued expression in culture of some intrinsic cellular differences. During their isolation from cartilage, the chondrocytes are completely denuded of their specialized matrix, and they are then placed under identical conditions of culture. However, they cannot be retained for a long period in the same milieu, because the chondrocytes themselves immediately begin to modify their microenvironments by elaborating a new extracellular matrix, and this in turn influences their metabolism. While subpopulations of chondrocytes from both superficial and deep zones continue to synthesize predominantly type II collagen and aggrecan in agarose gels, only the chondrocytes from deep in the tissue reestablish a highly organized matrix which closely resembles that in the deep zone of normal articular cartilage (4). The chondrocytes from the tangential zone of cartilage are normally enclosed within a dense matrix of fine collagen fibrils which has a relatively low concentration of proteoglycans, but these cells do not elaborate such a matrix under a variety of culture conditions so far tested.

Suspension within an agarose gel helps to preserve a spherical cell-shape which is important for normal phenotypic expression of chondrocytes, but even in this environment some cartilage cells eventually assume highly irregular contours with numerous processes. The zone I chondrocytes, in particular, are much more labile in their morphology than are deep cells, and they have a strong tendency to form monolayers and networks by spreading and migrating on any surfaces available within or around the agarose gel. Culture of chondrocytes suspended in liquid medium, and the absence of available surfaces for cellular attachment (apart from other chondrocytes), apparently resulted in better phenotypic stability of zone I chondrocytes (7). Nevertheless, in the culture environment, qualitative anabolic differences between populations from superficial and deep zones of human cartilage gradually diminished. Cells from both groups underwent an accelerated maturation and started to synthesize type X collagen and alkaline phosphatase (15). Thus, the conditions of culture which will induce cultured zone I chondrocytes to elaborate a matrix similar to that in the tangential zone of articular cartilage have not yet been realized. Furthermore, results of these experiments suggest that the heterogeneity of chondrocytes within articular cartilage stems to some degree from intrinsic cellular variation, but also results from differing environmental influences.

Within the joint, chondrocytes in the superficial zone are flattened and disc-shaped, oriented parallel to the articular surface. Perhaps this cell shape results partly from the forces of tension and compression in this part of the cartilage during development and growth of the epiphysis, and during normal loading with movement of the joint. Such a shape may also be a prerequisite for the normal phenotypic expression of superficial chondrocytes. It will be interesting to examine the morphology and metabolism of superficial chondrocytes, and to examine their capacity for reconstructing their characteristic matrix when cultured under tension, pressure, or other conditions which force the cells to retain a discoid shape. Such studies are planned, but the work is currently hampered by continuing difficulties in separating chondrocytes from the superficial zone in sufficient numbers, and with the least possible contamination with cells from deeper layers. If specific membrane markers for different groups of chondrocytes could be identified and prepared, these would facilitate more efficient cell separations.

The superficial zone of articular cartilage plays a vital role in the healthy joint by virtue of its unique location, structure, and material properties. It provides a smooth surface with low friction which withstands high tensile stresses, and it distributes the load over the surface of the joint, thereby protecting the underlying cartilage. However, the tangential layer is also the first region to show signs of deterioration in osteoarthritis; loss of integrity in this protective "skin" exposes the deeper cartilage to damaging stresses of loading during joint movement. Therefore, further attempts must be made to understand better the unique features of the superficial zone chondrocytes, to determine how their metabolism can be modulated to promote both the synthesis of appropriate macromolecules and the incorporation of these components into a strong, well-organized matrix.

If this goal could be attained for cultured chondrocytes, there would be better possibilities for understanding how the metabolism of these special cells could be manipulated within the intact joint in ways to maintain tissue integrity.

ACKNOWLEDGMENTS

We are grateful for support (for the preparation of this manuscript and for some of the studies described herein) from an Arthritis Research Grant of Werk Kalle-Albert of Hoechst Aktiengesellschaft (Germany) and from the National Institute of Arthritis and Musculoskeletal and Skin Diseases (NIH grant 1-P50 A-39239). We sincerely appreciate the expert technical assistance of Robert R. Greenhill and David H. Pearl.

REFERENCES

1. Aydelotte MB, Kuettner KE. Heterogeneity of articular chondrocytes and cartilage matrix. In: Woessner JF, Howell DS, eds. *Cartilage degradation: basic and clinical aspects.* New York: Marcel Dekker, 1991; in press.
2. Zanetti M, Ratcliffe A, Watt FM. Two subpopulations of differentiated chondrocytes identified with a monoclonal antibody to keratan sulfate. *J Cell Biol* 1985;101:53–59.
3. Aydelotte MB, Schleyerbach R, Zeck BJ, Kuettner KE. Articular chondrocytes cultured in agarose gel for study of chondrocytic chondrolysis. In: Kuettner KE, Schleyerbach R, Hascall VC, eds. *Articular cartilage biochemistry.* New York: Raven Press, 1986;235–256.
4. Aydelotte MB, Kuettner KE. Differences between sub-populations of cultured bovine articular chondrocytes. I. Morphology and cartilage matrix production. *Connect Tissue Res* 1988;18:205–222.
5. Aydelotte MB, Greenhill RR, Kuettner KE. Differences between sub-populations of cultured bovine articular chondrocytes. II. Proteoglycan metabolism. *Connect Tissue Res* 1988;18:223–234.
6. Siczkowski M, Watt FM. Subpopulations of chondrocytes from different zones of pig articular cartilage. Isolation, growth and proteoglycan synthesis in culture. *J Cell Sci* 1990;97:349–360.
7. Archer CW, McDowell J, Bayliss MT, Stephens MD, Bentley G. Phenotypic modulation in sub-populations of human articular chondrocytes *in vitro. J Cell Sci* 1990;97:361–371.
8. Maroudas A, Schneiderman R, Weinberg C, Grusko G. Choice of specimens in comparative studies involving human femoral head cartilage. In: Maroudas A, Kuettner K, eds. *Methods in cartilage research.* London: Academic Press, 1990;9–17.
9. Korver GHV, van de Stadt RJ, van Kampen GPJ, van der Korst JK. Composition of proteoglycans synthesized in different layers of cultured anatomically intact articular cartilage. *Matrix* 1990;10:394–401.
10. Benya PD, Shaffer JD. Dedifferentiated chondrocytes reexpress the differentiated collagen phenotype when cultured in agarose gels. *Cell* 1982;30:215–224.
11. Brown PD, Benya PD. Alterations in chondrocyte cytoskeletal architecture during phenotypic modulation by retinoic acid and dihydrocytochalasin B-induced reexpression. *J Cell Biol* 1988;106:171–179.
12. Archer CW, Bayliss MT. Phenotypic convergence of human articular chondrocytes *in vitro. Trans Orthop Res Soc* 1990;15:305.
13. Aydelotte MB, Thonar EJ-MA, Lenz RE, Schumacher BL, Kuettner KE. Differences in synthesis of keratan sulfate by sub-populations of cultured bovine articular chondrocytes. *Orthop Trans (J Bone Joint Surg)* 1989;13:273.
14. Aydelotte MB, Schmid TM, Greenhill RR, Luchene BL, Schumacher BL, Kuettner KE. Synthesis of collagen by cultured bovine chondrocytes derived from different depths of articular cartilage. *Trans Orthop Res Soc* 1991;16:26.
15. Stephens M, Kwan A, Bayliss M, Archer C. Human articular surface chondrocytes initiate alkaline phosphatase and type X collagen synthesis in suspension culture. *Trans Orthop Res Soc* 1991;16:101.

16. Murphy G, Hembry RM, Reynolds JJ. Characterization of a specific antiserum to rabbit stromelysin and demonstration of the synthesis of collagenase and stromelysin by stimulated rabbit articular chondrocytes. *Coll Relat Res* 1986;6:351–364.

17. Ratcliffe A, Tyler JA, Hardingham TE. Articular cartilage cultured with interleukin 1. Increased release of link protein, hyaluronate-binding region and other proteoglycan fragments. *Biochem J* 1986;238:571–580.

18. Benton HP, Tyler JA. Inhibition of cartilage proteoglycan synthesis by interleukin I. *Biochem Biophys Res Commun* 1988;154:421–428.

19. Morales TI, Hascall VC. Effects of interleukin-1 and lipopolysaccharides on protein and carbohydrate metabolism in bovine articular cartilage organ cultures. *Connect Tissue Res* 1989;19: 255–275.

20. Aydelotte MB, Raiss RX, Schleyerbach R, Kuettner KE. Effects of interleukin-1 on metabolism of proteoglycans by cultured bovine articular chondrocytes. *Orthop Trans (J Bone Joint Surg)* 1988;12:359.

21. Ollivierre F, Gubler U, Towle CA, Laurencin C, Treadwell BV. Expression of IL-1 genes in human and bovine chondrocytes: a mechanism for autocrine control of cartilage matrix degradation. *Biochem Biophys Res Commun* 1986;141:904–911.

22. Módis L. Factors involved in formation and maintenance of oriented microstructure of matrix constituents. In: Módis L, ed. *Organization of the extracellular matrix: a polarization microscope approach.* Boca Raton, FL: CRC Press, 1991;177–206.

DISCUSSION

Werb: What are the phenotypic differences between cells derived from the different zones?

Aydelotte: The cells from the superficial zone degrade proteoglycans more rapidly. That's the only way they seem to be more metabolically active than the cells from the deep zone; otherwise they synthesize less proteoglycans and less collagen.

Werb: But have they become more fibroblastic? For example, do they make type I collagen?

Aydelotte: I think they make some type I collagen when they flatten and attach to a surface. It would also be interesting to know if they make type IIA collagen rather than type IIB, because Linda Sandell stated that cells that make type IIA collagen do not accumulate matrix.

Kimura: We have a cell line from a human chondrosarcoma which morphologically exhibits many of the features that you see for these superficial cells, including cell processes. They make a large cartilage-type proteoglycan that has keratan sulfate on it. They stain positively with an antibody against type II collagen. Therefore, I am not sure one can correlate cell morphology with biochemical expression.

von der Mark: Do the chondrocyte–agarose cultures synthesize any type IX collagen? Furthermore, was there any type X synthesized in your long-term cultures?

Aydelotte: We have shown by immunohistochemistry that both type IX and type XI collagen are made. Their distribution is similar to that of type II collagen. SDS-PAGE analyses in a calcification study show that the cells from deep cartilage synthesize type X collagen, but not in great quantities.

Campion: Danger to cartilage integrity is thought to come from the synovial cavity, and it seems paradoxical that the superficial cells seem to be more responsive to cytokines such as IL-1, which are implicated in some joint diseases. Are we looking the wrong way round? Is the danger to cartilage coming from the bone side?

Aydelotte: No, not really! I think cells near the articular surface have special roles such as in controlling what passes through that zone to the deeper layers. I think some of Derek Cooke's work on deposition of immune complexes may illustrate this specialized function.

Articular Cartilage and Osteoarthritis,
edited by K. Kuettner et al.
Raven Press, Ltd., New York © 1992.

17

Mediators of Matrix Catabolism

Jenny A. Tyler, Shirley Bolis, John T. Dingle,
and James F. S. Middleton

Strangeways Research Laboratory, Cambridge CB1 4RN, England

RELATIONSHIP BETWEEN MATRIX STRUCTURE AND SUSCEPTIBILITY TO DEGRADATION

Articular chondrocytes synthesize, organize, and regulate the deposition of their complex extracellular matrix in a highly ordered and efficient manner. At each stage of growth and development the relative rates of synthesis and degradation are adjusted to achieve net growth, remodeling, or a balanced equilibrium. The two major structural components of the matrix, namely the collagen fibrils and the aggregating proteoglycans, have very different structures and rates of turnover, which reflect their different function within the joint. The type II collagen exists as a composite fibrillar structure together with types IX and XI collagen in a ratio of about 8:1:1 (1), and the three are bound together via covalent cross-links (2–5) (see chapter by Eyre et al.). The synthesis, secretion, and maturation of these molecules into insoluble fibers proceed via a series of complex processing stages (6), and the various intermediate forms vary considerably in their susceptibility to degradation. An important early intracellular step is the formation of a continuous triple helix by 96% of the type II protein. This portion of the molecule is digested by all neutral proteinases except for the specific collagenase. The formation of intermolecular cross-links within hours after fibril formation also dramatically increases the resistance of the helix to solubilization by collagenase (7). Even the vulnerable nonhelical telopeptide regions become protected as the fiber bundle increases in diameter.

Type XI collagen also consists mainly of a continuous helix, but lacks the specific site for collagenase cleavage (8,9), and it may act to stabilize the fibril structure. The insoluble, highly cross-linked collagen present in mature articular cartilage is therefore designed to have a very slow basal rate of turnover and provides a permanent inextensible framework which is essential for normal function and which provides the tensile strength of the tissue.

The aggregating proteoglycans are packed within this fibril network at a concentration of 50–80 mg/ml. The monomers can bind noncovalently to a single unbranched chain of hyaluronic acid (HA) to form large macromolecular aggregates (10) (see chapter by Hardingham et al.). The interaction is promoted and stabilized by link protein (11) as shown in Fig. 1. The core protein of the proteoglycan extends away from the HA into the matrix; in addition, the attached negatively charged glycosaminoglycans entrap solvent, thereby creating a high osmotic pressure which is restrained by the collagen. It is this swelling pressure, together with the low hydraulic permeability of the proteoglycan gel, that enables cartilage to resist compressive loads with minimal deformation. In contrast to the collagen, the core protein of the proteoglycan is extremely sensitive to proteolysis. Many active proteinases will preferentially cleave the region between the G1 and G2 globular domains, which is not protected sterically by either the HA or the glycosaminoglycans. A single cleavage leads to the irreversible loss of the functional part of the molecule which rapidly diffuses out of the tissue. These proteoglycans are therefore continually being degraded throughout the life of the cartilage.

Fortunately, normal chondrocytes are able to maintain the appropriate concentration of proteoglycan which is characteristic of the age, location, and species of the tissue. Following enzyme-induced (12) or interleukin-1 (IL-1)-induced (13) depletion, the proteoglycans are easily resynthesised and repacked within the fibrillar network to restore the balance back to the original level. It is not known how the chondrocytes regulate this equilibrium or why the cells lose the ability to do so in osteoarthritis.

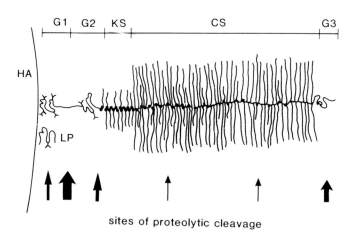

sites of proteolytic cleavage

FIG. 1. Diagram of cartilage proteoglycan molecule (10) to show the interaction of the G1 region of the core protein with hyaluronic acid (HA) and link protein (LP). The major sites sensitive to proteolytic attack are the three globular regions G3, G2, and G1, although cleavage can also occur within the chondroitin sulfate (CS) and keratan sulfate (KS) attachment regions and the link protein.

MEDIATORS OF MATRIX DEPLETION

The balance of matrix equilibrium in cartilage can be influenced experimentally by many different factors. One of the most important but least understood is mechanical loading (14); another is the induction of matrix resorption by products of synovial and mononuclear cells, most of which have been shown to be cytokines. Retinol, retinoic acid, and bacterial lipopolysaccharides will also induce rapid net loss of matrix (Fig. 2) (15–18). It is now widely accepted that cytokines induce proteoglycan depletion in cartilage by increasing the rate of degradation (19–25) and decreasing synthesis (26–29). Dose–response curves for pig articular cartilage cultured for 72 hr with a variety of cytokines are shown in Fig. 3a and 3b. When used alone, IL-1α is more potent (by at least an order of magnitude) than TNFα, but together they show a synergistic enhancement (27). The rate-limiting step for decreased matrix production is either transcription or translation of the core protein and procollagen chains. IL-1 had no significant effect on post-translational modification or secretion of proteoglycan (30) and did not alter the rate of intracellular degradation of newly synthesized collagen (31). The mRNA levels for types II, IX, and XI collagen were decreased in parallel in a dose-dependent manner in response to IL-1 (32). The potency of IL-1 can also be modified by the presence of growth factors such as insulin-like growth factor 1 (IGF-1) (Table 1) (33), transforming growth factor β (TGF-β) (34,35), and

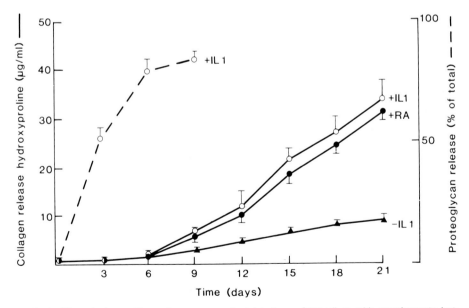

FIG. 2. Pig articular cartilage slices were cultured in Iscove's medium with supplements but without serum for 21 days in the presence or absence of human recombinant IL-1α (10 ng/ml) or retinoic acid (10^{-7} M). Cumulative release of collagen (measured as hydroxyproline) and proteoglycan (measured by reaction with 1,9-dimethylmethylene blue) into the medium is shown ($n = 4 \pm$ SEM).

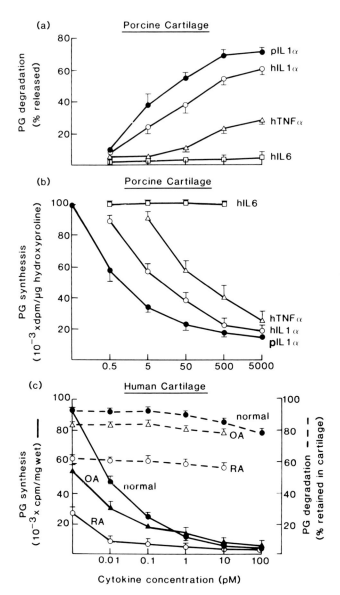

FIG. 3. a,b: The effects of different cytokines on cartilage proteoglycan (PG) synthesis and degradation. Pig articular cartilage slices were cultured for 72 hr in Iscove's medium with supplements but without serum, as described (26). The cultures contained increasing concentrations of human recombinant cytokines. Proteoglycan synthesis was estimated by incorporation of [^{35}S]sulfate (3-hr pulse) into glycosaminoglycan at the end of the culture period, and is shown as a proportion of the control value cultured in the absence of cytokines. Degradation was analyzed by reaction with 1,9-dimethylmethylene blue binding to glycosaminoglycans and is shown as the proportion of the total present in the medium ($n = 4 \pm$ SEM). **c:** Cartilage explants of equivalent size were taken postoperatively from disease-free (histologically normal) knee joints of patients undergoing lower-limb amputations or from osteoarthritic (OA) and rheumatoarthritic (RA) patients following total joint replacement. The slices were cultured in DMEM with 5% FCS for 8 days, with increasing concentrations of recombinant human IL-1α. Proteoglycan synthesis was estimated by incorporation of [^{35}S]sulfate (16-hr pulse) into glycosaminoglycan at the end of the culture period. Degradation was analyzed by reaction with 1,9-dimethylmethylene blue and is shown as the proportion of the total proteoglycan remaining in the cartilage ($n = 10 \pm$ SEM). pIL 1α, porcine interleukin-1α; hIL 1α, human interleukin-1α; hTNFα, human tumor necrosis factor α; hIL6, human interleukin-6.

TABLE 1. *Degradation of cartilage proteoglycan[a]*

	Medium (% of total)			Extract (% of total)		
	Control	IL-1	IL-1 + IGF-1	Control	IL-1	IL-1 + IGF-1
GAG	10	55	28	90	45	72
G1	3	34	8	97	20	92
G2	8	40	10	92	30	81
HA	7	21	6	93	79	94

[a] Pig articular cartilage explants were cultured in Iscove's medium without serum. The cultures contained no addition (control), human recombinant IL-1 (500 pM), or IL-1 and human recombinant IGF-1 (100 ng/ml) together. The amounts of glycosaminoglycan (GAG), hyaluronic acid (HA), and G1 or G2 globular regions of the core protein (see Fig. 1) were estimated by chemical or radioimmunoassay as described (56); these amounts are shown as the proportion of total present in the culture medium or in the cartilage extracts after 4 days.

fibroblast growth factor (FGF) (36), so the net activity observed will depend on the relative concentration of each mediator present.

Cartilage and chondrocytes cultured with IL-1 secrete both IL-6 and IL-8 into the medium (37,38; J. A. Tyler, *unpublished results*). It was not known whether these cytokines could influence cartilage metabolism. We therefore tested the action of IL-6 in several cartilage bioassays. Proteoglycan synthesis and degradation was unaffected at concentrations of up to 500 pM (Figure 3 a and 3b), and this cytokine did not induce production of stromelysin or prostaglandin E2 and did not alter collagen synthesis. There was also no effect of dexamethasone on IL-1-mediated proteoglycan degradation at doses which inhibit synthesis of IL-6 and IL-8, indicating that these cytokines do not potentiate the action of IL-1 on cartilage. IL-6 has been detected in the synovial fluid of patients with osteoarthritis (39,40) and could act locally to promote local antibody production. However, the main role of IL-6 *in vivo* is to stimulate hepatocytes as part of the acute-phase response to trauma (40). Unlike IL-1 which can also stimulate production of some acute-phase proteins, IL-6 specifically induces the synthesis of serum proteinase inhibitors such as $\alpha 2$ macroglobulin, $\alpha 1$ antitrypsin, and $\alpha 1$ proteinase inhibitor. This markedly increases the inhibitory capacity of the serum and synovial fluid, which can provide a valuable protection mechanism against rapid cartilage degradation.

Interferon γ also inhibits type II collagen synthesis in chondrocytes and induces the expression of class II major histocompatibility complex (MHC) antigens on the cell surface (41), although it is not clear whether chondrocytes stimulated in this way can present antigen or activate T lymphocytes.

THE ACTION OF IL-1 ON NORMAL AND DISEASED HUMAN CARTILAGE

The effects of increasing concentrations of IL-1 on proteoglycan metabolism in normal and diseased human cartilage are shown in Fig. 3. A dose-dependent inhibition of proteoglycan synthesis occurred in the normal tissue in a similar manner to that observed with pig and other animal cartilages. However, no release of proteoglycan degradation fragments was induced by IL-1 at concentrations of less than 500 pM. These effects are not age-dependent, because 10 cartilage specimens from a young group (6–18 years of age) and 10 from an older group (20–66 years of age) reacted in the same way. The initial rates of proteoglycan synthesis in the pathological specimens cultured without IL-1 was much less than those in the normal specimens (rheumatoarthritic < osteoarthritic), and the basal release of proteoglycan was higher (rheumatoarthritic > osteoarthritic); but again a similar inhibition of matrix synthesis was evident in response to IL-1, with little increase in the rate of degradation. The reason for the poor general catabolic response of human cartilage to IL-1 is not known and is under investigation. It is unlikely to result from an inability of degradation

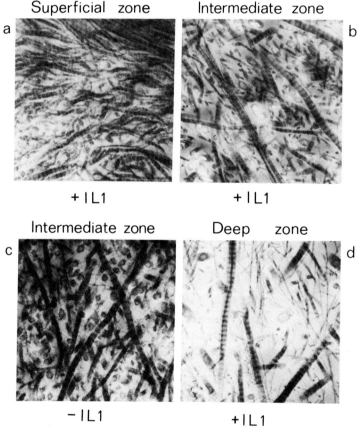

FIG. 4. Transmission electron micrographs showing the collagen fibrils in pig articular cartilage slices cultured in the presence (**a,b,d**) and absence (**c**) of human recombinant IL-1α (10 ng/ml) for 15 days as shown in Fig. 2.

fragments to diffuse out of the matrix, because we have shown that a few (<10%) specimens in previous samples (42) could be stimulated to resorb when cultured with IL-1; furthermore, explants similar to those used in the present study consistently show enhanced release of proteoglycan when cultured with retinol (43).

In complete contrast to cartilage injuries involving acute and transient loss of proteoglycan, any damage which involves mechanical disruption of the collagen network is usually irreversible, particularly if significant cell death also occurs (see ref. 61). If cultured cartilage is exposed to high concentrations of IL-1, a significant increase in the release of collagen can only be detected after 6–8 days (Fig. 2). This emphasizes the difference between collagen's susceptibility to degradation and that of proteoglycan, where increased release of fragments can be detected within 12 hr. A similar lag period for collagen resorption is seen using retinol as the catabolic mediator. Examination of the resorbing explants following 15 days of continuous exposure to IL-1 (10 ng/ml) demonstrated a major change in the fibril structure. In the superficial layers of the cartilage, electron micrographs revealed that instead of the usual tangential orientation parallel to the surface, the fibrils were often random and disorientated (Fig. 4a). In the deeper layers, a high proportion of fibrils had split parallel to their long axes and were frayed at the ends (Figs. 4b and 4d). These changes in collagen ultrastructure are similar to those observed in human and animal osteoarthritic articular cartilage (44,45). It is not yet known how collagen fragmentation is induced by IL-1, but it is possible that degradation of the type IX collagen or a change in the way these molecules are cross-linked within the composite fibril may promote swelling and permit access of proteinases to initiate degradation of the bulk of the type II collagen.

ENZYMES THAT CAN DEGRADE CARTILAGE MATRIX

Many proteinases that can degrade cartilage matrix components have been identified in connective tissues and inflammatory cells, and four main classes are recognized. The likely substrates of these enzymes and their modes of action on cartilage proteoglycan and collagen are shown in Table 2 and described in detail elsewhere (46). Genes specifying all of these enzymes have now been cloned and sequenced, and the synthesis of many of them has been shown to be altered by a variety of cytokines, growth factors, and hormones. All are produced initially as inactive proforms that are later converted to the active proteinases. These, in turn, are subject to inhibition by a range of specific protein inhibitors. The availability of proteolytic activity within cytokine-activated cartilage is therefore very carefully regulated at several stages (for recent reviews see refs. 46–51). The conversion of proenzymes to the active forms probably represents the key step in the degradative process. Knowledge of where and how this activation is achieved is essential in order to understand how the chondrocyte controls the turnover of its extracellular matrix.

TABLE 2. *Proteinases that can degrade cartilage proteoglycan and type II collagen*

Proteinase	Class	Inhibitors	pH range	Core protein[a]	Collagen telopeptides	Substrates Insoluble helical collagen	Solubilized helical collagen	Gelatin
Cathepsin B	Cysteine (EC 3.4.22)	Cystatins, α2M	3–5.5	1–2	Yes	Yes	Yes	Yes
Cathepsin L	Cysteine (EC 3.4.22)	Cystatins, α2M		5–12	Yes	Yes	Yes	Yes
Cathepsin H	Cysteine (EC 3.4.22)	Cystatins, α2M		?	Yes	Yes	Yes	Yes
Cathepsin D	Aspartic (EC 3.4.23)	α2M	4–6	5–12	Limited	No	No	No
Plasmin	Serine (EC 3.4.21)	α2M, α1AC, α1 PI	6–9	>15	?	No	No	
Elastase	Serine (EC 3.4.21)	α1 PI, α1AC, α2M	6–9	1–2	Yes[b]	No	No	
Cathepsin G	Serine	α1	6–9	5–12	Yes[b]	No	No	Yes
Stromelysin	Metallo (EC 3.4.24)	TIMP1, TIMP2, α2M	6–9	5–12	Yes[b]	No	No	Limited
Gelatinase	Metallo (EC 3.4.24)	TIMP1, TIMP2, α2M	7–8	?	Limited	No	No	Yes
Collagenase	Metallo (EC 3.4.24)	TIMP1, TIMP2, α2M	7–8	No	No	Limited	Yes	Limited/?

[a] Numbers represent the average number of glycosaminoglycan chains left attached to the core protein fragments.
[b] Active only at very high enzyme concentrations.

GROWTH FACTORS CAN ANTAGONIZE CYTOKINE ACTION AND DECREASE MATRIX CATABOLISM

Insulin-like growth factor 1 (IGF-1) has long been regarded as a major mediator of proteoglycan synthesis (52,53), and sulfation of proteoglycan in cultured cartilage explants has formed the basis of the somatomedin bioassay for many years (54,55). IGF-1 can promote proteoglycan synthesis even in the presence of quite high concentrations of cytokines and can partially alleviate the inhibition induced by IL-1 and tumor necrosis factor (TNF) (33). Surprisingly, IGF-1 also has a marked effect on matrix degradation. Glycosaminoglycans are released from cartilage exposed to IL-1 due to a cleavage of the core protein between G2 and the keratan sulfate attachment region and between G1 and G2. Some molecules are also cleaved within the chondroitin sulfate attachment region (Fig. 1). The large fragments bearing intact glycosaminoglycan chains rapidly diffuse out of the matrix. There is also a significant increase in the release of HA and of the G1 portion of the molecule, which remains functional in the sense that it can still bind to both HA and link protein. Thus, in cartilage cultured for 4 days with IL-1 (50 pM), 55% of the chondroitin sulfate and keratan sulfate, 21% of the HA, 34% of G1, and 40% of G2 are released into the medium (Table 1) compared to 10%, 7%, 3%, and 8%, respectively, in the controls cultured without IL-1. In addition, 46% of the G1 and 30% of the G2 epitope cannot be accounted for within the matrix and are presumed to be completely degraded. If IGF-1 (100 ng/ml) is included in the cultures together with IL-1, only half as many core protein molecules were cleaved to release glycosaminoglycan (28%), and release of HA, G1, and G2 decreased almost to the level of the controls. There was also complete protection from proteolysis of the G1 and G2 epitopes within the explant (56). IGF-1 is therefore able to protect the cartilage (to a considerable extent) from the effects of cytokines.

IGF-1 IS SYNTHESIZED BY ARTICULAR CHONDROCYTES IN OSTEOARTHRITIC CARTILAGE

It seemed likely that increased local concentrations of cytokines and growth factors within the joint could give rise to some of the altered features observed in osteoarthritic cartilage. We therefore prepared cartilage blocks from normal and osteoarthritic human tissue. The samples were graded according to depth from the surface and were taken from macroscopically intact areas of the joint and from mild and severe osteoarthritic lesions. cDNA encoding IGF-1 (57) was cloned in two orientations in pSP64 and pSP65 plasmid vectors, and sense or antisense [^{35}S]RNA probes were synthesized by *in vitro* transcription using the SP6 promoter. *In situ* hybridization using the radiolabeled antisense probe as a specific signal and the sense probe as a nonspecific control showed that some IGF-1 mRNA was present in most chondrocytes (Fig. 5a). No significant

IGF 1   Tropomyosin

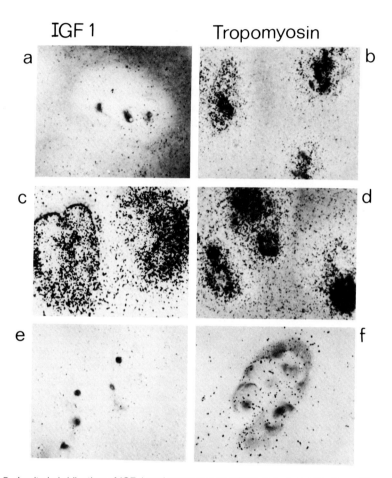

FIG. 5. *In situ* hybridization of IGF-1 and tropomyosin mRNA in human articular cartilage using ^{35}S-labeled RNA probes. **a,b:** Histologically normal region of osteoarthritic cartilage hybridized with antisense probes (the same pattern is seen for normal, nonosteoarthritic cartilage; *results not shown*). **c,d:** Fibrillated osteoarthritic cartilage with cell clones hybridized with antisense probes. **e,f:** As for **c,d,** but hybridized with control sense RNA probes to demonstrate specificity of binding.

difference was found between normal cartilage and histologically normal areas of osteoarthritic cartilage. Normal intact cartilage showed low message levels in the superficial zone and exhibited slightly higher message levels in the deeper zones. There was a striking increase in the amount of mRNA in chondrocytes from abnormal regions of osteoarthritic cartilage which were depleted of matrix. The highest level, four to five times that found in normal tissue, was demonstrated in clonal clusters of cells near the surface of fibrillated cartilage (Fig. 5c).

Immunolocalization with specific antibody (58) confirmed that the mRNA was also translated into protein. A quantitative analysis revealed that expression of the IGF-1 gene is increased in human articular chondrocytes in proportion to the severity of lesion in osteoarthritic cartilage (59). It is possible that a general increase in protein synthesis may accompany the cellular hypertrophy which occurs in osteoarthritic chondrocytes. To determine whether this is the case, we hybridized a variety of different RNA probes to the same range of tissues. In contrast to IGF-1, a high constant expression of tropomyosin (60) was detected in both normal and osteoarthritic chondrocytes (Fig. 5b and 5d) in parallel sections cut immediately adjacent to those shown for IGF-1 (Fig. 5a and 5c). We therefore concluded that up-regulation of IGF-1 expression in OA cartilage is a selective event.

CONCLUSIONS

The identity of mediators involved in the initiation and development of osteoarthritis has not yet been established, and it is not known why some joints progress to an irreversible degenerative condition while others can reverse the degradation process and even promote healing. It is proposed that the relative concentration of cytokines and growth factors acting locally on the chondrocytes at each stage may determine the rate of progress and final outcome of this type of disease.

ACKNOWLEDGMENTS

We thank Mrs. Yvonne Sawyer for expert technical assistance, and we are grateful to the Arthritis and Rheumatism Council and the Medical Research Council for financial support.

REFERENCES

1. Mayne R. Cartilage collagens. *Arthritis Rheum* 1989;32:241–246.
2. Eyre DR, Apon S, Wu J-J, Ericsson LH, Walsh KA. Collagen type IX: evidence for covalent cross-links to type II collagen in cartilage. *FEBS Lett* 1987;220:337–341.
3. van der Rest M, Mayne R. In: Mayne R, Burgeson RE, eds. *Structure and function in collagen types.* New York: Academic Press, 1987;195–221.
4. Vaughan L, Mendler M, Huber S, Bruckner P, Winterhalter KH, Irwin MI, Mayne R. D-periodic distribution of collagen type IX along cartilage fibrils. *J Cell Biol* 1988;106:991–997.
5. Mendler M, Eich-Bender SG, Vaughan L, Winterhalter KH, Bruckner P. Cartilage contains mixed fibrils of collagen types II, IX and XI. *J Cell Biol* 1989;108:191–197.
6. Kivirikko KI, Myllyla R. Biosynthesis of the collagens. In: Piez KA, Reddi AH, eds. *Extracellular matrix biochemistry.* New York: Elsevier, 1984;83–118.
7. Vator CA, Harris ED, Siegel RC. Native cross-links in collagen fibrils induced resistance to human synovial collagenase. *Biochem J* 1979;181:639–645.
8. Gadher SJ, Eyre DR, Wotton SF, Schmid TM, Woolley DE. Degradation of cartilage collagens type II, IX, X and XI by enzymes derived from human articular chondrocytes. *Matrix* 1990;110: 154–163.
9. Eyre DR, Wu J-J, Woolley DE. All three chains of 1α, 2α and 3α collagen from hyaline cartilage resist human cartilage. *Biochem Biophys Res Commun* 1984;118:724–729.

10. Hardingham TE, Beardmore-Grey M, Dunham DG, Ratcliffe A. Cartilage proteoglycans. *Ciba Found Symp* 1986;124:30–46.
11. Hardingham TE. The role of link protein in the structure of cartilage proteoglycan aggregates. *Biochem J* 1979;177:237–247.
12. Thomas L. Reversible collapse of rabbit ears after intravenous papain and prevention of recovery by cortisone. *J Exp Med* 1956;104:245–255.
13. Page Thomas DP, King B, Stephens T, Dingle JT. *In vivo* studies of cartilage regeneration after damage induced by catabolin/IL1. *Ann Rheum Dis* 1991;50:75–80.
14. Helminen HJ, Jurvelin J, Kiviranta I, Paukkonen K, Saamanen AM, Tammi M. Joint loading effects on articular cartilage. A historical review. In: Helminen HJ, ed. *Joint loading biology and health of articular structures*. Bristol: John Wright & Sons, 1987;1–46.
15. Hembry RM. Studies on the action of retinol on cartilage. *Biochem Soc Trans* 1973;1:383–384.
16. Brinkerhoff CE, Nagas H, Nagel JE, Harris ED Jr. Effects of all *trans* retinoic acid and 4-hydroxyphenyl retinamide on synovial cells and articular cartilage. *J Am Acad Dermatol* 1982;6: 591–602.
17. Morales TI. The effect of bacterial LPS on the biosynthesis and release of proteoglycans from calf articular cartilage cultures. *J Biol Chem* 1984;259:6720–6729.
18. Tyler JA. The influence of IL1 and IGF1 on the integrity of cartilage matrix. In: Glauert AM, ed. *The control of tissue damage*. Amsterdam: Elsevier 1988;197–219.
19. Dingle JT, Saklatvala J, Hembry RM, Tyler JA, Fell HB, Jubb RN. A cartilage catabolic factor from synovium. *Biochem J* 1979;184:177–180.
20. Gowen M, Wood DD, Ihrie EJ, Meats JE, Russell RGG. Stimulation by human IL1 of cartilage breakdown and production of collagenase and proteoglycanase by human chondrocytes but not by human osteoblasts *in vitro. Biochem J* 1984;797;186.
21. Krakauer T, Oppenheim JJ, Jasin HE. Human interleukin 1 mediates cartilage matrix degradation. *Cell Immunol* 1985;91:92–99.
22. Tyler JA. Chondrocyte-mediated depletion of articular cartilage *in vitro. Biochem J* 1985;225: 493–507.
23. Saklatvala J. Pig catabolin is a form of interleukin 1. *Biochem J* 1984;224:461–66.
24. Pettipher ER, Higgs GA, Henderson B. Interleukin 1 induces leucocyte infiltration and cartilage proteoglycan degradation in the synovial joint. *Proc Natl Acad Sci USA* 1986;83:8749–8753.
25. Hubbard JR, Steinberg JJ, Bednar MS, Sledge CB. Effect on purified human interleukin 1 in cartilage degradation. *J Orthop Res* 1988;6:180–187.
26. Tyler JA. Articular cartilage cultured with catabolin (pig interleukin 1) synthesizes a decreased number of normal proteoglycan molecules. *Biochem J* 1985;227:869–878.
27. Saklatvala J. Tumour necrosis factor stimulates resorption and inhibits synthesis of proteoglycan in cartilage. *Nature* 1986;322:547–549.
28. van de Loo FAJ, van Beuningen, van Lend, van den Berg WB. Direct effect of murine rIL1 on cartilage metabolism *in vivo. Agents Actions* 1989;26:153–156.
29. van den Berg WB, van de Loo FAJ, Zwarts WA, Otterness IG. Effects of murine recombinant IL1 on intact homologous articular cartilage. *Ann Rheum Dis* 1988;47:855–863.
30. Benton H, Tyler JA. Inhibition of cartilage proteoglycan synthesis by interleukin 1. *Biochem Biophys Res Commun* 1988;154:421–428.
31. Tyler JA, Benton H. Synthesis of type II collagen is decreased in cartilage cultured with interleukin 1 while the rate of intracellular degradation remains unchanged. *Coll Relat Res* 1988;8:393–405.
32. Tyler JA, Bird JLE, Giller T. IL1 inhibits the production of types II, IX and XI procollagen mRNA in cartilage. *Ann New York Acad Sci* 1990;580:512–513.
33. Tyler JA. IGF1 can decrease degradation and promote synthesis of proteoglycan in cartilage exposed to cytokines. *Biochem J* 1989;260:543–548.
34. Chandraskehar S, Harvey AK. TGFβ is a potent inhibitor of IL1 induced protease activity and proteoglycan degradation. *Biochem Biophys Res Commun* 1988;157:1352–1359.
35. Morales TI, Roberts AB. TGFβ regulates the metabolism of proteoglycans in bovine cartilage organ cultures. *J Biol Chem* 1988;263:12828–12831.
36. Chandraskehar S, Harvey AK. Induction of IL1 receptors on chondrocytes by fibroblast growth factor. *J Cell Physiol* 1989;138:236–246.
37. Shinmei M, Masuda K, Kikuchi T, Shimomura Y. Interleukin 1, tumour necrosis factor and interleukin 6 as mediators of cartilage destruction. *Semin Arthritis Rheum* 1988;18:27–32.
38. Guerne PA, Vaughan JH, Carson DA, Terkettaub R, Lotz M. Interleukin 6 and joint tissues. *Ann NY Acad Sci* 1989;557:558–611.

39. Kishimoto T, Taga R, Yamazaki K. Normal and abnormal regulation of human B cell differentiation by a new cytokine BSF.2/IL6. In: Gupta S, Paul WE, Franci AS, eds. *Mechanisms of lymphocyte activation and immune regulation.* New York: Plenum Press, 1989;167–181.
40. Gauldie J. Interleukin 6 in the inflammatory response. In: Lewis AJ, Doherty NF, Akerman NR, eds. *The therapeutic control of inflammatory diseases.* Amsterdam: Elsevier, 1989;36–46.
41. Goldring MB, Sandell LJ, Stephenson ML, Krane SM. Immune interferon suppresses levels of procollagen mRNA and type II collagen synthesis in cultured human articular chondrocytes. *J Biol Chem* 1986;261:9049–9056.
42. Tyler JA, Sawyer Y. Cartilage explant cultures: a model system for the analyses of matrix degradation. In: Maroudas A, Kuettner K, eds. *Methods in cartilage research.* New York: Academic Press, 1990;112–116.
43. Jubb RW. Differential responses of human articular cartilage to retinol. *Ann Rheum Dis* 1984;43: 833–40.
44. Curtin WA, Reville WJ. Collagen profiles in normal & fibrillated articular cartilage. *Proc R Microsc Soc [Suppl]* 1990;25(6):5.
45. Orford CR, Gardener DL, O'Connor P. Ultrastructural changes in dog femoral condylar cartilage following anterior cruciate ligament section *J Anat* 1983;137(4):653–663.
46. Tyler JA. Cartilage degradation. In: Hall BK, Newman SA, eds. *Cartilage molecular aspects.* Boca Raton, FL: CRC Press, 1991;213–256.
47. Docherty AJP, Murphy G. The tissue metalloproteinase family and the inhibitor TIMP a study using cDNAs and recombinant proteins *Ann Rheum Dis* 1990;49:469–479.
48. Matrisian LM. Metalloproteinases and their inhibitors in matrix remodelling. *TIG* 1990;6:121–125.
49. Murphy G., Docherty AJP, Hembry RM, Reynolds JJ. Metalloproteinases and tissue damage. *Br J Rheumatol* 1991;30(Suppl):25–31.
50. Barrett AJ. *Proteinase inhibitors.* Amsterdam: Elsevier, 1986.
51. Barrett AJ, Buttle DJ, Mason RW. Lysosomal cysteine proteinases. In: *ISI atlas of science: Biochemistry.* 1988;1:256–260.
52. Schoenle E, Zapf J, Humbel RE, Froesch ER. Insulin-like growth factor 1 stimulates growth in hypophysectomized rats. *Nature* 1982;296:252–253.
53. Guenther HL, Guenther HE, Froesch ER, Fleisch H. Effect of insulin-like growth factor 1 on collagen and glycosaminoglycan synthesis by rabbit articular chondrocytes in culture. *Experientia* 1982;38:979–980.
54. Salmon WD, Daughaday WH. A hormonally controlled serum factor which stimulates sulphate incorporation by cartilage *in vitro. J Lab Clin Med* 1957;49:825–836.
55. Daughaday WH, Hall K, Raben MS, Salmon WD Jr, van den Brande JL, van Wyk JJ. Somatomedin: proposed designation for sulphation factor. *Nature* 1972;255:107.
56. Fosang AJ, Tyler JA, Hardingham TE. Effect of IL1 and IGF1 on the release of proteoglycan components and hyaluronan from pig articular cartilage in explant cultures. *Matrix* 1991;11: 17–24.
57. Jansen M, van Schaik FMA, Ricker AT, Bullock B, Woods DE, Gabbay KH, Nussbaum AL, Sussenbach JS, van den Brande JL. Sequence of cDNA encoding human insulin-like growth factor 1 precursor. *Nature* 1983;306:609–611.
58. Furlanetto RW, Underwood LE, van Wyk JJ, D'Ercole AJ. Estimation of somatomedin-C levels in normals and patients with pituitary disease by radioimmunoassay. *J Clin Invest* 1977;60:647–648.
59. Middleton JF, Tyler JA, IGF1 gene expression by osteoarthritic and normal human articular chondrocytes. *Trans Orthop Res Soc* 1991;16:384.
60. MacLeod AR, Houlker C, Reinach FC, Smille LB, Talbot K, Modi G, Walsh FS. A muscle-type tropomysin in human fibroblasts: evidence for expression by an alternative RNA splicing mechanism. *Proc Natl Acad Sci USA* 1985;82:7835–7839.
61. Buckwalter J, Rosenberg L, Coutts R, et al. Articular cartilage: injury and repair. In: Woo S, Buckwalter JA, eds. *Injury and repair of the musculoskeletal soft tissues.* John Wright and Sons, Bristol, 1988;465–482.

DISCUSSION

Sandell: Have you looked at IGF-1 receptors or binding parameters for IGF-1 to evaluate how the cells actually respond?

Tyler: Yes, but there are problems. When we started binding studies for IGF-1, we realized that IGF-1 was interacting with cell-associated binding protein 3 (BP3), a specific IGF-1-binding protein. In fact, all bound BP3 can enhance IGF-1 activity. In terms of receptor numbers, cells that produce high levels of IGF-1 down-regulate their receptors. This can lead to a lower response to exogenously added IGF-1.

Roughley: When IGF-1 is used to counteract the IL-1 response, does metalloproteinase production decrease or is there less activation, or does TIMP production increase?

Tyler: IGF-1 does alter production of these molecules. All the metalloproteinases are in the proenzyme form and therefore is latent in the explant culture system. Measurements of the amount of inactive enzyme secreted into the medium may not reveal much about the degradation process. Retinoic acid, for example, is a good resorptive agent, but inhibits metalloproteinase production.

van den Berg: You showed that adult human cartilage is not sensitive to IL-1-mediated degradation. Would you speculate that IL-1 is not a main factor in cartilage degradation in human disease like rheumatoid arthritis or osteoarthritis?

Tyler: It may be a question of dose and time. Longer exposure and higher doses may induce responses. In fact, about 15% of human explants do readily respond to IL-1 by increasing degradation. The difference between the nonresponders and responders really is not known.

van den Berg: Could the mechanism be related to different degrees of inhibitors present in the tissues?

Tyler: I do not think so, because retinol induces resorption of these explants by a mechanism that is probably quite different.

Maroudas: The relative lack of response of human cartilage to IL-1 depends on IL-1 partition and diffusion through the matrix. Adult human cartilages, particularly the hips, contain very high concentrations of proteoglycans compared with those of other cartilages. Although solutes the size of IL-1 do penetrate into cartilage, the rate and level are dependent on "excluded volume" effects of the glycosaminoglycans.

Tyler: But the dose response for inhibition of synthesis is actually very sensitive even in explants that do not respond by increasing degradation. So the IL-1 is getting in.

Hirschelmann: Both glucocorticoids and IL-1 inhibit proteoglycan synthesis while on the other hand glucocorticoids inhibit IL-1 synthesis in cartilage. Is this paradoxical?

Tyler: In my experience, glucocorticoids are very poor inhibitors of IL-1 action in the explant system. *In vivo,* however, there is a marked effect due to the inhibition of IL-1 synthesis. But I really have not done any detailed experiments along these lines.

Articular Cartilage and Osteoarthritis,
edited by K. Kuettner et al.
Raven Press, Ltd., New York © 1992.

18

Polypeptide Regulators of Matrix Homeostasis in Articular Cartilage

Teresa I. Morales

*Bone Research Branch, National Institute of Dental Research,
National Institutes of Health, Bethesda, Maryland 20205*

Osteoarthritis is a joint disease hallmarked by degeneration of the resilient layer of articular cartilage that shields bone from the compressive and frictional forces of normal joint motion and weight-bearing (1). The disease has a high incidence in the world population and a devastating economic impact. In the United States alone, it has been estimated that more than 37 million people suffer from arthritis and related diseases, costing the U.S. economy an estimated $8.6 billion in lost earnings and medical care (2,3). Osteoarthritis is the most common form of arthritis, claiming 16 million victims (3). Prevalence increases with age (4), and it has been estimated that by the year 2000 the cost to society of musculoskeletal diseases will triple (3). Osteoarthritis is a disease of diverse etiology and obscure pathogenesis (1).

Although the complexities of the disease remain to be fully elucidated, interest in understanding this ailment has generated vigorous research efforts focused on the elucidation of the morphology, biochemistry, and biomechanics of normal and diseased articular cartilage. Progress in these areas is evident in many of the chapters of this book, and only selected areas are overviewed here to provide general background for a discussion of polypeptide mediators of articular cartilage metabolism.

Anatomically, osteoarthritis includes (a) fragmentation of the surface layer of cartilage and (b) fissures of the matrix that eventually reach the underlying bone (1). Ulcers that grow radially, with progressive erosion of surrounding matrix, are seen as the disease progresses. Finally, there is complete loss of the cartilage surface with exposure of eburnated, sclerotic bone. Biochemically, human and experimental osteoarthritis involve an early swelling of cartilage, which is believed to be due to a loosening of the fibrillar network of the tissue (1). Furthermore, the progression of the human disease is correlated with increased metalloproteinase activity (5,6), particularly around the edges of the growing ulcers and

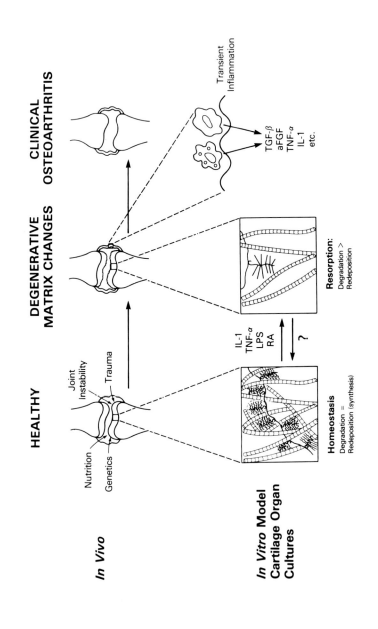

HEALTHY   **DEGENERATIVE MATRIX CHANGES**   **CLINICAL OSTEOARTHRITIS**

In Vivo

Genetics
Nutrition
Joint Instability
Trauma

Transient Inflammation

TGF-β
aFGF
TNF-α
IL-1
etc.

In Vitro Model Cartilage Organ Cultures

Homeostasis
Degradation =
Redeposition (synthesis)

IL-1
TNF-α
LPS
RA

?

Resorption:
Degradation >
Redeposition

with progressive loss of proteoglycans, collagen, and other matrix proteins (1). Thus, whether the trigger for matrix changes is biomechanical or biochemical, or both, this disease involves a common pathway that is characterized by extensive degeneration of the cartilage matrix (see Fig. 1).

The close interrelationships between structural design and biological function in articular cartilage suggest that changes in matrix structure can lead to further abnormalities in chondrocyte function. For example, it is clear that the swelling of the large anionic proteoglycan (aggrecan) complexes against the high tensile strength of the fibrillar collagen network creates an internal pressure within the tissue that opposes external compressive forces and that helps to restore cartilage to its initial shape upon removal of force (see ref. 7 for review). The collagen–proteoglycan architecture thus contributes to the protection of chondrocytes from the harsh mechanical environment of the joint and changes in matrix structure, if unrepaired, may lead to a vicious cycle of chondrocyte pathology and cartilage destruction.

Polypeptide mediators regulate matrix synthesis and structure, as well as tissue degradation (8,9). Thus, it is important to ask which polypeptides regulate the metabolism of normal articular chondrocytes, because this knowledge may lead to a mechanistic elucidation of derangements in osteoarthritis. Related questions pertaining to the potential role of polypeptide mediators as contributors and/or amplifiers of disease processes are relevant. For example, even though inflammation of the synovial membranes during early stages of osteoarthritis is believed to be minimal as compared to the severe, destructive inflammation that occurs during rheumatoid arthritis, it is likely that mediators released during transient inflammatory episodes contribute to the initiation and/or sustenance of matrix changes in osteoarthritic cartilage (1).

←———

FIG. 1. Schematic diagrams of degradative changes in the joint during the pathogenesis of osteoarthritis and of the *in vitro* model system used for evaluation of regulators of these processes. The etiology of osteoarthritis is diverse but commonly leads to degenerative matrix changes which evolve into complete erosion of the cartilage surface with exposure of eburnated bone. Cartilage slices maintained under suitable culture conditions provide a realistic *in vitro* model for the study of regulation of matrix metabolism, because: the cells remain embedded within the tissue architecture produced *in vivo;* they remain phenotypically stable for several weeks in culture; and they retain the ability to maintain tissue homeostasis. Shown in the lower diagrams are the two major matrix constituents: the collagen fibers and the aggrecans shown in association with a central hyaluronan strand. Interleukin-1 (IL-1), tumor necrosis factor α (TNF-α), bacterial lipopolysaccharides (LPS), and retinoic acid (RA) can induce resorption of matrix. Although it is not yet clear which regulators are able to repair degraded matrix by restoration of lost components, both insulin-like growth factor 1 (IGF-1) and transforming growth factor β (TGF-β) are able to halt resorption, preventing further matrix loss. Whether knowledge regarding these effectors can be used to create pharmaceutical agents to block degenerative matrix changes during osteoarthritis is a provocative question for further research. aFGF, acidic fibroblast growth factor.

THE ROLE OF POLYPEPTIDE MEDIATORS IN THE
REGULATION OF CARTILAGE METABOLISM

Historically, the important role of polypeptide mediators in the control of articular cartilage metabolism was heralded by the pioneering work of Fell and Jubb (10) which demonstrated for the first time that a polypeptide factor derived from synovium could induce pervasive cartilage destruction. The factor, termed *catabolin,* induced resident chondrocytes within cultured cartilage slices to produce lytic agents that rapidly hydrolyzed the proteoglycan and then the collagen matrix (11). It was later demonstrated that catabolin was identical to interleukin-1 (IL-1) and that it induced the release of metalloproteinases from chondrocytes (12). Furthermore, the polypeptide also had the ability to suppress synthesis of proteoglycans, thereby accelerating matrix loss by impeding redeposition of lost components (11,13). More recently, it was shown that the effects of tumor necrosis factor α on articular cartilage metabolism are similar to those of IL-1 (14). The role of catabolic factors in cartilage pathophysiology is discussed in the chapter by Tyler.

Matrix Homeostasis: Insulin-like Growth Factor 1
and Transforming Growth Factor β

The accelerated matrix resorption that characterizes osteoarthritis involves an uncoupling of the anabolic and catabolic pathways of aggrecan metabolism such that degradation outpaces the attempts of the chondrocyte to lay down new matrix. Although a pharmacologic agent to reestablish metabolic balance is not yet available, our understanding of the physiological polypeptides that regulate homeostasis has increased over the course of the past 5 years, and continued research along this avenue is likely to uncover insights into therapeutic modalities.

Studies of articular cartilage in organ culture have provided new information on the regulation of matrix metabolism. One of the most extensively studied system uses bovine cartilage from the metacarpalphalangeal joints (15). In the organ culture models, the chondrocytes remain embedded in a matrix synthesized *in vivo* and retain their phenotypic mode of expression, synthesizing aggrecans and type II collagen in either the presence or absence of serum (15,16). Furthermore, the cultured bovine tissues are able to maintain the initial amount of proteoglycan and collagen in the matrix for at least 5 weeks through a regulated interplay of the anabolic and catabolic pathways (15–18). Initial studies clearly indicated that chondrocytes required serum to maintain this homeostasis and that withdrawal of serum from the system led to a decrease in the anabolism and an increase in the catabolism of aggrecans, thereby resulting in progressive depletion of this component from the matrix (15). Whether effectors such as IL-1 are produced in the explanted tissue and contribute to this loss is not clear. Nevertheless, the organ culture models are well-suited for asking which specific mediators and/or combinations thereof are able to restore this resorbing system to a homeostatic mode.

Insulin-like growth factor 1 (IGF-1) and transforming growth factor β1 (TGF-β1), each added alone to spontaneously resorbing calf articular cartilage organ cultures, restore homeostasis of proteoglycans through an increase in anabolism and a decrease in catabolism (17,18). Neither IGF-1 nor TGF-β significantly increases the DNA content of the tissue after 3–5 weeks of culture, indicating that they act by modulating the metabolic activity of existing cells. The general chemistry, physiology, and regulation of IGF-1 and TGF-β have been covered in excellent reviews, and the interested reader is referred to these (8,9).

The definition of the effect of IGF-1 and TGF-β on the structure and function of the cartilage matrix as a whole is of critical importance not only for our understanding of the potential role of these effectors in normal physiology but also for their potential therapeutic use. In organ culture, IGF-1 increases synthesis of the aggrecan species characteristic of cartilage (19). The effects of exogenous TGF-β1 on the calf articular cartilage cultures have been explored in detail (20). Thus, it is clear that this polypeptide increases aggrecans and hyaluronic acid in a coordinated manner to form the aggregan–hyaluronic acid complex responsible for the resiliency of cartilage. In addition, TGF-β increases synthesis of the small interstitial proteoglycans resident in cartilage (20), which include decorin and biglycan. Decorin has been strongly implicated in the fibrillogenesis of collagen (21), and both proteoglycans have recently been shown to bind specifically to TGF-β (22). Our preliminary observations indicate that in calf cartilage, biglycan is selectively increased in response to this polypeptide as compared to decorin (T. I. Morales, *unpublished observations*). By contrast, IGF-1 does not increase the interstitial proteoglycans in calf or steer organ cultures (19).

In addition to increasing proteoglycan anabolism, TGF-β increases general protein synthesis (20). Furthermore, display of ^{3}H-labeled proteins synthesized in the presence of TGF-β on sodium dodecyl sulfate–polyacrylamide gel electrophoresis (SDS-PAGE) shows a protein pattern that closely resembles that of the proteins synthesized 2 weeks earlier on the day of tissue explant in the absence of added growth factors (T. I. Morales and A. B. Roberts, *unpublished observations*). The pattern also closely resembles that of 2-week-old basal cultures. Thus it appears that, in general, TGF-β increases synthesis of proteins typical for chondrocytes and does not significantly change phenotypic expression of the cells. Definitive proof of the overall beneficial effects of this polypeptide awaits the elucidation of (a) the pattern of collagens produced in the presence of TGF-β and (b) the biomechanical integrity of this tissue. Independent investigations carried out with dog articular cartilage cultures show that whereas IGF-1 increases synthesis of proteoglycans, it is not able to maintain high protein synthesis, but addition of TGF-β to the IGF-1-containing cultures does (23). Likewise, the effect of TGF-β on protein synthesis in human cartilage organ cultures was more pronounced than that of IGF-1 (24); the former polypeptide stimulated synthesis of the same spectrum of proteins synthesized in control cultures. The data support a specific role for IGF-1 in the maintenance of aggrecan metabolism, whereas TGF-β appears to have an overall regulatory effect on articular cartilage metabolism, including aggrecan pathways.

Interactions of Polypeptide Mediators in Articular Cartilage

TGF-β has the capacity to antagonize the action of two inducers of proteoglycan loss in articular cartilage: IL-1 (25,26) and retinoic acid (T. I. Morales and A. B. Roberts, *unpublished observations*). Therefore its role in the tissue might extend into a defense mechanism against resorbing stimuli. Recently, it has been shown that TGF-β decreases the number of receptors for IL-1 in monolayer cultures of chondrocytes (27). Likewise, IGF-1 antagonizes the effects of IL-1 and tumor necrosis factor α (28). Interestingly, TGF-β is released in large amounts by inflamed synovium (29). The critical question in the context of an inflammatory episode, then, is which and how much of the different polypeptide effectors released by the synovium reach and signal the chondrocyte. Clearly, factors other than those mentioned above will need to be considered. For example, acidic fibroblast growth factor (FGF) has recently been shown to be elevated in the synovial membranes of osteoarthritic joints (30).

Another question of importance is whether the effects of growth factors on articular cartilage are age-dependent. Barone-Varelas et al. (19) have recently reported that calf cartilage ($\sim$15 weeks old) is able to maintain elevated rates of synthesis of proteoglycans for more than 2 weeks in the presence of IGF-1 in culture, whereas rates decline in similar cultures of cartilage derived from older bovines (18–24 months old). A decrease in the ability of human articular cartilage organ cultures and isolated chondrocytes from patients older than 60 years of age to respond to IGF-1 and TGF-β has been reported (31). Further evaluation of this desensitization process is clearly important.

The discussion above has focused on the two polypeptides known to maintain matrix proteoglycan homeostasis, but it is relevant to point out that other polypeptide effectors may have mitogenic activity on chondrocytes *in situ,* and therefore can complement and/or synergize with the homeostasis-controlling factors. For example, platelet-derived growth factor synergizes with IGF-1 (32), and fibroblast growth factor synergizes with insulin to induce chondrocyte proliferation (33). It is quite possible that release of these factors during inflammation helps to promote the chondrocyte cloning characteristic of osteoarthritis—that is, the cellular division that leads to formation of tightly packed clusters of cells separated from each other by expanses of matrix.

Experimentally, it is important to distinguish between factors that elicit cell proliferation by inducing peripheral cells on the edges of the cut tissue to divide and those that induce chondrocyte proliferation within an intact matrix. In the latter case, the tightly woven "collagen basket" that encapsulates individual chondrocytes (see chapter by Hunziker) may present a barrier to cell division that needs to be weakened or remodeled for cloning to occur.

ENDOGENOUS PHYSIOLOGY OF POLYPEPTIDE MEDIATORS: REGULATORY MECHANISMS

Recent work has clearly shown that cultured calf articular cartilage synthesizes TGF-β and that levels of synthesis of the polypeptide decrease during the first week of culture in tandem with a decrease in proteoglycan synthesis (34). A working hypothesis is that newly synthesized TGF-β is activated and signals the producer cells through an autocrine loop. Although the validity of this hypothesis remains to be firmly established, further studies have suggested a more complex regulation of TGF-β activity within articular cartilage. In contrast to the declining levels of TGF-β and aggrecan biosynthesis in the cultures, the overall content of TGF-β in the tissue is remarkably constant during the first week in culture (34). An example is shown in Fig. 2 (34): The tissue extracts were analyzed for TGF-β content by a functional assay which quantitates the inhibitory effect of the polypeptide on growth of CCL-64 mink lung epithelial cells. The level of endogenous TGF-β during a week in culture, ~300 ng/g tissue, is in large excess to the levels of exogenous polypeptide required to induce a maximal increase in proteoglycan synthesis, 5–10 ng/ml. This problem was also investigated using a highly specific sandwich enzyme-linked immunosorbent assay (SELISA) for TGF-β1 and TGF-β2. Although the total levels of TGF-β measured by SELISA were lower than the TGF-β levels quantitated by the functional assay, the SELISA

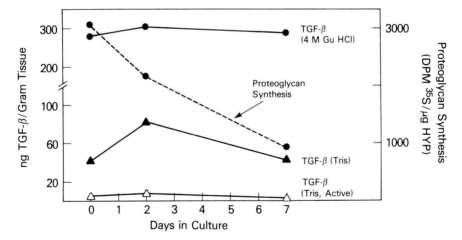

FIG. 2. Quantitation of TGF-β in articular cartilage. Cartilage was cultured under basal conditions (no added growth factors) and on the days indicated, cultures were extracted in buffer containing 4 M guanidine-HCl (Gu HCl) and dialyzed against 4 mM HCl containing 1 μg/ml each of pepstatin and leupeptin. Alternatively, cartilage was sliced into 30-μm sections and extracted in Tris buffer (without guanidine-HCl) by homogenization. The samples were assayed before and after acid activation to reveal latent forms of TGF-β. The activity of TGF-β was measured by inhibition of growth of CCL-64 mink lung epithelial cells (see ref. 34). Note that the maximal amount of exogenous TGF-β required for activation of these cultures is 5 ng/ml. (Reprinted from ref. 34.)

methodology confirmed the trends observed before (Fig. 2). Thus the endogenous TGF-β content was >10-fold in excess of the requirement for exogenous activation, and the TGF-β content was constant throughout the first week in culture. Clearly, there are large stores of TGF-β in the tissue which are unable to signal the chondrocytes, and, more importantly, these stores are present in the tissue at the time of explantation, suggesting a physiological role. Immunocytochemistry showed the presence of the polypeptide both intracellularly and extracellularly, but did not establish the location of the major storage sites (34). Low ($\sim$30%) extraction of TGF-β by homogenization of thin tissue slices in the presence of physiological buffers and detergents, as compared to effective extraction in denaturing solvents, led us to postulate that much, if not all, of the polypeptide is tightly bound in the extracellular matrix.

Binding of TGF-β to various isolated matrix and pericellular proteoglycans (betaglycan, decorin, and biglycan) (22,35) through their core proteins has been demonstrated. Although this type of binding has been assessed *in vitro* with isolated components, the existence of high levels of tightly bound polypeptide in the tissue help to substantiate the concept of matrix binding. Positive identification of physiologically relevant binding proteins and their interactive domains awaits specific binding studies carried out with these proteins *in situ* within tissue slices. In a network as complex as the cartilage matrix, polypeptide sequences available for binding in solution could be blocked while binding to other molecular structures may be facilitated. For example, decorin has been shown to be localized at specific sites along collagen fibrils *in vivo* (for review see ref. 36), and one may ask whether the molecule is able to bind TGF-β in this configuration. The significance of matrix stores of TGF-β is not clear, but such a system might provide a relay network that rapidly senses environmental changes and generates a cellular response. For example, compressive forces are capable of modulating the metabolic activities of the chondrocyte (37); one may ask experimentally whether such forces help to release signaling molecules from matrix stores. Another attractive possibility is that coupling of TGF-β to a key matrix component(s) provides a mechanism whereby catabolic activity in the matrix is quickly transmitted to the chondrocyte as a cue to restore homeostatic balance. Thus, proteolysis of a matrix component might release active TGF-β which diffuses to activate cellular receptors. If this scenario is true, then the metabolic parameters of the molecules in question should be coupled.

The concept of extracellular binding of growth factors is not limited to the TGF-β family of polypeptides. The binding of FGF to heparan sulfate proteoglycans has been known and studied for some time and provides further insights into the physiological dynamics of matrix binding of polypeptide effectors. This growth factor binds to heparan sulfate chains, and both a pericellular proteoglycan species and an extracellular one bind the growth factor, at least in smooth muscle cells (38). Interestingly, binding of the polypeptide to heparan sulfate protects it from degradation by proteolytic enzymes, and it has been postulated that hydrolytic enzymes, such as plasmin or heparanase, may release it from its immobilized storage form (38,39). Furthermore, the heparan sulfate–FGF complex diffuses more readily through negatively charged gels than does free FGF (40), indicating that a glycosaminoglycan carrier can efficiently transport cationic growth factors through negatively charged matrices. More recently it has been demonstrated that binding of FGF to a pericellular heparan sulfate is required for effective binding of the polypeptide to its signaling receptor (41). It was postulated that binding to the glycosaminoglycan changes the conformation of the growth factor, thereby unmasking its signaling activity (41).

The role of FGF in articular cartilage has gained interest with the recent finding that it is able to suppress the differentiation of proliferative chondrocytes to the hypertrophic stage and their subsequent mineralization (42). One may ask whether a decrease in active factor might lead to and/or permit mineralizing changes in articular cartilage. Such changes were proposed by Ali (43), who observed mineralized matrix vesicles in the middle-to-deep zones of human osteoarthritic cartilage. The subsequent identification of hydroxyapatite crystals in synovial fluids of osteoarthritic patients by Dieppe et al. (44) was consistent with this proposal. More recent observations that type X collagen, a marker for mineralizing cartilage, is present in osteoarthritic cartilage (see chapter by von der Mark et al.) further supports the concept that there is mineralization of cartilage during osteoarthritis and raises the question whether a phenotypic transition of an articular to a hypertrophic chondrocyte is a key event during osteoarthritis.

Control mechanisms for growth factor activity are not limited to extracellular and pericellular binding as discussed above. Human recombinant TGF-β is released from Chinese hamster ovary (CHO) cells as an $\sim$100-kD inactive precursor (45). The mature 25-kD polypeptide is cleaved from the 75-kD "latency" glycopeptide before release from the cell (8,45) (Fig. 3). However, this cleavage is insufficient to confer activity upon TGF-β, because it remains complexed to the latency peptide through noncovalent interactions (Fig. 3). Interestingly, platelet degranulation leads to the release of the latency-peptide–TGF-β complex in association with a third component, a "modulator" protein of $\sim$135 kD (8,45). Although the role of this protein remains shrouded by mystery, it is known that it contains EGF-like repeats and that it is covalently linked to the latency peptide via a disulfide bond (45). Possibly, the modulator protein helps to deliver TGF-β by preventing and/or promoting matrix interactions.

Various proteinases activate the latency-peptide–TGF-β complex *in vitro* (8). Plasmin cleaves the amino-terminal end of the latency peptide in the complex, and it is believed that this changes the conformation of the precursor portion releasing active TGF-β (47). A physiological role for plasmin in the activation of TGF-β has recently received support, at least in a coculture system of smooth muscle and endothelial cells, because it was shown that endogenous activation of the factor was blocked by the presence of plasminogen activator inhibitor (48). Because TGF-β increases synthesis of this inhibitor, a scheme was proposed in which activation of the factor leads to a feedback repression of further activation

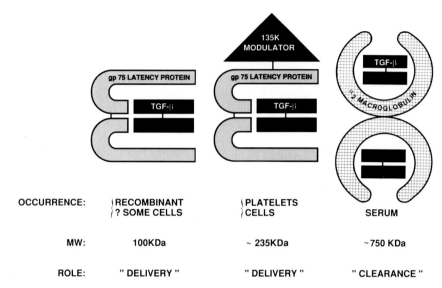

FIG. 3. Model of the latent TGF-β complex. Latent TGF-β is secreted by recombinant expression systems and some cells as a complex of a 75-kD glycoprotein corresponding to the TGF-β precursor "pro" region and the 25-kD TGF-β protein. Even though the complex has been cleaved, it remains associated through noncovalent interactions (see text). As released from platelets and many cultured cells, the complex contains an additional 135-kD "modulator" protein. The function of this protein is unknown. α2-Macroglobulin specifically binds TGF-β, forming a latent complex, and probably functions to clear the polypeptide. (Reprinted from ref. 46, with permission.)

through the control of the plasmin-generating system (47,48). Further work in the same system has shown that activation of latent TGF-β requires its binding to the IGF-II receptor (49); this may help to concentrate the precursor on the cell surface, thereby augmenting the effectiveness of catalytic action.

Although the mechanisms for activation of TGF-β in articular cartilage are unknown, at least 20% of the TGF-β stores in calf cartilage exist in latent form (34). This estimate may be low, because it is based on the fact that only 30% of the total tissue TGF-β was extractable under nondenaturing conditions (chaotropic agents activate TGF-β) (34,45). In any event, the results indicate that activation of latent forms of TGF-β is likely to be one of several mechanisms by which the endogenous activity of this polypeptide is regulated in articular cartilage.

IGF-1 is also stored in large amounts in the cartilage matrix (18), and its activity is probably subject to specific regulatory mechanisms as well. Thus, IGF-1 is present in serum, in biological fluids, and in several tissues in the form of complexes with binding proteins (9). At least three groups of binding proteins that seem to modulate the activity of IGF-1 have been cloned (9). Thus, the physiology and control of IGF-1 polypeptides and their related proteins in articular cartilage are exciting areas of future research.

Clearly, the biology and regulation of the growth factors in cartilage is complex, and much remains to be learned about the complement of factors that act in combination to carry out the functions of this tissue. Nevertheless, regulatory themes are beginning to emerge which may simplify experimentation and help resolve the complexities involved. For example, the concepts of matrix binding, growth factor presentation, and proteinase involvement may be used to guide studies of the physiology of the various factors within articular cartilage.

SUMMARY AND FUTURE DIRECTIONS

Two polypeptide effectors capable of shifting the metabolic synchrony of cartilage from a resorptive into a homeostatic mode, IGF-1 and TGF-β, have recently been identified. The synthesis of TGF-β by chondrocytes in articular cartilage implicates this polypeptide in the endogenous physiology of the tissue. The storage of "inert" pools of TGF-β within the tissue, probably involving both matrix sequestration and latency of the polypeptide, has been documented. Thus, the existence of complex regulatory mechanisms for TGF-β in cartilage are expected to be key controls of matrix metabolism and function. Although we have not yet explored the physiology of IGF-1 in cartilage in detail, its presence in the tissue suggests a role for this polypeptide as well.

As our knowledge of these two polypeptides and their interactions with other effectors in normal articular cartilage increases, it will be desirable to learn the dynamics of these regulators during experimental and human disease. For example, TGF-β is known to decrease synthesis of various proteinases and to increase synthesis of their corresponding inhibitors (8). Because the reverse pattern has been documented on the edges of growing ulcers in osteoarthritic cartilage (i.e., increased proteinase and decreased inhibitor activity), one may ask if a reduction in the activity of TGF-β can be documented in these sites. If so, is there a way of restimulating TGF-β synthesis to prevent further ulceration? A related question is whether osteoarthritic chondrocytes will respond to TGF-β in the same manner as normal chondrocytes.

Receptors for the relevant polypeptide effectors need to be investigated, particularly in view of the apparent "desensitization" of older tissues to IGF-1 and TGF-β action. Traditionally, this has been a difficult experimental problem, because receptors are studied not *in situ* but instead following release of cells from the tissues. Commonly, this involves the use of proteinases, and the effects of these activities on the complement and amount of the receptors and binding proteins on the cell surface are unknown. A recent elegant study of FGF receptors in growth-plate chondrocytes demonstrated a similar pattern of high-affinity binding in isolated cells and in thin tissue slices from the corresponding anatomical site (42). This study suggests that realistic approaches to the problem are feasible.

In conclusion, the field of growth factor research in general is progressing at a rapid pace, and its contribution to the field of clinical medicine is already apparent. The continued influx of this knowledge into the area of research on osteoarthritis cannot fail to increase our understanding of the physiopathological dynamics of articular cartilage.

ACKNOWLEDGMENTS

I would like to acknowledge my collaborators for providing invaluable input into the work on polypeptide mediators discussed here. Drs. F. Luyten, H. Reddi, P. Nissley, and V. Hascall collaborated in the IGF-1 studies, whereas Drs. A. Roberts, D. Danielpore, M. Joyce, and M. Soble collaborated on various aspects of the TGF-β work. Particular thanks to Drs. M. Sporn and A. Roberts, as well as to the staff of their laboratory, for sharing their state-of-the-art knowledge of TGF-β and other growth factors with me and for their continued support. Many thanks to Drs. Sharon Wahl, Vincent Hascall, and Klaus Kuettner for their critical and careful review of this chapter.

REFERENCES

1. Mankin HJ, Brandt KD, Shulman LE, eds. Workshop on etiopathogenesis of osteoarthritis. *J Rheumatol* 1986;13:1126–1160.
2. National Arthritis and Musculoskeletal and Skin Diseases Advisory Council. *Biennial report of the National Institutes of Health. Reports of the NIH advisory councils and boards, vol 2, 1987–1988.* NIH publication no. 89-2913. Bethesda, MD: National Institutes of Health, 1989.
3. Arthritis and Musculoskeletal Diseases Interagency Coordinating Committee. *1990 Annual report.* Bethesda, MD: Department of Health and Human Services, Public Health Service, National Institutes of Health, 1990;7.
4. Grazier KL, Holbrook TL, Kelsey JL, Stauffer RN. In: *The frequency of occurrence, impact, and cost of musculoskeletal conditions in the United States.* Chicago, IL: American Academy of Orthopedic Surgeons, 1984;28.
5. Dean DD, Azzo W, Martel-Pelletier J, Pelletier JP, Woessner JF. Levels of metalloproteases and tissue inhibitor of metalloproteases in human osteoarthritic cartilage. *J Rheumatol* 1987;14:33–43.
6. Dean DD, Martel-Pelletier J, Pelletier J-P, Howell DS, Woessner JF. Evidence for metalloproteinase and metalloproteinase inhibitor (TIMP) imbalance in human osteoarthritic cartilage. *J Clin Invest* 1989;84:678–685.
7. Hascall VC. Proteoglycans: The chondroitin sulfate/keratan sulfate proteoglycans of cartilage. *ISI Atlas of Science: Biochemistry* 1988;1:189–198.
8. Roberts AB, Sporn MB. The transforming growth factor-βs. In: Sporn MB, Roberts AB, eds. *Handbook of experimental pharmacology,* vol 95/I. Berlin: Springer-Verlag, 1990;419–472.
9. Rechler MM, Nissley PS. Insulin-like growth factors. In: Sporn MB, Roberts AB, eds. *Handbook of experimental pharmacology,* vol 95/I. Berlin: Springer-Verlag, 1990;263–346.
10. Fell HB, Jubb R. The effect of synovial tissue on the breakdown of articular cartilage in organ culture. *Arthritis Rheum* 1977;20:1371–1395.
11. Dingle JT, Tyler JA. Role of intercellular messengers in the control of cartilage matrix dynamics. In: Kuettner K, et al., eds. *Articular cartilage biochemistry.* New York: Raven Press, 1986;181–193.
12. Saklatvala J, Pilsworth LMC, Sarsfield SJ, Gavrilovic J, Heath JK. Pig catabolin is a form of interleukin-1. *Biochem J* 1984;224:461–466.
13. Morales TI, Hascall VC. Effects of interleukin-1 and lipopolysaccharides on protein and carbohydrate metabolism in bovine articular cartilage organ cultures. *Connect Tissue Res* 1989;19:255–275.

14. Saklatvala J. Tumour necrosis factor α stimulates resorption and inhibits synthesis of proteoglycans in cartilage. *Nature* 1986;322:547–549.
15. Hascall VC, Handley CJ, McQuillan DJ, Hascall GK, Robinson HC, Lowther DA. Effect of serum on biosynthesis of proteoglycans by bovine cartilage in culture. *Arch Biochem Biophys* 1983;224:206–223.
16. Morales TI, Hascall VC. Correlated metabolism of proteoglycans and hyaluronic acid in bovine cartilage organ cultures. *J Biol Chem* 1988;263:3632–3638.
17. Morales TI, Roberts AB. Transforming growth factor-β regulates the metabolism of proteoglycans in bovine cartilage organ cultures. *J Biol Chem* 1988;263:12828–12831.
18. Luyten FP, Hascall VC, Nissley SP, Morales TI, Reddi AH. Insulin-like growth factors maintain steady state metabolism of proteoglycans in bovine articular cartilage explants. *Arch Biochem Biophys* 1988;267:416–425.
19. Barone-Varelas J, Schnitzer TJ, Meng Q, Otten L, Thonar E. Age related differences in the metabolism of proteoglycans in bovine articular cartilage explants maintained in the presence of insulin-like growth factor-1. *Connect Tissue Res* 1991;26:101–120.
20. Morales TI. Transforming growth factor-β1 stimulates synthesis of proteoglycan aggregates in calf articular cartilage organ cultures. *Arch Biochem Biophys* 1991;286:99–106.
21. Vogel KG, Paulsson M, Heinegard D. Specific inhibition of type I and type II collagen fibrillogenesis by the low molecular mass proteoglycan of tendon. *Biochem J* 1984;223:587–597.
22. Yamagushi Y, Mann DM, Ruoslahti E. Negative regulation of transforming growth factor-β by the proteoglycan decorin. *Nature* 1990;346:281–284.
23. Burton-Wurster N, Lust G. Fibronectin and proteoglycan synthesis in long term cultures of cartilage explants in Ham's F_{12} supplemented with insulin and calcium: effects of the addition of TGF-β. *Arch Biochem Biophys* 1990;283:27–33.
24. Recklies AD, White C. Differential effects of transforming growth factor-β on matrix synthesis in cartilage explants and isolated chondrocytes. *Trans Orthop Res Soc* 1990;15:316.
25. Chandrasekhar S, Harvey AK. Transforming growth factor-β is a potent inhibitor of IL-1 induced protease activity and cartilage proteoglycan degradation. *Biochem Biophys Res Commun* 1988;157:1352–1355.
26. Andrews HJ, Edwards TA, Cawston TE, Hazleman BL. Transforming growth factor-β causes partial inhibition of interleukin-1 stimulated cartilage degradation *in vitro*. *Biochem Biophys Res Commun* 1989;162:150–155.
27. Harvey AK, Hrubey PS, Chandrasekhar S. Transforming growth factor-β inhibition of interleukin-1 activity involves down regulation of interleukin-1 receptors on chondrocytes. *Exp Cell Res* 1991;195(2):376–385.
28. Tyler JA. IGF-1 can decrease degradation and promote synthesis of proteoglycans in cartilage exposed to cytokines. *Biochem J* 1989;260:543–548.
29. Wahl SM, Allen JB, Wong HL, Dougherty SF, Ellingsworth LR. Antagonistic and agonistic effects of transforming growth factor-β and IL-1 in rheumatoid synovium. *J Immunol* 1990;145:2514–2519.
30. Sano H, Forough R, Maier JAM, Case JP, Jackson A, Engleka K, Maciag T, Wilder T. Detection of high levels of heparan binding growth factor-1 (acidic fibroblast growth factor) in inflammatory arthritic joints. *J Cell Biol* 1990;110:1417–1426.
31. Recklies AD, Roughley PJ, Bilimoria KM. Differential response of young and old human articular chondrocytes to IGF-1 and TGF-β. *Trans Orthop Res Soc* 1989;14:281.
32. Tyler J, Lawrence C, Giller T. IGF-1 alone can promote replacement of matrix but not clonal expansion of chondrocytes in cultured explants of depleted articular cartilage. *Trans Orthop Res Soc* 1990;15:137.
33. Osborn KD, Trippel SB, Mankin HJ. Growth factor stimulation of adult articular cartilage. *J Orthop Res* 1989;7:35–42.
34. Morales TI, Joyce ME, Soble ME, Danielpour D, Roberts AB. Transforming growth factor-β in calf articular cartilage organ cultures: synthesis and distribution. *Arch Biochem Biophys* 1991;288:397–405.
35. Andres JL, Stanley K, Cheifets S, Massague J. Membrane anchored and soluble forms of betaglycan, a polymorphic proteoglycan that binds transforming growth factor-β. *J Cell Biol* 1989;109:3137–3145.
36. Scott JE. Proteoglycan–fibrillar collagen interactions. *Biochem J* 1988;252:313–323.
37. Sah RLY, Kim YJ, Grodzinsky AJ. The effect of mechanical compression on cartilage metabolism.

In: Maroudas A, Kuettner K, eds. *Methods in cartilage research.* San Diego: Academic Press, 1990;116–119.

38. Saksela O, Rifkin DB. Release of basic fibroblast growth factor–heparan sulfate complexes from endothelial cells by plasminogen activator-mediated proteolytic activity. *J Cell Biol* 1990;110: 767–775.

39. Vlodavsky I, Fuks Z, Ishai-Michaeli R, Bashkin P, Levi E, Korner G, Bar-Shavit R, Klagsburn M. Extracellular matrix-resident basic fibroblast growth factor: implication for the control of angiogenesis. *J Cell Biochem* 1991;45:167–176.

40. Flaumenhaft R, Moscatelli D, Rifkin DB. Heparin and heparan sulfate increase the radius of diffusion and action of basic fibroblast growth factor. *J Cell Biol* 1991;11:1651–1659.

41. Yayon A, Klagsbrun M, Esko JD, Leder P, Ornitz DM. Cell surface, heparin-like molecules are required for binding of basic fibroblast growth factor to its high affinity receptor. *Cell* 1991;64: 841–848.

42. Iwamoto M, Shimazu A, Nakashima K, Suzudi F, Kato Y. Reduction in basic fibroblast growth factor receptor is coupled with terminal differentiation of chondrocytes. *J Biol Chem* 1991;266(1): 461–467.

43. Ali YS. Mineral-containing matrix vesicles in human osteoarthritic cartilage. In: Nuki G, ed. *The aetiopathogenesis of osteoarthrosis.* Kent, England: Pitman Medical Publishers, 1980;105–116.

44. Dieppe PA, Crocker P, Huskisson EC, Willoughby DA. Apatite deposition disease. A new arthropathy. *Lancet* 1976;266–269.

45. Wakefield LM, Smith DM, Flanders KC, Sporn MB. Latent transforming growth factor-β from human platelets. *J Biol Chem* 1988;263:7646–7654.

46. Wakefield LM, Smith DM, Broz S, Jackson M, Levinson AD, Sporn MB. *Growth Factors* 1989;1: 203–218.

47. Lyons RM, Gentry LE, Purchio AF, Moses HL. Mechanism of activation of latent recombinant transforming growth factor-β1 by plasmin. *J Cell Biol* 1990;110:1361–1367.

48. Sato Y, Tsuboi R, Lyons R, Moses H, Rifkin DB. Characterization of the activation of latent TGF-β by cultures of endothelial cells and pericytes or smooth muscle cells: a self regulating system. *J Cell Biol* 1990;111:757–763.

49. Dennis PA, Rifkin DB. Cellular activation of latent transforming growth factor-β requires binding to the cation independent mannose 6-phosphate insulin like growth factor type II receptor. *Proc Natl Acad Sci USA* 1991;88:580–584.

DISCUSSION

van der Berg: We have screened the effects of TGF-β and IGF-1 on cartilage proteoglycan synthesis and breakdown under normal conditions. We find that IGF-1 can substitute for TGF-β. If IGF-1 is present, however, it will obscure effects of TGF-β. You only see supplementary effects in pathologic conditions—for instance, IL-1-induced degradation. My speculation is that TGF-β is more important under pathologic conditions than in normal conditions.

Morales: I do agree that the effects of exogenous IGF-1 and TGF-β on normal cartilage are additive as long as neither is at a saturating level. However, we need to determine which factors are resident and active in normal cartilage to define their relative importance in the physiology of the tissue. In terms of pathology, your observations are provocative and may be indicative of a greater effectiveness of TGF-β than of IGF-1 as an antagonist of IL-1 action.

Kresse: There is a gradient of decorin with depth in articular cartilage. Does the distribution of TGF-β follow this gradient? A codistribution would support the concept of a growth-regulatory role for decorin.

Morales: I have initiated work with Larry Fisher using immunological probes for the small proteoglycans to address such questions.

Heinegard: Does TGF-β induce decorin synthesis, and can decorin bind TGF-β in this system?

Morales: Preliminary experiments show that TGF-β increases both decorin and biglycan synthesis, but biglycan is preferentially increased. This might suggest that biglycan binds TGF-β *in vivo,* but this is speculative.

Articular Cartilage and Osteoarthritis,
edited by K. Kuettner et al.
Raven Press, Ltd., New York © 1992.

19

Two Distinct Metabolic Pools of Proteoglycans in Articular Cartilage

G. P. Jos van Kampen, Robert J. van de Stadt,
Martin A. F. J. van de Laar, and Jan K. van der Korst

*Jan van Breemen Instituut, Dr. J. van Breemenstraat 2,
1056 AB Amsterdam, The Netherlands*

PROTEOGLYCANS IN ARTICULAR CARTILAGE

Proteoglycan Composition

Proteoglycans are huge macromolecules that consist of a large number of chondroitin sulfate (CS) and keratan sulfate (KS) glycosaminoglycans covalently bonded to a protein core. The protein core contains extended and globular domains. The extended domains form specialized glycosaminoglycan attachment regions; two for CS and one for KS. The globular domain at the N-terminal side forms a site for aggregation with hyaluronic acid (HA). HA is an unbranched glycosaminoglycan chain which can bind up to a hundred or more proteoglycans (1). Proteoglycans are synthesized and secreted as monomers that aggregate in the extracellular matrix when they encounter a free binding space on HA. The interaction is stabilized by a glycoprotein link molecule.

The proteoglycans in articular cartilage undergo marked transformations during life (2). The most predominant changes in the developmental phase of the tissue are an increase in the relative content of KS and an increase of the ratio of 6-sulfated to 4-sulfated CS. The hydrodynamic volume of the proteoglycans and the length of their CS chains remain the same.

In adult articular cartilage, the alterations in the proteoglycans are much smaller than in the developing tissue. The relative content of KS and the ratio of 6-sulfated to 4-sulfated CS further increase, but much more slowly and to a lesser extent (2). The major change is a slow decrease in hydrodynamic volume of the tissue proteoglycans. The changes in proteoglycan size and composition in adult tissue result from the accumulation in the tissue of proteoglycans from which parts of the C-terminal CS-rich regions have been lost. These molecules are thus correspondingly enriched in KS content, because this is more abundant toward the N-terminal domains.

Proteoglycan Turnover

The chondrocytes in articular cartilage are responsible for the synthesis of the cartilage matrix components. The two major components are collagen and proteoglycans. Collagen type II is synthesized at a low rate, and its turnover rate in adult cartilage is believed to be extremely low (3). Proteoglycans, on the other hand, are synthesized in considerable amounts (4), and it is generally believed that the turnover of the proteoglycans in the matrix takes place more rapidly.

The turnover of cartilage proteoglycans has been the subject of several studies both *in vitro* and *in vivo* (5). Labeled proteoglycans are released from explant cultures of bovine articular cartilage with a half-life of 11–40 days (6). Proteoglycans labeled *in vivo* are released from rabbit articular cartilage explants with a half-life of ~22 days (7). Half of the labeled proteoglycans in guinea-pig costal cartilage *in vivo* was lost from the tissue after 60–70 days (8). However, detailed comparisons between the structure of newly synthesized proteoglycans and that of tissue proteoglycans are lacking.

NEWLY SYNTHESIZED PROTEOGLYCANS VERSUS TISSUE PROTEOGLYCANS

Tissue Cultures

We have studied the composition of newly synthesized ^{35}S-labeled proteoglycans and compared the results with the corresponding tissue proteoglycans in several culture systems (9–11). The 4 M guanidine-HCl-extractable proteoglycans were chromatographed on an analytical Sepharose CL-2B column under dissociative conditions, and the fractions were analyzed for both radioactivity and dimethylmethylene blue (DMB)-positive material. This procedure allows the comparison of the hydrodynamic volume of both labeled and nonlabeled proteoglycans under exactly the same conditions. A typical Sepharose Cl-2B elution profile of a 4 M guanidine-HCl extract of articular cartilage is shown in Fig. 1. The solid line represents all extracted proteoglycans (detected with DMB) and shows two peaks. A peak of large proteoglycans ($K_{av} = 0.30$) and a peak of smaller proteoglycans ($K_{av} = 0.70$). The latter peak is formed by the dermatan sulfate proteoglycans and is not discussed.

Newly synthesized labeled proteoglycans always eluted in a monodisperse peak and coeluted with the front of the polydisperse peak of tissue proteoglycans (Fig. 1, dashed line). The CS glycosaminoglycan chains of the labeled proteoglycans were always a little longer than those of the tissue proteoglycans, but not enough to explain the differences in hydrodynamic volume of the proteoglycan molecules.

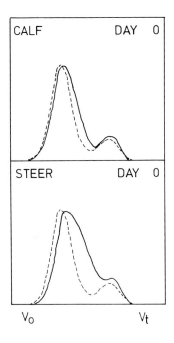

FIG. 1. Sepharose Cl-2B elution profile of 4 M guanidine-HCl extracts of cultured young and adult bovine articular cartilage (**upper panel** and **lower panel,** respectively). The solid line represents all extracted proteoglycans (detected with DMB) and shows a polydisperse peak of large proteoglycans ($K_{av} = 0.30$). The dashed line represents the newly synthesized proteoglycans (^{35}S) and shows large proteoglycans ($K_{av} = 0.28$) eluting in front of the peak of tissue proteoglycans. The small dermatan sulfate proteoglycans ($K_{av} = 0.70$) are not discussed. The elution buffer contained 4 M guanidine-HCl. V_0, void volume; V_t, total volume.

The labeled proteoglycans had a considerably higher galactosamine-to-glucosamine ratio than did the tissue proteoglycans, suggesting a high CS content in newly synthesized proteoglycans. The tissue proteoglycans extracted from adult steer cartilage were smaller than the tissue proteoglycans from calf cartilage. The hydrodynamic volume of the newly synthesized ^{35}S-labeled proteoglycans was, however, the same in both calf and steer. The observed differences between newly labeled and resident proteoglycans were therefore greater with increasing age of the tissue.

The labeled proteoglycans were rapidly lost from the tissue ($T_{1/2} \approx 20$ days). However, the characteristics of ^{35}S-labeled proteoglycans which were retained in the tissue did not change during chase *in vitro* for periods of up to 4 weeks, indicating that the newly synthesized proteoglycans did not transform to the smaller, endogenous proteoglycans. Transition of the large synthesized proteoglycans into the smaller tissue proteoglycans could not be demonstrated in cultured bovine articular cartilage.

Short-Term Chase *In Vivo*

Because we anticipated that the extracellular modification of proteoglycans was more likely to occur in older cartilage, we injected 75-week-old rabbits with [^{35}S]sulfate and [^{3}H]glucosamine into the knee joint cavities (7) and left the animals with normal cage activity for up to 3 weeks. The proteoglycans were extracted from the articular cartilage with 4 M guanidine-HCl. The amount of labeled proteoglycans in the tissue per dry weight decreased with time—from 100% on day 1, to 71% on day 8, to 67% on day 15, to 47% on day 22. These data suggest an *in vivo* half-life of approximately 20 days for the newly made proteoglycans. This value is very similar to that reported by Sandy and Plaas (7) and is relatively short compared to the life span of the rabbit. The hydrodynamic size distributions of the labeled proteoglycans remaining in the cartilage after the chase periods *in vivo* were assessed by analytical Sepharose Cl-2B chromatography (Fig. 2). The ^{35}S-labeled proteoglycans eluted in a sharp peak (Fig. 2, dashed line), with the front of the polydisperse peak of tissue proteoglycans detected by DMB (Fig. 2, solid line). No detectable change in size distribution of labeled large proteoglycans towards molecules of smaller hydrodynamic size was observed during chase *in vivo* for 3 weeks (Fig. 2, lower panel).

The ratio of galactosamine to glucosamine in the tissue proteoglycans in the front region of the peak exceeded that of the proteoglycans in the tail region. Thus, the large proteoglycans with a smaller hydrodynamic volume contain less CS. All labeled proteoglycans showed a markedly higher galactosamine-to-glucosamine ratio than did the unlabeled proteoglycans, indicating a relatively high CS content in the newly synthesized proteoglycans. The labeled proteoglycans also contained relatively more chondroitin-4-sulfate than did the unlabeled proteoglycans, independent of the time elapsed after the pulse-labeling.

We have demonstrated that the newly synthesized labeled proteoglycans are

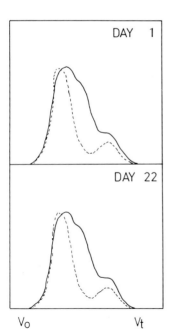

FIG. 2. Sepharose Cl-2B elution profile of 4 M guanidine-HCl extracts of articular cartilage of 75-week-old rabbits. The proteoglycans were labeled and chased *in vivo* for 1 and 22 days (**upper panel** and **lower panel,** respectively). The solid line represents all extracted proteoglycans (detected with DMB) and shows a polydisperse peak (K_{av} = 0.30) of large proteoglycans with a trailing shoulder. The dashed line represents the newly synthesized proteoglycans (^{35}S) that elute in front of the large proteoglycan peak (K_{av} = 0.28). The small dermatan sulfate proteoglycans (K_{av} = 0.70) are not discussed. The elution buffer contained 4 M guanidine-HCl. V_0, void volume; V_t, total volume.

monodisperse and are, on average, larger than the more polydisperse tissue proteoglycans. The same can be concluded from the work of Sandy et al. (12), who compared the labeled proteoglycans in immature, mature, and aged rabbits. The labeled monomers in mature and aged rabbits were nearly identical in hydrodynamic volume, but tissue proteoglycans appeared more polydisperse with increasing age.

Proteoglycans synthesized *in vivo* and chased for a period close to the apparent half-life of the labeled proteoglycans did not transform to the smaller tissue proteoglycans. These results were in agreement with our studies *in vitro* on bovine articular cartilage.

Long-Term Chase *In Vivo*

We expected changes to occur when the proteoglycans synthesized in the early stages of adolescence were studied and chased *in vivo* well into adulthood of the animals. In such an experiment younger, rabbits (24 weeks) were injected with [^{35}S]sulfate in the knee and chased for approximately 5 times the half-life of labeled proteoglycans. The proteoglycans from the articular cartilage were studied 1 and 15 weeks after injection of the label. One week after injection, the newly synthesized large proteoglycans eluted in a monodisperse peak, with the front of the polydisperse peak of tissue proteoglycans detected by DMB (Fig. 3, upper panel). After a chase *in vivo* for 15 weeks, the peak of labeled large proteoglycans

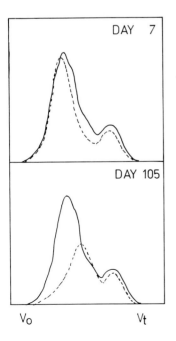

FIG. 3. Elution profiles of proteoglycans on Sepharose Cl-2B of 4 M guanidine-HCl extracts of articular cartilage of 24-week-old rabbits. The proteoglycans were labeled and chased *in vivo* for 1 and 15 weeks. The solid line represents all extracted proteoglycans (detected by DMB) and shows a polydisperse peak of large proteoglycans ($K_{av} = 0.30$). The dashed line represents the newly synthesized proteoglycans (^{35}S) and shows a shift in hydrodynamic volume of the labeled large proteoglycans from $K_{av} = 0.28$ (**upper panel**) to $K_{av} = 0.35$ after 15 weeks (**lower panel**). All small dermatan sulfate proteoglycans have the same hydrodynamic volume ($K_{av} = 0.70$). The elution buffer contained 4 M guanidine-HCl. V_0, void volume; V_t, total volume.

still was monodisperse but had shifted to the tail region of the peak of tissue proteoglycans (Fig. 3, lower panel). The labeled proteoglycans aggregated well with exogenously added HA, indicating that their HA-binding regions were still intact (data not shown). The transition of large CS-rich proteoglycans to smaller proteoglycans, poor in CS, was demonstrated *in vivo* after five times the apparent half-life of the large proteoglycans.

The articular cartilage of two rabbits that were sacrificed 1 week after injection of the label contained 133,000 and 149,000 dpm ^{35}S/mg dry weight, respectively. From the cartilage of the animals chased for 15 weeks, 40,700 (S.D. 9500, $n = 9$) dpm ^{35}S/mg dry weight were recovered. These data indicate that 29% of the synthesized proteoglycans were still present in the tissue after the chase for 15 weeks. This is nine times the amount expected assuming first-order kinetics of the release and a half-life of 20 days. This provides good evidence for a population of proteoglycans which is retained in the tissue much longer than the population with an apparent half-life of 20 days.

More Evidence for Two Populations of Proteoglycans

We think that proteoglycans are synthesized as large molecules, rich in CS. Most of the synthesized proteoglycans are lost from the tissue with a half-life of approximately 20 days. The modification of proteoglycans to smaller, CS-poor proteoglycans occurs slowly and on a population of molecules that reside in the matrix for a long time.

Other evidence for more than one population of proteoglycans in cartilage has been reported. Two proteoglycan populations can be observed in the extracts of cartilage of adult animals (13) on agarose–polyacrylamide composite gels. Proteoglycans in the faster migrating bands contain relatively less CS (14). Labeled proteoglycans migrate almost exclusively in the slower band and have a proportionally higher CS content (15). The labeled, newly synthesized proteoglycans in the slower band on the gels are very likely comparable to the proteoglycans that elute in front of the peak of the large proteoglycans on Sepharose Cl-2B in our experiments.

DESTINY OF SYNTHESIZED PROTEOGLYCANS IN ADULT ARTICULAR CARTILAGE: A MODEL

The chondrocytes in adult articular cartilage continuously produce proteoglycans that are rich in both KS and CS. These newly synthesized proteoglycans are able to aggregate shortly after extrusion from the cell. The proteoglycans diffuse through the matrix and will aggregate when a binding site on HA is available. The interaction between proteoglycans and HA can be stabilized by link protein. However, in adult articular cartilage, most of the synthesized proteoglycans seem to form "nonstabilized aggregates." These molecules are rapidly lost from the tissue. Cleavage in the CS-rich region does not occur during their relatively short stay in the cartilage matrix.

Link-stabilized proteoglycans remain in the matrix for a very long time and are slowly converted into the CS-poor (and KS-rich) proteoglycans found in aged tissue. Proteolytic cleavage of the core protein starting from the C-terminal end is often suggested (16). Cleavage is not necessarily a gradual process. One can imagine that there are regions in the core protein that are more susceptible for cleavage than others. The change from large CS-rich into large CS-poor proteoglycans might involve the loss of defined parts of the CS-rich region and might take place in discrete steps.

We have consistently observed that the newly synthesized CS chains are longer than the tissue glycosaminoglycans ($\Delta K_{av} \approx 0.04$, data not shown). The glycosaminoglycan chains also might undergo a fine-tuning resulting in shorter chains. Recently it has been reported that the CS residues located at the ends of the glycosaminoglycan chain contain more sulfates in the 4-position than in the 6-position (17). Loss of the peripheral residues will lead to an increase in the ratio of 6-sulfated to 4-sulfated residues which has been reported in aging tissue. It might be interesting to see whether the distribution of 4-sulfated and 6-sulfated glycosaminoglycans of the different regions on the core protein varies in a certain order. In view of the proposed model, one would expect the CS chains at the C-terminal end to be rich in 4-sulfated residues.

IMPACT ON RESEARCH AND UNDERSTANDING OF DISEASE

We present a new concept of homeostasis of large proteoglycans in adult articular cartilage. It is suggested that the majority of the synthesized proteoglycans is rapidly lost from the cartilage. Only when proteoglycans are entrapped in link-protein-stabilized aggregates do they remain in the matrix for a considerable time and are thus subject to a slow but progressive breakdown.

Alterations in proteoglycans which take place during development and maturation are caused by changes in *de novo* synthesis. A second phase of aging starts in early adulthood. The synthesized proteoglycans remain more or less the same, but the alterations take place primarily as the result of extracellular modification of proteoglycans that are already fixed in the matrix (Fig. 4).

With increasing age, the elasticity of human articular cartilage decreases and the chances to develop osteoarthritis increase markedly. These changes start to play a role in the tissue in late adolescence or early adulthood, and their significance increases when the cartilage becomes older. This phase is characterized by gradual loss of CS chains by specific degradation of the proteoglycans bound in the tissue as aggregates. In this phase the tissue loses water-binding capacity while the number of collagen cross-links increases, thereby making the cartilage less elastic. Therefore, it seems that not only aging of collagen, but also that of proteoglycans, might contribute to the increasing susceptibility to degenerative joint disease.

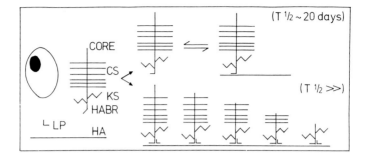

FIG. 4. Illustration of the destiny of the synthesized proteoglycans in articular cartilage. The proteoglycans in "nonstabilized aggregates" will diffuse through the matrix and will be lost from the tissue ($T_{1/2} \approx 20$ days). The proteoglycans in link-stabilized aggregates ($T_{1/2} \gg 20$ days) slowly change with increasing age. CORE, core protein; CS, chondroitin sulfate glycosaminoglycans; KS, keratan sulfate glycosaminoglycans; HABR, hyaluronic acid binding region; LP, link protein; HA, hyaluronic acid.

Furthermore, the reported findings suggest that the capacity of articular cartilage to repair osteoarthritic lesions is not so much determined by the capacity of the chondrocytes to synthesize large proteoglycans. The repair capacity might, in our opinion, be decisively determined by the ability of the cartilage to first remove degraded proteoglycan aggregates to make room for new ones.

ACKNOWLEDGMENT

This study was supported by grants from "Het National Reumafonds."

REFERENCES

1. Heinegard D, Oldberg A. Structure and biology of cartilage and bone matrix noncollagenous macromolecules. *FASEB J* 1989;3:2042–2051.
2. Kuijer R, van de Stadt RJ, van Kampen GPJ, de Koning MHMT, van de Voorde-Vissers E, van der Korst JK. Heterogeneity of proteoglycans extracted before and after collagenase treatment of human articular cartilage. II. Variations with age and tissue source. *Arthritis Rheum* 1986;29: 1248–1255.
3. Libby WF, Berger R, Mead JF, Alexander GV, Ross JF. Replacement rates for human tissue from atmospheric radiocarbon. *Science* 1964;146:1170–1172.
4. Hascall VC, Handley CJ, McQuillan DJ, Hascall GK, Robinson HC, Lowther DA. The effect of serum on biosynthesis of proteoglycans by bovine articular cartilage in culture. *Arch Biochem Biophys* 1983;224:206–223.
5. Maroudas A. Glycosaminoglycan turn-over in articular cartilage. *Philos Trans R Soc Lond* 1975;271:293–313.
6. Campbell MA, Handley CJ, Hascall VC, Campbell RA, Lowther DA. Turnover of proteoglycans in cultures of bovine articular cartilage. *Arch Biochem Biophys* 1984;234:275–289.
7. Sandy JD, Plaas AHK. Age-related changes in the kinetics of release of proteoglycans from normal rabbit cartilage explants. *J Orthop Res* 1986;4:263–272.
8. Lohmander S. Turnover of proteoglycans in guinea pig costal cartilage. *Arch Biochem Biophys* 1977;180:93–101.

9. van Kampen GPJ, van de Stadt RJ, Kiljan E, Brand HS, Kuijer R, Van der Korst JK. Effects of tissue disorganization on proteoglycan synthesis by articular chondrocytes *in vitro. Agents Actions* 1988;22:3–4.
10. Korver GHV, van de Stadt RJ, van Kampen GPJ, Kiljan E, van der Korst JK. Bovine sesamoid bones—a culture system for anatomically intact articular cartilage. *In Vitro Cell Dev Biol* 1989;25: 1099–1106.
11. Brand HS, Korver GHV, van de Stadt RJ, van Kampen GPJ, van der Korst JK. Studies on the extraction of different proteoglycan populations in bovine articular cartilage. *Biol Chem Hoppe-Seyler* 1990;371:581–587.
12. Sandy JD, O'Neill JR, Ratzlaff LC. Acquisition of hyaluronate-binding affinity *in vivo* by newly synthesized cartilage proteoglycans. *Biochem J* 1989;258:875–880.
13. Stanescu V, Maroteaux P, Sobczak E: Proteoglycan populations of baboon (*Papio papio*) articular cartilage. Gel-electrophoretic analyses of fractions obtained by density gradient centrifugation and sequential extraction. *Biochem J* 1977;163:103–109.
14. Roughley PJ, White RJ. Age-related changes in the structure of the proteoglycan subunits from human articular cartilage. *J Biol Chem* 1980;255:217–224.
15. Carney SL, Bayliss MT, Collier JM, Muir H. Electrophoresis of ^{35}S-labeled proteoglycans on polyacrylamide–agarose composite gels and their visualization by fluorography. *Anal Biochem* 1986;156:38–44.
16. Hardingham TE, Venn G, Bayliss MT. Chondrocyte responses in cartilage and experimental osteoarthritis. *Br J Rheumatol* 1991;30(S1):32–37.
17. Caterson B, Mahmoodian F, Sorrell JM, Hardingham TE, Bayliss MT, Carney SL, Ratcliffe A, Muir H. Modulation of native chondroitin sulphate structure in tissue development and disease. *J Cell Sci* 1990;97:441–447.

DISCUSSION

Hascall: The fact that there appear to be two metabolic pools can be related with the cartilage morphology discussed by Ernst Hunziker which defined the difference between the chondron, or the territorial matrix, and the interterritorial matrix. The metabolically active pool would be mainly in the chondron matrix, and the inactive one mainly in the interterritorial matrix. This may also relate to the interleukin-1 data presented by Jenny Tyler and the apparent lack of response of the human articular cartilage in the degradative aspects, which would be primarily localized to the interterritorial pool, while still having a rather marked effect on the biosynthetic pathways which would be more related to regulation and control by the chondrocyte of its territorial matrix. Ernst Hunziker showed that the relative ratio of territorial matrix to interterritorial matrix in the rabbit was much higher than that in the human cartilages. Thus, interleukin-1 would perhaps have a bigger net effect on degradation in the rabbit tissue because the chondrocyte regulates a higher proportion of the matrix.

van Kampen: We see the labeled proteoglycans confined to the vicinity of the chondrocytes, perhaps within the chondron. We see very little label diffusing through the matrix. I think that once the proteoglycan leaves the chondron, it rapidly diffuses through the matrix and leaves the tissue.

Muir: The delayed aggregation phenomenon would also be relevant here. It takes a finite time for newly synthesized proteoglycans to form stable aggregates with hyaluronic acid. This would allow the proteoglycans to diffuse some distance away from the cell.

Tyler: Coming back to what Vincent Hascall said, it has always surprised me that in cartilage from young animals the newly synthesized and the resident population of proteoglycans behave with very similar kinetics in response to mediators. However, in our adult human explants, the newly synthesized proteoglycans are more readily degraded than are those already resident in the matrix.

Articular Cartilage and Osteoarthritis,
edited by K. Kuettner et al.
Raven Press, Ltd., New York © 1992.

Part VI: Remodeling in Joint Tissues

Introduction

Helen M. Muir

Department of Biochemistry, Charing Cross Hospital,
Hammersmith, London W68RF, England

Remodeling of joint tissues is a normal process that is most rapid during growth, but it persists throughout life and involves the coordinated degradation and resynthesis of molecules of the extracellular matrix. How the normal process is coordinated is not understood, but coordination is progressively lost in osteoarthritis and hence becomes a major problem. It is notable that all components of joints (cartilage, bone, ligaments, synovium) function together as a mechanical unit. They differ, however, in structure, cell type, cell density, and composition, whereas their constituent matrix molecules turn over at different rates. Even within a given tissue such as cartilage, the cells at different depths from the articular surface are distinct and have different metabolic activities, some of which are retained by isolated cells in culture (see chapter by Aydelotte et al.). To maintain homeostasis, the continuous interplay between anabolic and catabolic processes has to be finely balanced. The latter, which have been studied the most, form the basis of chapters in the following section of this volume.

The complexity of degradative processes is well illustrated by Werb's chapter. Degradative processes are induced in cartilage by the cytokines interleukin-1 (IL-1) and tumor necrosis factor α (TNF-α), which stimulate the activation of a multigene family of metalloproteinases. These enzymes are produced locally by chondrocytes themselves, and are partly regulated by endogenous closely related inhibitors [the tissue inhibitors of metal proteinases (TIMPs)]. The metalloproteinases are initially produced as zymogens, and their activation by proteolytic cleavage provides a further point of control involving two pathways, one dependent and one independent of plasminogen. The cellular mechanisms regulating expression of genes and gene products involved in the degradative process is examined in detail. Various agents that affect cell adhesion influence collagenase induction in a complex manner. The processes are interactive, and there are multiple pathways for regulating gene expression of metalloproteinases. Hence, to examine any one factor in isolation could be misleading, which makes decisive experimental design difficult. The situation is further complicated by the fact that chondrocytes respond to changes in their pericellular environment. Metal-loproteinases may be induced by alteration of chondrocyte receptors for a variety of matrix proteins. On the other hand, corticoids and transforming growth factor β (TGF-β) reduce expression of collagenase and stromelysin.

Other agents may also participate in degradation, as pointed out in the chapter by Roughley et al. These include cathepsins B, G, and L and oxygen-generated free radicals. These suggestions are based on the use of endogenous link proteins in cartilage as a monitor of degradative reactions in human cartilage at different ages. A single-site cleavage in the neonate is compatible with the action of stro-melysin, whereas further cleavages at later ages suggest the action of other agents. The N-terminal immunoglobulin fold of link protein is attacked by free radicals.

In normal adult human articular cartilage, the levels of pro-stromelysin are greater than those of pro-collagenase, which may perhaps be one reason why proteoglycan turnover is relatively rapid compared with collagen turnover (which is exceedingly slow). The differences between these levels of the pro-enzymes diminishes in chondrocytes isolated from their matrix. Hence, results obtained with isolated chondrocyte cultures should not be extrapolated without caution to intact cartilage.

The remodeling of joint tissues is particularly evident in the zone of calcified cartilage as discussed in the chapter by Oegema and Thompson. This zone forms the interface between articular cartilage and bone, and although it is penetrated by a few blood vessels, it forms a subchondral barrier for diffusion for nutrients and waste material in adult articular cartilage. The zone of calcified cartilage may be regarded as a quiescent growth plate in adult joints which, in osteoarthritis, becomes activated with duplication of the tidemark, indicating movement of the zone into articular cartilage. The zone contains (a) enzymes associated with mineralization and (b) type X collagen, which is peculiar to this zone. Movement of the zone into articular cartilage allows remodeling of subchondral bone which occurs throughout life but which is normally extremely slow. When accelerated in osteoarthritis, this leads to the typical bone changes that are diagnostic. Mech-anisms of activation of the quiescent zone of calcified cartilage in osteoarthritis are not understood, but probably represent response to altered mechanical forces such as those induced in experimental models of osteoarthritis where similar changes occur.

Bone remodeling is a prominent feature of advanced osteoarthritis. The cellular mechanisms involved are discussed in the chapter by Oyajobi and Russell. The cytokines IL-1 and TNF-α are potent inducers of bone resorption and are pro-duced by bone cells themselves, which also produce transforming growth factor β (TGF-β) and insulin-like growth factor 1 (IGF-1), which stimulate synthesis of bone matrix proteins. Bone is a metabolically active tissue whose turnover and remodeling (including collagen and mineral, in contrast with cartilage) con-tinues throughout life. Whether the exaggerated remodeling of subchondral bone in osteoarthritis is harmful or beneficial is not known. It is presumably a response to altered mechanical forces and can sometimes act to stabilize the joint. In contrast, in inflammatory arthritis the production of IL-1 and TNF-α, by inflammatory and immune cells, leads to bone loss on a shorter time scale, which is opposite to the situation in osteoarthritis.

The interplay of all the factors, including mechanical force, that govern synthesis and degradation of joint tissues is a topic of great importance in osteoarthritis research, as illustrated by the following four chapters.

Articular Cartilage and Osteoarthritis,
edited by K. Kuettner et al.
Raven Press, Ltd., New York © 1992.

20

The Biologic Role of Metalloproteinases and Their Inhibitors

Zena Werb

Laboratory of Radiobiology and Environmental Health, University of California at San Francisco, San Francisco, California 94143

The destruction of normal tissue structures, replacement of these structures by inflammatory and fibrotic tissue, and, finally, loss of function are key elements of osteoarthritis. This chapter considers (a) the proteolytic events responsible for inflammation and connective tissue remodeling and (b) the cellular and molecular mechanisms controlling these processes.

EXTRACELLULAR MATRIX-DEGRADING PROTEINASES

The enzymes that are most important in the degradation of the extracellular matrix (ECM) macromolecules in connective tissues are the matrix metalloproteinases. The metalloproteinase gene family (reviewed in refs. 1–3) consists of eight well-characterized members in human tissues that have been cloned and that show sequence conservation (Fig. 1).

Collagenase

The interstitial collagenases [also called matrix metalloproteinase (MMP)-1] are specific for collagen as substrate and cleave all three chains of the triple helix at one susceptible point, between residues 775 and 776 of the α_1 (I) chain. The bonds cleaved are between residues of glycine and isoleucine of collagens of type I, II, and III (1–4). Collagenase also cleaves collagens of type VII and VIII and makes two cleavages in collagen type X, but does not degrade either (a) basement membrane collagen type IV or (b) types V or VI collagen. The primary sequence of collagenase consists of activation, catalytic, zinc-binding, and hemopexin/vitronectin homology domains (1–4).

About 95% of the inhibitory capacity of plasma for collagenase is due to α_2-macroglobulin, which reacts more slowly with polymorphonuclear (PMN) leu-

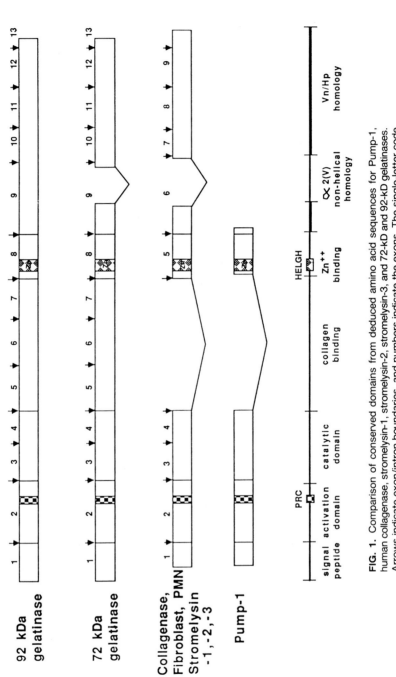

FIG. 1. Comparison of conserved domains from deduced amino acid sequences for Pump-1, human collagenase, stromelysin-1, stromelysin-2, stromelysin-3, and 72-kD and 92-kD gelatinases. Arrows indicate exon/intron boundaries, and numbers indicate the exons. The single-letter code for amino acids is used. Vn/Hp, vitronectin/hemopexin domain. (Modified from refs. 1, 3, 4, and 8.)

kocyte collagenase than with interstitial collagenase from other cells (4). The major tissue inhibitor is the tissue inhibitor of metalloproteinases (TIMP) of about 28 kD that can enter the interstitial spaces such as cartilage matrix, unlike α_2-macroglobulin. A new member of the TIMP family, TIMP-2, also inhibits collagenase (5). Collagenase and the other mammalian metalloproteinases are commonly found in culture and tissues in inactive proenzyme form. The 53- and 57-kD procollagenases are activated by a multienzyme cascade described below. Collagenase is inhibited by zinc chelating agents such as 1,10-phenanthroline. Interstitial collagenase is produced by a wide variety of cells, including macrophages, fibroblasts, synovial cells, osteoblasts, chondrocytes, and endothelial cells (4).

PMN Collagenase

There are two distinct human collagenases. PMN leukocytes have an enzyme that has a sequence different from that produced by cells of tissues such as the synovium, although sequence analysis indicates that it is closely related to collagenase (6). The PMN collagenase (also called MMP-8), whose molecular weight is about 75 kD, is stored in the specific granules of PMN leukocytes and secreted in response to appropriate stimuli (1). PMN collagenase degrades type I collagens more readily than type III collagen and prefers collagen in solution to fibrillar collagen. PMN collagenase occurs in much smaller amounts in the cells than do elastase and cathepsin G, and its significance in collagen degradation remains to be determined.

Stromelysin

The major metalloproteinase, other than collagenase, found in cultures of fibroblasts, synovium, and other cells is stromelysin (1–4), which has also been called proteoglycanase, MMP-3, transin, and neutral proteinase. It is produced as a proenzyme of about 51 kD that is activated to forms of 41 kD and further degraded to active enzymes of 21–25 kD. Stromelysin has a wide variety of connective tissue and plasma protein substrates, including: proteoglycans (decorin, fibromodulin, aggrecan, link protein); collagen of types IV, V, VII, IX, and XI; denatured type I collagen; laminin; fibronectin; elastin; α_1-proteinase inhibitor; immunoglobulins; and substance P. In addition, it has a significant function in the multienzyme cascade involved in activating procollagenase (7).

Stromelysin is inhibited by α_2-macroglobulin and TIMP. Stromelysin is produced by the same range of cells as collagenase. Although it is frequently synthesized and secreted coordinately with collagenase, it is clear in human fibroblasts, chondrocytes, and macrophages that collagenase and stromelysin may be regulated independently.

Stromelysin-2

A second enzyme closely related to stromelysin, called stromelysin-2 (also called MMP-10 and transin-2), with sequence identity of nearly 80%, has been cloned and characterized (1–4). It has nearly identical substrate specificity with stromelysin but has very distinct regulation, and its role in inflammatory diseases is unknown.

Stromelysin-3

Recently, a new member of the metalloproteinase family has been cloned as a stromal gene induced in human breast carcinoma (8). It is in the same size class and general domain structure of stromelysin and collagenase, although it is distantly related to both (about 40% sequence identity). It has been named stromelysin-3, although nothing is yet known about its substrates. Because it is also expressed in human embryonic fibroblasts after treatment with growth factors or phorbol esters, it may have significance in inflammatory diseases.

The 72-kD Gelatinase

A 72-kD gelatin-degrading proteinase (also called MMP-2, type IV collagenase, and matrilysin) that is secreted by many cells in culture, including fibroblasts and macrophages, has been characterized as an enzyme that degrades type IV collagen (1–4). The 72-kD gelatinase shows sequence homology with collagenase and stromelysin and even more so with the 92-kD gelatinase. The difference in size compared to collagenase is due to an additional domain homologous with the collagen-binding domain of fibronectin, inserted next to the zinc-binding pocket of the active site. It too requires proteolytic cleavage for activation and is inhibited by TIMP-1 and TIMP-2. The 72-kD gelatinase in proenzyme form binds one molecule of TIMP-2 (5). A second molecule is required to inhibit the activated enzyme. The TIMP-2 bound to the proenzyme may stabilize it against autoactivation.

In addition to denatured collagen and type IV collagen, it has significant proteolytic activity against fibronectin, elastin, and collagen types V, VII, and X, but not against collagen types I and VI (1–4).

The 92-kD Gelatinase

The 92-kD gelatinase (also called type IV collagenase, type V collagenase, MMP-9, and invasin) is a major secretion product of stimulated PMN leukocytes and macrophages (1–4). In PMN leukocytes this gelatinase is present in specific granules, although it was previously thought to be in a unique "C"-type granule because of release kinetics different from those of PMN collagenase and lactoferrin. In sequence it is related to the 72-kD gelatinase, characterized by a domain closely related to the binding sequence of fibronectin. It also has a sequence related to the nonhelical C-terminal domain of $\alpha2(V)$ collagen.

Like other metalloproteinases, the 92-kD gelatinase is a proenzyme that requires limited proteolytic cleavage for activation. However, the plasminogen activator/plasmin cascade does not activate this enzyme. The active forms of this gelatinase cleave denatured collagens, fibronectin, elastin, and collagens of type IV, V, VII, and XI (1–4). It is inhibited by TIMP-1, and, in parallel with 72-kD gelatinase and TIMP-2, the proenzyme form of the 92-kD enzyme binds one molecule of TIMP-1, requiring a second molecule for inhibition of the activated form. It does not cross-react immunologically with the 72-kD gelatinase.

Pump-1

Pump-1 (also known as punctuated metalloproteinase, small uterine metalloproteinase, and MMP-7) was initially described as a truncated cDNA with the proenzyme activation, catalytic, and zinc-binding sequences of metalloproteinases, but lacking the hemopexin domain found in all other members of the family (1–4). It has now been shown to have a substrate specificity like that of stromelysin, degrading fibronectin, proteoglycans, and gelatin. It also is a coactivator of collagenase. It is expressed in involuting uterus and certain tumors, and is induced in fibroblasts by concanavalin A.

CONTROL OF METALLOPROTEINASE GENE EXPRESSION

Although a range of ECM-degrading potential is exhibited by a variety of cells, many cells secrete little, if any, metalloproteinase unless appropriately triggered. Factors involved in the stimulation or suppression of metalloproteinase activity in tissue or cell culture are well described and appear to act directly on the enzyme-producing cells (Table 1).

Collagenase is expressed by cells cultured from a variety of cells and tissues. Synovial fibroblasts can be induced in culture to express collagenase and stromelysin transcripts, and collagenase and stromelysin mRNA and protein can be readily demonstrated in rheumatoid synovium by *in situ* methods (9,10). The rather broad tissue specificity and potentially high expression levels of metalloproteinases, in contrast to the low or undetectable collagen turnover rates observed in the normal organism, suggest a complex control of metalloproteinase activity *in vivo,* which is partially achieved at the level of proteinase gene expression.

Collagenase and stromelysin expression increase during fibroblast aging and in response to stress in culture, and, with increasing age, stromelysin can be extracted from human cartilage (11). Osteoarthritic cartilage contains (a) degraded

TABLE 1. *Regulation of collagenase expression*

Stimulatory factors	Inhibitory factors
Cell matrix interactions via integrins, fibronectin fragments, and soluble collagen	Glucocorticoids
Interleukin-1α and -1β, tumor necrosis factor-α	Retinoids
Growth factors (EGF, PDGF, FGF, TGF-α, NGF, relaxin)[a]	Increased production of endogenous inhibitors
Transformation (*src, ras*)	Hormones (estrogens, progesterone)
Proteinases	Indomethacin
Phagocytosis, formation of multinucleate giant cells	TGF-β
Prostaglandin E	Autocrine inhibitory factor
Phorbol diester tumor promoters	Interferon-γ
Cell aging	Transformation (Ela)
Serum amyloid A	
β_2-Microglobulin	

[a] EGF, epidermal growth factor; FGF, fibroblast growth factor; NGF, nerve growth factor; PDGF, platelet-derived growth factor; TGF, transforming growth factor.

type II collagen around chondrocytes and (b) fragments of cartilage link protein, both of which can be attributed to stromelysin action (12,13).

The fragments of fibronectin produced by plasmin and metalloproteinases may also amplify metalloproteinase expression by acting as agonistic ligands for the fibronectin receptor (14). This may play an important role in osteoarthritis because of the increase in fibronectin in cartilage. In addition to modifying cell–ECM interaction directly by targeting receptors of ECM, it is also possible to modify the interaction by modifying ECM. For example, polyclonal antibodies to fibronectin modify adhesion of fibroblasts to fibronectin and result in induction of collagenase and stromelysin, probably by a shape-dependent mechanism (P. Tremble and Z. Werb, *unpublished observation*). Several proteins have been reported to have antiadhesive properties (14). Secreted protein, acidic and rich in cysteine (SPARC), also called osteonectin, interferes with endothelial cell adhesion, and its regulation correlates with the formation of capillary sprouts in endothelial cell cultures. Tenascin (also called hexabrachion and cytotactin) is a multimeric protein enriched in cartilage that has antiadhesive properties for cells attaching to fibronectin. Decorin and biglycan also regulate cell adhesion. Tenascin is also expressed in situations where ECM–cell interactions are changing, such as mesenchyme–epithelial interactions and tissue repair. It was of interest to determine whether such a protein could regulate metalloproteinase expression by fibroblasts. Tenascin induced expression of collagenase by fibroblasts with rapid kinetics of induction (P. Tremble, H. Sage, and Z. Werb, *unpublished observation*). Thus, the changing composition of ECM that occurs during morphogenesis and tissue repair may also regulate ECM remodeling through its effects on cell adhesion through integrins. This paradigm for regulation of cellular genes by ECM molecules may be generalized to gene regulation in cartilage. Changes in gene transcription for ECM molecules in cartilage cells or precursors result in an altered ECM composition. Such ECM molecules may then interact with matrix receptors, change the cell cytoskeleton, or signal directly, and thus modulate genes to affect altered differentiated functions in cartilage.

EXTRACELLULAR REGULATION OF MATRIX DEGRADATION

One of the key factors in our understanding of connective tissue catabolism is the regulation of the activity of proteinases. Degradation of collagen is likely to be rate-limiting in most cases of ECM degradation. For collagens, one mechanism of regulation is the variation in susceptibility to collagenases by the genetic type of collagen in the tissue as well as by the degree of cross-linking of the collagen. Other proteinases may also be involved in the breakdown of collagen *in vivo* by removing proteoglycans and glycoproteins surrounding collagen fibrils, and by breaking collagen cross-links before the action of collagenase and the further degradation of the products of the initial cleavage. A second mechanism involved in the local control of metalloproteinase activity is that of inhibitors and activators. Metalloproteinase inhibitors, as well as proenzyme forms and putative activators, have been found in association with connective tissue.

CONTROL OF METALLOPROTEINASE ACTIVATION

It has been appreciated for many years that collagenase activation occurs by multiple pathways. There is a pathway involving initial cleavage by trypsin between amino acid residues 81 and 82, followed by a concentration-independent autocatalysis that can be achieved by organomercurial treatment alone (Fig. 2). Collagenase is activated in the absence of stromelysin; however, stromelysin-1 and -2, stromelysin-like Pump-1, or small forms of collagenase are required for the full activation of procollagenase by trypsin (7). Stromelysin is activated by the proteinases that activate collagenase, as well as by mast cell tryptase, PMN elastase, and cathepsin G. *In vivo,* the generation of plasmin by urokinase-type or tissue-type plasminogen activator is likely to be a significant activation mechanism for collagenase and stromelysin (4). The mechanism of activation of the 72-kD and 92-kD gelatinases *in vivo* is unknown. Plasmin does not activate these enzymes; however, neutrophil serine proteinases cathepsin G and elastase can activate the 72-kD gelatinase.

The degradation of ECM macromolecules is mediated by the availability of active proteolytic enzymes in the face of large amounts of proteinase inhibitors from plasma and local tissue sources. These inhibitors serve to control cascade activation reactions and limit proteolysis to areas where the enzyme–inhibitor balance is in favor of the enzyme. Tissues (such as cartilage) that are resistant to degradation and invasion by synovial pannus and blood vessels are rich in inhibitors such as TIMP and TIMP-2 (15).

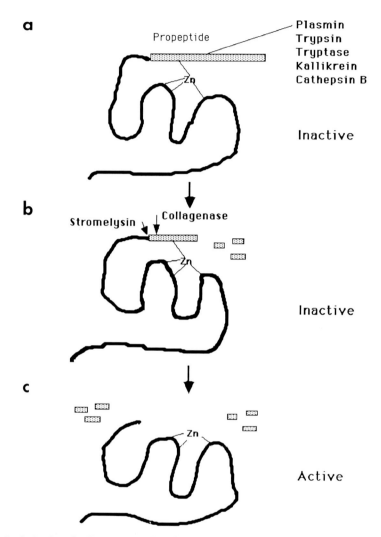

FIG. 2. Activation of collagenase. (a) Proteinases produce an initial cleavage at basic residues in the collagenase propeptide. (b) This produces a conformational change that renders the collagenase molecule active in a transautocatalytic cleavage, but inactive with respect to triple-helical collagen. (c) After this cleavage the collagenase molecule is catalytically active. Collagenase autoactivation results in a molecule that has several N-terminal amino acids more than that produced by stromelysin. The stromelysin-activated enzyme is 7–10 times more active (7). Organomercurials interact with the cysteine ligand of zinc in the propeptide, changing the conformation of the proenzyme (a) and allowing autoactivation (b) to take place.

ACKNOWLEDGMENTS

This work was supported by a contract from the Office of Health and Environmental Research [U.S. Department of Energy (DE-AC03-76-SF01012)] and by grants from the National Institutes of Health (HD 23539 and HD 26732).

REFERENCES

1. Matrisian LM. Metalloproteinases and their inhibitors in matrix remodeling. *Trends Genet* 1990;6: 121–125.
2. Matrisian LM, Hogan BLM. Growth factor-regulated proteases and extracellular matrix remodeling during mammalian development. *Curr Top Dev Biol* 1990;24:219–259.
3. Alexander CM, Werb Z. Proteinases and extracellular matrix remodeling. *Curr Opin Cell Biol* 1989;1:974–982.
4. Werb Z. Proteinases and matrix degradation. In: Kelley WN, Harris ED Jr, Ruddy S, Sledge CB, ed. *Textbook of Rheumatology,* 3rd ed. Philadelphia: WB Saunders, 1989;300–321.
5. Stetler-Stevenson WG, Krutzsch HC, Liotta LA. Tissue inhibitor of metalloproteinase (TIMP-2): a new member of the metalloproteinase inhibitor family. *J Biol Chem* 1989;264:17374–17378.
6. Hasty KA, Pourmotabbed TF, Goldberg GI, Thompson JP, Spinella DG, Stevens RM, Mainardi CL. Human neutrophil collagenase. A distinct gene product with homology to other matrix metalloproteinases. *J Biol Chem* 1990;265:11421–11424.
7. Murphy G, Cockett MI, Stephens PE, Smith BJ, Docherty AJP. Stromelysin is an activator of procollagenase. A study with natural and recombinant enzymes. *Biochem J* 1987;248:265–268.
8. Basset P, Bellocq JP, Wolf C, et al. A novel metalloproteinase gene specifically expressed in stromal cells of breast carcinomas. *Nature* 1990;348:699–704.
9. McCachren SS, Haynes BF, Niedel JE. Localisation of collagenase mRNA in rheumatoid arthritis synovium by *in situ* hybridization histochemistry. *J Clin Immunol* 1990;10:19–27.
10. Woolley DE, Crossley MJ, Evanston JM. Collagenase at sites of cartilage erosion in the rheumatoid joint. *Arthritis Rheum* 1977;20:1231–1239.
11. Gunja-Smith Z, Nagase H, Woessner JF Jr. Purification of the neutral proteoglycan-degrading metalloproteinase from human articular cartilage tissue and its identification as stromelysin/matrix metalloproteinase-3. *Biochem J* 1989;258:115–119.
12. Dodge GR, Poole AR. Immunohistochemical detection and immunochemical analysis of type II collagen degradation in human normal, rheumatoid, and osteoarthritic articular cartilages and in explants of bovine articular cartilage cultured with interleukin-1. *J Clin Invest* 1989;83:647–661.
13. Nguyen Q, Murphy G, Roughley PJ, Mort JS. Degradation of proteoglycan aggregate by a cartilage metalloproteinase. Evidence for the involvement of stromelysin in the generation of link protein heterogeneity *in situ. Biochem J* 1989;259:61–67.
14. Werb Z, Tremble P, Behrendtsen O, Crowley E, Damsky C. Signal transduction through the fibronectin receptor induces collagenase and stromelysin gene expression. *J Cell Biol* 1989;109:877–889.
15. Moses MA, Sudhalter J, Langer R. Identification of an inhibitor of neovascularization from cartilage. *Science* 1990;248:1408–1410.

DISCUSSION

Tyler: Do you think that synthesis of neutral metalloproteinases or their activation is the most important rate-limiting step in controlling matrix degradation?

Werb: In vivo, we have no evidence that enzyme activation is rate-limiting. In fact, we've made transgenic mice to address some problems of matrix remodeling in mammary glands with stromelysin constructs that are either self-activating or requiring activation. The ones requiring activation work just fine. So I do not understand how activation *in vivo* controls these processes.

Rosenberg: You mentioned that sulfhydryl groups are important in the cleavage at the N-terminus of stromelysin which converts it from a latent to an active form. Is that true? If those sulfhydryl groups are alkylated, does this inactivate the enzyme?

Werb: The zinc is coordinately complexed by four ligands, with the fourth going to a particular cysteine. If the cysteine is occupied with an organomercurial material like 4-aminophenylmercuric acetate, then it opens up and now allows a water molecule in. Then there can be catalysis.

Articular Cartilage and Osteoarthritis,
edited by K. Kuettner et al.
Raven Press, Ltd., New York © 1992.

21

The Role of Proteinases and Oxygen Radicals in the Degradation of Human Articular Cartilage

Peter J. Roughley,* Quang Nguyen,† and John S. Mort†

**Genetics Unit and †Joint Diseases Laboratory, Shriners Hospital
for Crippled Children, Montreal, Quebec H3G 1A6, Canada*

It is generally accepted that the articular cartilage degeneration which is observed during aging and which characterizes the osteoarthritic joint is the consequence of proteolysis. The need to justify such a statement may indeed appear superfluous, in view of the intimate role played by protein in the various structural elements of the extracellular matrix. However, the linkage between matrix degradation and proteolysis is in many ways circumstantial. The increased presence of matrix degradation products and the increased abundance of proteolytic agents have both been reported (1). However, definitive evidence linking a particular proteolytic agent directly with the observed damage in a cause–effect relationship is lacking. Such information is an essential prerequisite if a rational approach is to be used in the future development of therapeutic agents that may be able to counteract cartilage degeneration by preventing proteolytic action.

ARTICULAR CARTILAGE FUNCTION AND AGGREGATING PROTEOGLYCANS

Articular cartilage covers the surface of bones where they meet in movable joints. It serves two major functions: (i) facilitating smooth and painless joint motion and (ii) helping prevent excessive damage to the subchondral bone under load. This latter function is thought to be intimately related to the aggregating proteoglycan (aggrecan) content of the tissue. Two structural features of aggrecan are essential for its functional role. First, it has a very high anionic nature due to its abundance of sulfated glycosaminoglycan chains. Second, it forms large aggregates through association with hyaluronic acid. These features reside in distinct parts of the molecule, correlating with the division of the aggrecan core protein into separate structural domains. The core protein contains three globular domains (2): two at the amino terminus, termed G1 and G2, and one at the carboxy terminus, called G3. The N-terminal globular domain, G1, is responsible for the interaction of aggrecan with hyaluronic acid. This interaction is reversible under physiological conditions, but is stabilized by further interaction with a small glycoprotein, link protein (3). Each link protein interacts with both the G1 domain of aggrecan and the hyaluronic acid so that a highly stable complex is formed (4). Link protein shows considerable structural homology to the G1 domain of aggrecan (5,6). Between the G2 and G3 domains of aggrecan there is a long extended domain to which the numerous glycosaminoglycan chains are attached.

The glycosaminoglycan content of aggrecan provides the molecule with strong osmotic properties (4,7), so that in cartilage the molecule attempts to draw water into the tissue in order to expand its molecular domain. Under normal circumstances, aggrecan expansion is resisted by the surrounding inextensible network of collagen fibrils. Furthermore, in normal cartilage the aggrecan content is such that the molecules never attain their fully expanded state due to the resistance of the collagen network, but remain in an underhydrated state and thus provide the tissue with a positive swelling pressure. Upon loading, cartilage can be compressed to a limited degree by displacement of water. However, aggregation limits free diffusion of the aggrecan, and compression therefore increases the focal concentration of the proteoglycan, thereby increasing the focal swelling pressure and resisting further deformation. On removal of the load, the increased swelling pressure will be dissipated as the aggrecan expands its molecular domain by reimbibition of water.

This property of aggrecan may aid articular cartilage in a number of ways, including protecting the subchondral bone and enhancing the flow of nutrients. It is also possible that aggrecan protects the chondrocytes from being subjected to adverse compression. Such compression could potentially result in the release of proteolytic agents as an attempt to remodel the surrounding matrix, in order to relieve the physical constraints imposed on the cells. If uncontrolled, this would be deleterious to tissue function. There are a number of parameters that are essential for normal cartilage function based on the above model. In particular, aggrecan content should be high, and free diffusion of the molecule must be limited. The first criterion is compromised during the degenerative stages of osteoarthritis, when proteoglycan loss from the cartilage may occur. The second criterion is most readily breached by the action of proteolytic agents upon the aggrecan core protein or the fibrillar collagen network. Every proteolytic cleavage within the aggrecan molecule generates one proteoglycan fragment which is no longer able to interact with hyaluronic acid and which can be readily lost from the cartilage matrix, thereby leading to the long-held view that proteolysis and osteoarthritis are tightly associated.

PROTEOLYTIC AGENTS AND OSTEOARTHRITIS

The changes in proteoglycan structure that accompany osteoarthritis have been well described (8), though the interpretation of these changes has often proved confusing. This situation now appears to be due to the fact that osteo-arthritis can involve both reparative and degenerative phases; hence, depending on the stage at which analysis of the joint cartilage is performed, one may detect evidence of both new synthesis and proteolysis. It is generally believed that in areas where cartilage erosion will eventually occur, proteolysis ultimately pre-dominates over synthesis, and depletion of proteoglycans from the matrix occurs as a prelude to overt tissue degeneration. The identities of the proteolytic agents responsible for this depletion are, however, less clear. Traditionally, enzymic mechanisms via the action of proteinases have been deemed responsible (9), though one cannot categorically exclude the participation of nonenzymatic agents, such as reactive oxygen metabolites, which are also capable of causing protein degradation (10).

Of the tissue proteinases present in the body, those produced by the chondro-cytes themselves have been considered prime candidates for mediating cartilage degradation in both normal turnover and pathological states, because of their ready access to the cartilage matrix. Foremost amongst these are the secreted metalloproteinases, including collagenase and stromelysin (11). Stromelysin has a wide range of protein substrates among which are the cartilage proteoglycans, whereas collagenase appears to be the only enzyme capable of cleaving the triple-helical region of type II collagen. However, these metalloproteinases are produced as inactive proenzymes, and while a variety of mechanisms, including proteolytic processing, can generate activity, the identity of the *in situ* activator is still un-resolved. Other chondrocyte-derived proteinases that may potentially participate in proteoglycan degradation are the lysosomal enzymes cathepsins B, D, and L. Lysosomal proteinases have been identified within the cartilage matrix (9), though their participation in matrix degradation has been thought unlikely due to their requirement of an acidic environment for activity. Under inflammatory con-ditions, proteinases derived from leukocytes or blood plasma may gain access to the joint. Likely candidates from inflammatory cells to be involved in cartilage degradation are polymorphonuclear leukocyte elastase and cathepsin G (9), and among the plasma proteinases plasmin has received considerable attention be-cause of its ability to activate the latent metalloproteinases. However, with the exception of the aspartic proteinases, specific inhibitors are present in plasma, synovial fluid, and the cartilage extracellular matrix for all the proteinases listed above (9). Thus, in order to be able to damage the cartilage matrix these pro-teinases must first be able to escape the action of the proteinase inhibitors present.

Another mediator of cartilage matrix degradation could be reactive oxygen metabolites (12). These include the superoxide anion, hydrogen peroxide, and the hydroxyl radical. The hydroxyl radical is the most reactive of these species, and in the presence of transition metal ions it can be derived from either hydrogen peroxide or superoxide. The most abundant source of extracellular reactive ox-ygen metabolites is phagocytic cells, such as macrophages and polymorphonuclear leukocytes. Whether the agents released from such cells can actually gain access to the joint is debatable in view of the scavenging potential of the synovial fluid. However, it has recently been shown that chondrocytes themselves are capable of producing hydrogen peroxide (13), and hence this potential mechanism of matrix degradation cannot be discounted.

AGE CHANGES AND THE ROLE OF PROTEOLYSIS

The structure of aggrecan and link protein change considerably throughout life, and many of these changes are indicative of degradative processes. The structural changes in aggrecan include variation in both glycosaminoglycan and core protein composition (1). The changes in glycosaminoglycan include variation in both chain length and sulfation position, and are likely the result of changes in synthesis by the cell. In contrast, the core protein changes are likely due to degradative events taking place in the extracellular matrix. These changes result in the production of core proteins of shorter length, still possessing the ability to interact with hyaluronic acid. Such molecules are thought to arise by proteolytic action within the glycosaminoglycan attachment region, thereby removing the carboxy-terminal portion of the aggrecan with the globular G3 domain. Proteolytic cleavage also appears to take place between the globular G1 and G2 domains, because isolated G1 domains, presumably still bound to hyaluronic acid, abound in adult cartilage. It is not surprising that aggrecan undergoes extensive proteolytic processing within the extracellular matrix, because it appears to be a substrate for most proteinases and can be modified by hydroxyl radicals.

Link protein undergoes less extensive modification than does aggrecan, and all the changes appear to be due to proteolysis. In the newborn, human link protein exists in three forms, termed LP1, LP2, and LP3 (14). LP1 is the largest form and consists of an intact core protein to which two N-linked oligosaccharide chains are attached at amino acid residues 6 and 41 (Fig. 1). LP2 shares the same core protein as LP1, but has an N-linked oligosaccharide only at residue 41. LP3 appears to be derived from either of the two larger link protein components by proteolytic cleavage within the N-terminal region between the two N-linked oligosaccharide attachment sites. *In vitro,* many proteinases and hydroxyl radicals are able to act within this N-terminal region of the link proteins (15) and therefore could potentially be responsible for LP3 generation. However, all three link protein forms possess the three disulfide-bonded loops that are associated with link protein function, and therefore it is unlikely that the stability of the proteoglycan aggregate is affected by LP3 generation.

In the adult, the abundance of LP3 increases at the expense of LP1 and LP2, and additional sites of proteolytic cleavage become apparent (16). These additional sites reside within one of the disulfide-bonded loops, because upon reduction of disulfide bonds a series of smaller link protein fragments are produced. The size of these fragments, and their ability to be recognized by a monoclonal antibody with specificity for sequence within the two carboxy-terminal disulfide-bonded loops, suggests that fragmentation is occurring within the amino-terminal disulfide-bonded loop, which appears to be responsible for the interaction of link protein with aggrecan (17). Such fragmentation occurs within all three forms

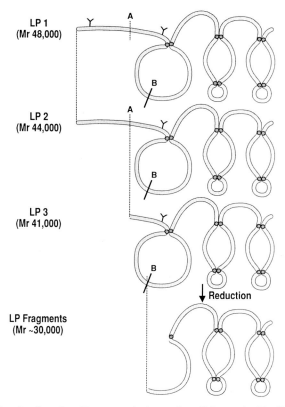

FIG. 1. The molecular diversity of human articular cartilage link protein. The link protein can be separated into three molecular forms under nonreducing conditions, termed LP1, LP2, and LP3, which have molecular weights of 48,000, 44,000, and 41,000, respectively. LP1 and LP2 possess the same protein core but differ in their substitution by N-linked oligosaccharides. LP3 is derived from either LP1 or LP2 by proteolytic cleavage at sites within the N-terminal region (A). Under reducing conditions, LP fragments may be generated from either LP1, LP2, or LP3, owing to proteolytic cleavage that can occur in the N-terminal disulfide-bonded loop (B). The LP fragments have molecular weights of about 30,000.

of link protein, and as with LP3 formation it increases progressively with age. The continued ability of fragmented link proteins to interact with hyaluronic acid probably reflects the absence of proteolytic modification within the carboxy-terminal disulfide-bonded loops, where the sites responsible for this interaction reside (17). Unlike the generation of LP3, very few proteolytic agents can cleave within the disulfide-bonded loops, and of the physiologically relevant agents only cathepsin L and hydroxyl radicals can fulfill the role (15).

LINK PROTEIN AS A MONITOR OF PROTEOLYSIS

In order to identify which proteolytic agents are actually responsible for protein degradation within the extracellular matrix of cartilage, it would be ideal if a native protein could act as a monitor of endogenous proteolysis. To be useful in such a role, the protein should fulfill a number of criteria: (a) It must be relatively resistant to proteolysis, such that a stable major degradation product results, (b) the major degradation product must be retained within the cartilage matrix over long periods of time, and (c) the cleavage site responsible for the generation of the major degradation product must be characteristic of the proteinase used in its generation. Link protein, when present in a proteoglycan aggregate, fulfills these criteria. Most proteinases are only able to cleave near the amino terminus of the molecule, and no proteinase appears able to cleave within the regions responsible for binding to hyaluronate. Furthermore, it is known that the degraded forms of the molecule accumulate within the cartilage matrix with age, probably because the protein domains responsible for the interaction with hyaluronic acid remain intact.

It is also apparent that the cleavage sites responsible for the generation of these degraded forms of link protein are characteristic for the proteinase of origin, at least for the physiologically relevant agents. Stromelysin, cathepsin D, cathepsin B, cathepsin L, plasmin, cathepsin G, and polymorphonuclear leukocyte elastase are all capable of generating LP3 forms of link protein *in vitro* having distinct amino-terminal sequences (18). All the forms have their amino termini within the region between residues 14 and 29 of the intact link proteins (Fig. 2), and in most cases only a single amino terminus is observed. The exceptions are cathepsin B and cathepsin L, which show three and two amino termini, respectively. Of the above proteinases, only cathepsin L is able to cleave elsewhere in the link protein, and this is within the amino-terminal disulfide-bonded loop. Interestingly, hydroxyl radicals also show similar limited cleavage sites: There is a single site of action in the amino-terminal region prior to residue 14 (10), and there are two sites in the disulfide-bonded loop near the site of action of cathepsin L (18). Thus the above agents are ideal candidates for the *in situ* generation of both LP3 and link-protein fragments, and analysis of the native sites of link-protein modification has the potential to distinguish the agent of its origin.

In the case of LP3, only a single amino terminus is present in the newborn, compatible with cleavage at the bond between residues 16/17 (His/Ile) of the intact link protein (15,18). The only physiologically relevant proteinase able to cleave at this site is stromelysin. In the adult, the LP3 component possesses three amino termini (15,18), compatible with cleavage between residues 16/17 (His/Ile), 18/19 (Gln/Ala), and 23/24 (Pro/His) in the intact link protein (Fig. 2). Although stromelysin action can account for the first site, it cannot account for the others, indicating that additional proteolytic agents must be involved. Cleavage prior to residue 19 is a property of both cathepsin B and cathepsin G, and therefore it is feasible that one or both of these proteinases have been active within the cartilage matrix. In contrast, none of the proteinases tested, at least when acting in isolation, were able to cleave prior to residue 24. Whether this cleavage is due to the cooperative action of several proteinases or to the action of an additional proteinase is not known at present.

In the case of link-protein fragments, two major sites of cleavage appear to be responsible for their generation in the adult (15,18). These sites are both within

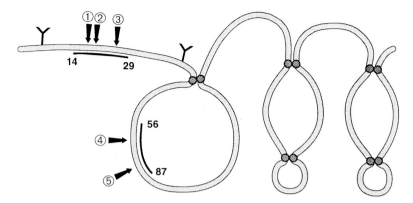

FIG. 2. The sites of proteolytic modification in human articular cartilage link protein. Many proteolytic agents are able to cleave the link proteins *in vitro* within the N-terminal region between amino acid residues 14 and 29, to produce LP3 forms of the molecule. In contrast, only a few proteolytic agents can cleave the link protein *in vitro* within the N-terminal disulfide-bonded loop between amino acid residues 56 and 87, to produce LP fragments upon reduction. The sites for LP3 generation (1,2, and 3) and LP fragment generation (4 and 5) *in vivo* occur within the same regions that are susceptible to *in vitro* proteolysis.

the N-terminal disulfide-bonded loop and occur between residues 65/66 (Lys/ Trp) and 72/73 (Asp/Tyr) (Fig. 2). None of the proteinases tested, acting in isolation, were able to cleave at these sites. Furthermore, the sites are situated in between the *in vitro* cleavage sites of cathepsin L and hydroxyl radicals. Although it cannot be discounted that an as yet unidentified proteolytic agent is responsible for the direct generation of the native cleavage sites, it is also possible that either cathepsin L or hydroxyl radicals could perform an initial cleavage within the disulfide-bonded loop, thereby altering its conformation and permitting the further action of one of the other proteinases.

When the cartilage remaining on osteoarthritic joints was examined in a similar manner, cleavage sites identical to those present in the normal adult were observed, suggesting that the same proteolytic agents were acting in the pathological and normal cartilage matrices. However, the pattern of link-protein heterogeneity in the osteoarthritic cartilage showed differences from the normal adult, with a lower abundance of both LP3 and link protein fragments (15,18). Such a pattern is compatible with new matrix synthesis having taken place in the osteoarthritic cartilage, and therefore the tissue may reflect more of the hypertrophic repair phase than of the degradative phase of the disease. If so, then it is possible that additional proteolytic agents could have been acting at sites which have already undergone erosion.

THE ROLE OF STROMELYSIN IN AGING
AND OSTEOARTHRITIS

At all ages the action of stromelysin is evident as a major factor involved in the generation of LP3, and therefore it is not unreasonable to assume that this metalloproteinase may be a major mediator of matrix turnover in general. Upon [^{35}S]methionine labeling of proteins synthesized by human articular cartilage in organ culture, it is evident that prostromelysin is a major secreted product, particularly when the cells are stimulated with interleukin-1 (14). Perhaps surprisingly, there is a much lower level of secretion of procollagenase into the culture medium, even in the presence of interleukin-1. This deficit is not due to a selective retention of procollagenase within the cartilage matrix, but rather to its lower level of synthesis.

The conclusions reached at the protein level are also apparent at the mRNA level, because the steady-state level of prostromelysin mRNA commonly exceeds that of procollagenase mRNA (19). Furthermore, the level of prostromelysin mRNA is considerably higher in the adult than in the newborn, making the difference between prostromelysin and procollagenase mRNA levels most apparent in the adult (Fig. 3). Although, it should be pointed out that this high level of prostromelysin production in the adult need not necessarily reflect increased proteolysis, because essentially all the product in the culture medium is in the inactive proenzyme form. However, the presence of large amounts of proenzyme in the adult certainly gives the tissue a potential for disaster.

When prostromelysin mRNA was localized in adult cartilage using the technique of *in situ* hybridization, expression was found to be predominant within the superficial chondrocytes (20), with little evidence of production within the chondrocytes of the deeper zones (Fig. 4). This site of expression corresponds to that region of the cartilage where safranin O staining is deplete, indicating a deficit in proteoglycan. It is possible that low levels of stromelysin activation could give rise to proteoglycan degradation in this region. Although general matrix staining was maintained beneath the superficial region, there was an apparent absence of staining immediately around the chondrocytes, suggesting possible pericellular degradation of proteoglycans. Because prostromelysin

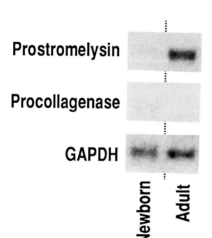

FIG. 3. The expression of prostromelysin and procollagenase mRNA by human articular cartilage. Total cellular RNA was isolated from chondrocytes that had been liberated from cartilage by enzyme digestion. Levels of mRNA for prostromelysin and procollagenase were estimated by Northern blotting using specific cDNA probes. Loading of RNA was assessed by monitoring the level of glyceraldehyde-3-phosphate dehydrogenase (GAPDH) mRNA.

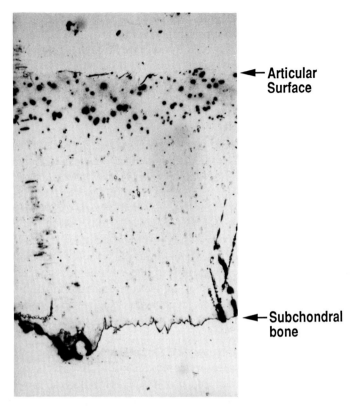

FIG. 4. The tissue localization of prostromelysin mRNA in adult human articular cartilage. Prostromelysin mRNA was localized in the chondrocytes by the technique of *in situ* hybridization using a specific ^{35}S-labeled cRNA probe. Cartilage pieces attached to subchondral bone were fixed and decalcified in formalin/EDTA prior to hybridization, so that mRNA expression throughout the full tissue thickness could be evaluated.

mRNA levels are low in these chondrocytes, it is feasible that agents other than stromelysin may be responsible. Ideal candidates for such a site of action would be lysosomal proteinases, such as cathepsin B or cathepsin L, whose action is compatible with the degradative changes in link protein, and whose instability at physiological pH would limit their site of action once outside the chondrocyte.

The reason for the predominance of prostromelysin expression in the superficial region of the articular cartilage is not clear. However, procollagenase expression shows a similar distribution, albeit at a lower level. It is possible that cytokines, such as interleukin-1 or tumor necrosis factor α, present in the synovial fluid could stimulate a superficial expression of metalloproteinase production due to a concentration gradient of their activity, decreasing with depth from the articular surface. Certainly, there is no inherent deficit in the ability of the deeper chondrocytes to produce both prostromelysin and procollagenase mRNA in response to exogenous cytokine in organ culture (20). Alternatively, however, mechanical stresses unique to the superficial regions of the joint cartilage during motion could influence gene expression by the cells within this region. Both explanations are compatible with the decreased expression of prostromelysin mRNA observed when cartilage is maintained in organ culture in the absence of cytokines. Irrespective of its origin, the increased production of proenzymes by the superficial region of normal cartilage can be viewed as a potential hazard, because it gives the propensity for tissue destruction should activation occur.

When the cartilage remaining on osteoarthritic joints at the time of surgery for joint replacement was examined by Northern blotting, there was usually a lower level of prostromelysin mRNA than in normal cartilage. However, by *in situ* hybridization its localization was still predominantly in the superficial regions of the tissue. At first sight, both of these observations would seem unexpected. First, tissues undergoing degenerative disease might be expected to be producing more proteinase. Second, global activation of chondrocytes by inflammatory cytokines might have been expected. Certainly neither scenario was true in the tissue under investigation. It should, however, be remembered that the link-protein data provided evidence suggestive of hypertrophic repair in the cartilage remaining on the osteoarthritic joints. This conclusion is supported by the abundant safranin O staining seen in the deeper zones of the cartilage, indicating that proteoglycan is not being depleted in these regions. Under conditions where new matrix synthesis is taking place, it is quite likely that expression of the metalloproteinase genes will be down-regulated. Agents such as transforming growth factor β, which induce the expression of collagen and proteoglycan, also suppress the expression of prostromelysin and procollagenase. Alternative explanations may exist, however. For example, it is possible that decreased metalloproteinase expression occurs generally within osteoarthritic joints as a consequence of drug therapy. Whether a similar down-regulation of metalloproteinase production could have occurred in the cartilage that was present at the erosive sites is not known. If this is the case, then one assumes that proenzyme activation rather than proenzyme production plays a major role in regulating the degradative phase of the disease, and that this process is focal in nature.

CONCLUSIONS

If one assumes that link protein is not unique in its susceptibility or accessibility to proteolysis compared to other matrix proteins, then it would appear that much of the noncollagenous matrix protein turnover in the neonate is mediated by stromelysin. This is not too surprising in view of (a) the active remodeling presumably taking place in this tissue during growth and (b) the need for regulation of such a process by the chondrocytes. The action of additional proteolytic agents is apparent in the adult, and in some cases these may be derived from cells other than the chondrocytes. Some evidence for the action of cathepsin G is presented, which presumably would arise from polymorphonuclear leukocytes that may gain access to the joint during minor inflammatory episodes throughout life. At present, one cannot state whether the degradative processes are carried out entirely by proteinases, because the data on link-protein fragmentation are also compatible with the action of hydroxyl radicals. However, if such agents are participating, their action would appear to involve site-selective generation.

The abundance of prostromelysin in the adult is both surprising and of concern. It is surprising why a tissue that has presumably completed the remodeling process associated with growth and development would need such a degradative potential. It is of concern that in many normal adults the superficial regions of their articular cartilage may contain a vast pool of latent proteinase that may become activated by endogenous agents outside the control of the chondrocytes. It is not inconceivable that those individuals in whom such activation occurred would be at risk for the development of the degenerative proteolytic changes associated with osteoarthritis.

ACKNOWLEDGMENTS

We would like to thank the Shriners of North America and the Arthritis Society of Canada for financial support. Thanks are also due to the pathology departments at the Royal Victoria Hospital, Montreal General Hospital, and l'Hôpital Sainte-Justine for the provision of cartilage specimens from autopsy, and to Drs. E. Brookes, W. Fisher, and D. Zukor for the provision of cartilage specimens from joint replacement. We are also grateful to Ms. N. Nikolajew for typing the manuscript and to Ms. J. Wishart for preparing the figures.

REFERENCES

1. Roughley PJ, Mort JS. Ageing and the aggregating proteoglycans of human articular cartilage. *Clin Sci* 1986;71:337–344.
2. Paulsson M, Mörgelin M, Wiedemann M, et al. Extended and globular protein domains in cartilage proteoglycans. *Biochem J* 1987;245:763–772.
3. Hardingham TE. The role of link-protein in the structure of cartilage proteoglycan aggregates. *Biochem J* 1979;177:237–247.
4. Hascall VC. Interaction of cartilage proteoglycans with hyaluronic acid. *J Supramol Struct* 1977;7: 101–120.
5. Doege K, Sasaki M, Horigan E, Hassell JR, Yamada Y. Complete primary structure of the rat cartilage proteoglycan core protein deduced from cDNA clones. *J Biol Chem* 1987;262:17757–17767.
6. Doege K, Sasaki M, Kimura T, Yamada Y. Complete coding sequence and deduced primary structure of the human cartilage large aggregating proteoglycan, aggrecan. *J Biol Chem* 1991;266: 894–902.
7. Maroudas A, Ziv I, Weisman N, Venn M. Studies of hydration and swelling pressure in normal and osteoarthritic cartilage. *Biorheology* 1985;22:159–169.
8. Bayliss MT. Proteoglycan structure in normal and osteoarthritic human cartilage. In: Kuettner KE, Schleyerbach R, Hascall VC, eds. *Articular cartilage biochemistry.* New York: Raven Press, 1986;295–310.
9. Poole AR. Changes in the collagen and proteoglycan of articular cartilage in arthritis. In: Kühn K, Krieg T, eds. *Rheumatology,* vol 10, Basel: Karger, 1986;316–371.

10. Roberts CR, Roughley PJ, Mort JS. Degradation of human proteoglycan aggregate induced by hydrogen peroxide. Protein fragmentation, amino acid modification and hyaluronic acid cleavage. *Biochem J* 1989;259:805–811.
11. Matrisian LM. Metalloproteinases and their inhibitors in matrix remodeling. *Trends Genet* 1990;6: 121–125.
12. Brunori M, Rotillo G. Biochemistry of oxygen radical species. *Methods Enzymol* 1984;105:22–35.
13. Tiku ML, Liesch JB, Robertson FM. Production of hydrogen peroxide by rabbit articular chondrocytes. Enhancement by cytokines. *J Immunol* 1990;145:690–696.
14. Nguyen Q, Murphy G, Roughley PJ, Mort JS. Degradation of proteoglycan aggregate by a cartilage metalloproteinase. Evidence for the involvement of stromelysin in the generation of link protein heterogeneity *in situ. Biochem J* 1989;259:61–67.
15. Roughley PJ, Nguyen Q, Mort JS. Mechanisms of proteoglycan degradation in human articular cartilage. *J Rheumatol* 1991;18(suppl 27):52–54.
16. Mort JS, Poole AR, Roughley PJ. Age-related changes in the structure of proteoglycan link proteins present in normal human articular cartilage. *Biochem J* 1983;214:269–272.
17. Périn JP, Bonnet F, Thurieau C, Jollés P. Link protein interactions with hyaluronate and proteoglycans. Characterization of two distinct domains in bovine cartilage link proteins. *J Biol Chem* 1987;262:13269–13272.
18. Nguyen Q, Liu J, Roughley PJ, Mort, JS. Link protein as an *in situ* monitor of endogenous proteolysis in adult human articular cartilage. *Biochem J* 1991;278:143–147.
19. Nguyen Q, Roughley PJ, Mort JS. Preferential expression of prostromelysin relative to procollagenase in human articular cartilage. *Trans Orthop Res Soc* 1991;16:196.
20. Nguyen Q, Mort JS, Roughley PJ. Preferential mRNA expression of prostromelysin relative to procollagenase and *in situ* localization in human articular cartilage. Submitted for publication, 1991.

DISCUSSION

Sandell: Somebody once said that link protein was born to be cleaved in its N-terminal peptide. Is intact link protein really a proform?

Roughley: The LP3 form appears to stabilize aggregates just as well as the LP1 or LP2 forms. If a cleavage at the N-terminal peptide does not affect link-protein function, then the intact link protein cannot be viewed as a traditional proform. However, the N-terminal region is the only part of the link protein that is not highly conserved in different species, and its function, if any, is unclear.

Sandell: The cleavage sites are conserved, aren't they?

Roughley: Yes and no. The stromelysin site may be conserved because the histidine and isoleucine residues that surround this site occur in all species. For other enzymes the sites are not always conserved. The region with the proline–histidine sequence occurs in humans, but not in other species. This region becomes sensitive to trypsin in other species because of the replacement of histidine by arginine.

Sandell: Is LP3 always present?

Roughley: Strangely enough, humans may be unique. In no other species that we have looked at do we find a marked accumulation of LP3 with age. Thus, humans seem to produce these proteolytic products as we mature, and they are presumably retained within the tissue allowing a greater accumulation with age. Such an accumulation would only be expected in animals that live to the age we do.

Muir: Look at elephants. They have a similar life span.

Roughley: We have never tried elephants. We have tried horses after 28 years and we have tried mature bovines, but never elephants.

Howell: We found elevated levels of stromelysin, especially the latent form, in osteo-arthritic lesions of cartilage compared with cartilage from age-matched auto and motorcycle accident victims. In human and Pond Nuki osteoarthritis, samples with Mankin grades indicative of early- or middle-stage osteoarthritis had higher-than-normal enzyme levels. In cartilage graded as having highly severe osteoarthritis, enzyme levels were not elevated.

Muir: Yes, I think that's an important point because late-stage osteoarthritis is clearly different from early- and middle-stage osteoarthritis.

Articular Cartilage and Osteoarthritis,
edited by K. Kuettner et al.
Raven Press, Ltd., New York © 1992.

22

The Zone of Calcified Cartilage

Its Role in Osteoarthritis

Theodore R. Oegema, Jr.*† and Roby C. Thompson, Jr.*

*Departments of Orthopaedic Surgery and †Biochemistry, University of Minnesota,
Minneapolis, Minnesota 55455*

The zone of calcified cartilage represents a unique region in mature articular cartilage. Basic biology and biochemistry of the zone of calcified cartilage (ZCC) have recently been reviewed (1). This region has biologic significance because it forms the unique bridge between the underlying bone and the nonmineralized cushioning articular cartilage above it and is a barrier to nutrition. Additionally, alterations in its biology have been implicated in the pathogenesis of osteoarthritis (OA) as exemplified by such observations as duplication of the tidemark at the calcified cartilage–cartilage interface during the development of OA.

ANATOMICAL DESCRIPTION

The "tidemark" on the nonmineralized-cartilage–calcified-cartilage interface is relatively smooth, with a gentle undulation in two dimensions (Fig. 1). This calcified–noncalcified interface of the ZCC was originally characterized as a unique histologic entity and called the "tidemark" because of its unusual affinity for a wide variety of stains. Although the interface is real, there is still some controversy as to whether "tidemark" represents a biologic entity or is just a fixation artifact (2). The presence of multiple tidemarks has been a marker for a number of biologic processes, including OA. Data collected from a wide variety of animal species and from joints within the human support not only the concept that the total height of articular cartilage is proportional to the forces placed upon it, but also the fact that the ratio of the ZCC to the total cartilage height is relatively constant, 6–8% (3). This suggests that the ZCC plays some critical role in cartilage function.

With the recent development of gentler techniques for dissection, there have been improved descriptions of the morphology of the ZCC. Digestion with papain

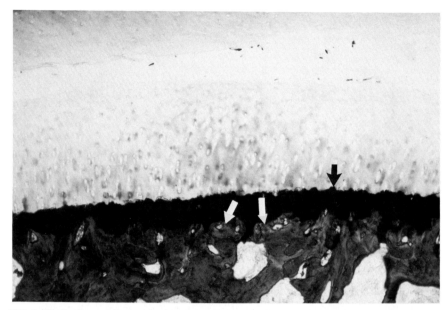

FIG. 1. Photomicrograph of canine facet joint. The intact joint was fixed in 70% ethanol, embedded in methyl methacrylate, sectioned at 100 μm with a diamond saw, and polished, and the surface was stained with toluidine blue–basic fuscin. The zone of calcified cartilage stains intensely blue. The tidemark (*black arrow*) shows gentle undulations, whereas the cement line (*white arrows*) is highly irregular. Small blood vessels are present in the subchondral bone below the ZCC.

at neutral pH to remove the overlying cartilage, followed by scanning electron microscopy, has revealed a very gentle, undulating surface with depressions corresponding to a cell diameter with occasional larger openings (Fig. 2) which represent the blood vessels that occasionally go all the way through the ZCC (4).

The chondrocytes that are present within the ZCC are still in the well-aligned lacunae or chondrons that are characteristic of the deeper layers of mature articular cartilage. There is some question as to their viability. They certainly are viable at the time of mineralization and remain so for at least a while in the mineralized tissue. Histologically, there is evidence of the continued presence of proteoglycans within the ZCC after mineralization, and mineralization does not extend all the way up to the cell membrane. By transmission electron microscopy, the collagen fibril bundles are large, well-aligned, and perpendicular to the surface (1,2).

The interface with bone, or cement line, is much more convoluted than the tidemark. Thus, the ZCC provides a highly interdigitated surface with the bone. There are no fibers crossing this interface, so that interdigitation forms the only method of attachment of the bone to cartilage. Blood vessels lined with endothelial cells will occasionally penetrate into the ZCC. They can originate from the marrow cavity and, when followed, do not form capillary loops. Within the joint, the number of blood vessels changes with location and with age and disease

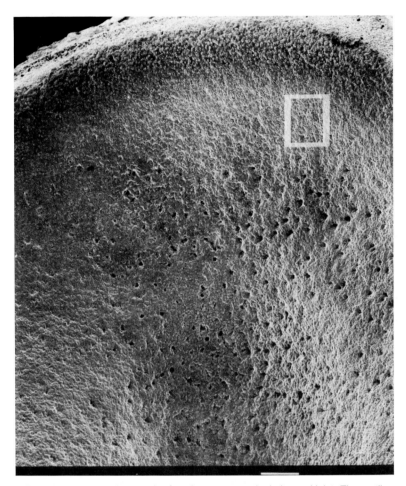

FIG. 2. Scanning electron micrograph of canine metacarpal–phalangeal joint. The cartilage was removed by digestion with papain, and the joint was dried in acetone and was processed for scanning electron microscopy. There is a very regional distribution of penetrating blood vessels. Numerous chondrocyte lacunae are present on the surface. The bar indicates 500 μm. (Courtesy of Dr. Michael Venner.)

(1,2,4). An example of highly regional penetration of capillaries coming through the ZCC is shown for a canine digit (Fig. 2). Some areas have almost no crossing blood vessels, whereas others are frequently penetrated. Many more enter the ZCC but do not cross to the tidemark.

BIOCHEMICAL CHARACTERIZATION

Lovell and Eyre (5) have shown that the ZCC from 2-year-old bovine steer contains about half the proteoglycans found within the mature articular cartilage deep zones. As expected, the major collagen is type II. In addition, they were able to isolate and characterize type X collagen [Col(X)]. This is a product characteristic of hypertrophic chondrocytes in the mineralizing growth plate. These investigators have also reported the presence of osteonectin as well as a unique protein seen only in the ZCC. The mineral present in the ZCC has the characteristic 1.67 calcium-to-phosphate ratio of hydroxyapatite. The mineral content does not change with age but does vary between species (see ref. 1 and references therein).

BIOMECHANICS

Redler et al. (6) have examined the proposed biomechanics of the ZCC. The ZCC serves as a mechanism for diffusing forces and providing the bone–cartilage interface. The perpendicular orientation of the major collagen fibrils would cause the forces to dissipate at the interface because of the gentle undulation and change in tissue properties—that is, in going from the soft resilient cartilage to the rigid underlying bone. Because of the geometry, if there was a fracture caused by these forces, it would be parallel to the interface and caused by sheer along the interface. Such splits have been seen occasionally in osteoarthritic tissue.

ORIGIN

The ZCC arises after the secondary center of ossification forms. The cells above the secondary center of ossification have growth-plate-like characteristics and continue to divide until near-maturation. Mankin (7) followed the rates of cell division in this region in rabbits and determined that mitosis essentially stops in the region just above the area that will become the ZCC slightly before maturation of the zone. With calcification, the ZCC then forms, and bone remodeling approaches from the secondary center of ossification. This is then subsequently remodeled into the subchondral bony plate. Blood vessels or outpouching of the marrow space penetrate through the subchondral plate into the ZCC but usually do not cross or even touch the interface. This means that the ZCC becomes a barrier to nutrition, and, in fact, in the thick adult articular cartilage, the deep cells then become largely dependent on diffusion from the synovial fluid for their nutrition. Lack of adequate nutrition has been proposed to be a potential mechanism for alterations of the deep zone during the aging process and in disease states such as osteoarthritis. The processes of calcification into the unmineralized overlying deep zone and vascular invasion from below are carefully balanced in the growth plate, and a similar balance is thought to be important in the ZCC. There is still a major controversy over whether movement of the ZCC is an active, ongoing process in mature cartilage (2).

Cells from the deep zone of articular cartilage retain some of the properties of hypertrophic-like chondrocytes, and particularly in osteoarthritis these characteristics are accentuated. The properties in common with the hypertropic chondrocytes include the increased expression of alkaline phosphatase and the presence of matrix vesicles (8). As shown below, synthesis of Col(X) is also a common property. Col(X) is recognized as a marker of hypertrophic chondrocytes, and in a normal situation it is uniquely present in the lower portion of the growth plate just before mineralization. This nonfibrillar, short-chained collagen has globular domains on both the amino and carboxy termini, and its structure has been determined for several species both biochemically and from the deduced sequences from cDNAs. The majority of the immunolocalization and functional studies on Col(X) have been done in the chick; recently, however, observations on several mammalian species have confirmed that the presence of Col(X) is unique to hypertrophic chondrocytes and is present just before mineralization (see ref. 9 and references therein).

With an understanding of this basic biology of the ZCC, the current controversy can be stated. The question is whether the ZCC is a stable, nonactive entity in mature cartilage or whether it undergoes continuous remodeling in the adult and can be "activated" in osteoarthritis. Arguments for a continuously remodeling system are (a) the observed gradual change in shape of joints with age (2) and (b) tetracycline labeling results which show ZCC movement in old rabbits (10). In the latter experiment, Lemperg (10) found that in mature (9 months old) rabbits given tetracycline, some regions of the tidemark were labeled; 7 months later, this label was clearly in the mid-body of the ZCC. This could only have happened if the tidemark and the ZCC had moved toward the surface. It was not clear if there was a corresponding decrease in cartilage height.

TYPE X COLLAGEN AND THE ZONE OF CALCIFIED CARTILAGE

In osteoarthritis, the movement of the tidemark has been postulated based on the presence of multiple tidemarks within the tissue. Thus, the following questions arise: Exactly how analogous are the ZCC and the growth plate, and how is the ZCC activated?

We have generated a goat polyclonal antisera as well as mouse monoclonal antibodies to canine Col(X). These antibodies were directed against pepsinized Col(X) and detected Col(X) in histological sections, on Western blots, and by enzyme-linked immunosorbent assay (ELISA). Polyclonal antisera raised against purified canine Col(X) were absorbed against affinity columns of pepsinized native Col(X) and denatured Col(X), as well as against a positive absorption step on a Col(X) column. Binding of antisera was then detected in tissues by indirect immunoperoxidase techniques. We used formalin-fixed, paraffin-embedded tissues, and the endogenous peroxidase activation was quenched with methanol–hydrogen peroxide. In mature 2 to 4-year-old canine patellar cartilages, the ZCC

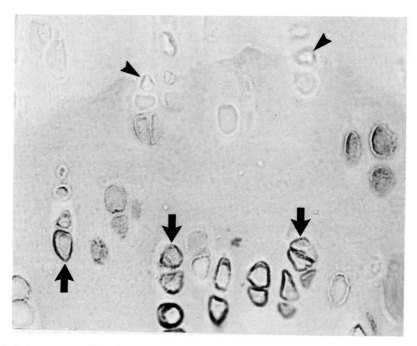

FIG. 3. Immunoperoxidase localization of Col(X) in the ZCC (*arrows*) and immediately above the tidemark (*arrowheads*) in mature dogs. (From ref. 9, reprinted with permission of the *Journal of Orthopaedic Research.*)

contained Col(X) which is located immediately around the chondrocytes (Fig. 3, *arrows*). The first cells that express detectable Col(X) are just above the tidemark (*arrowheads*). These cells immediately above the tidemark would be the same cells that would be positive for alkaline phosphatase, which can be demonstrated by histochemistry in unfixed citrate-decalcified samples. This information suggests that in mature animals, Col(X) is a normal constituent of the ZCC, and that chondrocytes involved in mineralization at the tidemark are expressing Col(X). This is consistent with the information on the isolation of Col(X) by Lovell and Eyre (5) from 2-year-old steer ZCC. It does not, however, answer the question whether this is an active, ongoing process or whether this represents Col(X) that remained there from the initial formation of the ZCC.

MOVEMENT OF THE ZONE OF CALCIFIED CARTILAGE

We have recently determined the rate of the movement of the ZCC during the process of maturation. To do this, we have used rabbits, in which Mankin (7) previously studied the rates of cell division, or the number of mitoses seen in the articular cartilage with age. In this model, animals of known birth date were given intra-articular injections of 2,4-bis[*N,N*-di(carboxymethyl)-

aminomethyl]fluorescein (DCAF), a calcium-seeking chromophore, and then the patellae were harvested after various time periods depending on the age of the animals. There was a rapid movement of the ZCC in immature animals; the rate was sufficient to remove an entire thickness of the ZCC in 3 weeks in the 3-month-old animals. The rate of movement decreased precipitously to less than 10% of this value by 6 months of age. In 7-month-old animals the rate was even slower but still detectable (1).

Because the DCAF-labeling technique has potential for measuring the ZCC movement, we have tried to optimize the retention of the dye. In mature rabbits and dogs, we have noticed that 6 weeks after dye labeling, there are areas (particularly where the two joints have more contact) where the dye is lost. One explanation for this is that if the ZCC does not move, crystals at the interface may alternately dissolve and recrystalize, resulting in the loss of dye. We have tried two methods for improving dye retention. We have injected the dye intra-articularly into mature rabbits, which gives even staining across the surface. The animals were then exposed to either (a) sodium fluoride at 50 ppm in the drinking water for a week or (b) sodium etidronate (disodium 1-hydroxyethylidene-diphosphonate) at 20 mg/kg/day for a week, and the results were evaluated 6 weeks later. The fluoride treatment did not give improved retention, but the sodium etidronate did. The results of this study in mature rabbits were promising. If brief exposure to diphosphonate does not alter the disease process investigated, this presents an excellent way of fixing the fluorescent dye.

We have compared single- and double-labeled tissues, and unless the separation is greater than 10–20 μm, it was easier to back-light the sample partially to detect the tidemark. Considerable overlap occurred if two dyes were used when the band width was greater than 10 μm and the rate of movement small.

THE ZONE OF CALCIFIED CARTILAGE IN OSTEOARTHRITIS

In a preliminary study using the rabbit model of osteoarthritis where the anterior cruciate and medial collateral ligaments were severed and a partial meniscectomy was performed, we were able to show acceleration in movement of the ZCC. The ZCC in the patellae of the operated leg had moved 45 μm in 6 weeks, whereas that in the opposite leg moved less than 5 μm. Although additional experimental evidence needs to be gathered to see if these results hold up, this observation would represent the first time such accelerated movement of the ZCC has been documented. Since this was measured on the patellae, it would be consistent with the entire joint being involved in the disease process. This is not humeral since the opposite leg showed no movement. This could be explained if instability of the joint also affects the biomechanical stability of the patellae within the joint complex.

In summary, even in the mature animal, there may be a slow progression of the ZCC toward the surface. This could potentially be accelerated in a number of pathologic states. The mechanical or biochemical parameters responsible for the acceleration are unknown. However, some simple manipulations such as matrix depletion may not be sufficient for acceleration. The complex environment present in the osteoarthritic joint allows activation. Whether the acceleration takes place at a rate that is sufficient to compromise the joint integrity is unknown at this time. However, it should be noted that many of the parameters, such as the forces across the joint and the way they are dissipated by the articular cartilage, are critically dependent on the cartilage height. Thus relatively subtle, 10–15% changes in the cartilage thickness, without other changes in properties of the cartilage, could alter the stress pattern and the way the cells respond to these forces.

ACUTE TRANSARTICULAR LOADING MODEL
OF OSTEOARTHRITIS

In an attempt to look at repair or degeneration in osteoarthritis, we have been working for several years to develop an alternate model for osteoarthritis that involves injuring the ZCC–cartilage interface. In this model, the canine patellae is given a single acute transarticular load, with the joint closed at 100° flexion (11). The force used rises to a maximum within 1 msec, remains constant for about 2 msec, and then falls. Initially, we had examined states which did not produce fractures in the ZCC, subchondral bone, or cartilage but which seemed to produce an initial increase in water content of the cartilage. In our more recent study, we have now increased the impaction so that we get characteristic multiple stair-step fractures in the ZCC. In the majority of cases, there is a partial lesion into the deep layers of cartilage, with an occasional surface lesion. In a recently published study (11), we investigated three different time frames (2, 12, and 24 weeks). Immediately after impaction, the surface of the patellae has a characteristic, slightly pleated pattern which is visible with India ink staining. This does not generally represent a tear within the cartilage but seems to correspond to the underlying pathology of the ZCC. The ZCC, after digestion with papain to remove the overlying cartilage, has a pleated accordion pattern running perpendicular to the long poles of the patellae (Fig. 4). Occasionally, animals will have full-thickness fractures of the cartilage or in the deep regions of the bone. By 2 weeks, there is evidence of active repair processes at the base of fractures of the ZCC–cartilage interface. Some cells in the overlying cartilage are dead, and the matrix shows loss of proteoglycan. By 3 months, there is extensive loss of proteoglycan in the overlying matrix in an area of the lesion, and subchondal bone is remodeling. By 6 months, cells that had survived in the overlying cartilage have now started to form clones (Fig. 5, *arrows*). The sites of fracture appeared to communicate with subchondral vessels when the fractures were traced through five or six serial sections. There was extensive loss of the safranin-O staining and fibrillation. No gross joint pathology of the synovium, ligament, or meniscus was noted.

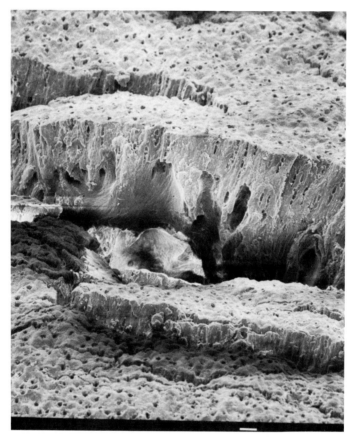

FIG. 4. Scanning electron photomicrograph of canine patella immediately after acute transarticular loading. The sample was processed as in Fig. 2. There is extensive parallel branching fractures. Columns of cells and long-range ordered collagen are visible. (Courtesy of Dr. Michael Venner.)

In the acute transarticular loading system, we have significantly changed the loading parameters from those of our previous protocol. There is now extensive damage to the ZCC. It is clear that this new impacting format generates forces exceeding those previously recorded in the other system. Previous work with a totally disrupted ZCC has focused on the ability to heal and suggested that the healing tissues came from cells penetrating from the underlying marrow space. However, direct damage to the cartilaginous surface without penetration of the ZCC has failed to produce repair or progression (see ref. 11 for discussion).

The canine acute transarticular damage model has several advantages over the anterior cruciate models in that the joint is not invaded, avoiding artifactual tissue response. The initiating event can then be well characterized, and the initial mechanical changes can be determined. Initial damage is reasonably reproducible, is controlled, and can be graded to severity. After the initial damage,

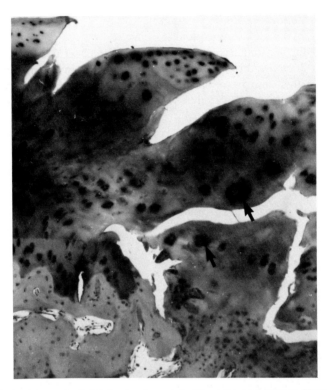

FIG. 5. Photomicrograph of distal pole of a patella 24 weeks post-loading. There are surface clefts and fractures in the ZCC. Some clefts are from the surface into the transition zone, and others are confined to the zone of calcified cartilage. New bone formation is present below these clefts. Clones (*arrows*) of cells are present in the radial zone of cartilage, and there is a significant loss of safranin-O stain. (From ref. 11, reprinted with the permission of the *Journal of Bone and Joint Surgery.*)

animals can be kept in normal conditions without special restrictions. The major disadvantage is that the time frame requires at least 6 months to a year to produce identifiable osteoarthritic lesions. We are in the process of scaling down to a smaller animal size which may accelerate the process and cut down the cost.

These experiments suggest that cartilage degeneration would be a consequence of damage to the ZCC and subchondral bone if sufficient damage was done at the time of injury. More importantly, this underscores the possibility that subchondral fractures which do not disrupt the cartilage can play a role in the development of osteoarthritis. Such an entity has recently been identified as a cohort of those that receive anterior cruciate ligament injuries. Magnetic resonance imaging studies by Vellet et al. (12) documented the presence of acute and hidden post-traumatic osteochondral lesions in 86 out of 120 patients with acute hemarthrosis, but who still had normal cartilage surfaces by arthroscopic examination. This would be equivalent to damage seen in the present model. Subchondral fractures could be a common feature of musculoskeletal trauma and a significant source of subsequent arthritis.

This study further underscores the potential role the ZCC could play in the development of osteoarthritis. Much of the information involving the ZCC has come from indirect sources. Because of its thinness, small size, and irregularity, it has been difficult to dissect directly to obtain good chemical parameters. Because of the need to decalcify the ZCC before applying many of the immunochemical and histochemical techniques, very little has been learned about its composition. The responses of the ZCC to outside forces or to exposure to various biochemical and mechanical insults are largely unknown. It is very clear that the ZCC arises from a growth-plate-like process. Many of the studies that have been done to date suggest that at least some aspects of these persist through maturity and can be activated under certain disease states. Because osteoarthritis affects the entire joint, not only does the ZCC in the affected area have to be considered, but so do the distal regions of the joint which often give rise to other sets of pathology.

CURRENT QUESTIONS CONCERNING THE ZONE OF CALCIFIED CARTILAGE

Current questions that need to be investigated are whether or not under normal circumstances the ZCC movement is of a sufficient magnitude to be involved in the change of thickness of the uncalcified cartilage. Such changes in height would make the joint much more vulnerable to mechanical processes, especially if they are coupled with a dramatic change in the cartilage properties that alter the stress distribution and stiffness. Such changes in cartilage properties have been postulated from published data on aging. Whether or not the ZCC can be activated and significantly change its response is something else that has to be evaluated with more sensitive methodology. Whether the overlying cartilage can actually participate in a slow but reproducible production of matrix and thickening is something that has been speculated upon (see ref. 1 and references therein; also see refs. 2–4 and 10) but for which there is no direct evidence. If cells in normal cartilage divide slowly, beyond most normal ranges of detection by [^{3}H]thymidine labeling, can the more recently devised 5-bromodeoxyuridine labeling techniques, which have long labeling windows, be used? The actual mechanism for calcification would appear to be different than that seen in the growth plate. The magnitude of the cell-to-matrix calcification ratio is much greater in the ZCC than in the growth plate, and the cells in articular cartilage are not undergoing the large volume changes that have been shown to occur in the growth plate.

Additionally, the same careful interplay between vascular invasion and mineralization that is seen in the growth plate must also play a significant role in maintaining the stability of the ZCC. This balance is thought to involve both

(a) the presence of an inhibitor of vascular invasion synthesized by cells higher in the growth column and (b) the actual production of enhancers for angiogenesis by the more terminal hypertropic chondrocytes. Such an interplay would be critically important in mature cartilage.

Finally, there is significant question as to the activation of the ZCC. This would have to be initiated by the cells above the ZCC in the deep layer. Current information is consistent with the proposal that they are indeed a different population of cells and correspond in osteoarthritis by increased alkaline phosphatase production, vesicle formation, properties consistent with mineralization, and the expression of Col(X). This enforces the analogy with hypertropic chondrocytes. Investigation of the mechanisms of the ZCC perturbation and maintenance of steady state should yield valuable information in the normal and osteoarthritic process. Regulation of this process throughout the joint may lead to better understanding of the processes of maintaining or changing joint shape that involve maintaining the cartilage–bone interface.

ACKNOWLEDGMENTS

This work was supported by NIH AR39255 (SCOR on osteoarthritis), NIH AR07555 (training grant), and Bristol-Meyer Squibb/Zimmer O.R.E.F. 89-492. The expert technical help of Randall J. Carpenter, Toni Meglitsch, Francine Hofmeister, Michael Venner, and Gordon Walker, as well as the preparation of the manuscript by Andrea Chatfield, is gratefully acknowledged. The ongoing collaboration with Jack Lewis and Larry Wallace is much appreciated.

REFERENCES

1. Oegema TR Jr, Thompson RC Jr. Cartilage–bone interface (tidemark). In: Brandt K, ed. *Cartilage changes in osteoarthritis.* Indiana School of Medicine publication. Basel: Ciba-Geigy, 1990;43–52.
2. Bullough PG, Jagannath A. The morphology of the calcification front in articular cartilage: its significance in joint function. *J Bone Joint Surg* 1983;65A:72–78.
3. Müller-Gerbl M, Schulte E, Putz R. The thickness of the calcified layer in different joints of a single individual. *Acta Morphol Neerl Scand* 1987;25:41–49.
4. Clark JM, Huber JD. The structure of the human subchondral plate. *J Bone Joint Surg* 1990;72B: 866–873.
5. Lovell TP, Eyre DR. Unique biochemical characteristics of the calcified zone of articular cartilage. *Trans Orthop Res Soc* 1988;13:511.
6. Redler I, Mow VC, Zimny ML, Mansell J. The ultrastructure and biomechanical significance of the tidemark of articular cartilage. *Clin Orthop* 1975;112:357–362.
7. Mankin HJ. Mitosis in articular cartilage of immature rabbits. *Clin Orthop* 1964;34:170–183.
8. Einhorn TA, Gordon SL, Siegel SA, Hummel GF, Auitable MJ, Carty RP. Matrix vesicle enzymes in human osteoarthritis. *J Orthop Res* 1985;3:160–169.
9. Gannon JW, Walker G, Fischer M, Carpenter R, Thompson RC Jr, Oegema TR Jr. Localization of type X collagen in canine growth plate and adult articular cartilage. *J Orthop Res* 1991;9: 485–494.
10. Lemperg R. The subchondral bone plate of the femoral head in adult rabbits. I. Spontaneous

remodeling studied by microradiography and tetracycline labeling. *Virchows Arch* 1971;352: 1–13.

11. Thompson RC Jr, Oegema TR Jr, Lewis JL, Wallace L. Osteoarthritic changes following acute transarticular load: an animal model. *J Bone Joint Surg* 1991;73-A:990–1001.

12. Vollet AD, Marks P, Fowler P, Mururo T. MRI of occult post-traumatic osteochondral lesion. *Radiology* 1991;178:271–276.

DISCUSSION

Handley: Where do chondrocytes in the transition zone of the tidemark derive their nutrition?

Oegema: Others have shown that when the zone of calcified cartilage forms, nutrition from underneath drops off dramatically, probably to only about 10% of what it was before the zone forms, so nutrition is mainly by diffusion from the synovium.

Dieppe: Scintigraphy in human osteoarthritis shows increased uptake in the subchondral bone region, and this is our best predictor of subsequent destruction of the joint. Have you done any scintigraphic work with your model?

Oegema: No, we haven't had a chance to do that with our model yet.

Peyron: Is the tidemark involvement specific to particular subsets of arthritis, such as the post-traumatic type after impact loading?

Oegema: We have not made a general survey. The problem is that some post-traumatic patients do not have an overt fracture and are read as normal, even though they have a sore joint for a long time. This important subclass has not been looked at. With the advent of MRI and scintigraphy, we should be able to identify more of these patients.

Cooke: With respect to the relationship between trauma and osteoarthritic patterns, I think that in patients with anterior ligament cruciate disruption or with direct force and impact injury to the patella, tidemark damage will be involved. But I still do not think that many of the patients that come with osteoarthritic knees have subchondral fractures or that trauma was the primary basis of the disease. With regard to the point raised by Paul Dieppe about bone scan positivity, there are some data from orthopedic surgeons interested in osteotomy. They looked at changes in bone scan responses after osteotomy and showed that they correlated strongly with changes in loading patterns.

Buckland-Wright: Regarding this last point, we have studied changes in subchondral bone and have observed advancing tidemarks which occur immediately where load is applied. Where there is no load in the joint, we see no advance in the tidemark at all. So there is a good correlation between load and the advancing tidemark. Can you suggest what might be causing this marked advance of the tidemark into the cartilage?

Oegema: So far in our model of osteoarthritis, we only see tidemark movement in areas where changes in forces or loading would be predicted because of the altered joint patterns. It is not seen in the unchanged areas.

Mason: The intermediary metabolism of cells in the calcified zone may be rather different from that of cells in the cartilage above. For example, the oxygen tension may be much higher in the calcified zone. Electron-microscopic pictures show very few mitochondria in chondrocytes of hyaline cartilage. Have you observed mitochondria in your pictures of chondrocytes in the calcified zone?

Oegema: We have not yet looked for that. If alkaline phosphatase is any indication, this enzyme is only expressed up to the first layer of cells above the zone of calcified cartilage.

Articular Cartilage and Osteoarthritis,
edited by K. Kuettner et al.
Raven Press, Ltd., New York © 1992.

23

Bone Remodeling, Cytokines, and Joint Disease

Babatunde O. Oyajobi and R. G. G. Russell

Departments of Human Metabolism and Clinical Biochemistry, University of Sheffield Medical School, Sheffield S10 2RX, England

The predictable and organized sequence of events at discrete sites throughout the skeleton that involves the coordinated actions of osteoclasts and osteoblasts is termed *bone remodeling.* The initial event in bone remodeling is osteoclastic resorption. This is almost always followed by new bone formation mediated by osteoblasts (Fig. 1). Bone resorption can be enhanced by increasing the activity of mature osteoclasts as well as by increasing the total number of osteoclasts via stimulation of recruitment, proliferation, and fusion of osteoclast precursors. Likewise, bone formation can be enhanced by two mechanisms: (i) stimulation of proliferation of cells of osteoblastic lineage and (ii) induction of differentiation of commited osteoblast precursors into mature osteoblasts. It is likely that the factors that regulate bone remodeling do so by one or more of the above mechanisms.

Individual remodeling sites are spatially and temporally separated, and this suggests that the cellular events in the remodeling process are coordinated locally. Peptide regulatory factors are emerging as important autocrine and paracrine regulators of various cell functions in several tissues. These include the classical lymphokines, monokines, growth factors, colony-stimulating factors, and neuropeptides. Several of these peptide factors are known to be released by the inflammatory cells that infiltrate arthritic joints. In addition, enhanced production of cytokines in patients with arthritis is well documented. Some of these cytokines, as well as growth factors, have been shown to be present, and to be biologically active, in the synovia and synovial fluid of patients with arthritis (1,2). Surprisingly, a large number of these growth factors are sequestered in bone matrix, and these are listed in Table 1. There is evidence that some, but not all, of these peptide regulatory factors may be synthesized and released by osteoblast-like cells constitutively or in response to various stimuli (Fig. 2). Furthermore, some of these biologically active molecules may be produced in or around bone by marrow constituents (e.g., lymphocytes, monocyte/macrophages, and platelets),

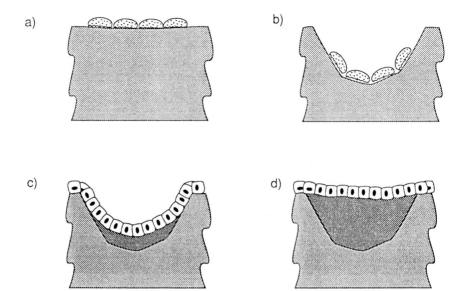

FIG. 1. The sequence of remodeling of bone. Osteoclasts are recruited to the bone surface **(a)** and resorb a cavity **(b)**. Osteoblasts then replace the osteoclasts and proceed to form new bone to fill the resorption cavity **(c)** until the amount of bone replaced matches that removed during the resorptive phase **(d)**.

TABLE 1. *Bone-active cytokines and growth factors*

Cytokines and growth factors[a]	Present in bone matrix	Produced by osteoblasts
IGF-1 and IGF-2	+	+
TGF-β_1 and TGF-β_2	+	+
PDGF (AA, AB, BB)	+	+
BMPs (e.g., 1 and 3)	+	+
TGF-α	+	?
FGF (basic and acidic)	+	+
BDGF (β_2-microglobulin)	+	?
PTH-rP	?	+
GM-CSF, M-CSF	?	+
IL-1α and IL-1β	+	+
IL-6	?	+
IL-8	?	+
TNF-α	?	+

[a] IGF, insulin-like growth factor; TGF, transforming growth factor; PDGF, platelet-derived growth factor; BMP, bone morphogenic protein; FGF, fibroblast growth factor; BDGF, bone-derived growth factor; PTH-rP, parathyroid hormone-related peptide; GM-CSF, granulocyte/macrophage colony-stimulating factor; M-CSF, macrophage colony-stimulating factor; IL, interleukin; TNF, tumor necrosis factor.

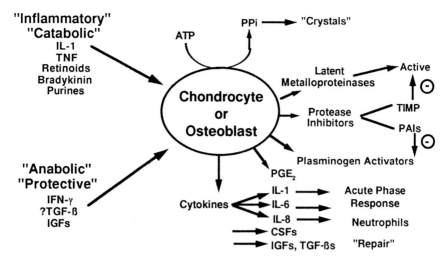

FIG. 2. Scheme showing some of the many responses that may occur in chondrocytes and osteoblasts during physiological and pathological activation. IL-1, interleukin-1; TNF, tumor necrosis factor; IFN-γ, interferon-γ; TGF-β, transforming growth factor β; IGFs, insulin-like growth factors; PGE$_2$, prostaglandin E$_2$; IL-6, interleukin-6; IL-8, interleukin-8; CSF, colony-stimulating factor; TIMP, tissue inhibitor of metalloproteinases; PAIs, plasminogen-activator inhibitors; ATP, adenosine triphosphate; PPi, inorganic pyrophosphate phosphate.

whereas some are produced at distant extraosseous sites and reach bone via the circulation. Many of these peptide factors modulate the growth and differentiation of bone cells and may therefore play important regulatory roles in normal bone remodeling. There is increasing evidence to suggest that these factors interact with each other such that one factor may influence the production and/or biological effects of others. Furthermore, natural and specific inhibitors of some of these factors appear to exist, and these may exert a balancing effect on their overall effects. Consequently, the net effect of each peptide factor in bone turnover may depend, in part, on its concentration and on the relative amount of other potentially synergistic and antagonistic factors in the immediate microenvironment of individual bone remodeling units.

In addition to peptide regulatory factors, osteotrophic hormones such as parathyroid hormone (PTH), 1,25-dihydroxyvitamin D$_3$, glucocorticoids, calcitonin, estrogens, and androgens are likely to play key roles in remodeling, especially as the synthesis and release of several cytokines are known to be modulated by some of these hormones. The degree of receptor modulation by other factors and by osteotrophic hormones is also likely to be an important determinant of the actual effect of each individual factor *in vivo*.

The potent effects of these cytokines and growth factors on bone metabolism, as well as the presence of large numbers of cells capable of producing them in and around affected joints, indicate an important role for these factors in the connective tissue destruction that accompanies inflammatory joint diseases. It is probable that in chronic inflammatory joint diseases such as osteoarthritis, these factors may be involved not only in the sclerosis of underlying subchondral bone, but also in the development of osteophytes. Until the precise mechanisms by which cytokines and growth factors regulate bone remodeling in physiological circumstances are fully elucidated, it will not be possible to understand fully the changes that may occur in pathological conditions such as the arthritides.

In this brief overview, the major cytokines and growth factors that modulate osteoclastic bone resorption and osteoblast-mediated bone formation will be discussed, especially as these may relate to joint diseases. Some of the mechanisms by which these local mediators of bone cell responses may regulate normal bone remodeling, and bone remodeling in joint diseases, will also be discussed. We will outline some of the current concepts about the intercellular interactions that may occur within bone and within the joint.

LOCAL FACTORS THAT MAY BE INVOLVED IN BONE MATRIX DEGRADATION (FIG. 3)

Of the polypeptide factors presently identified, perhaps the two most potent mediators of bone and cartilage degradation are the interleukins-1 and the tumor necrosis factors (TNFs). It is generally accepted that the destruction of articular cartilage and subchondral bone that occurs during inflammatory processes in joints results from the concerted actions of tissue proteases (e.g., collagenase,

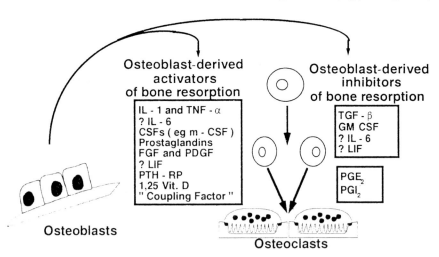

FIG. 3. Osteoblasts can produce a variety of cytokines and growth factors that can, in turn, influence bone resorption under physiological and pathological conditions. IL-1, interleukin-1; TNF-α, tumor necrosis factor α; CSFs, colony-stimulating factors; m-CSF, monocyte colony-stimulating factor; FGF, fibroblast growth factor; PDGF, platelet-derived growth factor; 1,25 Vit. D, 1,25-dihydroxyvitamin D_3; TGF-β, transforming growth factor β; GM CSF, granulocyte/macrophage colony-stimulating factor; IL-6, interleukin-6; PGE$_2$, prostaglandin E$_2$; PGI$_2$, prostaglandin I$_2$; LIF, leukemia inhibitory factor; PTH-RP, parathyroid hormone-related peptide.

stromelysin, and plasminogen activators). These enzymes have been shown, individually and collectively, to degrade various extracellular matrices, including those in bone and cartilage. The interleukins and TNFs can stimulate all the connective tissue cell types present in joints (synovial cells, articular chondrocytes, and osteoblasts) to produce these collagenolytic and proteolytic enzymes as well as prostaglandins. Clearly, the production of these cytokines, prostaglandins, and some of the tissue proteases by inflammatory cells associated with synovitis are important in mediating bone destruction in arthritis.

Interleukin-1

There are two species of interleukin-1 (IL-1), both of which are products of separate genes and which exhibit a limited structural homology. The two forms, IL-1α and IL-1β, which represent acidic and neutral forms respectively, are synthesized as 31-kD precursor molecules which are then cleaved to the mature 17-kD molecules. Both IL-1 species bind with similar affinity to the same cell-surface receptors in connective tissues, and both have been shown in several systems (*in vitro* and *in vivo*) to have virtually identical biological activity. IL-1 was originally described as a product of activated cells of the monocyte/macrophage lineage, but it is now well recognized that IL-1 is also produced by a wide variety of nonimmune cells, including connective tissue cells. IL-1 is produced by bone organ cultures and isolated bone cells *in vitro* (3).

IL-1 is a potent inducer of bone resorption *in vitro* (4), and it is the most powerful natural bone-resorbing agent described to date. IL-1 is also a powerful stimulator of bone resorption *in vivo* (5,6). It stimulates osteoclastic resorption, in part, by increasing formation of new osteoclasts from mononuclear cells in marrow. Because isolated osteoclasts are not affected by IL-1, intermediate cells such as osteoblasts primed by IL-1 may, in turn, activate mature osteoclasts, enabling them to resorb bone (4).

IL-1 is a potent co-mitogen for osteoblast-like cells *in vitro,* and it inhibits osteoblastic alkaline phosphatase expression and osteocalcin production (7–9). High doses and long-term incubation with IL-1 also inhibit collagen synthesis by bone organ cultures and by cultured osteoblast-like cells (8). Interestingly, IL-1-stimulated osteoclastic bone resorption is followed by increased bone formation *in vivo* (5), an observation which points to a possible role for IL-1 in the coordination of the remodeling cycle.

The mechanism of action of IL-1 in bone remodeling remains unclear. Many of its actions appear to be due to production of other factors. For example, IL-1 stimulation of prostaglandin E production by connective tissue cells and mononuclear cells *in vitro* is well documented. IL-1 also induces its own production, as well as the production of other cytokines and growth factors (e.g., TNF-α and the colony-stimulating factors), from a wide variety of cell types. Conversely, several of these factors modulate IL-1 synthesis and release from several cell types, including connective tissue cells. These include TNF-α and -β, transforming growth factor β (TGF-β), colony-stimulating factors, and neuropeptides such as substance P. Furthermore, IL-1 stimulates several connective tissue cell types (including osteoblasts) to secrete tissue proteases (e.g., collagenase and plasminogen activators) (7,8).

There is considerable evidence to suggest that IL-1 may be an important mediator of connective tissue degradation in various arthritic conditions. It is produced by infiltrating inflammatory cells and synoviocytes in rheumatoid arthritis (RA), and IL-1 bioactivity has also been detected in synovial fluid from affected joints in RA. IL-1 is also produced spontaneously by RA synovial fibroblasts (1,2).

There are known natural inhibitors of IL-1. Changes in these peptides in juvenile RA have been described which suggest that it may be clinically important (10).

Tumor Necrosis Factors

Tumor necrosis factors (TNFs) exist in two forms that have a high degree of sequence homology. TNF-α (cachectin) is a 17-kD peptide produced mainly by activated macrophages/monocytes, and TNF-β (lymphotoxin) is a structurally related 18-kD peptide produced by activated T lymphocytes. Both forms exhibit a spectrum of activity similar to that of each other and to that of IL-1, although they are not structurally related to either species of IL-1 and bind to separate cell-surface receptors (11). Like IL-1, the TNFs are potent inducers of bone resorption *in vitro* and *in vivo* (4,6). IL-1 acts synergistically with TNF-α as well as with other bone-resorbing cytokines [TGF-α and epidermal growth factor (EGF)] and systemic bone-resorbing hormones to induce osteoclastic resorption (4,8). As with IL-1, the bone resorptive activity of TNF is mediated via stimulation of the proliferation of osteoclastic progenitors as well as via osteoblast-mediated activation of mature isolated osteoclasts (4). Other effects of TNF-α on bone cells and other connective tissue cells are very similar to those of IL-1, including the inhibition of collagen and osteocalcin synthesis, induction of synthesis of prostaglandins and metalloproteinases, and stimulation of the production of colony-stimulating factors (8).

TNF-α is produced spontaneously by synovial tissue cells in certain arthritic conditions, and TNF-α bioactivity has also been detected in RA synovial fluid (1,2). TNF-α is also produced by osteoblast-like cells *in vitro* (12), and it may therefore be an autocrine modulator of normal bone remodeling. The effects of TNF-α on bone remodeling in various arthritic conditions may be mediated, in part, by IL-1, because TNF-α induces the release of IL-1 by mononuclear cells and macrophages (8). The presence of both IL-1 and TNF-α in synovial fluid in inflammatory joint diseases, along with their synergistic interactions, may be a significant factor in the destruction of articular cartilage and the underlying subchondral bone characteristic of the late stages of these conditions. Furthermore, it has been reported that TNF-α is a potent stimulator of angiogenesis, and this may be relevant in the vascularization of the invading pannus, which would enhance entry of macrophages and T lymphocytes into the synovium.

Interleukin-6

Several diverse biological activities previously attributed to a variety of factors are now recognized to reside in one distinct protein now termed interleukin-6 (IL-6) (13). This multifunctional cytokine is produced by many different cell types of lymphoid and nonlymphoid origin. These include: activated T lymphocytes, monocytes/macrophages, and plasma cells. IL-6 is produced in bone and by osteoblast-like cells constitutively, as well as in response to IL-1. TNF-α and bacterial lipopolysaccharides (endotoxins) are also strong inducers of IL-6 gene expression and IL-6 production by several cell types, including bone cells (14,15). IL-6 production in bone is also strongly modulated by osteotrophic hormones. It is not yet clear what the function of the large amount of IL-6 produced in bone is (16). IL-6 stimulates proliferation of some, but not all, osteoblast-like cells (17). IL-6 appears to have no bone-resorptive activity when tested in *in vitro* organ cultures, but it partially inhibits bone resorption induced by calcitrophic hormones (e.g., PTH and 1,25 dihydroxyvitamin D_3) (14,18). The significance of this is as yet unknown. IL-6 has constitutive granulocyte/macrophage colony-stimulating factor (GM-CSF) activity, and GM-CSF has been shown to stimulate formation of osteoclast-like cells in long-term marrow cultures. Thus, IL-6 secreted by mature osteoblasts in response to various cytokines and osteotrophic hormones may act as a signal for recruitment of osteoclast progenitors (16), and by so doing modulate bone resorption as well as mediate distant responses to local inflammatory events.

IL-6 is produced spontaneously by rheumatoid synovial cells, and this can be enhanced by IL-1 and TNF-α. IL-6 bioactivity also has been detected in synovial fluid in various inflammatory joint diseases.

Interleukin-8

Interleukin-8 (IL-8) is a recently characterized polypeptide factor also known as *neutrophil activating factor* (NAF) (19). It is a member of a larger family of inflammatory mediators, which includes MCP-1 (monocyte chemotactic peptide). IL-8 is a potent attractant and activator of neutrophils. It is of interest in relation to arthritis and other inflammatory skeletal diseases, because it appears to be produced by a variety of cell types. IL-8 is produced spontaneously by unstimulated mononuclear cells, and this production is enhanced in mononuclear cells derived from patients with RA. Treatments with IL-1, TNF-α, and lipopolysaccharide stimulate IL-8 production by monocytes more effectively in RA patients than in healthy subjects. IL-8 is also produced constitutively by endothelial cells and other connective tissue cells, including bone cells. IL-8 production can be induced in human articular chondrocytes (A. Fraser, *personal communication*). IL-8 and MCP may therefore be other locally active mediators released at sites of inflammation or tissue damage in joints.

Colony-Stimulating Factors

Several members of a family of glycoproteins, the hematopoietic growth factors, have been described which directly stimulate differentiation of a broad spectrum of myeloid progenitor cells resulting in colony formation. They include multi-CSF (IL-3), GM-CSF, G-CSF, M-CSF (CSF-1), IL-5, and erythropoetin. GM-CSF and M-CSF are growth and differentiation factors for cells of the monocyte/macrophage lineage and probably play a key role in hemopoeitic differentiation (20), as does IL-1.

GM-CSF and M-CSF stimulate bone resorption *in vitro,* and this may be attributable to their effects on osteoclast generation, because both factors stimulate the formation of osteoclast-like cells in long-term bone marrow cultures. Osteoblast-like cells produce both GM-CSF and M-CSF constitutively and in response to several bone-resorbing cytokines (e.g., IL-1, TNF-α, and PTH) (8). Direct effects of CSFs on osteoblast-like cells, such as stimulation of proliferation, inhibition of alkaline phosphatase activity, and reduction in osteocalcin production, have been demonstrated (21).

Both IL-1 and TNF stimulate the production of CSFs from osteoblastic cells *in vitro* (8), and this could be a mechanism of hemopoetic response to inflammation and tissue destruction.

Prostaglandins

The exact role of prostanoids in bone remodeling remains unclear. It is well known that prostaglandins, particularly those of the E series (PGE), stimulate osteoclastic resorption (22). However, the physiological and pathological significance is still not fully resolved. Many factors that stimulate bone resorption seem to do so by generation of endogenous prostaglandin production in bone cultures. This accounts for some or all of the bone resorptive activity of IL-1, EGF, TNF, platelet-derived growth factor (PDGF) and TGF-α (4). Prostaglandins promote formation of osteoclast-like cells in marrow cultures. There is enhanced prostaglandin release from monocytes in RA (2). Although IL-1 stimulates PGE production by monocytes and bone cells, there is evidence to suggest that IL-1-induced osteoclastic bone resorption is mediated, only in part, by PGE (5). Under certain conditions, prostaglandins may indeed stimulate new bone formation, particularly at endosteal and periosteal surfaces.

Neuropeptides

Several neuropeptides have effects on bone and cartilage metabolism which may be of clinical significance in neuropathic joints. These include substances P and K, neuropeptide Y, bradykinin, vasoactive intestinal peptide (VIP), and the calcitonin-gene-related peptides (CGRPs). VIP and bradykinin stimulate bone resorption *in vitro,* whereas CGRPs inhibit it (23). More recently, some of the neuropeptides have been shown to modulate cytokine production by human connective tissue cells and peripheral blood mononuclear cells. For example, substance P enhances interferon-γ production by peripheral blood mononuclear cells, and bradykinin stimulates IL-6 production by osteoblast-like cells, articular chondrocytes, synoviocytes, and peripheral blood mononuclear cells. Substance P has been detected in synovial fluid exudates in certain arthritic conditions.

Interferon γ

Interferon γ (IFN-γ) is a member of a large family of peptides, originally defined by their ability to inhibit viral replication and classified as α, β, or γ, depending on their origin (24). Along with TNF, IFN-γ is one of the major products of activated T lymphocytes and natural killer cells. IFN-γ, while sharing some properties with other interferons, appears to differ from IFN-α and IFN-β in terms of its effects on connective tissues. Although it is not known whether IFN-γ is produced in bone, it appears to have distinct osteotrophic effects. Broadly speaking, these effects are opposite to those of IL-1 and TNF-α. Thus, IFN-γ inhibits IL-1 and TNF-α and prostaglandin-induced bone resorption (8), an action probably mediated via inhibition of both (a) proliferation of osteoclast precursors and (b) formation of mature osteoclasts from these precursors (4). However, IFN-γ has a much less inhibitory effect on resorption induced by classical calciotropic hormones, PTH, or 1,25-dihydroxyvitamin D_3 (8). IFN-γ also opposes other actions of IL-1 and TNF-α on connective tissue cells. For example, it inhibits IL-1 and TNF-α-induced proliferation of human articular chondrocytes and osteoblast-like cells. It also antagonizes IL-1- and TNF-α-induced suppression of both basal and 1,25-dihydroxyvitamin D_3-stimulated alkaline phosphatase activity in osteoblastic cells. Furthermore, IFN-γ inhibits production of collagenase by osteoblasts induced by resorbing cytokines and hormones such as IL-1, TNF-α, PTH and 1,25-dihydroxyvitamin D_3 (8). However, like TNF-α and IL-1, IFN-γ inhibits collagen synthesis in bone organ cultures (8).

IFN-γ inhibition of IL-1 production by activated immune cells has been reported. IFN-γ is present in synovial fluid from affected joints in a variety of inflammatory joint diseases (2,3). IFN-γ production appears to be diminished in RA (3). However, the significance of this remains unclear.

LOCAL FACTORS THAT MAY BE INVOLVED IN BONE MATRIX FORMATION (FIG. 4)

Transforming Growth Factor β

The TGF-β isoforms are members of a distinct superfamily of ubiquitous polypeptide growth factors that regulate cell growth and differentiation. The list of growth factors belonging to this superfamily, which includes the bone morphogenetic proteins, has been increasing steadily. Four isoforms of TGF-β (TGF-β_1 through TGF-β_4) have been identified and cloned, but only TGFβ_1 through TGFβ_3 have been detected in mammals (25). Although the primary sequences of the four isoforms differ, they have very similar spectra of biological activity (26,27). The primary sequence of each isoform appears to be very highly conserved across species (28), suggesting that it has a fundamental biological role. The TGF-β isoforms are thought to be important in embryological development and differentiation as well as in connective tissue repair and fibrosis (29).

TGF-β was originally purified from human platelets. Apart from platelets, bone matrix is the richest source of TGF-β. TGF-β_1 and TGF-β_2 are responsible for the activities previously ascribed to bovine bone matrix-derived cartilage-inducing factors A and B, respectively (30). TGF-β is produced by a variety of cells and tissues which include T cells, macrophages, platelets, and bone as a 25-kD, disulfide-linked homodimeric peptide. TGF-β mRNA has been detected in developing human calvarial bones and bovine osteoblastic cells, and transcript levels were several times greater in bone-forming cells than in any other mammalian cells. TGF-β is produced and secreted constitutively by osteoblast-like cells and bone organ cultures (8,28), and also by monocytes and activated T lymphocytes. This may be relevant in inflammatory joint diseases where these cells are known to infiltrate, because TGF-β inhibits proliferation of activated T lymphocyte as well as monocytic IL-1 production (30,31).

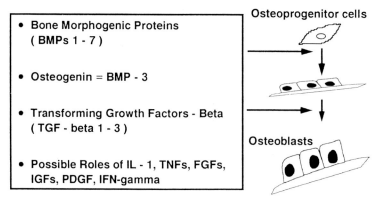

FIG. 4. Scheme showing some of the factors that may be involved in stimulating the formation of new bone as may occur in fracture repair and the formation of osteophytes in osteoarthritis.

TGF-β is a powerful multipotential regulator of cellular activity, and it has profound effects on the growth and differentiated function of cells of mesenchymal origin, including bone-derived cells *in vitro.* TGF-β stimulates proliferation of a variety of connective tissue cell types, including human osteoblastic bone cells. TGF-β also stimulates differentiated functions (including the syntheses of both collagen and noncollagenous proteins) in connective tissue cells, including osteoblast-like cells *in vitro* (8,28). When injected in or around existing bone, TGF-β induces extensive new bone formation (29). The effect of TGF-β on osteoclastic bone resorption is not clear. Depending on the conditions, TGF-β exhibits inhibitory or stimulatory effects on bone resorption *in vitro* (8). When injected *in vivo,* TGF-β induces a wound repair response which includes fibrosis and angiogenesis (27).

The maintenance of the integrity of various extracellular matrices is dependent on the activity of proteolytic enzymes such as plasminogen activators (PAs), which can degrade collagen directly or indirectly via a plasminogen–plasmin–collagenase activation cascade. These enzymes are, in turn, regulated by plasminogen activator inhibitors (PAIs). PA and PAI control the activation of plasmin, a protease which is capable of degrading extracellular matrices directly or indirectly by activating latent collagenase secreted by osteoblasts. Collagenase is, in turn, regulated directly by its natural inhibitor, tissue inhibitor of metalloproteinases (TIMPs), and indirectly by plasmin (30). TGF-β is released as an inactive propeptide, bound to a high-molecular-weight protein, during osteoclastic resorption. This latent TGF-β can be activated by proteolytic or acid-induced dissociation of this "inhibitory" protein (4,29). It is particularly interesting that active TGF-β is one of the few agents known to inhibit the production from osteoblasts and articular chondrocytes of PAs and other tissue proteases such as stromelysin. Active TGF-β also stimulates the production of the natural inhibitors of these proteases such as PAI and TIMP (5).

Given the powerful inhibitory effects of activated TGF-β on osteoclastic activity and its inhibition of proteolytic degradation of the matrix, release of sequestered TGF-β from bone matrix during resorption would provide a negative feedback mechanism to limit the extent of osteoclastic excavations. This suggests that TGF-β may be of crucial importance in the maintenance of the integrity of bone extracellular matrix and, in concert with its effects on synthesis of matrix proteins, may promote tissue repair.

TGF-β also inhibits endothelial cell proliferation (32), thus opposing the effect of TNF-α on neovascularization. This may serve to reduce the influx of inflammatory cells into surrounding tissues. TGF-β also modulates its own production as well as that of other cytokines by several cell types, including osteoblastic cells (31).

Bone Morphogenetic Proteins

One of the most interesting aspects of the transforming growth factors beta is their relationship to bone morphogenetic proteins (BMPs). BMP was originally defined as an activity within the growth factor complex in bone matrix that can induce new cartilage and bone formation when implanted *in vivo,* at a non-bony site. It is now well recognized that bone-derived BMP activity resides in not one, but several, distinct peptides. There are now seven BMPs described, six of which are members of the TGF-β superfamily (30). Subgroups of the BMP family exhibit varying degrees of homology with each other and with TGF-β. The sequence of events seen when new bone/cartilage is induced by BMP closely approximates that seen during embryonic long bone development. Various growth factors and hormones augment growth of preexisting bone, but, to date, it is only BMP that induces bone morphogenesis. At present, very few of the BMPs are available as recombinant molecules, and this has hampered the study of their role in bone metabolism.

An unrelated molecule, osteoinductive factor (OIF), also exhibits BMP activity, but only in the presence of TGF-β_1 or TGF-β_2. OIF is a 22- to 28-kD, highly glycosylated protein that was initially thought to induce bone and cartilage formation. There is no sequence identity between the primary amino acid structure of OIF and any of the BMPs or any other known growth factor.

Insulin-like Growth Factors

Insulin-like growth factors (IGFs), or somatomedins, are a family of growth stimulatory peptides with biological activity similar to that of insulin. There are two major circulating forms, IGF-1 and IGF-2, both of which are structurally related. Both IGF-1 and IGF-2 also have a strong structural homology to insulin, and many of their actions on bone are similar to those of insulin (31,32).

IGF-1 and IGF-2 are both produced within bone itself and by isolated osteoblastic cells, and this production is regulated by growth hormone (31,32). The activity of both IGF-1 and IGF-2 are modulated by specific binding proteins in serum, which in the case of IGF-1 are under the control of growth hormone and cortisol (32).

Both IGF-1, also known as somatomedin C, and IGF-2, previously known as skeletal growth factor, stimulate the replication of bone cells. Although several of the growth factors found within the bone matrix are mitogenic for osteoblasts, apart from TGF-β, only IGF-1 and IGF-2 consistently stimulate osteoblastic differentiation and enhance production of matrix constituents, especially collagen and osteocalcin (31,32).

Platelet-Derived Growth Factor

Platelet-derived growth factor (PDGF) was originally isolated from platelets but is now known to be produced by other cell types (33). Human PDGF is a 31-kD protein which exists as a heterodimer or homodimer of two structurally related peptide chains, A and B. At least three isoforms of PDGF are known:

AA, AB, and BB. The B-chain homodimer appears to be the most potent. PDGF is probably also important in development and is one of the most potent growth factors known. PDGF has been isolated from bone matrix, and PDGF-like activities are produced by human osteoblastic osteosarcoma cell lines. Isolated osteoblasts express PDGF receptor mRNA (34). PDGF is mitogenic for both differentiated and undifferentiated bone cells (31,32) and may mediate the mitogenic effect of IL-1. This suggests that PDGF, stored locally within bone or released from aggregated platelets, may stimulate proliferation of osteoblasts and their precursors. In addition to increasing the number of cells synthesizing collagen and noncollagenous proteins in bone, PDGF also has a direct stimulatory effect on bone collagen synthesis (32).

Fibroblast Growth Factors (Acidic and Basic)

Apart from the above growth factors, bone matrix also contains acidic fibroblast growth factor (FGF) and basic FGF, both of which stimulate replication of osteoblastic cells and inhibit collagen synthesis in bone organ cultures and cultured osteoblast-like cells (31,32).

Mast Cell Products

Mast cell products such as heparin and histamine may be important, because these cells are present in excess in inflammatory arthritis (35,36). Heparin is known to inhibit both the proliferation and the differentiated function of osteoblastic cells *in vitro* (37).

RELEVANCE TO OSTEOARTHRITIS; CONCLUSIONS

Osteoarthritis is a clinically heterogeneous condition. It is well known that the alterations in joint structure and function that accompany certain endocrinopathies or other diseases associated with excessive bone remodeling (e.g., Paget's disease) may predispose to osteoarthritis. Similarly, metabolic changes as seen in chondrocalcinosis and ochronosis also predispose to osteoarthritis. Usually, by the time osteoarthritis is diagnosed clinically, joint damage is extensive and the associated bone lesions are well defined. Notably, the underlying subchondral bone is sclerotic and osteophytes protrude into the joint space. It is still not clear what factor(s) initiate these changes.

Although osteoarthritis is not always considered to be an inflammatory disease, acute inflammatory episodes do occur (e.g., in response to trauma), and the associated production of cytokines such as IL-1 and TNF-α may be involved in the initiation and progression of cartilage damage. It seems very likely that the chondrocytes themselves play a major role in the degradation and repair of the surrounding cartilage matrix. Increased remodeling of underlying subchondral bone is a feature of osteoarthritis, and it may influence the progression of the disease by altering the mechanical compliance of the overlying cartilage but may also be a secondary response to damage to the articular cartilage. Once arthritis is established, there is usually a marked increase in osteoblastic new bone formation in osteochondral regions of the joint, and this is associated with the developments of osteophytes. It is possible that growth factors such as TGF-β and the IGFs play an important role in osteophyte formation.

In RA the picture is perhaps clearer. The well-demarcated erosions of bone and cartilage seen in rheumatoid joints occur typically in areas contiguous with the inflammatory pannus. It is therefore likely that the potentially large amounts of cytokines with resorptive activity produced by infiltrating monocytes and immune cells may mediate not only destruction of articular cartilage but also the extensive destruction of underlying subchondral bone. This tissue destruction may be further aggravated because many of these cytokines can then induce their own production or the production of other bone-resorptive factors, namely, prostaglandins and tissue proteases. Thus bone cells can actively participate in the degradation of their own extracellular matrix. Furthermore, the various cytokines released by synoviocytes into the synovial fluid may function to expand the population of inflammatory cells within the joint as well as that of synoviocytes, chondrocytes, and bone cells. One of the consequences of this, at least temporally, would be a further increase in cytokine production and further degradation of bone matrix.

Because there are so many factors that have demonstrable effects on bone, a major task in contemporary research is to determine how these agents interact and which are the most important under physiological conditions and in different disease states. It appears that some of these factors are "natural" inhibitors of others. Most notably, the effects of IFN-γ counterbalance the effects of IL-1 and TNF-α. Although it has been suggested that IFN-γ production may be reduced in RA, it remains to be seen whether changes in the production of various cytokines and growth regulatory molecules by bone cells and inflammatory cells and/or abnormalities in the responsiveness of bone cells to these agents may be involved in connective tissue turnover in arthritis.

REFERENCES

1. Duff GW. Peptide regulatory factors in non-malignant disease. *Lancet* 1989;1:1432–1434.
2. Lipsky PE, David LS, Cush JJ, et al. The role of cytokines in the pathogenesis of rheumatoid arthritis. *Springer Semin Immunopathol* 1989;11:123–162.
3. Lorenzo JA, Sousa SL, VanDenBrink-Webb SE, et al. Production of interleukin-1α and β by newborn mouse calvaria. *J Bone Miner Res* 1990;5:77–84.
4. Mundy GR. Local factors in bone remodeling. *Recent Prog Horm Res* 1989;45:507–531.
5. Boyce BF, Aufdemorte TB, Garrett IR, et al. Effects of interleukin-1 on bone turnover in normal mice. *Endocrinology* 1989;125:1142–1150.
6. Konig A, Muhlbauer RC, Fleisch H. Tumor necrosis factor alpha and interleukin-1 stimulate

bone resorption *in vivo* as measured by urinary [³H]tetracycline excretion from prelabeled mice. *J Bone Miner Res* 1988;3:621–627.

7. Evans DB, Bunning RAD, Russell RGG. The effects of human interleukin-1β on cellular proliferation, and the production of prostaglandin E₂, plasminogen activator, osteocalcin and alkaline phosphatase by osteoblast-like cells derived from human. *Biochem Biophys Res Commun* 1990;166:208–216.

8. Goldring MB, Goldring SR. Skeletal tissue response to cytokines. *Clin Orthop* 1990;258:245–278.

9. Gowen M. Actions of IL-1 and TNF on human osteoblast-like cells: similarities and synergism. In: Oppenheim J, Dinarello C, Kluger M, et al., eds. *Monocytes and other non-lymphocytic cytokines.* New York: Alan R Liss, 1988;261–266.

10. Prieur A-M, Kaufmann M-T, Griscelli C, et al. Specific interleukin-1 inhibitor in serum and urine of children with systemic juvenile chronic arthritis. *Lancet* 1987;2:1240–1242.

11. Le J, Vilcek J. Tumour necrosis factor and interleukin-1: cytokines with multiple overlapping biological activities. *Lab Invest* 1987;56:234–248.

12. Gowen M, Chapman K, Littlewood A, et al. Production of tumour necrosis factor by human osteoblasts is modulated by other cytokines but not by osteotrophic hormones. *Endocrinology* 1990;126:1250–1255.

13. Wong GG, Clark SC. Multiple actions of interleukin-6 within a cytokine network. *Immunol Today* 1988;9:137–139.

14. Feyen JHM, Elford P, DiPadova FE, et al. Interleukin-6 is produced by bone and modulated by parathyroid hormone. *J Bone Miner Res* 1989;4:633–638.

15. Littlewood AJ, Aarden LA, Evans DB, et al. Human osteoblastlike cells do not respond to interleukin-6. *J Bone Miner Res* 1991;6:141–148.

16. Lowik C, van der Plujim G, Boys H, et al. IL-6 produced by PTH-stimulated osteogenic cells can be a mediator in osteoclast recruitment. In: Cohn DV, Glorieux FH, Martin TJ, eds. *Calcium regulation and bone metabolism: basic and clinical aspects,* vol 10. Amsterdam: Excerpta Medica, 1990;336–343.

17. Fang MA, Hahn TJ. Effects of interleukin-6 on UMR 106-01 osteoblastlike cells. *J Bone Miner Res* 1991;6:133–139.

18. Al-Humidan A, Ralston SH, Hughes DE, et al. Interleukin-6 does not stimulate bone resorption in neonatal mouse calvariae. *J Bone Miner Res* 1991;6:3–8.

19. Peveri P, Walz A, Dewald B, et al. A novel neutrophil activating factor produced by human mononuclear phagocytes. *J Exp Med* 1988;167:1547–1559.

20. Sieff CA. Biology and clinical aspects of the hematopoietic growth factors. *Annu Rev Med* 1990;41:483–496.

21. Evans DB, Bunning RAD, Russell RGG. The effects of recombinant human granulocyte macrophage colony-stimulating factor (rhGM-CSF) on human osteoblast-like cells. *Biochem Biophys Res Commun* 1989;160:588–595.

22. Raisz LG. Role of prostaglandins in the local regulation of bone metabolism. *Prog Clin Biol Res* 1990;332:195–203.

23. Russell RGG, Boysen M, Chapman K, et al. The possible role of cytokines, growth factors and their inhibitors. In: Russell RGG, Dieppe P, eds. *Osteoarthritis: current research and prospects for pharmacological intervention.* London: IBC Technical Services 1991;65–84.

24. Balkwill FR. Peptide regulatory factors. Interferons. *Lancet* 1989;1:1060–1063.

25. Sporn MB, Roberts AB. TGF-β: problems and prospects. *Cell Regul* 1990;1:875–882.

26. Sporn MB, Roberts AB, Wakefield LM, et al. Some recent advances in the chemistry and biology of transforming growth factor-beta. *J Cell Biol* 1987;105:1039–1045.

27. Sporn MB, Roberts AB. Peptide growth factors and inflammation, tissue repair and cancer. *J Clin Invest* 1986;78:329–332.

28. Bonewald LF, Mundy GR. Role of transforming growth factor-beta in bone remodeling. *Clin Orthop* 1990;250:261–276.

29. Mackie EJ, Treschel U. Stimulation of bone formation *in vivo* by transforming growth factor-β: remodeling of woven bone and lack of inhibition by indomethacin. *Bone* 1990;11:295–300.

30. Mundy GR, Bonewald LF. Role of TGFB in bone remodeling. *Ann NY Acad Sci* 1990;593:91–96.

31. Wozney JM. Bone morphogenetic proteins. *Prog Growth Factor Res* 1989;1:267–280.

32. Canalis EM. Regulation of bone formation by local growth factors. In: Peck WA, ed. *Bone and mineral research,* annual 6. Amsterdam: Elsevier, 1989;27–56.
33. Canalis E, McCarthy T, Centrella M. The role of growth factors in skeletal remodeling. *Endocrinol Metab Clin North Am* 1989;18:903–918.
34. Ross R. Platelet-derived growth factors. *Lancet* 1989;1:1179–1182.
35. McKenna MJ, Frame B. The mast cell and bone. *Clin Orthop* 1985;200:226–233.
36. Wooley DE. Mast cell: chondrocyte interactions in relation to osteoarthritis. In: Russell RGG, Dieppe P, eds. *Osteoarthritis: current research and prospects for pharmacological intervention.* London: IBC Technical Services 1991;129–135.
37. Hurley MM, Gronowicz G, Kream BE, et al. Effect of heparin on bone formation in cultured fetal rat calvaria. *Calcif Tissue Int* 1990;46:183–188.

DISCUSSION

Morales: You mentioned that transforming growth factor beta increases the production of metalloproteinases in your bone system. Are inhibitors of plasminogen activator (PAI) also increased?

Oyajobi: We have not been able to measure the PAI reproducibly because the chromogenic assay for PAI is very unreliable. We are able to separate them with SDS-PAGE, however, and actually show that bone cells produce PAI and PA2. TGF-β appears to stimulate the production of these inhibitors.

Heinegard: What proteins bind the TGF-β in bone?

Oyajobi: TGF-β is abundant in the bone matrix. When bone is resorbed by osteoclasts, TGF-β is released still bound to a high-molecular-weight protein which inhibits its activity. To obtain biological activity, this complex must be dissociated by proteolysis or by decreasing the pH.

Articular Cartilage and Osteoarthritis,
edited by K. Kuettner et al.
Raven Press, Ltd., New York © 1992.

24

General Discussion for Chapters 16–23

Hirschelmann: We have studied possible roles for oxygen radicals in inflammation-induced tissue damage for about 15 years and have become more and more skeptical. Thus we think active oxygen radicals may be more a consequence of, than a cause for inflammation and tissue damage. Dr. Roughley, how important do you think the generation of hydroxyl and oxygen radicals is *in vivo?*

Roughley: We have no evidence at all that human cartilage or human chondrocytes can actually make free radicals. However, it has been shown in rabbit articular cartilage that hydrogen peroxide can be made. So the possibility still exists that radicals may play a role. We have no direct evidence that even if these radicals are made *in vivo,* that they are actually causing damage to the protein part of the proteoglycan. They may cause damage to hyaluronic acid in proteoglycan aggregates, however.

Cooke: Dr. Aydelotte, do the superficial cells make more or less decorin than do the deeper cells?

Aydelotte: Although the cells from the superficial and the deep zones are both making primarily aggrecan, there is a higher percentage of small proteoglycans made by the cells from the superficial cartilage than by those from the deep zones. These proteoglycans diffuse into the medium more readily than does aggrecan.

Okyayuz-Baklouti: In the deeper layers of cartilage, chondrocytes are sparsely distributed, but they synthesize lots of matrix. So they should be very active metabolically. On the other hand, they are cut off from a blood supply and are functioning in a hypoxic environment. How do they generate the energy for their metabolism? Do they have mitochondria which are working more efficiently than in other cells? In these avascular conditions there should be lactate accumulation, pH decrease, and even a pH gradient throughout the cartilage. Can some of the biochemical heterogeneity reported be related to this pH gradient?

Mason: We have studied bovine articular cartilage in explant cultures. There are about 11 million cells per gram of wet tissue, producing 8 μm lactate per hour. These cultures produce virtually no $^{14}CO_2$ from [6-^{14}C]glucose, indicating that oxidation via the tricarboxylic acid cycle is negligible.

Hascall: With regard to the pH problem, chondrocytes are in fact remarkably tolerant to quite a range of pH in terms of their ability to metabolize proteoglycans and matrix molecules.

Muir: Do you want to expand on that, Alice?

Maroudas: No, but can I make a very brief comment about nutrition in general?

Muir: No, I think not! We are all thinking about nutrition ourselves!

Hascall: That was perhaps the liveliest discussion we have had. Maybe everyone is hungry and getting a little light-headed, but we will try and get as much of this discussion as possible into the book.

Articular Cartilage and Osteoarthritis,
edited by K. Kuettner et al.
Raven Press, Ltd., New York © 1992.

Part VII: Some Thoughts on the Physical Properties of Cartilage

Introduction

James H. Kimura

Breech Research Laboratory, Bone and Joint Center,
Henry Ford Hospital, Detroit, Michigan 48202

The chapters that follow provide the detail and depth on the physical chemistry of cartilage which are absent from this brief summary. Current work on the mechanical and physical properties of cartilage focuses not only on the tissue itself but also on the effect of these physical parameters on the chondrocytes of cartilage. The blending of physical chemistry and engineering with the biological responses of the tissue provides an exciting continuum likely to lead to a new understanding of cartilage biology.

The extracellular matrix of cartilage is a resilient material able to disperse compressive loads. Its properties are largely a consequence of the organization of fibrous collagen around anionic proteoglycans, effectively trapping high concentrations of negative charges within the tissue. The tendency of systems to move toward osmotic equilibrium and electrical neutrality gives rise to the swelling pressures of cartilage. Thus, the tissue will attract water in an attempt to dilute the high concentration of negative charges. The network of collagen fibers restricts the volume which can be occupied by proteoglycans to substantially less than they would otherwise occupy in solution. The imbalance is made greater by the presence of high concentrations of fixed negative charges (up to about 0.2 M sulfate ester) which makes the matrix an effective cation exchanger. As a consequence, there is not only a driving force for water to enter the tissue but there is also the tendency for small diffusible, positive counterions to be concentrated there.

During load, the tissue resists compression largely through its resistance to fluid flow. The tight network of collagen and high concentrations of solute offer considerable resistance of water movement. Understanding this process is important to understanding the relationship between matrix organization and tissue function. When water does leave, leading to compression, higher concentrations of negative charges result, and this leads proportionally to a greater resistance to further deformation. Upon removal of the load, the system can again imbibe water, leading to a recovery of tissue size and form as dictated by the collagen organization.

Even from this brief and oversimplified description of the physical–chemical considerations of cartilage function, it should be apparent that nature has created an elegant method to capitalize on the osmotic properties of highly charged macromolecules.

Although, by necessity, the structure of cartilage can be examined only at discrete time points, the tissue actually exists as a continuum over time. After its creation during embryogenesis, cartilage grows and develops; then it normally maintains itself during adulthood. The biogenesis and maintenance of this important structure is the province of the chondrocytes embedded in the extracellular matrix. Indeed, much current research is directed towards understanding how these cells respond to the changing structural requirements of the tissue. Chondrocytes are responsible for the synthesis of the collagens, proteoglycans, and other macromolecules which are part of cartilage. They must work in an osmotically and mechanically active environment, obtaining nutrients and eliminating waste products in the absence of a capillary network. Thus, diffusion and perhaps the periodic mechanical expulsion of fluid are the primary means of logistical support for these cells.

Yet, a consequence of the requisite organization of cartilage matrix is the restrictive nature of the matrix to fluid flow and to the movement of solutes. The hindrance to movement is not great for small ions which can diffuse into the tissue with relative ease. The difficulty is in the movement of larger molecules such as cytokines, which may play critical roles in activating or repressing cellular response to changing metabolic needs. The vital contributions of cytokines to cartilage metabolism have been clearly demonstrated, even though they are sufficiently large to be restricted in their entry into cartilage. Thus, learning how tissue structure and mechanics affects the movement of these cellular mediators in the tissue is important to our understanding of how chondrocytes might receive signals which modulate their metabolism.

Chondrocytes also respond to alterations in their mechanical environment. This is true during connective tissue embryogenesis, as in the theory articulated by Pauwels (1), where physical forces were regarded as specific stimuli for connective tissue differentiation. It continues to be true in the mature individual, where it has been known both experimentally and anecdotally that the cartilage of immobilized joints undergoes a dramatic alteration in composition, primarily due to a loss of proteoglycans. Restoration of normal loading results in a recovery of much of the material which was lost. Understanding the relationship between the physical and mechanical forces acting on the cells becomes of interest to aid in the development of a conceptual framework in which positive and negative modifiers can be identified.

Such an identification is not an easy task. The mechanical situation in cartilage is very complex. Deformational forces act during compression, giving rise to shear, tension, and compression in various parts of the tissue. Arguments for the primacy of a particular type of mechanical perturbation are full of controversy and cannot easily be dealt with. Additionally, there are changes in hydrostatic pressure and in the ionic composition of the medium surrounding the chondrocytes which may also affect their behavior. Perhaps a simpler way of dealing with the mechanical complexities is to resolve the signals to which the cells may respond into hydrostatic and deformational components.

It is simpler to study hydrostatic pressure free from other mechanical influences. Cells respond to increases in hydrostatic pressures in the physiological range by increasing their anabolic rates, even when exposed for only a few seconds. However, deformational changes also clearly occur, and, in addition to affecting cells directly, they can also affect cellular metabolism indirectly via alterations in solute transport.

Additional complexity is added, depending on whether the deformation is static or dynamic. Although static loading of cartilage tends to restrict nutrient transport, and especially that of cytokines, there are also clearly identified alterations in the extracellular ionic environment occurring as a consequence of the presence of the extensive extracellular matrix. Two examples are (i) an increase in the extracellular sodium concentration and (ii) a decrease in the extracellular pH. These changes appear to be inhibitory to matrix synthesis. Similar results are obtained *in vitro* by raising the concentration of sodium or lowering the pH in the external culture medium. Conversely, raising the pH or raising the extracellular potassium concentration has a positive effect on matrix synthesis. It should be pointed out that deformational changes accompany both the ionic and compressional perturbation of the matrix. Changes in the ionic environment, especially those which change the osmolarity of the culture medium, will also result in a change in the size or shape of the cell.

Dynamic changes are even more complex. Superimposed upon the changes produced during static compression are changes arising from transient movement of fluid and accompanying ions during the addition and removal of the load. Such changes include streaming currents, leading to streaming potentials, which can be considerable during compression. These arise as a consequence of the movement of water past immobilized polyanionic proteoglycans. The positive counterions are not firmly bound to the proteoglycan and hence can move with the moving fluid. The result is a streaming of ions which produces a local current. If given sufficient time, this potential dissipates as the counterions diffuse back into the tissue. Additional complexity is also present in the dynamic changes in cell deformation which produces periodic distortions in chondrocytes and their cytoskeletons. An additional variable which also should be taken into consideration is the change in bulk transport of material including nutrients and cytokines which may occur during the cycling.

An important consideration underlying many studies of the physical–chemical perturbations of cartilage is to understand the mechanism by which such changes are recognized by chondrocytes and how such signals are transduced into complex metabolic responses. Chondrocytes, in particular, are sensitive to cell shape. It has been well documented that chondrocytes prefer a rounded cell shape to maintain their phenotype. It is tempting therefore to focus on deformational mechanisms for the transduction of mechanical signals by chondrocytes. This implies the presence of some sort of a mechanoreceptor in the cells. The nature of this receptor is not known. However, arguments for its presence come from a number of studies, nicely summarized in a recent review by Watson (2), who argues that such a receptor would be a membrane protein that could alter its own activity as a result of conformational distortions transmitted from the extracellular matrix, or by the cell via integral membrane proteins coupled to the cytoskeleton. Such mechanoreceptors or stretch-activated ion channels have been described for other cell types. It is interesting to note that many of the intracellular ionic changes which might occur in response to the extracellular perturbations described above can be produced in this scheme by differential activation of specific ion-transport systems in the cell membrane.

Whether any of these speculations will prove to be correct must await experimental evidence. It is interesting, however, to note that our knowledge of the mechanism for the transmittal of mechanical information into biochemical action by cells is fast approaching a substantive level of understanding. One can envision a time in the foreseeable future in which we will understand how chondrocytes can "sense" physical and mechanical changes about them. Such knowledge can lead to alternative manipulation of injured or diseased cartilage, perhaps permitting one to mimic healthy mechanical activity while avoiding the damaging stresses associated with the actual activity by substituting chemical for mechanical signals.

REFERENCES

1. Pauwels F. A new theory concerning the influence of mechanical stimuli on the differentiation of the supporting tissues. In: *Biomechanics of the locomotor apparatus.* Berlin: Springer-Verlag, 1980;375–407.
2. Watson PA. Function follows form: generation of intracellular signals by cell deformation. *FASEB J* 1991;5:2013–2019.

Articular Cartilage and Osteoarthritis,
edited by K. Kuettner et al.
Raven Press, Ltd., New York © 1992.

25

The Role of Water, Proteoglycan, and Collagen in Solute Transport in Cartilage

Alice Maroudas, Rosa Schneiderman, and Orna Popper

*Department of Biomedical Engineering, Julius Silver Institute,
Technion-Israel Institute of Technology, Haifa 32000, Israel*

Knowledge of solute transport through the cartilage matrix is essential to our understanding of many physiological phenomena in this tissue. Chondrocytes situated far away from direct access to blood or synovial fluid depend for their needs on a supply of nutrients and different substrates which diffuse through the matrix. In addition to common nutrients, various regulatory substances, such as growth hormones and cytokines, also have to reach the cell. These substances are often required in extremely small amounts which, however, need to be rigorously controlled. This, again, depends on transport through the extracellular space. At the same time, metabolic waste products are secreted by the cells into the matrix and have to pass through the latter in order to reach the synovial fluid for removal from the joint space. The same must happen to matrix macromolecules degraded in the course of normal turnover, whether the degradation happens intra- or extracellularly. Finally, macromolecules, newly synthesized by the cells, are secreted into the matrix and must move through it before being assembled at some distance from the cell.

The concentration of a solute within the matrix, apart from being an important factor in determining the rate of transport, is also able to modify the properties of the matrix itself. Thus, ionic concentrations are largely responsible for determining the level of the osmotic pressure within the cartilage matrix in general, and in the immediate environment of the cell in particular. The osmotic pressure of the matrix is, in turn, responsible for the resistance of cartilage to fluid loss and hence to compressive stresses. Together with the hydraulic permeability of the pore space, it is also an important determinant of the rate of fluid movement out of and into the tissue. In addition, the high ionic concentration and osmotic pressure in the immediate environment of the chondrocyte have been shown to affect their synthetic processes (1,2).

The subject of solute and fluid transport in cartilage was described in some detail 12 years ago (3). Recently, methods for measuring solute transport have been evaluated (4). The purpose of the present chapter is to discuss the solute and fluid transport dependence on the three main cartilage constituents (i.e., the proteoglycans, water, and collagen) and on their organization within the tissue. The effects of matrix compression on transport properties will be examined to assess the conditions prevailing under load-bearing and to determine their influence on both tissue and cellular functions.

TWO-COMPARTMENT MODEL OF THE CARTILAGE MATRIX

Figure 1 shows our two-compartment model of the cartilage matrix, based on the concepts of intra- and extrafibrillar spaces. The matrix is shown in native cartilage (Fig. 1A), as well as in cartilage from which the proteoglycans (PGs) have been removed (Fig. 1B). It can be seen that in native tissue the PGs are confined to the extrafibrillar space. However, through their osmotic pressure acting across the surface of the collagen fibrils, they affect the amount of fluid retained within the fibrils (compare the intrafibrillar spaces in Fig. 1A and 1B).

Fluid flow takes place through both compartments in parallel, though it is even slower in the intrafibrillar than in the extrafibrillar space. In the extrafibrillar compartment it is the proteoglycans which control the effective pore size and hence the rate at which fluid will flow; fluid flows much more rapidly in the absence of PGs than in PG-rich tissue (compare Fig. 1A and 1B).

Solute penetration and partition is regulated by the effective pore size and exclusion volume of the macromolecules making up the two compartments and

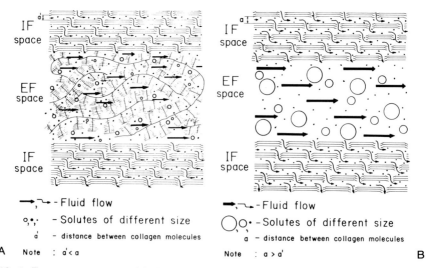

FIG. 1. Two-compartment model of the cartilage matrix. **A:** Native cartilage. **B:** Proteoglycan-free cartilage.

will be discussed in detail in the remainder of the chapter. Briefly, the intrafibrillar space is available to small solutes only; as for the extrafibrillar, PG-rich compartment, while even large solutes are not totally excluded from it, their partition coefficients are very low. In the absence of PGs, in principle, solutes are present in the extrafibrillar space at the same concentrations as in the equilibrating outside solution. However, collagen fibrils themselves may exhibit some "excluded volume" effects with respect to large solute molecules.

RELATIVE MAGNITUDES OF THE INTRA- AND EXTRAFIBRILLAR COMPARTMENTS

The PG component is present in the matrix of cartilaginous tissues at a very high concentration, and is responsible for some of the most important physicochemical and biomechanical properties of these tissues. However, because of their size the proteoglycans are restricted to the extrafibrillar, noncollagenous compartment. Thus, it is not their overall concentration in the matrix which is relevant, but rather their actual concentration in the extrafibrillar space. This effective concentration, in turn, depends on the proportions of water in the extra- and intrafibrillar compartments. Calculations based on total water can be seriously in error, particularly for compressed cartilage. However, it has been shown recently (5) that it is possible to estimate the relative proportions of water present in the two compartments under defined experimental conditions. We

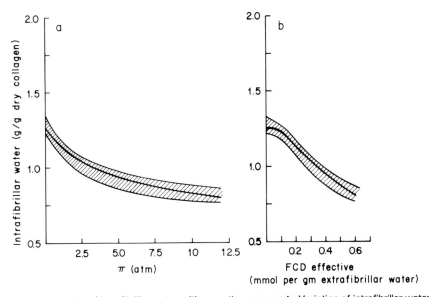

FIG. 2. a: Variation of intrafibrillar water with osmotic pressure. **b:** Variation of intrafibrillar water with effective FCD.

have shown that these proportions vary and are themselves regulated by the osmotic pressure and hence the PG content in the extrafibrillar compartment. This provides an additional complexity for estimating effective PG concentration or fixed charge densities (FCDs). Figure 2a shows the relationship between the intrafibrillar water (as calculated from x-ray diffraction data) and the osmotic pressure in the extrafibrillar space. Significant variations exist in the intrafibrillar water content over the range of osmotic pressures that correspond to the variations in PG content such as can occur in normal cartilage with distance from articular surface and with topography (2,3) or as a result of PG loss under pathological conditions. This range of values is further extended during weight-bearing, when cartilage is subjected to pressures which lead to fluid loss and a resultant increase in PG concentration. Importantly, the extrafibrillar compartment constitutes the "outer phase" of the cartilage matrix. Thus, the interactions of the matrix with both the external environment (i.e., synovial fluid or blood) and the chondrocytes are determined by the properties of this extrafibrillar compartment.

CALCULATIONS OF EFFECTIVE FIXED CHARGE DENSITY

In order to calculate the effective FCD of a given specimen, we need to know the fraction of extrafibrillar water. In order to calculate this, the intrafibrillar water per gram of collagen has to be determined. The intrafibrillar compartment contains a small quantity of "bound" water. The rest consists of free water, the quantity of which is controlled in part by (a) intermolecular repulsion forces (the precise nature of which is not clear at present) and (b) the osmotic pressure gradients between the outside and the inside of the fibrils.

The relationship between the FCD based on total tissue water (i.e., $FCD_{overall}$) and the FCD in the extrafibrillar compartment (i.e., FCD_{EF}) is given by the following expression:

$$FCD_{EF} = FCD_{overall}\left(\frac{W_{H_2O}}{W_{EF}}\right) = \frac{FCD_{overall} \times W_{H_2O}}{W_{H_2O} - W_{IF}} \qquad [1a]$$

where

$$W_{IF} = H_2O_{IF} \times C_{coll} \times W_0 \qquad [1b]$$

In Eqs. 1a and 1b the symbols have the following meanings: W_0 is the total initial wet weight of the specimen; W_{H_2O} is the weight of total water in the specimen either initially or under pressure; W_{EF} is the weight of extrafibrillar water; C_{coll} is the weight of collagen per gram of initial specimen weight; $FCD_{overall}$ is the fixed charge density based on initial total weight of specimen water; and H_2O_{IF} is the weight of intrafibrillar water per gram of dry collagen.

The intrafibrillar water (W_{IF}) can be obtained from Fig. 1A for any given value of extrafibrillar osmotic pressure, π (5). Furthermore, the relationship between π and PG concentration as expressed by FCD is given by Urban et al. (6):

$$\pi = B(\text{FCD})^2 \tag{2}$$

According to recent data on the osmotic pressures of PEG solutions (7) and the data of Urban et al. (6) for PG solutions, the value of the coefficient B is 26.6 at 4°C and 29 at 37°C.

Because π is determined by FCD_{EF}, there is a unique relationship between the latter and W_{IF}, which is shown in Fig. 2b.

MECHANISM OF SOLUTE TRANSPORT

The transport of a solute within cartilage is described by a general equation of the form

$$J = -D\left(\frac{d\bar{C}}{dx}\right) + \bar{C}u + Qdx \tag{3}$$

This equation expresses the dependence of the rate of transport (J) of a solute through the matrix and the local concentration of the solute at any point within the matrix, $\bar{C}$, on the solute diffusion coefficient, $\bar{D}$, on the rate of fluid flow, u, and on the rate of production or consumption of the given solute by the cells, Q (Q is positive in the case of production and negative in the case of consumption). It should be noted that the rate of fluid flow u in Eq. 3 can be replaced by the product of the hydraulic permeability K and the pressure gradient dP/dx.

When solute transport is considered between synovial fluid and cartilage or, under conditions *in vitro,* between an external solution and a cartilage specimen, the boundary condition of equilibrium at the interface defines the concentration of the solute in cartilage at that location, namely, $\bar{C}_0$. $\bar{C}_0$ is given by the following expression:

$$\bar{C}_0 = KC \tag{4}$$

where C is the solute concentration in solution and K is the partition coefficient of the solute between cartilage and the external solution.

Under steady-state conditions in the tissue, there is no change in solute concentration with time at any location, and the concentration gradients which exist are solely due to the utilization or production of the solute by the cells. This can be expressed by the equation

$$D\frac{d^2\bar{C}}{dx^2} = Q \tag{5}$$

Equation 5 can be integrated with respect to x in order to yield concentration profiles of solutes for which Q is known or can be estimated. Thus, for instance, for cartilage of thickness l, the concentration of a metabolite diffusing in from synovial fluid will be given at the cartilage–bone interface by the expression

$$\bar{C}_1 = \bar{C}_0 - \frac{Ql^2}{2\bar{D}} \tag{6}$$

PARTITION COEFFICIENTS

The partition coefficient of a solute has been defined as the maximum concentration of the unbound solute in the matrix relative to its concentration in the external contacting fluid, such as synovial fluid or plasma (3). It depends on the size and charge of the solute and on the properties of the matrix—in particular, its charge and excluded volume.

In the past, the partition coefficients were usually calculated with respect to the total matrix water. However, it is obvious that for some substances the partition coefficient will be very different, depending on whether one is considering the intra- or the extrafibrillar compartment. Thus, because the intrafibrillar space has no overall charge at physiological pH, whereas the extrafibrillar space has a strong negative charge, it is particularly important to note the existence of the two compartments when calculating the partition coefficients of ionic solutes. Again, larger solutes are only partially excluded from the extrafibrillar compartment because of the "excluded volume" properties of the PGs, whereas they are completely excluded from the intrafibrillar compartment into which they simply cannot fit.

Small Noncharged Solutes

These solutes [e.g., oxygen or amino acids (such as proline)] distribute themselves equally between the external solution and cartilage water, whether the latter is present in the extrafibrillar or intrafibrillar space. The partition coefficient of these substances is equal to unity.

Cations and Anions

In order to calculate the partition coefficients for the extrafibrillar compartment from the overall experimentally obtained partition data, we need to know (as for the calculation of the effective FCD) the magnitudes of the intra- and extrafibrillar compartments. In addition, we obviously need to know the ionic concentrations in the intrafibrillar space.

It is possible to investigate the concentrations of various solutes in the intrafibrillar compartment by using cartilage from which all PGs have been enzymatically removed (8) (see Fig. 2b). In such cartilage, the extrafibrillar space is uncharged and can be assumed to have the same properties as the equilibrating solution. Thus, any difference between the concentration of a solute in PG-free cartilage as a whole and its concentration in the outside solution is due to the difference between the latter and the concentration in the intrafibrillar compartment.

Table 1 shows the partition coefficients of Na^+, Ca^{2+}, Cl^-, and SO_4^{2-} in the intrafibrillar compartment, as deduced from the studies in PG-free bovine car-

TABLE 1. *Experimental partition coefficients of Na^+, Ca^{2+}, Cl^-, and SO_4^{2-} between PG-free bovine articular cartilage and external solution[a,b]*

Fixed charge density	$K_{total\ H_2O}$				$K_{extrafibrillar}$ (assumed)				$K_{intrafibrillar}$			
	Na^+	Ca^{2+}	Cl^-	SO_4^{2-}	Na^+	Ca^{2+}	Cl^-	SO_4^{2-}	Na^+	Ca^{2+}	Cl^-	SO_4^{2-}
~0.001	1.00	2.34	1.00	1.00	1.00	1.00	1.00	1.00	1.00	7.09	1.00	1.00

[a] External solution: 0.15 M NaCl + 2.5 mM $CaCl_2$ + 0.8 mM Na_2SO_4, pH 7.4.
[b] Note that the collagen compartment shows considerable selectivity towards Ca^{2+}.

tilage (C. Weinberg and A. Maroudas, *unpublished data*). The partition coefficients of Na^+, Cl^-, and SO_4^{2-} are clearly unity within experimental error, but K_{Ca} is high, indicating a selective uptake of Ca^{2+}, for reasons yet to be determined.

From the values for the intrafibrillar space and the overall experimentally determined partition coefficients for Na^+, Ca^{2+}, Cl^-, and SO_4^{2-} in native cartilage, we can now calculate the effective partition coefficients (and hence ionic concentrations) in the extrafibrillar compartment. By comparing these partition coefficients with those predicted from the theoretical Donnan equilibrium, we can also calculate the activity and selectivity coefficients for the above ions.

Table 2 shows typical values for Na^+, Ca^{2+}, Cl^-, and SO_4^{2-}. The activity and selectivity coefficients in the extrafibrillar compartment are similar to those measured for glycosaminoglycan and PG solutions at physiological concentrations (9). Assuming that the activity (γ) and the selectivity (K_b^q) coefficients are independent of hydration, and using the values determined for uncompressed cartilage (see Table 2), we can calculate the partition coefficients at hydrations corresponding to different degrees of compression.

Using the methods described above, we estimated the range of partition coefficients (and hence concentrations of Na^+, Ca^{2+}, H^+, Cl^-, and SO_4^{2-}) corresponding to the range of the effective FCDs resulting from compression up to approximately 10 atm, equivalent to volume changes in the specimens up to 30–50%. These calculated values are shown in Table 3. It can be seen that compression results in considerable changes in the concentrations of various ions in cartilage, particularly when they are expressed on the basis of extrafibrillar water. For the range of FCDs and final water contents assumed here, the maximum changes

TABLE 2. *Experimental partition coefficients of Na^+, Ca^{2+}, Cl^- and SO_4^{2-} between normal adult human articular cartilage and external solution[a]*

	K_{Na^+}	$K_{Ca^{2+}}$	K_{Cl^-}	$K_{SO_4^{2-}}$	$\sqrt{K_{Na^+} \cdot K_{Cl^-}}$ [b]	$\sqrt{K_{Ca^{2+}}/K_{Na^+}}$	$\sqrt{K_{SO_4^{2-}}/K_{Cl^-}}$
Per total H_2O [c]	2.00	8.98	0.64	0.48	1.13	1.50	1.08
Per intrafibrillar H_2O	1.00	7.09	1.00	1.00	1.0	2.66	1.00
Per extrafibrillar H_2O (calculated)	2.39	9.72	0.50	0.28	1.09	1.30	1.06

[a] External solution: 0.15 M NaCl + 2.5 mM $CaCl_2$ + 0.8 mM Na_2SO_4, pH 7.4.
[b] $\gamma_\pm = \sqrt{K_{Na^+} \cdot K_{Cl^-}}$.
[c] Intrafibrillar H_2O/total H_2O = 0.28.

TABLE 3. Predicted variations in partition coefficients of Na^+, Ca^{2+}, H^+, Cl^-, and SO_4^{2-} with cartilage compression

Conditions	FCD$_{initial}$ (mEq per g tissue)	FCD$_{effective}$ (mEq per g extrafibrillar water)	Water content (g H$_2$O per g dry wt)	W_{EF}/W_o	K_{Na^+} per W_o	K_{Na^+} per W_{EF}	$K_{Ca^{2+}}$ per W_o	$K_{Ca^{2+}}$ per W_{EF}	pH per W_o	pH per W_{EF}	K_{Cl^-} per W_o	K_{Cl^-} per W_{EF}	$K_{SO_4^{2-}}$ per W_o	$K_{SO_4^{2-}}$ per W_{EF}
Uncompressed	0.10	0.192	2.57	0.72	1.68	1.90	6.41	6.14	7.22	7.16	0.73	0.62	0.53	0.34
	0.17	0.310	2.57	0.75	2.16	2.54	10.01	10.98	7.11	7.04	0.60	0.47	0.40	0.20
2.6 atm	0.10	0.310	1.81	0.64	1.98	2.54	9.58	10.98	7.14	7.04	0.66	0.47	0.49	0.20
	0.17	0.310	2.57	0.75	2.16	2.54	10.01	10.98	7.11	7.04	0.60	0.47	0.40	0.20
4.70 atm	0.10	0.420	1.46	0.58	2.26	3.17	12.90	17.10	7.09	6.96	0.64	0.37	0.49	0.12
	0.17	0.420	2.06	0.70	2.52	3.17	14.10	17.10	7.05	6.96	0.56	0.37	0.38	0.12
6.00 atm	0.10	0.475	1.34	0.56	2.41	3.51	14.86	20.96	7.07	6.92	0.63	0.34	0.50	0.10
	0.17	0.475	1.86	0.69	2.73	3.51	16.66	20.96	7.02	6.92	0.54	0.34	0.38	0.10
7.50 atm	0.10	0.530	1.23	0.55	2.56	3.84	16.99	25.09	7.04	6.99	0.62	0.31	0.50	0.09
	0.17	0.530	1.70	0.67	2.90	3.84	19.15	25.09	6.88	6.88	0.54	0.31	0.39	0.09
10.20 atm	0.10	0.620	1.10	0.52	2.77	4.40	20.53	32.94	7.02	6.96	0.62	0.27	0.51	0.07
	0.17	0.620	1.51	0.65	3.21	4.40	23.89	32.94	6.83	6.83	0.53	0.27	0.40	0.07

range from a twofold increase in the case of Na^+, to a fivefold increase in the case of Ca^{2+} and a fivefold decrease in the case of SO_4^{2-}. It should be noted that these changes represent the actual changes in the ionic environment of the cell when cartilage is compressed.

Higher-Molecular-Weight Solutes

Intrafibrillar Compartment

The intrafibrillar space consists of two regions: the so-called "overlap" and "gap" regions. If one assumes a pseudohexagonal lattice for the collagen molecules (5), the pores in the overlap region are approximately 0.6 nm in radius. Thus, globular molecules of this size (i.e., of molecular weight larger than approximately 1000 daltons) are excluded from the "overlap" region. In the "gap" region of the fibril, somewhat larger molecules may be accommodated. Their sizes, which are probably shape-dependent, are not known at present. However, at least 80% of the intrafibrillar space consists of the overlap region. Thus, it is the latter which is mainly responsible for the exclusion properties of the intrafibrillar compartment.

From experimental work involving PG-free cartilage, it is possible, by methods mentioned above for ionic solutes, to determine the partition coefficients of large molecules for the intrafibrillar space. We found experimentally (5; also A. Maroudas et al., *unpublished data*) that the intrafibrillar compartment excludes molecules such as (a) polyethylene glycols of molecular weights 6000 and 20,000 daltons and (b) serum albumin.

Extrafibrillar Compartment

The partition coefficients of larger solutes in the extrafibrillar space can be reasonably accurately predicted, using Ogston's theory of excluded volume. In this theory, adopted for cartilage by Snowden and Maroudas (10), the partition coefficient is given by

$$K = \exp[-AC_X(r_r + r_s)^2] \qquad [7]$$

where C_X is the concentration of linear rod-like macromolecules (here glycos-aminoglycans), r_r is the radius of the rod-like macromolecule, r_s is the radius of globular solute, and A is a constant.

From Eq. 7 it is obvious that K decreases very steeply with increase in the size of the solute. Even for a relatively small solute, such as glucose, the partition coefficient is already slightly less than unity ($\sim$0.85); for proteins of the size of serum albumin, K can be as low as 0.001.

It is also clear from Eq. 7 that K decreases rapidly with increase in glycos-aminoglycan content (expressed here by FCD).

Recently (11), we have been interested in the penetration into cartilage of insulin-like growth factor (IGF-1) and its complexes with binding proteins. We have determined the partition coefficient of IGF-1 between buffer solutions (pH = 7) containing physiological concentrations of the hormone and femoral head cartilage of different glycosaminoglycan contents. ^{125}I-labeled IGF-1 was used for this purpose. The values obtained ($\sim$0.4–0.9 based on extrafibrillar space) are consistent with the predictions based on Ogston's "excluded volume" theory for a solute whose Stokes radius is $\sim$1.4 nm.

In some of our experiments, we included fetal calf serum in ^{125}I-labeled IGF-1-containing solutions in order to form labeled IGF-1–protein complexes, and then we measured their partition coefficients. Using gel chromatography, we found that complexes of different molecular weight were formed in the solution. The penetration into cartilage of the largest of these complexes (of size equal to or larger than that of serum albumin) was virtually nil. The mean partition coefficient for all the IGF-1–protein complexes combined was found to be around 0.04–0.06 (i.e., one order of magnitude lower than that for IGF-1 alone). These recent findings are of considerable relevance to the local variations in the effects of IGF-1 on PG metabolism in cartilage.

Figure 3 shows the variation of K with FCD, in the case of both serum albumin and IGF-1. It can be seen that the larger the solute, the greater the sensitivity of K to the PG content, in accordance with Eq. 7.

Compression leads to a decrease in hydration and hence an increase in effective FCD. One might, therefore, anticipate a decreased penetration of the larger solutes

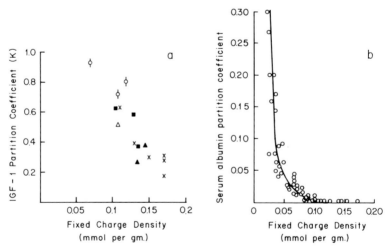

FIG. 3. Partition coefficients of (**a**) IGF-1 and (**b**) serum albumin as a function of FCD. (O) Serum albumin, ages 30–90 years; (⬡) IGF-1, 30 years old, 4°C; (×) IGF-1, 80 years old, 4°C; (■) IGF-1, 30 years old, 37°C; (▲) IGF-1, 80 years old, 37°C. (Part b reprinted from ref. 3 with publisher's permission.)

into compressed cartilage in accordance with the excluded volume principle. In fact, experiments have shown that an additional factor comes into play (12). Thus, in the case of laterally unconfined cartilage plugs subjected to either static or dynamic compression, there is actually an increase in the partition coefficients in relation to what might be expected. This has been explained by the hypothesis that matrix expansion may lead to the formation of a small number of wider channels in a plane normal to load application. Such channels would be able to accommodate additional numbers of large solute molecules in spite of the overall decrease in the available pore volume resulting from loss of fluid.

DIFFUSION COEFFICIENTS

Small Solutes

Diffusion coefficients of a number of solutes have been studied experimentally by Urban (13) in disc, and by Maroudas in cartilage (as summarized in ref. 3). The ratio D_{tissue}/D_{water} is similar for all small solutes tested in cartilage or in disc, whether uncharged (tritiated water), cationic (Na^+, Ca^{2+}), or anionic (Cl^- and SO_4^{2-}). The mean value of this ratio is 0.45.

The fact that solutes diffuse more slowly in cartilage than in free solution is due to several reasons: (a) The effective area for diffusion is less than that in free solution, and the diffusion paths are longer; (b) frictional effects can retard molecules which are moving through pores of diameter similar to that of their own; and (c) interactions with fixed groups may slow down counterion diffusion. It has been shown that for both cartilage and the intervertebral disc, the reduction in the diffusion coefficients of small solutes can be explained in terms of geometric factors alone. Thus, the formula of Mackie and Meares (14), which is based on steric considerations alone, can account for the reduction in the diffusion coefficients in both cartilage and disc (3,13) as well as in glycosaminoglycan–water solutions (9). This formula is

$$\frac{\bar{D}_{tissue}}{D_{water}} \frac{(1 - V_s)^2}{(1 + V_s)^2} \qquad [8]$$

where V_s is a volume fraction of solids in the tissue. The fact that there is no retardation of Na^+ or Ca^{2+} relative to tritiated H_2O or Cl^- shows that under physiological conditions the cations are in no way "bound" or "localized" by the negatively charged groups. This is consistent with the results recently obtained by Maroudas et al. (9) for chondroitin sulfate and hyaluronic acid–water gels in solutions of physiological ionic strength.

The variations in the values of the diffusion coefficient with hydration within the physiological hydration range for uncompressed cartilage were not found to be very large (15). But when cartilage loses larger amounts of water under applied load, the effective free space decreases and diffusion coefficients decrease strongly in accordance with Eq. 8.

Higher-Molecular-Weight Solutes

Because the mobilities of molecules decrease with their size, the diffusion coefficients in aqueous solution of solutes such as serum albumin or immunoglobulin (IgG) are much lower than those of small solutes. In addition, while small solutes diffuse through both extra- and intrafibrillar space, larger solutes, which cannot fit in the spaces between the collagen molecules, see the fibril as an impenetrable, solid space. This results in a bigger effective value of V_s in Eq. 7 and a lower value of $\bar{D}_{tissue}/D_{water}$.

Moreover, for molecules whose dimensions are not negligible in relation to average pore size, the diffusion coefficients may also be dependent on the friction between the solute molecules and the solid elements in the matrix.

Direct measurements of the diffusion coefficients of large solutes in uncompressed cartilage have been made. Data obtained by Maroudas on articular cartilage give $\bar{D}/D$ ratios of around 0.25–0.3. No measurements of $\bar{D}$ in compressed tissue are available, but on the basis of Eq. 8, $\bar{D}$ should be dramatically reduced. For a 50% loss in water content, the predicted reduction in $\bar{D}$ would be 15-fold.

CONCENTRATION OF METABOLITES IN CARTILAGE: EFFECT OF COMPRESSION

The knowledge of the partition coefficient of a solute enables one to calculate its concentration ($\bar{C}_0$) at the interface between cartilage and the synovial fluid. In the case of a metabolite, the concentration changes as one moves into the tissue further from the source of supply; Eq. 6 makes it possible to calculate the concentration of the metabolite farthest from the supply route. This minimum concentration ($\bar{C}_1$) can then be assumed to occur at the interface with the subchondral bone, which in the adult is usually impermeable to solutes.

If the water content of the cartilage changes, all the parameters in Eq. 6 will change in value, and the concentration profiles of the metabolites must change accordingly. Table 4 shows measured or estimated values of $\bar{C}_0$, Q, l, and $\bar{D}$, both for fully hydrated cartilage and for cartilage in which the water content has been reduced by 50%. The corresponding calculated values of $\bar{C}_1$ are also given.

The situation is different according to the metabolite considered. The concentration of SO_4^{2-} decreases in the deep zone only because of the higher FCD in that zone; the rate of sulfate consumption is so low that it is negligible in relation to the rate of diffusion. For this reason there is no difference in the profile for a fivefold range of Q values which correspond to the experimental results obtained in the presence or absence of fetal calf serum (16). Compression also has an effect through its influence on the partition coefficient.

In contrast to the sulfate ion, both glucose and oxygen show a considerable drop in the concentration in the deep zone; compression significantly enhances this decrease. The effect is particularly pronounced in the case of glucose. Thus, static compression, resulting in a significant decrease in the water content, may

TABLE 4. *Calculated results of diffusion coefficients, concentrations, and consumption rates for compressed and uncompressed cartilage*

Parameter	SO_4^{2-}		Glucose		Oxygen	
	Uncompressed	Compressed	Uncompressed	Compressed	Uncompressed	Compressed
Q (μmol/ml/hr)						
Per total tissue volume	$0.20\text{–}1.00] \times 10^{-2}$	$0.10\text{–}0.50] \times 10^{-2}$	2.53	4.18	0.23	0.38
Per extrafibrillar H_2O	$0.30\text{–}2.00]$	$0.20\text{–}1.00]$	4.32	10.00	0.40	0.91
Cartilage thickness l (cm)	0.200	0.121	0.200	0.121	0.200	0.121
Volume fraction of cartilage occupied by solids, V_s	0.21	0.35	0.21	0.35	0.21	0.35
$D = (1 - V_s/1 + V_s)^2 \times D_0$ (cm^2/hr)	10.8×10^{-3}	5.72×10^{-3}	9.0×10^{-3}	4.77×10^{-3}	46.0×10^{-3}	24.38×10^{-3}
Concentration at the surface (μmol/ml)						
Per total tissue volume	0.40	0.17	4.40	3.64	0.141	0.117
Per extrafibrillar H_2O	0.40	0.088	5.56	5.56	0.179	0.179
Concentration in deep zone (μmol/ml)						
Per total tissue volume	0.29	0.13	0	0	0.046	0
Per extrafibrillar H_2O	0.20	0.088	0[a]	0[b]	0.012	0[c]

[a] Glucose concentration drops to zero at a depth of 0.152 cm from the surface in uncompressed cartilage.
[b] Glucose concentration drops to zero at a depth of 0.073 cm from the surface in compressed cartilage.
[c] Oxygen concentration drops to zero at a depth of 0.096 cm from the surface in compressed cartilage.

lead to inadequate supplies of some nutrients to the cells in the deep zone. It should be noted that Q was assumed to be independent of the hydration itself, which in the case of SO_4^{2-}, for instance, is clearly not true (1,2).

The actual changes in concentrations with hydration are smaller than the changes in the individual parameters l, Q, and $\bar{D}$ accompanying loss of water. This is because the decrease in the diffusion coefficient $\bar{D}$ and the increase in Q (the latter due to an increased cell density) are compensated for by the decrease in thickness, which appears as a square term in Eq. 5.

For larger solutes, which would be excluded from intrafibrillar space and for which $\bar{D}$ would, therefore, be even more sensitive to hydration changes, the decrease in l will not make up for the drastic decrease in D. Moreover, the partition coefficient of a larger solute will also be more sensitive to changes in hydration than will that of a small solute. Thus, both the absolute concentration and the concentration profile of a metabolite of larger molecular weight (e.g., IGF-1) will be more affected by a decrease in hydration than will be the case for a small solute. However, at present we cannot calculate such profiles because we do not have data relating compression to Q.

INFLUENCE OF CYCLIC COMPRESSION ON SOLUTE TRANSPORT

Solutes may move through the cartilage matrix not only by diffusion, but also by being carried along with fluid which flows through the tissue when it is loaded. The relative influence of fluid flow on solute transport will depend on the ratio of the solute diffusion coefficient to the fluid transport coefficient. Solute transport will thus depend on solute size, because in general the value of the diffusion coefficient, D, decreases as solute size increases. Whether convective flow influences solute transport or not will also depend on tissue composition and on how the tissue is loaded, because these factors influence the value of the transport coefficient. The magnitude of the latter is greatest (i.e., fluid flow is fastest) where the pressure gradient is high and where the cartilage samples are low in PG content. The direction of fluid flow may also be important, because under some conditions fluid movement may oppose solute transport rather than assist it.

Recently it has been shown (17) that fluid movement does not contribute significantly to the rate of movement of small solutes through cartilage plugs, either when fluid movement opposes transport or when it assists it. These experimental findings are not surprising when the relative coefficients for fluid movement and diffusion are compared. The diffusion coefficients, $\bar{D}$, for small solutes in cartilage (e.g., oxygen, glucose, lactate, urea, inorganic ions) are in the range $2–6 \times 10^{-6}$ cm^2/sec, whereas the fluid transport coefficient, $D(H)$, for physiological loading conditions lies between 0.2×10^{-7} and 2×10^{-7} cm^2/sec and is thus 10–100 times smaller than $\bar{D}$. For large solutes, such as serum albumin, however, the value of $\bar{D}$ is about 2×10^{-7} cm^2/sec. Because it is of magnitude similar to that of $D(H)$, even allowing for viscous and fractional retardation, fluid flow would be expected to contribute significantly to the transport of such solutes. This has indeed been borne out by our experimental findings (17).

In summary, it can be said that although cyclic loading is not effective in speeding up transport of small solutes through the matrix, it is likely to increase the rate at which larger solutes such as growth factors, hormones, enzymes and their inhibitors, and cytokines reach the cells. Pumping may also influence the rate at which newly synthesized matrix macromolecules themselves move through the matrix, and it might influence the rate of loss of matrix breakdown products into the surrounding fluid (18).

Although our results indicate that loading does not influence the movement of small nutrients through the matrix itself, cyclic load application may none-theless be important for nutrition in other ways: Without movement, droplets of stagnant synovial fluid may be depleted of their supply of nutrients, and may accumulate acidic wastes such as lactate and carbon dioxide. In this way, lack of movement may cause inadequate "nutrition" of cartilage and inadequate removal of waste products.

CONCLUSION

The ability to quantify the distribution of water between the extra- and intra-fibrillar spaces in tissues under different physiological conditions renders it possible for us to estimate the concentration of different solutes in the cells' environment and to try and assess the effects of these concentrations on the metabolism of the chondrocytes.

In general, the more detailed the knowledge of the mechanisms involved in the transport of different types of solutes through cartilaginous tissues, the better our understanding of the mutual cell–matrix relationships and their interactions under both normal physiological and pathological conditions.

REFERENCES

1. Urban JPG, Bayliss MT. Regulation of proteoglycan synthesis rate in cartilage *in vitro:* influence of extracellular ionic composition. *Biochim Biophys Acta* 1989;992:59–65.
2. Schneiderman R, Keret D, Maroudas A. The effects of mechanical and osmotic pressure on the rate of glycosaminoglycan synthesis in the human adult femoral head. *J Orthop Res* 1986;4: 393–408.
3. Maroudas A. Physico-chemical properties of articular cartilage. In: Freeman MAR, ed. *Adult articular cartilage,* 2nd ed. London: Pitman Medical Publishers, 1979;215–290.
4. Urban JPG. Solute transport between tissue and environment. In: Maroudas A, Kuettner K, eds. *Methods in cartilage research.* London: Academic Press, 1990;241–273.
5. Maroudas A, Wachtel E, Grushko G, Katz EP, Weinberg P. The effect of osmotic and mechanical pressures on water partitioning in articular cartilage. *Biochim Biophys Acta* 1991;1093:285–294.
6. Urban J, Maroudas A, Bayliss MT, Dillon J. Swelling pressures of proteoglycans at the concentrations found in cartilaginous tissues. *Biorheology* 1979;16:447–464.
7. Maroudas A, Grushko G. Measurement of swelling pressure of cartilage. In: Maroudas A, Kuettner K, eds. *Methods in cartilage research.* London: Academic Press, 1990;298–301.

8. Chun LE, Koob TJ, Eyre DR. Sequential enzymic dissection of the proteoglycan complex from articular cartilage. Transactions of the 32nd annual meeting, *Orthop Res Soc* 1986;11:96.
9. Maroudas A, Weinberg PD, Parker KH, Winlove CP. The distributions and diffusivities of small ions in chrondroitin sulphate, hyaluronate and some proteoglycan solutions. *Biophys Chem* 1988;32:257–270.
10. Snowden JMcK, Maroudas A. The distribution of serum albumin in human normal and degenerate articular cartilage. *Biochim Biophys Acta* 1976;428:726–740.
11. Maroudas A, Popper O. Partition coefficients of IGF-1 between cartilage and external medium in the presence and absence of FCS. Transactions of the 37th annual meeting. *Orthop Res Soc* 1991;16:398.
12. O'Hara B, Tomlinson N, Maroudas A, Urban J. Manuscript in preparation, 1991.
13. Urban JPG. Fluid and solute transport in the intervertebral disc. Ph.D. thesis, University of London.
14. Mackie JS, Meares P. The diffusion of electrolytes in a cation-exchange resin membrane. *Proc R Soc Lond [A]* 1955;232:498–509.
15. Maroudas A, Venn M. Swelling of normal and osteoarthritic femoral head cartilage. *Ann Rheum Dis* 1977;36:399–406.
16. Maroudas A, Schneiderman R, Weinberg C, Grushko G. Choice of specimens in comparative studies involving human femoral head cartilage. In: Maroudas A, Kuettner K, eds. *Methods in cartilage research.* London: Academic Press, 1990;9–17.
17. O'Hara B, Urban J, Maroudas A. Influence of cyclic loading on the nutrition of articular cartilage. *Ann Rheum Dis* 1990;49:536–539.
18. Dvirin V, Maroudas A. Manuscript in preparation, 1991.

DISCUSSION

Cooke: What volumes of fluid flow in an individual who is not weight-bearing at the knee compared with an individual who is weight-bearing at the knee?

Maroudas: If one stands without any weight on the leg, presumably there should be no fluid flow in the tissue itself. If you move your leg without putting a load on it, the synovial fluid will be stirred. The agitation of synovial fluid in the synovial cavity is very important for eliminating stagnant liquid films at the cartilage interface and for ensuring that the liquid there does not become impoverished in metabolites. Synovial fluid movement is essential for cartilage nutrition. However, in order to get fluid flow through the matrix itself, cyclic load application is required.

Cooke: How much water would move out of the knee cartilage when, for example, a 200-pound man is standing?

Maroudas: Probably about 50% of the cartilage water—that is, about 0.35 grams per gram of cartilage.

Cooke: We have compared joint space distance in standing-knee radiographs of healthy young adults with and without loading. We could not show any significant joint-space change. If one loses as much as a third or half of the water volume, one would expect to see a change.

Maroudas: For how long did your subjects bear weight on the knee?

Cooke: To take the x-rays requires about 20 min altogether.

Maroudas: Apart from being a function of applied pressure, cartilage permeability, and osmotic pressure, expression depends on the length of the fluid flow paths within cartilage. If the loaded area is large in relation to the unloaded area, the fluid has to go a long way. Therefore, in the whole joint it may take several hours for cartilage to show a significant volume decrease and hence joint-space change. This is entirely unlike the geometry of small isolated cartilage plugs, such as we have used in our laboratory experiments. One must remember that fluid loss depends very much on the relationship between the size of the high-pressure zone and the low-pressure area through which the fluid can escape.

Glant: During the aging of the articular cartilage or during the degradation, large fragments from aggrecan molecules are released. Are cyclic loading patterns and fluid flow rates in the matrix great enough to remove these large fragments which are much larger than BSA molecules, for example? What is the mechanism in other nonarticular cartilages which do not undergo such biomechanical changes?

Maroudas: In the course of very slow turnover, even intact subunits can actually diffuse out of the tissue. Work that Mike Bayliss has done with thin cartilage slices bears this out. It should also be remembered that there is a fairly large proportion of nonaggregated proteoglycans in cartilage. The results of some preliminary experiments suggest that cyclic compression does enhance the rate at which proteoglycans move through cartilage. So I think that there is passive movement of some species of proteoglycans in the matrix, and that cyclic compression enhances it. With regard to aging in nonfibrillated human cartilage, we do not observe any loss of glycosaminoglycans with age. On the contrary, there is actually an increase in fixed charge density with age, leading to an increase in the osmotic pressure. Aging is thus not a deleterious process for cartilage function and is distinct from osteoarthritis.

Articular Cartilage and Osteoarthritis,
edited by K. Kuettner et al.
Raven Press, Ltd., New York © 1992.

26

Effects of Static and Dynamic Compression on Matrix Metabolism in Cartilage Explants

Robert L.-Y. Sah,* Alan J. Grodzinsky,* Anna H. K. Plaas,†
and John D. Sandy†

Continuum Electromechanics Group, Laboratory for Electromagnetic and Electronic Systems, Department of Electrical Engineering and Computer Science, Massachusetts Institute of Technology and the Harvard–M.I.T. Division of Health Sciences and Technology, Cambridge, Massachusetts 02139 and †Department of Orthopaedic Research, Shriners Hospital for Crippled Children, Tampa, Florida 33612

Articular cartilage functions as a weight-bearing, wear-resistant material in synovial joints. The ability of cartilage to withstand compressive, tensile, and shear forces depends critically on the composition and structural integrity of its extracellular matrix (1). While collagen fibrils are strong in tension, proteoglycans resist compression due to their bulk compressive stiffness and to electrostatic repulsive interactions between glycosaminoglycan chains (2–5). The maintenance of adequate concentrations of matrix components and the preservation of a structurally intact matrix require the coordinated synthesis, assembly, degradation, and loss of proteoglycan, collagen, and other matrix molecules (Fig. 1A). The regulation of these metabolic processes may involve a combination of cell biological and physical mechanisms.

Clinical observations and studies *in vivo* suggest that joint loading and motion can induce a wide range of metabolic responses in cartilage. Immobilization or reduced loading led to a decrease in proteoglycan synthesis and content (6,7). Increased dynamic loading led to an increase in proteoglycan synthesis and content (6,7). More severe static (8) or impact (9) loading caused cartilage deterioration. Anterior cruciate ligament transection in dogs led to increases in both synthesis and release of extracellular matrix constituents progressing to osteoarthritis (10). Thus, while some degree of "normal" joint loading appears to promote structural adaptation, "abnormal" mechanical forces predispose cartilage to degeneration. The physical phenomena and biological processes responsible for these alterations are difficult to identify *in vivo*. Complexities include: quantifying the biomechanics of loading, and distinguishing between (a) the direct effect of loading on cartilage metabolism and (b) indirect effects on other

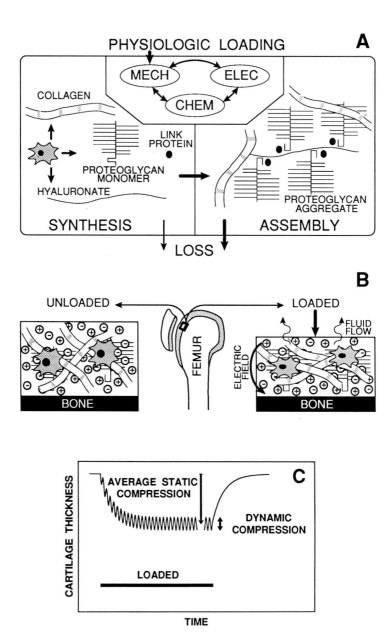

FIG. 1. Biophysical regulation of cartilage metabolism during mechanical loading. **A:** Chondrocytes synthesize matrix components such as the structurally important collagens, proteoglycans, hyaluronate, and link protein. These components assemble into a stable extracellular matrix; subsequent catabolic processes cause the release of certain components from the tissue. Alternatively, some biosynthetic products may never become incorporated into the matrix, but instead are immediately lost from the tissue. These metabolic processes may be influenced by mechanical, chemical, or electrical phenomena that are induced by physiological levels of loading. **B:** Schematic of joint loading showing physical phenomena: chondrocyte deformation, hydrostatic pressurization, fluid flow, electric fields (streaming potentials and currents), matrix consolidation, and physico-chemical alterations (altered ion concentrations and osmotic pressure). **C:** Simplified interpretation of compression of cartilage during dynamic joint loading. At steady state, there is a time-averaged static compression, on which is superimposed a dynamic compression.

mediators such as growth factors in synovial fluid (11) or vascularity of subchondral bone (12).

The physical properties of cartilage can be determined *in vitro* by testing explants in well-defined geometries. A number of physical phenomena which occur naturally during loading have been identified and quantified (Fig. 1B). Compression of cartilage results in deformation of cells and extracellular matrix (13), hydrostatic pressure gradients, fluid flow, streaming potentials and currents (5,14,15), and physicochemical changes such as altered matrix water content, fixed charge density, mobile ion concentrations, and osmotic pressure (4,16,17). Any of these mechanical, chemical, or electrical phenomena may modulate matrix metabolism (Fig. 1A). However, because these phenomena are naturally coupled during compression, it may be difficult to determine the involvement of an isolated physical stimulus in an observed metabolic response. Here, theoretical models for the poroviscoelastic mechanical (14,18) and electromechanical (19,20) behavior of cartilage can provide a useful framework for establishing protocols for *static* and *dynamic* testing of explants during culture and for distinguishing the results of these different stimuli.

Cartilage explants can be maintained *in vitro* in a stable and controlled biochemical and physical environment. The balance between synthesis and release of matrix components has been studied extensively in free-swelling explants (21,22). Calf and adult bovine articular cartilage explants attain steady-state levels of proteoglycan synthesis (21). Newly synthesized proteoglycans undergo an extracellular maturation process, eventually forming aggregates with hyaluronate and link protein (23). Cartilage matrix proteoglycans are susceptible to degradation by several classes of proteinases (24). Once cleaved to the nonaggregating form, proteoglycans are preferentially lost into the medium (23,25,26), with the overall loss of proteoglycan occurring approximately as a steady first-order rate process (22). The cell-dependent metabolism of proteoglycan and other matrix molecules can be greatly affected by growth factors; medium supplementation with fetal bovine serum (21), insulin-like growth factor 1 (IGF-1) (27), or transforming growth factor β (TGF-β) (25) stimulates proteoglycan synthesis and inhibits proteoglycan degradation and loss. Explant culture of cartilage also preserves the characteristic chondrocyte biosynthetic phenotype (28) as well as potentially important interactions between cells and extracellular matrix. Thus, many previous studies *in vitro* on the metabolic effects of mechanical compression have utilized cartilage explants (16,17,29–43).

In this chapter, we describe how static and dynamic testing protocols *in vitro* may relate to joint biomechanics *in vivo* and address the role of putative physical regulatory mechanisms. We then describe our studies where cartilage disks were subjected to mechanical compression during explant culture to (a) characterize and compare effects of static and dynamic compression on cartilage metabolism and (b) relate effects to possible biophysical regulatory mechanisms. By identifying mechanisms by which specific physical forces regulate cartilage matrix metabolism, it may be possible to infer how various mechanical loads contribute to the maintenance of healthy articular cartilage and to the degeneration of osteo-arthritic tissue.

MECHANICAL MODULATION OF CARTILAGE METABOLISM *IN VITRO*

Compression protocols *in vitro* are motivated, in part, by the range of loading magnitudes and frequencies relevant to joint motion *in vivo*. For example, peak contact pressures in the human femoropatellar and hip joint are 3–18 MPa (44–46) and result in average compression amplitudes of greater than 13% (47). However, joint loading *in vivo* would be expected to induce complex forces, fields, and flows varying in direction, space, and time within cartilage. Physical boundary conditions (discontinuities in material properties) and tissue inhomo-geneities that are difficult to assess complicate the distribution of forces and flows. Thus, protocols *in vitro* that can lessen these complexities are helpful.

A useful simplified interpretation of cartilage compression during repetitive joint loading is that fluid is exuded from cartilage and then imbibed during each cycle (Fig. 1C) (3,48). At early times, more fluid is exuded during each loading cycle than is imbibed, and there is a gradual net exudation of fluid. At steady state, the amount of fluid exuded during each cycle is exactly that reimbibed. When loading is discontinued, there is a gradual net influx of fluid. Thus, the resulting cartilage compression can be considered to consist of a time-varying *dynamic* component superimposed on a slowly evolving time-averaged *static* component. At higher frequencies [e.g., 1 cycle/sec (Hz)], there may be very little exudation/imbibition during each cycle, with elastic-like deformation (49). In contrast, at lower frequencies, fluid flow could be more significant during each cycle. For testing *in vitro*, the choice between alternatives such as imposed displacement versus imposed load may be motivated by the objective of isolating the effects of the specific static or dynamic component on matrix metabolism.

To date, most studies *in vitro* have focused on the metabolic responses: (a) during the onset and after the release of a static compression (29,30,33,35,38), (b) during static compression (16,17,29,33,35,38,40,41), and (c) during dynamic compression (38,50). During static compression of cartilage explants, proteogly-can synthesis is inhibited (16,17,29,33,38). With compression and fluid exudation, the density of fixed negative charges in the matrix is increased, resulting in at-traction and concentration of positive counterions such as H^+ and Na^+. Thus, it has been hypothesized that the physical initiator of the biosynthetic inhibition during compression may be physicochemical changes (e.g., extracellular ion concentrations and osmotic pressure) that accompany fluid loss (16,17,33,36). A theoretical model based on Donnan equilibrium and electroneutrality predicts the dependence of a given ion concentration on compression, and has been used to test such a hypothesis (3,17,36). Indeed, proteoglycan biosynthesis was similarly inhibited by equivalent increases in the intratissue concentration of H^+ (i.e., decreased pH) (17) or Na^+ (36) brought about by either (a) tissue compression or (b) incubation in bathing medium of low pH or high NaCl in the absence of compression.

Dynamic compression of cartilage explants has had variable effects on biosynthesis, depending on the specific loading protocol and whether synthesis was measured during or following compression. Dynamic compressive loads (60 sec on/60 sec off, and 4 sec on/11 sec off) for 2 hr led to a decrease and increase, respectively, in proteoglycan biosynthesis in the 2 hr following compression (30). The compression that occurred during loading was not measured, and the peak applied stress was relatively low (0.001–0.011 MPa). In another study, cyclic tensile stretching (5.5%) of high-density chick chondrocyte cultures at 0.2 Hz for 24 hr was accompanied by an increase in proteoglycan synthesis during the last 4 hr of stretching (50).

With increasing frequency (strain rates), dynamic compression of cartilage induces increasing levels of hydrostatic pressure within the tissue (18). The effect of hydrostatic pressure on cartilage metabolism could be studied via direct mechanical compression of cartilage, or by pressurizing the fluid in a vessel containing chondrocyte cultures (34) or cartilage explants (32). The latter approach can involve pressurizing the gas phase over the culture medium. This, however, would cause an increase in the partial pressure of gas in the incubation medium, which could alter matrix metabolism by mechanisms independent of hydrostatic pressure. To focus on effects due to hydrostatic pressure, investigators have sealed cultures in gas-impermeable containers (31); others have designed pressure vessels to eliminate an overlying gas phase (42).

Previous studies on the effects of mechanical compression on cartilage explant metabolism have focused primarily on anabolic processes. Few studies have examined the possibility that physical forces may be an important determinant of matrix assembly or catabolism. Release of radioactivity from disks prelabeled with [^{35}S]sulfate was not altered during 2 hours of low-amplitude static and dynamic loading protocols (with peak loads of 0.011 MPa) (30). However, release of radioactivity was decreased during 1–4 days of high-amplitude static loading (3 MPa) (29). After 1–2 days of static compression, unloading led to a subsequent increase in the rate of release of radioactivity above nonloaded control levels. However, the ^{35}S-labeled constituents lost into the medium were not characterized, and no interpretation of loss patterns in terms of physical and biochemical mechanisms or of structural alterations in the cartilage matrix was made.

COMPRESSION OF CARTILAGE DISKS

All experiments summarized below were done with 1-mm-thick, 3-mm-diameter cartilage disks that were explanted from the femoropatellar grooves of 1- to 2-week-old calves and cultured in DMEM supplemented with 10 mM HEPES, 0.1 mM nonessential amino acids, an additional 0.4 mM L-proline, 20

μg/ml ascorbate, and 10% fetal bovine serum (0.5 or 1.0 ml medium/disk) in a humidified 5% CO_2–95% air incubator at 37°C (38). All medium was prepared by temperature and CO_2 equilibration in the incubator for 1–2 hr just before use. Cartilage disks swelled to a thickness of ≥ 1.25 mm after 2–6 days of culture.

Compression was applied via polysulfone chambers in which cartilage disks were sandwiched between two fluid-impermeable platens (38,39). By varying the distance between the platens, cartilage disks were compressed in a uniaxial, radially unconfined configuration. One chamber was designed for a mechanical spectrometer so that arbitrary displacement functions could be applied while simultaneously monitoring the imposed load. With this chamber, up to 12 cartilage disks could be tested in parallel. A somewhat similar device has been developed to test individual cartilage disks affixed to culture dishes (37).

EFFECTS OF STATIC AND OSCILLATORY COMPRESSION ON CARTILAGE EXPLANT BIOSYNTHESIS

The differential effects of static and dynamic oscillatory compression on biosynthesis by cartilage explants were examined (38). Proteoglycan synthesis was assessed by [35S]sulfate incorporation, and protein synthesis was assessed by L-[5-3H]proline incorporation. Disks were typically incubated with 5–20 μCi/ml isotope for 8–12 hr during compression, serially washed with 1 ml phosphate-buffered saline (PBS) at 4°C six times over 1.5 hr, and analyzed for total incorporated radioactivity, as well as, in some cases, for macromolecular components. Radiolabel uptake by chondrocytes in cartilage explants reflects a combination of processes, including diffusion of radiolabel to the cell surface, transport across the cell membrane, metabolic conversion to high-energy precursors (i.e., proline to prolyl-tRNA and sulfate to 3'-phosphoadenosine 5'-phosphosulfate), mixing with endogenous precursor pools, and incorporation into protein or proteoglycan (38). Thus, compression could affect radiolabel incorporation by modulating any of several biological or physical processes.

The form of the 3H- and 35S-labeled products synthesized by cartilage explants was characterized in biophysical and biochemical control studies (38). Radiolabeling periods were 8–12 hr during the static and oscillatory compression protocols described here. This was sufficiently long to minimize possible effects of compression on radiolabel equilibration within the cartilage disk. The 90% radiolabel equilibration time for 3-mm-diameter disks is ~ 1 hr (51). Also, this incubation period was long enough such that most of the incorporated radioactivity was in the form of biosynthetic products (essentially all of the incorporated [35S]sulfate was in macromolecular proteoglycan, and $\sim 75\%$ of the incorporated [3H]proline was in macromolecular protein) (38). Furthermore, in our studies with explants of young calf cartilage, incorporation of [3H]proline was relatively specific for collagen formation, because [3H]hydroxyproline analysis indicated that $\sim 83\%$ of the 3H macromolecules could be accounted for by [3H]collagen.

The incubation medium was not routinely analyzed for newly synthesized macromolecules, because >90% of the ^{3}H macromolecules and >95% of the ^{35}S macromolecules were typically retained within the cartilage disks. Together, these control studies indicated that [^{35}S]sulfate incorporation into calf cartilage disks was a specific indicator of chondrocyte synthesis of proteoglycan, whereas [^{3}H]proline incorporation reflected chondrocyte uptake of amino acid precursor, as well as synthesis of collagens and other proteins.

The dose-dependence of the effect of static (12-hr) compression was determined (Fig. 2A). There was no significant difference between incorporation into disks freely swelling in 24-well culture dishes and that into disks compressed to 1.25–1.00 mm ($p > 0.15$). Thus, the compression chambers appeared biologically inert, and occlusion at the cartilage–platen interfaces did not appear to restrict nutrient supply at minimal compressions. At compression to 0.75 mm, [^{35}S]sulfate and [^{3}H]proline (not shown) incorporation was decreased by 22% and 17%, respectively (both $p < 0.001$), when compared to that with disks compressed to 1.00 mm (the original cut thickness). This trend is consistent with results from previous studies of mechanical and osmotic compression of cartilage explants where loading was for 4–12 hr (16,17,29,33). Kinetic studies indicated that radiolabel incorporation rates had decreased to lower steady-state values early during the compression (within ∼1 hr) (35,38). Mechanical measurements showed that stress relaxation of the 3-mm-diameter disks was 90% complete within 15 min. Thus, the period to reach mechanical equilibrium and biosynthetic steady state was short relative to the 12 hr of compression. As described above, the biosynthetic inhibition during compression appears to involve physicochemical phenomena (16,17,33,36).

With the dosimetry of static effects on biosynthesis established for 3-mm-diameter disks of calf cartilage, the effects of low-amplitude oscillatory compression over a wide range of frequencies were examined. Experimental groups were compressed to 1.0 mm, with a superimposed oscillatory compression of 1–2%; control disks were held statically at 1.0 mm. Experimental and control disks were radiolabeled during the last 8 hr of 23-hr compression protocols. Such oscillatory compression at frequencies (f) of 0.01–1 Hz stimulated incorporation of [^{35}S]sulfate (Fig. 2B) and [^{3}H]proline (not shown) by ∼30–40%, but had no effect at lower f. The low amplitude (1–2%) of such oscillations ensured that there was little change in tissue hydration and fixed charge density; thus, the biosynthetic effects of such oscillations could not have been induced by static physicochemical phenomena (compare Fig. 2A).

The mechanisms responsible for this stimulation may involve other biophysical phenomena occurring at the higher frequencies. During oscillatory compression, load and displacement measurements enabled dynamic stiffness to be computed (Fig. 2C). The frequency response of stiffness is qualitatively consistent with certain trends predicted by a linear poroelastic (biphasic) model (18,52) in the sinusoidal steady state (see refs. 38 and 52 for details). The dynamic stiffness amplitude increased sharply at ∼0.001 Hz and plateaued at ∼0.1 Hz; the theo-

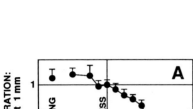
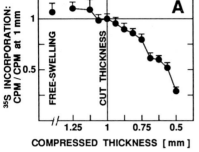
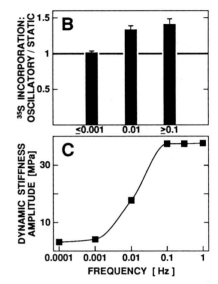

FIG. 2. Effect of static and oscillatory compression on [³⁵S]sulfate incorporation into cartilage disks, with correlation of frequency-dependence of oscillatory effect to dynamic stiffness. **A:** Disks were radiolabeled during 12 hr of static compression. Incorporation is expressed relative to incorporation into disks held at 1 mm (the initial cartilage explant thickness). Data are expressed as mean ± SEM (n = 9–12). **B:** Disks were radiolabeled during the last 8 hr of 23-hr oscillatory compression protocols. Experimental disks were statically compressed to 1 mm, with a superimposed oscillatory strain of 1–2% at frequencies of 0.0001–1.0 Hz; control disks were statically held at 1 mm. Incorporation data are expressed as oscillatory/static (n = 12–72). **C:** During oscillatory compression experiments, dynamic stiffness amplitude was measured. (Data adapted from refs. 38 and 39.)

retical transition frequency is of order $1/\tau_m$, where $\tau_m = a^2/H_a k$ is the characteristic unconfined compression stress relaxation time constant (18) (where a is the disk radius, H_a is the equilibrium confined compression modulus, and k is the hydraulic permeability). For $a = 1.5$ mm, $H_a \sim 0.5$ MPa, and $k \sim 2 \times 10^{-15}$ m²/Pa·sec, the characteristic frequency is $\sim 1/\tau_m$, or ~ 0.001 Hz. At the higher frequencies, there will be a concomitant increase in (a) hydrostatic pressure in the central region of the cartilage disk and (b) pressure gradients, fluid velocity, and streaming potential near the periphery. Recent experiments correlating biosynthesis with radial distance from the center of the disk indicate a greater biosynthetic stimulation near the disk periphery than in the central region (43). Nevertheless, the slight biosynthetic stimulation in the central region together with measured peak dynamic loads of ~ 0.5–1 MPa at the higher frequencies would be consistent with recent findings that hydrostatic pressure can stimulate biosynthesis (42).

EFFECTS OF STATIC AND OSCILLATORY COMPRESSION ON THE HYALURONATE-BINDING PROPERTIES OF NEWLY SYNTHESIZED PROTEOGLYCAN IN CARTILAGE EXPLANTS

In cartilage, most large proteoglycans (60–85%) appear to exist in aggregates, in which monomers are noncovalently bound to hyaluronate in an interaction stabilized by link protein (see ref. 23 for review). Such aggregates are macromolecular complexes that can consist of 30–100 proteoglycan monomers affixed to a hyaluronate backbone up to ~ 5 μm long. The size of the aggregate effectively immobilizes proteoglycans within the collagenous meshwork, preventing monomers from diffusing out of the tissue. The mechanism by which proteoglycan aggregates are assembled biosynthetically (23,40) has been extensively studied in chondrocyte culture and in solutions after proteoglycan purification (53). In cartilage explants as well as in articular cartilage *in vivo,* monomers, once secreted from chondrocytes, appear to undergo a maturation process in the extracellular matrix whereby their binding affinity for hyaluronate increases. With purified monomer solutions, the conversion process can be catalyzed by mild base (53,54). Within cartilage explants, the process appears to occur in the absence of continued cellular activity and can be slowed by low temperature, but is promoted by a low partial pressure of oxygen. The conversion appears to be blocked by *N*-ethylmaleimide and may involve free thiol groups and disulfide bonding.

The effects of compression on the hyaluronate-binding properties of newly synthesized proteoglycan were examined in pulse-chase experiments (40). Cartilage disks were pulse-radiolabeled with 100 μCi/ml [^{35}S]sulfate for 1.5 hr and washed three times over a total of 0.5 hr with culture medium (pH 7.45). Disks were then subjected to the following chase protocols: (a) 0–24 hr of static compression (1.25, 1.00, 0.75, or 0.50 mm) or (b) 8.5 hr of oscillatory compression (a 2% strain, superimposed on a static compression to a thickness of 1.00 mm) at 0.001, 0.01 or 0.1 Hz. After chase, disks were rinsed with a PBS solution containing proteinase inhibitors at 4°C. Control experiments indicated that during radiolabeling and up to 24 hr of chase, virtually all newly synthesized [^{35}S]proteoglycan were retained in the explant (<3% of ^{35}S macromolecules in the medium). Groups of four to six disks from each pulse-chase condition were then cryostat-sectioned to 20 μm and extracted with a 4 M guanidine-HCl solution containing proteinase inhibitors. Analysis of the cartilage residues confirmed that this achieved a high degree of extraction of both total tissue proteoglycans and [^{35}S]proteoglycan (both >93%). Finally, high-buoyant-density proteoglycans were isolated from the extract as the D1 fraction on CsCl dissociative density-gradient centrifugation and were then dialyzed exhaustively against 0.15 M sodium acetate (pH 6.8) at 4°C.

The hyaluronate-binding properties of D1 proteoglycans were analyzed by fractionating samples on Sephacryl S-1000 in 0.5 M sodium acetate/0.1% (v/v) Triton X-100/0.02% NaN$_3$ (pH 6.8) to separate proteoglycan eluting as monomers and aggregates. Fractionation of portions of D1 samples alone showed that >92% of the tissue proteoglycan and [^{35}S]proteoglycan were eluted in the free-monomer position, confirming their isolation from endogenous hyaluronate. The hyaluronate-binding affinity of the monomers was assessed by mixing portions of D1 samples with limiting amounts (1.6% w/w) of hyaluronate in associative conditions. The mixtures were then analyzed by chromatography. Proteoglycan monomers (total tissue or radiolabeled) which elute as aggregates under these conditions are defined as high-affinity, and those which fail to form aggregates are referred to as low-affinity (see ref. 53).

Newly synthesized proteoglycans in the pulse sample contained a small percentage of high-affinity monomers (Fig. 3C). With chase time, there was a conversion from the low-affinity form into the high-affinity form. On the other hand, the percentage of total tissue proteoglycan in the high-affinity form was not markedly altered during the chase period. Thus, a half-life ($t_{1/2}$) of the conversion process was computed as the extrapolated time at which the ratio of percentage of [^{35}S]proteoglycan in the high-affinity form to the percentage of total tissue proteoglycan in the high-affinity form reached half of the maximum. This yielded a $t_{1/2}$ of 5.7 hr for 1.25-mm control cartilage disks at pH 7.45 in two separate experiments (Fig. 3).

Static compression during chase slowed the conversion of the newly synthesized monomers into the high-affinity form (Fig. 3A). With increasing compression to 1.00, 0.75, and 0.50 mm, the conversion $t_{1/2}$ was lengthened to 6.9, 7.4, and 11.6 hr, respectively. Furthermore, even maximally compressed samples were fully converted into the high-affinity form by 48 hr of chase, indicating that compression delayed, but did not prevent, conversion. In contrast, 2% oscillatory compression at a frequency of 0.001, 0.01, or 0.1 Hz superimposed on a static compression to 1.00 mm did not alter the conversion compared to static compression of control samples at 1.00 mm (data not shown).

Because tissue compression would lead to a physicochemical decrease of intratissue pH (17), the effect of altered medium pH on affinity conversion was determined while holding the cartilage thickness constant at 1.25 mm (Fig. 3B). Medium at acidic pH markedly delayed the conversion relative to medium at normal pH (7.45), whereas medium at basic pH accelerated the conversion. With decreasing medium pH of 7.70, 7.45, 7.24, and 6.99, the conversion $t_{1/2}$ was increased to 3.3, 5.7, 8.3, and 10.6 hr, respectively. Thus, the effect of graded decreases in intratissue pH on conversion kinetics was similar whether acidification was due to static compression (Fig. 3A) or to medium titration (Fig. 3B). This decrease in affinity of [^{35}S]proteoglycans for hyaluronate with intratissue acidification was not due to degradation of hyaluronate-binding sites, because neither compression nor low pH during chase affected the maximum capacity of tissue monomers or ^{35}S monomers to form aggregates, with 77–86% eluting as aggregates after mixture with excess (5% w/w) hyaluronate and excess (5% w/w) link protein.

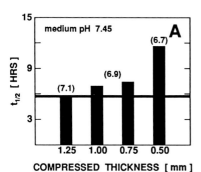

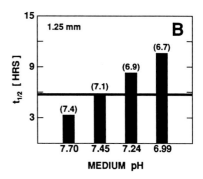

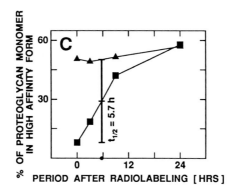

FIG. 3. Effect of static compression and altered medium pH on the hyaluronate-binding properties of radiolabeled proteoglycans from cartilage disks. Cartilage disks were radiolabeled with [^{35}S]sulfate for 1.5 hr and then chase-incubated for 0–24 hr while: **A:** compressed to a thickness of 0.50, 0.75, 1.00, or 1.25 mm (the initial cartilage explant thickness) while in medium at pH 7.45 or **B:** bathed in HCl- or NaOH-titrated medium at pH 6.99, 7.24, 7.45, or 7.70 while held at a thickness of 1.25 mm. Values in parentheses are estimates of interstitial pH, computed from the medium pH and charge density of compressed cartilage disks (17). After the chase period, high-buoyant density proteoglycan monomers were purified. **C:** Example of subsequent analysis to determine the characteristic time ($t_{1/2}$) for conversion of low-affinity ^{35}S monomers to the high-affinity form in control disks held at 1.25 mm in medium at pH 7.45. Portions of monomers were allowed to react with 1.6% (w/w) hyaluronate and then fractionated by Sephacryl S-1000 chromatography to determine the percentage of ^{35}S monomers (■) and total tissue monomers (▲) with a high affinity for hyaluronate. The ratio of percentages was computed, and $t_{1/2}$ is defined as the extrapolated chase time at which the ratio has increased to half of the maximum. (Data adapted from ref. 40.)

EFFECTS OF CYCLIC COMPRESSION ON THE LOSS OF NEWLY SYNTHESIZED PROTEIN AND PROTEOGLYCAN FROM CARTILAGE EXPLANTS

The rate of loss of proteoglycans from cartilage is modulated, in part, by enzymatic degradation (23). Proteoglycans are cleaved between the G1 and G2 globular domains, rendering the large G2-containing fragment unable to aggregate with hyaluronate and, consequently, able to diffuse within the matrix more rapidly than do intact aggregated monomers. Thus, catabolized monomers are preferentially released from thin cartilage slices *in vitro,* and the proteoglycans in the medium are more polydisperse and of smaller average size than are the proteoglycans remaining in the tissue.

The effects of compression on the degradation and loss of newly synthesized proteoglycan and collagenous protein from cartilage explants were examined (41). Cartilage disks were radiolabeled with 100 μCi/ml [^{35}S]sulfate and 160 μCi/ml L-[5-^{3}H]proline for $\sim$24 hr and were then washed with four to six changes of medium over $\sim$2 hr. Disks were then incubated free-swelling for another 1.5–2 days. This time was sufficient to allow newly synthesized proteoglycans to be converted to the high-affinity form (Fig. 3), and to allow newly synthesized collagens to become enriched in [^{3}H]hydroxyproline residues: $\sim$35% of the ^{3}H radioactivity was in the form of [^{3}H]hydroxyproline, and $\sim$80% of the [^{3}H]proline incorporated into the cartilage explants could be accounted for as ^{3}H radioactivity in collagen (41). Groups of 12 disks were then transferred to fresh medium for 24 hr of cyclic compression: 2 hr of compression to 1.00, 0.75, or 0.50 mm (2 hr on), followed by a release to 1.25 mm (2 hr off); control disks were held at 1.25 mm. After compression, disks were returned to the free-swelling state and either analyzed for wet and dry weights or incubated for an additional 5 days. The latter disks were guanidine-HCl-extracted or papain-digested, as described above, to quantitate ^{35}S and ^{3}H radioactivity, proteoglycan, and [^{3}H]-hydroxyproline constituents and to isolate and characterize cartilage proteoglycan. Throughout the culture period, medium was changed every 12–24 hr, and spent medium was stored at $-20°$C with proteinase inhibitors. Portions of the spent medium were analyzed for ^{35}S and ^{3}H radioactivity, ^{35}S macromolecules (by gel filtration chromatography on Sephadex G-25), total proteoglycan, and [^{3}H]hydroxyproline constituents.

The total ^{35}S and ^{3}H radioactivity was calculated as that remaining in the disks at the termination of the experiment plus all the radioactivity lost into the medium after the first day of chase. Control studies indicated that subsequent to this initial chase, the total ^{35}S and ^{3}H radioactivity as well as the total [^{3}H]hydroxyproline constituents in the culture system (i.e., remaining in the disks and lost into the medium) were constant. The cumulative loss from the tissue of ^{35}S macromolecules and [^{3}H]hydroxyproline components was determined. As in previous studies (e.g., refs. 25 and 26), the majority ($\sim$80%) of the ^{35}S radioactivity in the medium was macromolecular; the time ($t_{1/2}$) for half of the ^{35}S radioactivity to be released was extrapolated from the release of ^{35}S during the 5 days following compression.

During the 24 hr of cyclic (2 hr on/2 hr off) compression, the loss of [^{35}S]proteoglycan (Fig. 4A) was increased when compared to 1.25-mm control rates (+23%, +32%, and +124%, respectively). Over the following 5 days of incubation, the rates of loss from highly compressed disks remained somewhat

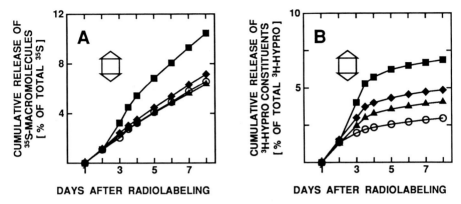

FIG. 4. Effect of 24 hr of cyclic compression on loss of ^{35}S-labeled macromolecules and [3H]hydroxyproline constituents from cartilage explants. Cartilage disks were radiolabeled with ^{35}S]sulfate and [3H]proline, washed, incubated free-swelling for 1.5–2 days, and then subjected to cyclic 2-hr-on/2-hr-off compression from 1.25 mm to 0.50 mm (■), 0.75 mm (◆), or 1.00 mm (▲) or subjected to static maintenance at a thickness of 1.25 mm (○). The double-headed arrows indicate the 24-hr period during which cyclic compression was applied. Disks were then incubated free-swelling for five more days. Medium from individual disks (12 per treatment group) was collected daily, pooled, and analyzed along with the cartilage disks to determine the cumulative loss into the medium of ^{35}S-labeled macromolecules (**A**) and [3H]hydroxyproline constituents (**B**). (Data adapted from ref. 41.)

elevated whereas rates from less compressed disks were similar to controls; the extrapolated $t_{1/2}$ values for disks cycled to 1.00, 0.75, and 0.50 mm were 72, 63, and 47 days, respectively, compared to a $t_{1/2}$ of 68 days in controls. Therefore, the net effect of 24-hr cyclic compression was a graded increase in the cumulative loss (during 7 days) of ^{35}S]proteoglycan, from 6.6% in 1.25-mm control disks to 7.2% and 10.5% in samples subjected to cyclic compression to 0.75 and 0.50 mm, respectively. The loss of total tissue proteoglycan (not shown) paralleled the loss of ^{35}S]proteoglycan during and following cyclic compression.

The effect of 24-hr cyclic (2 hr on/2 hr off) compression on release of collagenous [3H]hydroxyproline-containing molecules was even more pronounced. During cyclic compression to 1.00, 0.75, and 0.50 mm, there was a graded increase in release of [3H]hydroxyproline constituents (Fig. 4B). The rate of release of [3H]hydroxyproline constituents remained substantially elevated in compressed disks (relative to that of controls) throughout the remainder of the incubation. The net effect of 24-hr cyclic compression was a graded increase in the cumulative loss (during 7 days) of [3H]hydroxyproline constituents, from 3.0% in 1.25-mm control disks to 4.1%, 4.9%, and 6.9% in samples subjected to cyclic compression to 1.00, 0.75, and 0.50 mm, respectively.

The increased release during cyclic compression appeared to be associated with the dynamic fluid exudation phase of compression rather than with the time-averaged static component of compression. Independent experiments indicated that loss of radiolabeled macromolecules was enhanced during the initial

2 hr of compression (41). In contrast, once fluid exudation had ceased and static compaction was achieved [e.g., during longer 12-hr (41) or 1- to 4-day compression (29)], the rates of loss of [^{35}S]proteoglycans were decreased. Other experiments indicated that loss rates from radiolabeled disks were not greatly altered by incubation in acid-titrated medium. Thus, intratissue acidification during cyclic compression did not appear to be responsible for the accelerated loss of radiolabeled macromolecules from the tissue (41). The increased loss during compression appeared to be independent of possible cellular release or activation of proteinases, because cyclic compression also stimulated matrix loss from biosynthetically inactive cartilage disks bathed in a 4°C PBS solution in the presence of proteinase inhibitors (data not shown). Furthermore, although the [^{35}S]-proteoglycans lost during cyclic compression to 0.50 mm were of smaller average size than those from controls, cyclic compression did not affect the high aggregability ($\sim 70\%$) of the [^{35}S]proteoglycans remaining in the tissue, nor did it affect the low aggregability ($\sim 15\%$) of the [^{35}S]proteoglycans released into the medium (41). Yet, high-amplitude cyclic compression did appear to alter matrix structure. Immediately after cyclic compression, highly compressed samples were more swollen than the controls (84.0 ± 0.5% water in 0.50-mm cycled samples versus 82.8 ± 0.5% in controls, $p < 0.05$).

CONCLUDING REMARKS

The results described here demonstrate that static, oscillatory, and high-amplitude cyclic mechanical compression can markedly alter chondrocyte and matrix metabolism in cartilage explants. The induced biophysical phenomena are highly dependent on the amplitude and frequency of loading, as are the metabolic effects, as summarized in Fig. 5. In this section, we speculate on the role of biophysical regulation of matrix metabolism in the maintenance of normal cartilage or, alternatively, in the initiation and progression of cartilage degeneration.

The static physicochemical mechanisms involved in the inhibition of proteoglycan synthesis and the prolongation of subsequent extracellular processing may play a physiological role in the development and remodeling of an ordered, proteoglycan-rich matrix (Fig. 5A and 5B). On a microstructural level, chondrocytes in proteoglycan-depleted regions and of low fixed charge density would synthesize proteoglycan at a relatively high rate relative to that of chondrocytes in proteoglycan-rich regions (17). Once secreted, newly synthesized proteoglycan with a low affinity for hyaluronate may be able to diffuse through the proteoglycan-rich regions (of relatively low intratissue pH), preferentially reaching proteoglycan-poor regions (of relatively high pH), where they are functionally required (Fig. 5A). There, these proteoglycans are converted into the high-affinity form (Fig. 3A and 3B) (40) and stabilized into aggregates with hyaluronate (Fig. 5B). Also, during static compression (relatively low intratissue pH), newly synthesized proteoglycan may remain for a relatively long time in the low-affinity

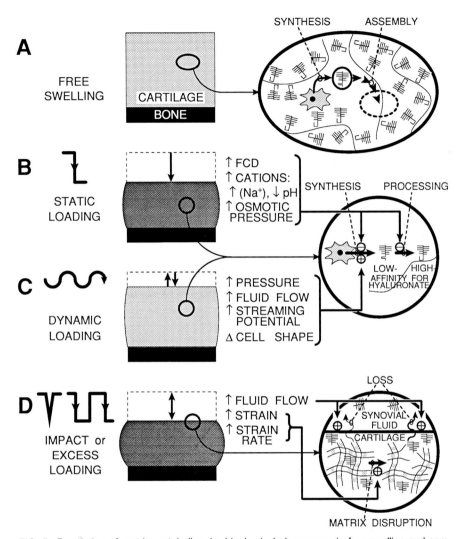

FIG. 5. Regulation of matrix metabolism by biophysical phenomena in free-swelling and compressed cartilage. Interstitial ion concentrations regulate the synthesis and subsequent extracellular processing of proteoglycan. In free-swelling cartilage (**A**), local regions of low proteoglycan content [and low fixed charge density (FCD)] attract a relatively low concentration of positive counterions (Na^+, H^+). Such a milieu stimulates chondrocyte synthesis of proteoglycan (17) and accelerates the conversion of newly formed proteoglycan with a low-affinity for hyaluronate to the form with a high-affinity for hyaluronate (Fig. 3) (40). Thus, proteoglycan formation and deposition would be favored in regions relatively lacking in proteoglycan. During static compression (**B**), regions have an increased FCD, an increased concentration of positive counterions, and an increased osmotic pressure; such factors inhibit proteoglycan synthesis (16,17,36) and processing (Fig. 3) (40). Dynamic compression can alter matrix metabolism through biophysical mechanisms other than physicochemical phenomena. During oscillatory compression (**C**), hydrostatic pressure, fluid flow, streaming potentials, and altered cell shape may stimulate biosynthesis (Fig. 2) (38,42). During excess or impact loading (**D**), fluid convection can increase loss of matrix macromolecules from cartilage into the bathing fluid, whereas high levels of strain or strain rate may cause matrix disruption, tissue swelling, and accentuated diffusion within cartilage (Fig. 4) (41).

form (with freedom to diffuse through the compacted matrix meshwork) before being stabilized in the high-affinity form. On a more macroscopic level, a differential growth of tissue could mold an efficient joint structure where applied loads are distributed over a broad contact area. Inhibition of proteoglycan synthesis and processing in regions where tissue is highly compressed would allow surrounding regions where tissue is less compressed to build up more matrix; these surrounding regions would then share the burden of applied load.

Low-displacement high-frequency oscillatory compression of cartilage explants can stimulate matrix biosynthesis, perhaps by generating high hydrostatic pressure, high fluid velocity, and high streaming potential but little deformation of cells and matrix (Fig. 5C). The frequency-dependence (Fig. 2B and 2C) (38) and spatial distribution (43) of the biosynthetic response *in vitro* may reflect the spatial and temporal distribution of these physical stimuli associated with the mechanical test configuration. Such dependencies allow further examination of the role of hypothesized physical regulators. For example, with the same applied compression amplitude and frequency, the resulting pressurization at the center of a disk is relatively greater for larger-diameter specimens (52). On the other hand, it is interesting that studies of continuous passive motion *in vivo* have utilized a frequency of 0.025 Hz (55), which is within the frequency range of biosynthetic stimulation *in vitro* (Fig. 2B). More detailed studies of the metabolic effects of low-displacement oscillatory compression, including the onset and duration of biosynthetic effects as well as matrix degradation and loss into the medium, would be important in making further physiologic interpretations. Biosynthetic stimulation during oscillatory compression *in vitro* may be related to the long-term increase in proteoglycan content with increased loading *in vivo* (6,7) or, conversely, related to the net loss of proteoglycan with the reduction or absence of dynamic loading (6,7).

High-amplitude 24-hr cyclic compression of cartilage explants can induce immediate increases in tissue swelling as well as prolonged increases in the rate of release of matrix macromolecules, while generating high levels of compressive or shear stresses, strains, or strain rates (Fig. 5D). Such mechanical forces may have disrupted the collagen meshwork and thereby led to the subsequent increase of the diffusion of macromolecules within and out of the cartilage matrix (Fig. 4A and 4B) (41). Diffusion of macromolecules also appeared to be an important mechanism during prolonged static compression when loss of matrix molecules was impeded (29,41). In the uniaxially compressed configuration, the impermeable compression platens form physical barriers at the cartilage surfaces and thus constrain mobile matrix molecules to travel over a longer distance to escape from the tissue. In addition, matrix compaction forces molecules to take a more tortuous path, effectively decreasing the diffusivity of molecules within the matrix. Both of these factors would increase the characteristic time of proteoglycan diffusion out of the cartilage disk during static compression (3). In addition, high-amplitude 2-hr-on/2-hr-off cyclic compression induces fluid exudation and imbibition (38). Such fluid flow appeared to entrain radiolabeled macromolecules and to thereby cause a convective redistribution of molecules within, and transport from, cartilage (Fig. 4A and 4B) (41). Compressive strain and fluid flow would be particularly high in tissue that is partially damaged (e.g., swollen due to matrix disruption or unable to resist compression for lack of proteoglycan). These physical mechanisms may relate to (a) matrix disruption *in vivo* following repeated impact loading (56,57) and (b) the initiation and possible progression of osteoarthritis (10).

These studies provide a framework for further examining the biophysical mechanisms involved in modulating synthesis, assembly, degradation, and loss of matrix molecules in cartilage during dynamic loading. Studies on the metabolism and transport of specific molecules, such as growth factors, small proteoglycans, and minor collagens, may be particularly relevant to cartilage structure and function. In addition, precise but disruptive long-term mechanical loading of adult cartilage explants in various culture configurations may yield insights into the direct role of biophysical mechanisms in cartilage degeneration. A model of controlled mechanically induced cartilage degeneration *in vitro* may allow testing of physical protocols or pharmacologic agents designed to limit or reverse cartilage disease processes.

ACKNOWLEDGMENT

This work was supported by NIH grant AR33236 and fellowships to RLS from the NIH Medical Science Training Program and Whitaker Health Sciences Fund.

REFERENCES

1. Buckwalter J, Hunziker E, Rosenberg L, Coutts R, Adams M, Eyre D. Articular cartilage: injury and repair. In: Woo SY, Buckwalter JA, eds. *Injury and repair of the musculoskeletal soft tissues.* Park Ridge, IL: American Academy of Orthopaedic Surgeons, 1988;405–425.
2. Kempson GE. Mechanical properties of articular cartilage. In: Freeman MAR, ed. *Adult articular cartilage,* 2nd ed. Tunbridge Wells, England: Pitman, 1979;333–414.
3. Maroudas A. Physico-chemical properties of articular cartilage. In: Freeman MAR, ed. *Adult articular cartilage.* 2nd ed. Tunbridge Wells, England: Pitman, 1979;215–290.
4. Grodzinsky AJ. Electromechanical and physicochemical properties of connective tissue. *CRC Crit Rev Bioeng* 1983;9:133–199.
5. Mow VC, Holmes MH, Lai WM. Fluid transport and mechanical properties of articular cartilage: a review. *J Biomech* 1984;17:377–394.
6. Caterson B, Lowther DA. Changes in the metabolism of the proteoglycans from sheep articular cartilage in response to mechanical stress. *Biochim Biophys Acta* 1978;540:412–422.
7. Kiviranta I, Jurvelin J, Tammi M, Saamanen AM, Helminen HJ. Weight bearing controls glycosaminoglycan concentration and articular cartilage thickness in the knee joints of young beagle dogs. *Arthritis Rheum* 1987;30:801–809.
8. Gritzka TL, Fry LR, Cheesman RL, Lavigne A. Deterioration of articular cartilage caused by continuous compression in a moving rabbit joint. *J Bone Joint Surg* 1973;55A:1698–1720.
9. Radin EL, Martin RB, Burr DB, Caterson B, Boyd RD, Goodwin C. Effects of mechanical loading on the tissues of the rabbit knee. *J Orthop Res* 1984;2:221–234.
10. Muir IHM. Current and future trends in articular cartilage research and osteoarthritis. In: Kuettner K, Schleyerbach R, Hascall VC, eds. *Articular cartilage biochemistry,* New York: Raven Press, 1986;423–440.
11. Schalkwijk J, Joosten LAB, van den Berg WB, van Wyk JJ, van de Putte LBA. Insulin-like

growth factor stimulation of chondrocyte proteoglycan synthesis by human synovial fluid. *Arthritis Rheum* 1989;32:66–71.

12. Farkas T, Boyd RD, Schaffler MB, Radin EL, Burr DB. Early vascular changes in rabbit subchondral bone after repetitive impulsive loading. *Clin Orthop* 1987;219:259–267.

13. Poole CA, Flint MH, Beaumont BW. Morphological and functional interrelationships of articular cartilage matrices. *J Anat* 1984;138:113–138.

14. Mak AF. Unconfined compression of hydrated viscoelastic tissues: a biphasic poroviscoelastic analysis. *Biorheology* 1986;23:371–383.

15. Frank EH, Grodzinsky AJ. Cartilage electromechanics. I. electrokinetic transduction and the effects of electrolyte pH and ionic strength. *J Biomechanics* 1987;20:615–627.

16. Schneiderman R, Kevet D, Maroudas A. Effects of mechanical and osmotic pressure on the rate of glycosaminoglycan synthesis in the human adult femoral head cartilage: an *in vitro* study. *J Orthop Res* 1986;4:393–408.

17. Gray ML, Pizzanelli AM, Grodzinsky AJ, Lee RC. Mechanical and physicochemical determinants of the chondrocyte biosynthetic response. *J Orthop Res* 1988;6:777–792.

18. Armstrong CG, Lai WM, Mow VC. An analysis of the unconfined compression of articular cartilage. *J Biomech Eng* 1984;106:165–173.

19. Eisenberg SR, Grodzinsky AJ. The kinetics of chemically induced nonequilibrium swelling of articular cartilage and corneal stroma. *J Biomech Eng* 1987;109:79–89.

20. Frank EH, Grodzinsky AJ. Cartilage electromechanics. II. A continuum model of cartilage electrokinetics and correlation with experiments. *J Biomech* 1987;20:629–639.

21. Hascall VC, Handley CJ, McQuillan DJ, Hascall GK, Robinson HC, Lowther DA. The effect of serum on biosynthesis of proteoglycans by bovine articular cartilage in culture. *Arch Biochem Biophys* 1983;224:206–223.

22. Hascall VC, Luyten FP, Plaas AHK, Sandy JD. Steady-state metabolism of proteoglycans in bovine articular cartilage. In: Maroudas A, Kuettner K, eds. *Methods in cartilage research.* San Diego: Academic Press, 1990;108–112.

23. Hardingham T, Bayliss M. Proteoglycans of articular cartilage: changes in aging and in joint disease. *Semin Arthritis Rheum* 1990;20S:12–33.

24. Poole AR. Enzymatic degradation: cartilage destruction. In: Brandt KD, ed. *Cartilage changes in osteoarthritis.* Indianapolis, IN: Indiana University School of Medicine, 1990;63–72.

25. Morales T, Roberts A. Transforming growth factor β regulates the metabolism of proteoglycans in bovine cartilage organ cultures. *J Biol Chem* 1988;263:12828–12831.

26. Morales TI, Hascall VC. Effects of interleukin-1 and lipopolysaccharides on protein and carbohydrate metabolism in bovine articular cartilage organ cultures. *Connect Tissue Res* 1989;10:255–275.

27. Luyten FP, Hascall VC, Nissley SP, Morales TI, Reddi AH. Insulin-like growth factors maintain steady-state metabolism of proteoglycans in bovine articular cartilage explants. *Arch Biochem Biophys* 1988;267:416–425.

28. Sokoloff L. *In vitro* culture of joints and articular tissues. In: Sokoloff L, ed. *The joints and synovial fluid.* New York: Academic Press, 1980;1–27.

29. Jones IL, Klamfeldt DDS, Sandstrom T. The effect of continuous mechanical pressure upon the turnover of articular cartilage proteoglycans *in vitro. Clin Orthop* 1982;165:283–289.

30. Palmoski MJ, Brandt KD. Effects of static and cyclic compressive loading on articular cartilage plugs in vitro. *Arthritis Rheum* 1984;27:675–681.

31. Kimura JH, Schipplein OD, Kuettner KE, Andriacchi TP. Effects of hydrostatic loading on extracellular matrix formation. *Trans Orthop Res Soc* 1984;9:365.

32. van Kampen GPJ, Veldhuijzen R, Kuijer R, van de Stadt RJ, Schipper CA. Cartilage response to mechanical force in high-density chondrocyte cultures. *Arthritis Rheum* 1985;28:419–424.

33. Bayliss MT, Urban JPG, Johnstone B, Holm S. *In vitro* method for measuring synthesis rates in the intervertebral disc. *J Orthop Res* 1986;4:10–17.

34. Klein-Nulend J, Veldhuijzen JP, van de Stadt RJ, van Kampen GPJ, Kuijer R, Burger EH. Influence of intermittent compressive force on proteoglycan content in calcifying growth plate cartilage *in vitro. J Biol Chem* 1987;262:15490–15495.

35. Gray ML, Pizzanelli AM, Lee RC, Grodzinsky AJ, Swann DA. Kinetics of the chondrocyte biosynthetic response to compressive load and release. *Biochim Biophys Acta* 1989;991:415–425.

36. Urban JPG, Bayliss MT. Regulation of proteoglycan synthesis rate in cartilage *in vitro:* influence of extracellular ionic composition. *Biochem Biophys Acta* 1989;992:59–65.

37. Parkkinen JJ, Lammi MJ, Karjalainen S, Laakkonen J, Hyvarinen E, Tiihonen A, Helminen HJ, Tammi M. A mechanical apparatus with microprocessor controlled stress profile for cyclic compression of cultured articular cartilage explants. *J Biomech* 1989;22:1285–1291.
38. Sah RL, Kim YJ, Doong JH, Grodzinsky AJ, Plaas AHK, Sandy JD. Biosynthetic response of cartilage explants to dynamic compression. *J Orthop Res* 1989;7:619–636.
39. Sah RL, Kim YJ, Grodzinsky AJ. The effect of mechanical compression on cartilage metabolism. In: Maroudas A, Kuettner KE, eds. *Methods for cartilage research.* New York: Academic Press, 1990;116–119.
40. Sah RL, Grodzinsky AJ, Plaas AHK, Sandy JD. Effects of tissue compression on the hyaluronate binding properties of newly synthesized proteoglycans in cartilage explants. *Biochem J* 1990;267:803–808.
41. Sah RL, Doong JYH, Grodzinsky AJ, Plaas AHK, Sandy JD. Effects of compression on the loss of newly synthesized proteoglycans and proteins from cartilage explants. *Arch Biochem Biophys* 1991;286:20–29.
42. Hall AC, Urban JPG, Gehl KA. The effects of hydrostatic pressure on matrix synthesis in articular cartilage. *J Orthop Res* 1991;9:1–10.
43. Kim YJ, Sah RL, Grodzinsky AJ, Plaas AHK, Sandy JD. Stimulation of cartilage biosynthesis by dynamic compression: physical mechanisms. *Trans Orthop Res Soc* 1991;16:53.
44. Afoke NYP, Byers PD, Hutton WC. Contact pressures in the human hip joint. *J Bone Joint Surg* 1987;69B:536–541.
45. Hodge WA, Fijan RS, Carlson KL, Burgess RG, Harris WH, Mann RW. Contact pressures in the human hip joint measured *in vivo*. *Proc Natl Acad Sci USA* 1986;83:2879–2883.
46. Huberti HH, Hayes WC. Patellofemoral contact pressures: the influence of *q*-angle and tendo-femoral contact. *J Bone Joint Surg* 1984;66A:715–724.
47. Armstrong CG, Bahrani AS, Gardner DL. Changes in the deformational behavior of human hip cartilage with age. *J Biomech Eng* 1980;102:214–220.
48. Weightman B, Kempson GE. Load carriage. In: Freeman MAR, ed. *Adult articular cartilage,* 2nd ed. Tunbridge Wells, England: Pitman, 1979;291–332.
49. Eberhardt AW, Keer LM, Lewis JL, Vithoontien V. An analytical model of joint contact. *J Biomech Eng* 1990;112:407–413.
50. DeWitt MT, Handley CJ, Oakes BW, Lowther DA. *In vitro* response of chondrocytes to mechanical loading: the effect of short term mechanical tension. *Connect Tissue Res* 1984;12:97–109.
51. Maroudas A, Evans H. Sulphate diffusion and incorporation into human articular cartilage. *Biochim Biophys Acta* 1974;338:265–279.
52. Kim Y. Radially unconfined compression of poroelastic media with axisymmetric boundary condition. Master's thesis, Massachusetts Institute of Technology, Cambridge, MA, 1989.
53. Sandy JD, Plaas AHK. Studies on the hyaluronate binding properties of newly synthesized proteoglycans purified from articular chondrocyte cultures. *Arch Biochem Biophys* 1989;271:300–314.
54. Plaas AHK, Sandy JD. The affinity of newly synthesized proteoglycan for hyaluronic acid can be enhanced by exposure to mild alkali. *Biochem J* 1986;234:221–223.
55. Salter RB, Simmonds DF, Malcolm BW, Rumble EJ, MacMichael D, Clements ND. The biological effect of continuous passive motion on the healing of full-thickness defects in articular cartilage. *J Bone Joint Surg* 1980;62A:1232–1251.
56. Repo RU, Finlay JB. Survival of articular cartilage after controlled impact. *J Bone Joint Surg* 1977;59A:1068–1076.
57. Donohue JM, Buss D, Oegema TR, Thompson RC. The effects of indirect blunt trauma on adult canine articular cartilage. *J Bone Joint Surg* 1983;65A:948–957.

DISCUSSION

Lust: Can you speculate whether cyclic loading or static loading would be more deleterious at force levels that may damage the tissue?

Grodzinsky: Low-amplitude dynamic compression can stimulate synthesis of matrix macromolecules at forces that are relevant to those used in animal studies. However, large-amplitude compressions applied for 2 hr but initiated at a high enough rate could damage the collagen network. It is possible that such techniques might enable us to detect mechanical initiation of damage versus enzymatic initiation of damage. This might help identify families of diseases that involve mechanical induction of matrix damage.

Lust: Would a static load for a long time be likely to cause collagen fibril damage?

Grodzinsky: We cannot answer that based on the data we have. Large enough amplitude on/off loads do appear to induce such damage, however.

Lohmander: Your experiments showed that prelabeled proteoglycans are released from the matrix at an increased rate after initiating certain low-amplitude force protocols, at least during the first several hours. Is this because of a stimulation of degradation pathways or the facilitated loss of predegraded molecules?

Grodzinsky: We found with plugs maintained at 4°C with protease inhibitors during the 24-hr loading period also exhibited this enhanced loss of labeled proteoglycans into the medium. However, the loss that occurred during 5–8 days of chase under normal culture conditions may reflect both mechanisms.

Hascall: In the case where you observed a correlation between dynamic stiffness and proteoglycan synthesis, what happens if you decrease stiffness by modifying the proteoglycan phase, with chondroitinase for example?

Grodzinsky: The cells may modulate synthesis in response to biomechanical or streaming potential changes which depend upon the proteoglycan phase. One of the problems is that the stimuli are coupled. That is, whenever there is fluid flow, there is streaming potential. We have been able to look at which of these components may be more important. Young-Jo Kim cored plugs from cartilage disks after dynamic loading to divide them into regions where there would be preferentially higher hydrostatic pressure versus higher fluid flow and streaming potential. For example, at a high enough frequency in the unconfined compression system there would be higher fluid flow at the periphery, but little elevation in hydrostatic pressure, whereas in the central region of the disk there would be high hydrostatic pressure and much lower fluid velocities. Young-Jo observed that there was stimulation of synthesis in both regions, but synthesis was slightly higher in the periphery. This suggests that fluid transport may play a very important role but that hydrostatic pressure may also be important.

Articular Cartilage and Osteoarthritis,
edited by K. Kuettner et al.
Raven Press, Ltd., New York © 1992.

27

Physical Modifiers of Cartilage Metabolism

Jill Urban and Andrew Hall

University Laboratory of Physiology, Oxford University, Oxford OX1 3PT, England

It has long been established that one of the factors regulating matrix synthesis in cartilage is feedback from the matrix itself (1). Turnover may be mediated via cellular receptors for matrix components (2). However, changes in matrix composition affect the environment of the cells in other ways: For example, a fall in proteoglycan concentration lowers extracellular osmolarity by affecting the ionic composition of the matrix (3). Cartilage stiffness is thus decreased, and consequently tissue deformation and fluid loss under mechanical loads increase. These physical changes to the chondrocyte's environment may also signal changes in cartilage composition and thus may be important in regulating matrix turnover. In this chapter we discuss the influence of the matrix on the physical environment of the chondrocytes and also discuss how changes to this environment affect cell behavior.

THE PHYSICAL ENVIRONMENT OF THE CHONDROCYTE

Chondrocytes live in an unusual environment for a mammalian cell. They usually lie isolated from one another and are enclosed in a dense extracellular matrix containing a high concentration of proteoglycans (4). The fixed negative charges on the proteoglycans dictate the extracellular ionic composition, which in accordance with the Gibbs–Donnan equilibrium equations contains a high concentration of free cations and a low concentration of anions (3). As shown by these equations, the concentration of any ion in the tissue depends on the concentration of that ion in the bathing medium. Ion concentrations are also very sensitive to the concentration of proteoglycans and will follow proteoglycan concentration, varying with position on the joint and from the surface to the deep zone (3). From studies of isolated "chondrons" and from x-ray probe microanalysis (5) there is also some suggestion that the immediate ionic environment of the chondrocyte may differ from that of the bulk matrix. As shown by Grushko et al. (6; also see chapter by Maroudas et al.), it is the effective proteoglycan concentration (i.e., the concentration in the interfibrillar space) which determines ion distributions, and to calculate these correctly it is also necessary to know the fraction of fluid in the collagen fibers which is unavailable to proteoglycans. Table 1 gives values of the ranges of free ion concentrations found in various cartilages, estimated from the Gibbs–Donnan equilibrium conditions and from the proteoglycan and collagen contents of the tissue. Where tested, the calculated values are in agreement with those determined experimentally (6).

As shown in Table 1, the concentration of inorganic ions in the matrix imparts a high osmotic pressure to the tissue, considerably higher than that of the surrounding plasma or synovial fluid. As a result of this osmotic pressure difference, fluid tends to be imbibed by the matrix, thereby setting the collagen fiber system into tension and creating hydrostatic pressure in the tissue. Fluid equilibrium is achieved when the hydrostatic pressure in the tissue balances the osmotic pressure difference between the matrix and the surrounding fluid. The hydrostatic pressure in unloaded articular cartilage is thus around 1–2 atm, as has been demonstrated experimentally (6). The chondrocytes in resting articular cartilage are thus normally under hydrostatic pressures of this magnitude.

As well as determining the distribution of major ions which contribute to the osmotic pressure around the cell, the fixed negative charge of the matrix also determines the distribution of hydrogen ions and thus the pH. From the Donnan equilibrium, the hydrogen ion concentrations must always be higher in the tissue than in the external solution, and the pH in cartilage consequently is lower (3). In living cartilage an additional factor, lactate, affects extracellular pH. Weight-bearing cartilages are avascular, so that some chondrocytes, such as those in the center of the nucleus of the human disc, are as much as 8–9 mm from the nearest blood vessels, whereas in adult human cartilage some chondrocytes are 1–2 mm from their nutrient supply. Steep gradients in nutrient concentrations develop, and because metabolism is mainly anaerobic, lactate levels in the center of the tissue may be up to 10 times greater than those in the surrounding plasma or synovial fluid (7). Gradients in pH consequently exist, and values as low as pH 6.5 have been measured in human discs *in vivo*.

The chondrocytes of weight-bearing cartilages are routinely exposed to large

TABLE 1. *Estimated ranges of free pericellular ion concentrations in cartilage*

Tissue	Region	[Na] (mM)	[K] (mM)	[Cl] (mM)	[Ca] (mM)	[π] (mOsm)	References
Human adult femoral head (40–50 years old)	Surface	240–270	7–9	60–90	6–9	310–370	3,6
	Deep	300–350	9–12	50–100	14–19	370–480	
Human adult disc (40–70 years old)	Nucleus	330–400	11–14	30–70	13–21	380–500	3,7
	Outer annulus	220–280	6–9	50–110	4–8	280–400	
	End-plate	230–280	6–8	80–110	3–7	320–400	
Bovine metacarpal (2 years old)	Full depth	220–260	6–9	70–100	7–10	310–380	12
DMEM, plasma, synovial fluid		120–140	5	140–150	1.5–2.5	250–300	

and varying mechanical loads. Loading deforms the matrix and increases the hydrostatic pressure of the tissue, and thus of the chondrocyte. The pressures *in vivo* may rise to 100–200 atm within milliseconds on standing, and may cycle between resting values and 40–50 atm when walking (8). If the load is maintained for any length of time, fluid is expressed, thereby increasing proteoglycan concentration and fixed charge density and consequently affecting the concentration of ions in the matrix and around the cell.

The chondrocyte in cartilage is thus surrounded by a high-extracellular-osmolarity, low-pH fluid that contains a high concentration of cations and a low concentration of anions and is under a resting pressure of around 2 atm. It routinely experiences changes to this environment when loads are applied. Chondrocytes in this changing environment maintain the composition of the cartilage matrix at quasi-steady-state values. How is this achieved? Are chondrocytes insensitive to alterations in their physical environment, especially within the physiological range, or, alternatively, is the steady-state composition of cartilage the net result of the response of the chondrocyte to these changes? If so, what are the signals linking the chondrocyte's response to its physical environment?

EFFECT OF CHANGES IN THE PHYSICAL ENVIRONMENT ON CHONDROCYTE BEHAVIOR

Matrix turnover certainly appears to be affected by changes to the physical environment of the chondrocyte. This has been most clearly seen in *in vivo* studies on the effects of mechanical load on cartilage synthesis and composition. In the long term, increasing load on one area of cartilage appears to increase cartilage thickness and proteoglycan concentration, whereas in unloaded cartilage the matrix thins and the proteoglycans are lost (9). Studies *in vitro* show that chondrocytes in cartilage respond directly to changes in load. The response is fast (within an hour), and the response depends critically on the nature of the load applied. As discussed in the studies of Sah et al. (10), loads which tend to raise hydrostatic pressure and cause fluid movement without significant fluid loss lead to an increase in matrix synthesis rates, whereas loading regimes which cause fluid loss decrease synthesis rates. The effects of load thus appear to be mediated mainly by these changes in the physical environment of the chondrocyte.

Chondrocytes in the Cartilage Matrix

The Effect of Changes in Hydrostatic Pressure on Synthesis Rates

When load is applied to cartilage, the hydrostatic pressure rises. Because, as shown below, hydrostatic pressure can affect many cellular processes, it is likely that the chondrocyte would also respond to changes in hydrostatic pressure. It is possible to study the direct effect of hydrostatic pressure on behavior of cartilage and chondrocytes, independently of other changes to the tissue. This is because hydrostatic pressure can be applied uniformly, does not cause fluid flow, and does not deform the tissue macroscopically, since water, the major component of cartilage, is virtually incompressible over the physiological range of pressure.

The influence of hydrostatic pressure has been examined in embryonic epiphyseal chondrocytes and cartilage (11). Low levels of pressure, around 0.1 MPa (1 atm above ambient), were found to have a noticeable effect on chondrocyte behavior. The experimental system used in these studies included a gas phase, and thus the consequent rise in pO_2 and pCO_2 complicates interpretation of these experiments. However, by whatever means the effect was mediated, it is clear that alterations to the physical environment affected synthesis, calcification, and proteoglycan production in these tests.

Physiological levels of hydrostatic pressure appear to have a significant effect on matrix synthesis rates in articular cartilage. In general, hydrostatic pressures between 5 and 15 MPa (50–150 atm) lead to an increase in the rate of sulfate and amino acid incorporation (12); these levels of stimulation are similar to those reported by others during studies of cartilage loading *in vitro* (10), suggesting that this pressure rise may be the cause of stimulation seen in loading. This stimulation is seen even if the pressure is applied for only the first 20 sec of a 2-hr incubation (Fig. 1). A short mechanical stimulus that leads to a prolonged cellular response has also been reported in bone (13) and in the compression-resistant zone of the flexor tendon (14). If, on the other hand, the same levels of pressure are applied continuously for 2 hr, stimulation still occurs but is less marked. Pressures above physiological levels have no effect if applied for 20 sec, but depress synthesis if applied for 2 hr (Fig. 1). These results suggest that hydrostatic pressure has at least two different effects on the synthetic pathway which lead to changes in tracer incorporation rates. The first effect is stimulatory and only requires a single short application of pressure, whereas the other is inhibitory and dependent on the magnitude of the applied pressure. The net effect of pressure application depends on the relative effect of each component. For example, if 15 MPa is applied for 20 sec or 5 min, synthesis is stimulated by 40%, and 20%, respectively, whereas 15 MPa applied for 2 hr has no effect.

Effect of Fluid Loss on Matrix Synthesis Rates

When a static load is applied to cartilage, fluid is expressed from the tissue, and the amount is directly related to the magnitude of the load and to the composition of the tissue. The invariable finding in studies *in vitro* has been that fluid expression decreases synthesis rates proportionately. It does not appear to matter whether the fluid is expressed as a result of an osmotic load or through a directional mechanical load. The extent of suppression of matrix synthesis is

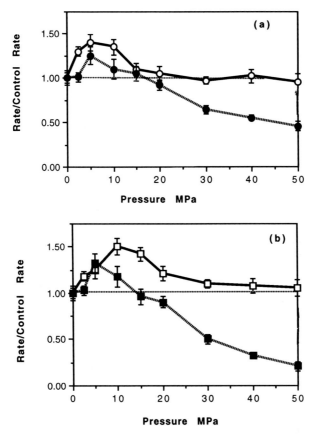

FIG. 1. The effect of exposures to different levels of hydrostatic pressure on proline (a) and sulfate (b) incorporation rates in bovine articular cartilage. (○, □) 20-sec exposure to pressure; (●, ■) 2-hr exposure to pressure. (Adapted from ref. 12.)

similar, and the effect seems to result directly from the changes in tissue hydration (10,15).

Changes in hydration have a number of separate effects on the pericellular environment. Proteoglycan concentration itself is altered by changes in hydration, as is the concentration of any other macromolecule in the chondrocyte's environment. Because of the polyelectrolyte nature of the proteoglycans, a change in proteoglycan concentration leads to alterations in the ionic composition and the pH of the matrix. Because cartilage osmotic pressure is mainly ionic in origin, the osmotic environment of the chondrocyte is also affected.

It is possible to examine the effect of changes in pericellular ionic concentrations on synthesis rates independently of changes in proteoglycan concentration by altering the composition of the bathing medium while keeping hydration, and thus proteoglycan concentration, constant. When cartilage is maintained at its normal hydration and the concentration of ions in the medium is changed from physiological to twice physiological levels, sulfate incorporation rates fall as intracellular ionic strength and osmolarity increase (16). It is apparent that the fall in synthesis rate induced by increasing medium ion concentrations is very similar to that induced by compressing the cartilage (Fig. 2). Similar results are seen if extracellular osmolarity is increased with sucrose (*unpublished data*) or mannose (15). Similarly, as shown by Gray et al. (17), the effect on synthesis rates of a fall in extracellular pH induced by compression in epiphyseal cartilage is comparable to that resulting from a change in medium pH. It can thus be argued that a major factor causing the fall in synthesis rate under static load is the consequent increase in pericellular ionic and osmotic strength accompanied by a decrease in the pH.

This argument is supported by another experiment where cartilage was compressed and fluid was lost, thus increasing the fixed charge density. In standard incubation medium, the internal cation concentration and osmolarity were higher than those in uncompressed conditions, and the synthesis rate was lower than that in the uncompressed control. Synthesis rates, however, rose toward control values if the tissue was incubated in medium of low ionic strength—that is, in an ionic strength which returned the cation concentration in the matrix to control conditions (16).

Isolated Chondrocytes

While such studies on cartilage explants have demonstrated that changes to the physical environment of the chondrocyte can influence its behavior, the

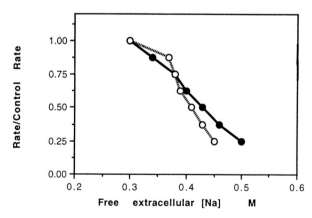

FIG. 2. Effect of changes in extracellular ion concentrations on synthesis rates in adult human articular cartilage using sodium as the reference ion (calculated from refs. 15 and 16). Extracellular ions changed by compression (proteoglycan concentration increases; sucrose addition) (●) or through changes in medium composition (proteoglycan concentration constant; sodium addition) (○).

ionic composition, pH, and osmolarity surrounding the chondrocytes in the tissue depend on the pericellular proteoglycan concentration and can only be estimated. In chondrocytes which have been isolated from their matrix, however, the extracellular ionic and hydrostatic environment can be precisely controlled. By changing medium ionic composition and pressure, the effects of such changes on these isolated cells can then be examined directly.

Effect of Changes in Osmolarity on Chondrocyte Volume

Water readily crosses the plasma membrane of most cells. Any change in external osmolarity thus leads to a rapid flux of water across the cell membrane and a change in cell volume in order to maintain osmotic equilibrium. Figure 3 shows that, as in other cells, the volume of chondrocytes varies with external osmolarity.

Effect of Changes in Extracellular Ions on Synthesis Rates

In chondrocytes incubated without serum, the synthesis rate per cell is only 5–15% that of chondrocytes in the matrix (*unpublished data*). That some of this fall in synthesis rates results from the change in the ionic environment can be seen when isolated chondrocytes are incubated for a few hours in medium whose osmolarity or ionic strength is varied by adding ions or sucrose to standard culture medium. As shown in Fig. 4, a change in the extracellular ion concentration has a significant effect on synthesis rates. The sulfate incorporation rate increases 50–80% when extracellular osmolarity is increased from 250 to 400 mOsm (i.e., back to the osmolarity the cell experienced in the tissue), and then it falls as the osmolarity is further increased.

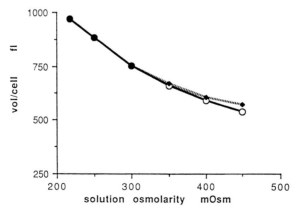

FIG. 3. Relationship between extracellular osmolarity and chondrocyte cell volume measured using a Coulter counter. (●) Sodium; (○) sucrose.

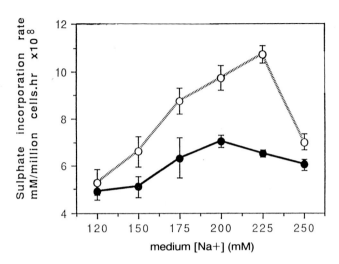

FIG. 4. Effect of extracellular osmolarity on synthesis rates at atmospheric pressure and 25 atm hydrostatic pressure in isolated chondrocytes. (●) Control; (○) pressure. (Unpublished data.)

The effect of an individual ionic species can be examined by altering its composition in media which are maintained iso-osmotic by sucrose addition. In long-term culture, it has been shown that high potassium concentrations affect the formation of the extracellular matrix (18). Potassium can also be seen to have an immediate effect on synthesis rates. Removing potassium from the medium causes the synthesis rate to fall to about 30% of control values; furthermore, synthesis increases as potassium concentration increases, reaching a maximum when [K] is 10–15 mM, a value similar to that seen in the tissue (19). Changing external calcium concentrations, on the other hand, appears to have no immediate effect on synthesis rates in articular chondrocytes; synthesis rates remain constant over the concentration range 50 μM to 15 mM calcium (*unpublished observations*).

Effect of Changes in Hydrostatic Pressure on Synthesis Rates

If hydrostatic pressure is applied to isolated chondrocytes, the effects are rather different from those seen in cartilage. Under conditions where stimulation of synthesis is seen in cartilage *in vitro,* synthesis in isolated chondrocytes is generally depressed. Thus a pressure of 5 MPa will stimulate synthesis in cartilage but depress it in chondrocytes. Lower pressures (i.e., 1 or 2.5 MPa) appear to have little effect on chondrocytes incubated in standard medium. However, if the osmolarity or ionic strength of the medium is increased, such hydrostatic pressures stimulate synthesis in these isolated chondrocytes as shown in Fig. 4. Pressures of this magnitude, however, appear to have no effect on synthesis in articular cartilage (Fig. 1). It thus appears that the effect of hydrostatic pressure on the

TABLE 2. *Some effects of hydrostatic pressure on physiological processes*[a]

Physiological process	Example	Pressure effect
Cell morphology	Cultured human amnion cells	Cell rounding (>50% at 47 MPa)
Exocytosis	Bovine adrenal cells/mast cells	Reduced 50% at 10 MPa
Structural proteins	F-actin/tubulin	Dissociates (>65% at 32 MPa)
Macromolecular synthesis	DNA synthesis (*Tetrahymena*)	Reduced 20% at 33 MPa
Macromolecular synthesis	RNA and protein synthesis	Reduced 20% at 13 MPa
Enzyme activity	Red-cell Na,K-ATPase	Increased 40% at 5 MPa
Membrane transport	Red-cell amino acid (Gly, Ala, Lys)	Inhibits 50% at 40 MPa
Membrane transport	Glucose, anions, (SO₄, HPO₄, Cl, etc.)	Inhibits 30–60% at 40 MPa

[a] For comprehensive reference, see ref. 24.

cell is mediated to some extent by the external ionic environment of the chondrocyte. However, there are other factors involved in the pressure response which are also altered when the chondrocyte is removed from its matrix. These factors are unknown; however, changes in cell shape may be involved, because pressure affects cytoskeletal elements (Table 2), and chondrocytes swell and change shape when isolated from cartilage (Fig. 3).

POSSIBLE MECHANISMS FOR THE EFFECTS OF PHYSICAL FACTORS ON CELL BEHAVIOR

Effect of Extracellular Ionic Environment on Intracellular Composition

It is apparent that changes to the hydrostatic and ionic environment of the chondrocyte affect the rate at which matrix is synthesized, and the response is rapid. One possible way in which these changes could affect cell behavior is by altering the intracellular ionic composition. In most mammalian cells, the internal composition of the cytoplasm is different from that of the surrounding extracellular fluid. Internal potassium, $[K]_i$, is usually held at around 140 mM, compared to an extracellular concentration of 5 mM, whereas for sodium the reverse holds (20). Internal calcium, $[Ca]_i$, is in the nanomolar range, compared to an extracellular concentration of around 2 mM. The small amount of information available suggests that the intracellular ionic composition of chondrocytes incubated in standard medium is similar to that of other cells (21) (Fig. 5). Cells maintain tight control of this internal composition because many cellular processes such as protein synthesis, glycolysis, intracellular transport, and endocytosis are critically dependent on $[K]_i$, pH_i, and $[Ca]_i$.

The intracellular concentration of permeant solutes (such as ions) depends on

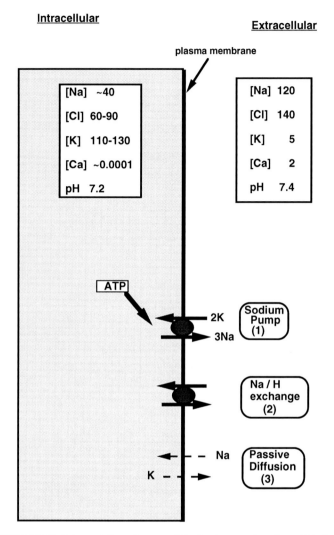

FIG. 5. A diagrammatic representation of some of the ion transporters thought to be present in the chondrocyte plasma membrane, and estimates of intra- and extracellular ion concentrations. Ion concentrations are given in millimoles, and extracellular values are those typically present in standard tissue culture media. The transport systems shown are as follows: (1) the 3Na/2K pump, a "primary active" transporter which uses the energy obtained from ATP hydrolysis to move Na and K ions *against* their concentration gradients, (2) the Na/H exchanger, which uses the Na gradient into the cell generated by the 3Na/2K pump to move H ions out of the cell, and (3) electrodiffusion, where ions move passively down their respective gradients. There are a range of other transporters which have been omitted for clarity (see ref. 20 for further details). From this diagram it can be seen that, for example, raising the external Na concentration will increase the Na gradient into the cell and will raise the internal Na concentration via pathway 3. Consequently, this will increase the activity of the 3Na/2K pump, leading to a rise in intracellular K concentration. In addition, changes to the Na gradient will influence the intracellular pH via pathway 2.

their electrochemical gradient across the cell membrane (20). Sodium and calcium thus tend to move into the cell, and potassium tends to move out of it. In order to maintain these ion imbalances, the cell expends energy. Most of the energy used by the cell is used by active transport systems such as the sodium and calcium pumps, which move these ions against their electrochemical gradients. Intracellular composition thus depends on the balance of movement of solutes such as sodium and potassium into and out of the cell and thus also depends on the relative ease (permeability) with which these solutes cross the cell membrane.

The permeability of the cell membrane to biologically relevant substances varies over many orders of magnitude. For example, water and nonpolar small solutes such as gases and sugars are very permeable and equilibrate across the cell membrane within seconds. At the other end of the spectrum, monovalent cations such as Na^+ and K^+ are extremely impermeable and require hours to equilibrate across the plasma membrane itself. Membrane transport proteins, often of high specificity, can increase the transport of such solutes, especially cations, into and out of the cell (20). The membrane transport systems which control the internal ion concentrations of the cell have been studied in detail in other cell types, and the information available shows that the main transport systems found in other mammalian cells are also present in chondrocytes (*unpublished data*). The action of some of the main K^+ and Na^+ membrane transport systems are summarized in Fig. 5.

Any change in external composition alters the electrochemical gradient and thus the intracellular composition. Our initial results show that when the volume of chondrocytes, incubated in standard medium, is decreased by placing them in medium of 350–400 mOsm [i.e., the extracellular osmolarity in the matrix (Table 1)], $[Na]_i$ increases from 30–40 mM to 80–100 mM. Similar changes have been seen in fibroblasts (22). If the extracellular pH falls to pH 6.5, intracellular pH falls from 7.2 to 6.3–6.5 (23). It is thus likely that the effect of the extracellular ionic environment on synthesis rates is, at least in part, directly related to its effect on internal composition.

That internal composition affects synthesis rates has been seen in other cells (22). It can be tested by altering membrane transport systems; inhibiting the activity of the sodium pump with ouabain (20) will, for example, lead to a fall in $[K]_i$ and a rise in $[Na]_i$, because these ions will move down their concentration gradients to equilibrate eventually with the external solution across the cell membrane. Under these conditions, synthesis rates in chondrocytes fall by 40–50%. It is also of interest to note that glycolysis rates in ouabain-treated chondrocytes fall by 50–60%, showing that, as in other cells, most of the energy required by the cell is used to drive the sodium pump.

Hydrostatic Pressure May Also Alter Intracellular Composition

It is not known how the effects of pressure are mediated, but in Table 2 it can be seen that hydrostatic pressure is known to influence a variety of systems in other cell types. When pressure is applied to cartilage and chondrocytes, it is possible that changes in synthesis are mediated by one or more of these systems.

Some clues to the mechanism of action of hydrostatic pressure may be obtained from Fig. 4, which shows that the effect of pressure on isolated chondrocytes depends on the ionic environment of the cell. Hydrostatic pressure increases sodium pump activity in chondrocytes, as in other cells (Table 2), but only if cell volume is close to that found in the tissue. Pressure also decreases passive K transport systems, thus slowing the rate of loss of K from the cell (*unpublished observations*). Pressure would thus tend to increase $[K]_i$, and the stimulation observed may arise because an increase in $[K]_i$ and decrease in $[Na]_i$, provides a more favorable environment for protein synthesis.

Although a change in internal ionic composition can explain some of the effects of long-term exposure to hydrostatic pressure, it is unlikely to provide the explanation for the stimulation seen after a 20-sec exposure to pressure, because no significant change in intracellular composition would occur in so short a time. We do not know how this stimulation occurs, but it is likely that second messenger systems are involved because an increase in cAMP levels occurs after such short pressure applications and endures for tens of minutes. An increase in cAMP has also been seen after pressure application to epiphyseal chondrocytes, and has been shown to correlate with an increase in synthesis rates (11).

SUMMARY AND CONCLUSIONS

The extracellular matrix of cartilage is constantly turned over, and its composition will thus depend on the balance between the rates of synthesis and loss. A change to one or both of these rates may lead to a change in matrix composition and properties. It appears that synthesis rates respond proportionately and quickly to changes in some physical parameters such as extracellular ion concentrations, osmotic pressure, or hydrostatic pressure: Any change in the ionic environment tends to depress synthesis, whereas physiological levels of hydrostatic pressure tend to stimulate it. The normal cartilage matrix is thus the product of cells whose synthesis rates vary in response to the changes in their microenvironment routinely experienced.

If the physical environment alters outside these limits, the net synthesis rate would be expected to change, at least in the short term. Such abnormal changes to the physical environment occur in osteoarthritis, for example. One of the first signs of osteoarthritis in human cartilage or in animal models of osteoarthritis is cartilage swelling before there is any noticeable loss of proteoglycans (6). Swelling alters tissue composition, diluting the proteoglycans and thus leading to a fall in fixed charge density, an alteration in the concentration of pericellular ions, and a decrease in pericellular osmolarity. These changes would be expected to lead to a short-term decrease in the synthesis rate. However, such changes to the matrix will also affect the hydrostatic pressure developed under load, which may also affect synthesis rate. The net effect cannot yet be predicted. At later stages of degeneration in osteoarthritis, proteoglycans are lost from the matrix, leading to a further fall in fixed charge density, change in ionic composition, and fall in osmotic and swelling pressures. It is not known how chondrocytes will adapt to this altered environment.

ACKNOWLEDGMENT

This work was carried out with the support of the Arthritis and Rheumatism Council (United Kingdom).

REFERENCES

1. Muir IH. The chemistry of the ground substance of joint cartilage. In: Sokoloff L, ed. *The joints and synovial fluid.* New York: Academic Press, 1981;28–94.
2. Sommarin Y, Larsson T, Heinegard D. Chondrocyte matrix interaction. *Exp Cell Res* 1989;184: 181–192.
3. Maroudas A. Physical chemistry of articular cartilage and the intervertebral disc. In: Sokoloff L, ed. *The joints and synovial fluid.* New York: Academic Press, 1981;240–291.
4. Stockwell R. *Biology of cartilage cells.* Cambridge, England: Cambridge University Press, 1979.
5. Maroudas A. X-ray microprobe analysis of cartilage. *Connect Tissue Res* 1972;1:153–163.
6. Grushko G, Schneiderman R, Maroudas A. Some biochemical and biophysical parameters for the study of the pathogenesis of osteoarthritis. A comparison between the processes of ageing and degeneration. *Connect Tissue Res* 1989;19:149–176.
7. Holm S, Maroudas A, Urban JPG, Selstam G, Nachemson A. Nutrition of the intervertebral disc. *Connect Tissue Res* 1981;8:101–119.
8. Afoke NYP, Byers PD, Hutton WC. Contact pressures in the human hip joint. *J Bone Joint Surg* 1987;69B:536–542.
9. Tammi M, Paukkonen K, Kiviranta I, Jurvelin J, Helminen HJ. Joint-loading induced alterations in articular cartilage. In: *Joint loading.* Bristol, England: John Wright, 1987;64–88.
10. Sah RL, Kim YL, Doong JYH, Grodzinsky AJ, Plaas AJ, Sandy JD. Biosynthetic response of cartilage explants to dynamic compression. *J Orthop Res* 1989;7:619–639.
11. Bourrett LA, Rodan GA. The role of calcium in the inhibition of cAMP accumulation in epiphyseal cartilage cells exposed to physiological forces. *J Cell Physiol* 1976;88:353–361.
12. Hall A, Urban JPG, Gehl K. The effects of hydrostatic pressure on matrix synthesis in articular cartilage. *J Orthop Res* 1991;9:1–10.
13. Rubin CT, Lanyon LE. Osteoregulatory nature of mechanical stimuli: function as a determinant for remodelling in bone. *J Orthop Res* 1987;5:300–310.
14. Koob TJ, Vogel KG, Thurmond FA. Compression loading *in vitro* regulates proteoglycan synthesis by fibrocartilage in tendon. *Trans Orthop Res Soc* 1991;16:49.
15. Schneiderman R, Keret D, Maroudas A. Effect of mechanical and osmotic pressure on the rate of glycosaminoglycan synthesis in the human adult femoral head. *J Orthop Res* 1986;4:393–408.
16. Urban JPG, Bayliss MT. Regulation of proteoglycan synthesis rate in cartilage *in vitro;* influence of extracellular ionic composition. *Biochim Biophys Acta* 1989;992:59–65.
17. Gray ML, Pizzanelli AM, Grodzinsky AJ, Lee RC. Mechanical and physicochemical determinants of chondrocyte biosynthetic response. *J Orthop Res* 1988;6:777–792.
18. Daniel JC, Kosher RA, Hamos JE, Lash JW. The influence of extracellular potassium on synthesis and deposition of matrix components by chondrocytes. *J Cell Biol* 1974;63:843–854.
19. Hall A, Urban JPG. Is membrane transport involved in the response to pressure of articular cartilage? *Trans Orthop Res Soc* 15:340.
20. Stein WD. *Transport and diffusion across cell membranes.* London: Academic Press, 1986.

21. Middleton JFS, Hunt S, Oates K. Electron microprobe x-ray analysis of the composition of hyaline articular and non-articular cartilage in young and aged rats. *Cell Tissue Res* 1988;253: 469–475.
22. Petronini PG, Tracamere M, Mazzini A, Kay JE, Borghetti AF. (1989) Control of protein synthesis by extracellular Na$^+$ in cultured fibroblasts. *J Cell Physiol* 1989;140:202–211.
23. Wilkins RJ, Hall AC, Urban JPG. Some factors involved in the control of intracellular pH in chondrocytes isolated from bovine articular cartilage. *J Physiol* (Lond). 1991 (in press).
24. Jannasch HW, Marquis RE, Zimmerman AM, eds. *Current perspectives in high pressure biology.* London: Academic Press, 1987.

DISCUSSION

Brune: Can you comment on the chloride concentration in the extracellular space of chondrocytes?

Urban: In cartilage the chloride concentration is much lower than that in the surrounding plasma or medium—about 60–100 mM compared to 150 mM. The cells are seeing a low concentration of all anions, including chloride. Chloride crosses the cell membrane relatively fast.

Hascall: You showed that changes in sodium ion concentrations modulate proteoglycan synthesis. Do changes in chloride also affect synthesis?

Urban: We have tried to substitute other anions such as sulfate for chloride, but did not see an effect on synthesis. I do not know how to adjust the chloride except by substitution. If anyone has any suggestions how to have a low anion concentration around cells except by having proteoglycans there, or other large polyanions, I would be grateful to hear about it.

Articular Cartilage and Osteoarthritis,
edited by K. Kuettner et al.
Raven Press, Ltd., New York © 1992.

28

General Discussion for Chapters 25–27

Kimura: Dr. Urban, you have shown that the chondrocytes respond to intracellular ion changes. How similar are these changes to those induced by cytokine or growth factor receptor binding? Might they be activating the same intermediary processes?

Urban: One of the effects of growth factors is to up-regulate exchangers like the sodium–hydrogen exchanger, probably to maintain internal environment while other changes occur. But I certainly do not think that all the effects of growth factors are in any way related to changes in intracellular ion composition, such as those I have studied.

Hascall: I am intrigued by Dr. Grodzinsky's hypothesis about the role of pH in regulating both proteoglycan metabolism and matrix organization. There is a further complication because there is a gradient in cells from the articular surface. If the cells rely primarily on anaerobic metabolism, they will produce lactic acid and probably create pH gradients metabolically. It would be unusual to choose a primary regulatory factor that is greatly influenced by other processes, which the cells cannot always control.

Grodzinsky: It is hard to be absolutely certain that there is a cause-and-effect relationship, even though responses to changes in load and in pH can be correlated. It is possible that the microenvironment within a very localized region of matrix may still dominate such physicochemical effects and superimpose them on the broader lactate or pH gradients that may exist.

Benya: Dr. Grodzinsky demonstrated a nice correlation between increasing frequency in dynamic loading and increasing pressurization. He suggested that pressurization was an explanation for increased synthesis. Perhaps there are alternative explanations. Many growth factors stimulate changes in intracellular Ca^{2+}, Na^+, and other small molecules which are transient, even when the growth factor is continuously present. If each loading cycle caused such a transient signal without growth factor intervention, then loading at higher frequency might cause the signals to add up before each could decay. This might generate a signal-versus-frequency curve similar to the pressure-versus-frequency curve. Such signals might then be responsible for increased synthesis.

Brune: What is known about the resting potential and the action potentials of chondrocytes? Based on the ion composition of the extracellular space, there should be a high resting potential. Do the chondrocytes have ion pumps, and are they influenced by drugs?

Urban: It is very difficult to measure the membrane properties of a chondrocyte in its matrix. You can measure the membrane potential of a cartilage cell in medium, but cannot simulate the correct extracellular composition easily. The membrane potentials that have been measured in isolated chondrocytes have all been measured in ordinary medium and are very similar to those found in other cells, around −40 mV. As far as sodium pumps are concerned, there are many in a chondrocyte, about 100,000 per cell, compared to about 3000 in an erythrocyte. There are also calcium pumps, but we don't know about their density.

Caterson: On the subject of pumps, the only ones I know about pour beer out! Does anybody know about sulfate pumps? In cystic fibrosis, there are problems with the chloride pump, and patients produce oversulfated mucins and proteoglycans.

Hascall: Jeff Esko's group has identified a CHO cell mutant which fully sulfates proteoglycans but which cannot use extracellular sulfate as a source. The cells have defective sulfate transporters and use cysteine as a sulfate source. So there must be active transport of sulfate into most cells.

Urban: Kathy Whittaker, who works on sulfate transport in chondrocytes, has found that ordinary sulfate enters the cell very easily and quickly at a rate well above that needed for proteoglycan synthesis. However, the concentration of sulfate appears to depend on the membrane potential. So, if you change extracellular potassium in particular, and thus alter membrane potential, the level of sulfate inside the chondrocyte changes and this may affect sulfation. Low extracellular sulfate concentrations, which begin to decrease sulfation, probably result from a fall in intracellular concentration rather than a fall in the rate at which sulfate enters the cell.

Maroudas: Because sulfate is a divalent anion, its concentration is much lower in the cartilage matrix than in the external medium. In uncompressed cartilage, the sulfate concentration lies in a range in which its rate of incorporation into glycosaminoglycan is independent of free sulfate concentration. When cartilage is compressed, its water content is decreased and free sulfate concentrations fall to values such that the rate of sulfate incorporation may become concentration-dependent.

Bruckner: Alice Maroudas has pointed out that the concentration of calcium, a divalent cation, is sensitive to mechanical loads and that calcium concentrations around chondrocytes in cartilage must be very high compared to that in culture medium. Is there an influence of calcium concentration on the synthetic rates?

Maroudas: We found no change in the rate of sulfate incorporation on increasing calcium concentrations up to 10-fold.

Urban: We find the same. If medium calcium is increased up to about 20 mM, there is no effect on synthesis rate. However, if calcium is depleted with EGTA, then synthesis rates fall very dramatically in a very short time.

Pritzker: I will offer a data-free contrarian view to the opinion that bulk effects such as pressure or osmolarity control chondrocyte metabolism. Chondrocytes are highly oriented. The surface cells are in a horizontal alignment, while the deeper cells are anisotropic spheroids oriented vertically. There are also external organelles on the cells, such as solitary cilia, which may mediate responses to pressures or to chemical environmental changes. Cartilage cells in a given area are probably exposed to a relatively constant environment of pressures and fluid flows.

Cooke: I think that the surface zone of the cartilage is much more compressible than the deeper zone. Does Dr. Grodzinsky observe differences in deformation and/or cell response if the slices are taken from the surface versus the middle or low zones? The flow of fluid should be far greater in the upper zone.

Grodzinsky: It is clear from the biomechanical studies in many laboratories that the flows are very different at the surface versus the deeper layers. Our explant studies did not address this question.

Tammi: We have done some cyclic loading experiments on calf articular cartilage explants similar to those used by Dr. Grodzinsky, except that we left surface layers intact. We analyzed the compression effects on sulfate incorporation separately in the different zones. With increasing pressure, the stimulation of synthesis, which is observed in all zones at low pressures, is first lost from the superficial layer at high pressures. We think that the superficial layer is more susceptible to excessive load because it has a smaller concentration of proteoglycans. So there is certainly a different response in different layers.

Maroudas: We also looked at the response of the different zones to static compression. We thought that compression of the surface layer would make it less hydrated, hence richer in proteoglycans and more similar in that respect to the middle zone. However, this did not increase proteoglycan synthesis, since each layer has its own characteristic rate of metabolism, which decreases with compression to a different extent. The middle zone chondrocytes show the greatest drop in sulfate incorporation when subjected to mechanical or osmotic compression.

Articular Cartilage and Osteoarthritis,
edited by K. Kuettner et al.
Raven Press, Ltd., New York © 1992.

Part VIII: Experimental Osteoarthritis in Relation to Human Pathology

Introduction

Christopher J. Handley

Department of Biochemistry, Monash University, Clayton, Victoria 3168, Australia

The molecular composition and organization of the extracellular matrix of articular cartilage gives this tissue a nearly frictionless surface as well as the ability to withstand and distribute compressive loads over the subchondral bone. The tensile properties of articular cartilage come from the collagen network of the tissue. The highly negative fixed charge of the proteoglycan aggregate is responsible for the compressive load-bearing properties of the tissue. Over the past 5 years, other components of the extracellular matrix of cartilage have been recognized, and they include small proteoglycans [PG I (biglycan), PG II (decorin)] and noncollagenous proteins such as fibronectin, link protein, and fibromodulin. Little is known about the exact function of these molecules in the maintenance and organization of the extracellular matrix of cartilage, but it is very likely that they are involved in cell–matrix or matrix–matrix interactions.

In normal adult articular cartilage the macromolecular components of the extracellular matrix are maintained at constant levels, which is reflected in stable biomechanical properties of the tissue. This is achieved by the chondrocytes synthesizing these macromolecules at a rate equal to their loss from the matrix. The loss of these components of the extracellular matrix is achieved in a precise manner usually through the action of proteinases originating from chondrocytes and, to a much lesser extent, by mechanical or passive means.

In osteoarthritis, a disease of unknown pathogenesis, there is a slow degeneration of the articular cartilage, resulting in the gradual loss of the biomechanical function of the tissue. Ultimately this leads to the loss of articular cartilage from the diarthrodial joint. The change in the biomechanical properties of articular cartilage in osteoarthritis appears to be the consequence of a change in the metabolism of the chondrocytes, as no other cell type appears to be involved. This perturbation in the metabolism of chondrocytes may be reflected in the synthesis and/or the catabolism of macromolecular constituents of the extracellular matrix of the tissue. Changes in the synthetic processes may lead to either the expression of new macromolecules by cartilage, an alteration in the amount of a macromolecule in the extracellular matrix of the tissue, or variations in the pattern of post-translational modifications to these macromolecules. Alterations in the catabolism of articular cartilage may result in either (a) changes in tissue levels of the various macromolecules or (b) damage to the macromolecules retained within the matrix of this tissue. These situations will lead to alterations in the architecture of the extracellular matrix of the tissue, and ultimately may be reflected in the biomechanical properties of the tissue.

The following four chapters investigate changes in the metabolism and structure of the macromolecules of the extracellular matrix of articular cartilage during the onset of osteoarthritis. In the chapter by Caterson et al., the expression of antibody epitopes not usually present in articular cartilage is investigated. These epitopes occur as the consequence of changes in the sulfation pattern of chondroitin sulfate chains and thus reflect an alteration in the regulation of the cellular processes involved in the post-translational modification of proteoglycans. Other epitopes studied in this chapter are derived from the action of proteinases on cartilage proteoglycan creating new C- and N-terminal sequences in the core protein. The importance of this work is the identification of epitopes that may act as markers not only for the diagnosis of osteoarthritis, but also for monitoring the progression or regression of the disease during therapy. The elucidation of the molecular structure of such epitopes will give an insight into changes in the molecular and cellular events associated with osteoarthritis.

The chapter by Thonar et al. also investigates the appearance of an epitope as the result of osteoarthritis. These authors show that in osteoarthritis in humans there are elevated serum levels of keratan sulfate, and that surgical replacement of the diseased joint does not significantly affect the serum levels of this epitope. Thonar et al. suggest that the elevated serum keratan sulfate level is due to a change in the rate of catabolism of the large, aggregating proteoglycan of cartilage from both unaffected and diseased joints. Clearly the elucidation of the mechanism of the induction of this systemic increase in the rate of catabolism of cartilage, as a result of osteoarthritis, is important in the understanding and treatment of the disease.

As pointed out above, the extracellular matrix of articular cartilage contains structural macromolecules other than collagen and proteoglycan. The chapter by Lust and Burton-Wurster shows that in both human and canine osteoarthritic cartilage there are elevated levels of the glycoprotein fibronectin. The fibronectin derived from cartilage appears to be chemically different from the molecule present in serum. Fibronectin is a multifunctional glycoprotein capable of participating in cell–matrix and matrix–matrix interactions. Changes in the levels of this macromolecule in cartilage may itself be a marker of the disease. It is also expected that changes in tissue levels of fibronectin will eventually affect the organization of the extracellular matrix.

The proteoglycan aggregate in the extracellular matrix of cartilage is responsible for the compressive load-bearing properties of the tissue. Changes in the level and composition of this complex in cartilage will result in the perturbation in the biomechanical properties of the tissue. In the last chapter in this section, Dr. Manicourt and colleagues investigate changes in the molecular composition and physical nature of proteoglycan aggregate in cartilage from osteoarthritic cartilage and from immobilized joints. The significance of the latter is that immobilization of a synovial joint results in degenerative changes similar to that observed in osteoarthritis but that with gentle exercise, proteoglycan loss can be reversed. This reversal in proteoglycan loss is not observed in osteoarthritic cartilage. These authors suggest that this reversibility of proteoglycan content in cartilage is partly due to changes in the hyaluronan content of the tissue.

Articular Cartilage and Osteoarthritis,
edited by K. Kuettner et al.
Raven Press, Ltd., New York © 1992.

29

Immunological Markers of Cartilage Proteoglycan Metabolism in Animal and Human Osteoarthritis

Bruce Caterson,* Clare E. Hughes,* Brian Johnstone,*
and John S. Mort†

*Division of Orthopaedic Surgery, University of North Carolina School of Medicine,
Chapel Hill, North Carolina 27599 and †Joint Diseases Laboratory, Shriners
Hospital for Crippled Children, Montreal, Quebec H3G 1A6, Canada

Over the past two decades there have been a considerable number of basic research studies that have investigated the pathogenesis of osteoarthritis (see ref. 1 and 2 for review). However, the potential biological mechanisms that initiate and perpetuate this disease are still not known. Research into the etiology of this disease has been complicated by the multitude of biological, biomechanical, genetic, and environmental factors that can initiate the disease and by the multiple tissues involved (bone, cartilage, synovium, meniscus). Consequently, it is difficult to establish experimental conditions that mimic the disease situation. Furthermore, the protracted development of the disease in humans and our inability to detect the disease at an early stage have hampered studies of its pathogenesis. Postmortem and surgical human material has provided some information on factors involved in the development of osteoarthritis, but generally this concerns changes that occur in the latter stages of the disease process.

The development and use of animal models has provided investigators the opportunity to study the various stages of the disease process. Several different species have been used (including dogs, rabbits, sheep, guinea pigs, and mice) utilizing genetic (inbred) predispositions as well as biomechanical and/or surgical procedures to facilitate the development of this disease process. The advantages of these models are that osteoarthritis-like changes usually develop more quickly than those observed in humans and, importantly, that early stages of disease can be studied more easily. Disadvantages of these models are that they often only mimic certain parts of the disease process and that, when surgical intervention is used, postoperative inflammation (which is not usually observed in early osteoarthritis) may be a significant contributing factor. In addition, there is always a question of animal-to-animal variation in the pathogenesis of the disease. These factors are important considerations when extrapolating conclusions and therapies to the analogous situation in humans. Nonetheless, recent studies using animal models of osteoarthritis have considerably advanced our knowledge of factors that are involved in its pathogenesis. These models offer probably the best opportunity for the researcher to unravel the biological mechanisms that are involved in the different stages of the disease process. They provide useful experimental systems for much-needed drug development and subsequent therapeutic intervention, which may eventually be used to prevent or arrest the early stages of the disease process.

Studies of animal models and analysis of human osteoarthritic specimens have indicated that several changes occur in the articular cartilage morphology, biochemical composition, and cellular metabolism that differ from those observed in normal cartilage with aging (1,2). In the early stages of osteoarthritis the following events occur: (a) an increase in tissue hydration, (b) changes in the cartilage biomechanics, (c) an increase in the chondroitin sulfate chain size and overall content in the proteoglycans, and (d) an increase in proteoglycan and collagen biosynthesis. In the latter stages of the disease there are changes in cartilage morphology; chondrocyte clusters occur with increased cell division and there is an extensive loss of proteoglycan from the extracellular matrix, which eventually leads to fibrillation and destruction of the cartilage from mechanical wear and tear.

The observation of the progressive loss of components from the cartilage extracellular matrix has prompted many researchers to develop techniques for measuring their release into body fluids, with a view toward developing diagnostic methods for monitoring the rate of disease progression. Immunological methods have the potential of providing specific means of quantifying the biochemical changes that occur in cartilage during development, in aging, and in pathology. The primary focus of research in our laboratory has been the production, characterization, and use of monoclonal antibodies with specificities directed against proteoglycan epitopes that can be used to study proteoglycan structure, function, and metabolism in connective tissues. The use of these antibodies for studies investigating the pathogenesis of osteoarthritis in humans and animal models is the subject of the present chapter.

MONOCLONAL ANTIBODIES AGAINST EPITOPES IN CHONDROITIN SULFATE GLYCOSAMINOGLYCANS

Chondroitin sulfate (CS) proteoglycans are major components of cartilage but are lesser constituents of many other connective tissues. Until recently, the biochemical functions of the polyanionic CS glycosaminoglycan chains were thought to be limited to (a) their contribution towards maintaining a Donnan osmotic pressure within the cartilage, (b) their participation in excluded volume effects, and (c) their contributions to the viscoelastic properties of the tissue (3–5). Recent studies from this laboratory have changed our thoughts on this matter. Biochemical analysis of the CS glycosaminoglycans present on cartilage proteoglycans indicates that different isomeric forms of CS occur during normal growth and development, as well as in pathology (6–9). The function of the differential expression of these CS isomers is not known. However, recent studies from this laboratory (10–12) have indicated that sulfation patterns in CS glycosaminoglycans are a more highly controlled and cell-regulated process than was previously thought. These studies involved the use of a panel of monoclonal antibodies that recognize different epitopes in CS glycosaminoglycans (see Fig. 1). They demonstrated that macromolecules with CS glycosaminoglycans contained different isomer combinations that are highly compartmentalized in connective tissues and that are also synthesized by specific cell types within these tissues.

Details of what is known about the specifics of the antibodies shown in Fig. 1 have been recently described (13). They can be divided into two general categories: (i) those that recognize epitopes present in the "native" CS glycosami-

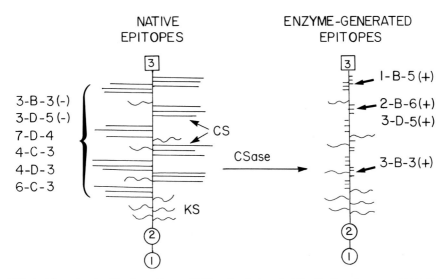

FIG. 1. Monoclonal antibodies with specificities directed against "native" and enzyme-generated CS epitopes. Monoclonal antibodies 3-B-3 (−), 3-D-5 (−), 7-D-4, 4-C-3, 4-D-3, and 6-C-3 all recognize epitopes in the native CS glycosaminoglycan chains. Antibodies 3-B-3 (−) and 3-D-5 (−) recognize epitopes at the nonreducing termini of CS chains that contain a terminal saturated hexuronate residue adjacent to a 6-sulfated or 4-sulfated *N*-acetylgalactosamine residue, respectively. Antibodies 7-D-4, 4-C-3, 4-D-3, and 6-C-3 recognize more complex epitopes that reside within the CS glycosaminoglycan chains. Monoclonal antibodies 1-B-5 (+), 2-B-6 (+), 3-D-5 (+), and 3-B-3 (+) all require either endo- or exo-glycosidase pretreatment to generate their epitopes that consist of unsulfated (1-B-5), 4-sulfated (2-B-6 and 3-D-5), or 6-sulfated (3-B-3) disaccharides of the monosulfated CS isomers. (+) and (−) indicate whether or not enzyme pretreatment is required in order to produce the epitope recognized by specific monoclonal antibodies; 1, 2, and 3 denote the G1, G2, and G3 domains of the proteoglycan core protein; CS and KS denote chondroitin sulfate and keratan sulfate glycosaminoglycans, respectively; CSase denotes chondroitinase pretreatment.

noglycan chains and (ii) those that require predigestion of the CS glycosaminoglycan with endo- or exoglycosidases to generate their nonreducing terminal epitopes. Two of these antibodies (3-B-3 and 3-D-5) recognize epitopes that fall into both of these categories. Monoclonal antibody 3-B-3 recognizes an epitope in native CS glycosaminoglycan chains when the chain possesses a saturated hexuronic acid residue adjacent to 6-sulfated N-acetyl galactosamine at the nonreducing terminus of the CS glycosaminoglycan. The 3-B-3 monoclonal antibody also recognizes a similar epitope that is generated by enzyme pretreatment of 6-sulfated CS glycosaminoglycans with mammalian hyaluronidase, which produces similar terminal nonreducing disaccharides, or with chondroitinase in which a related epitope that contains a 4,5-delta-unsaturated hexuronic acid moiety is present at nonreducing termini (13). The presence of a (−) or (+) after the antibody name is used to denote whether or not an enzyme pretreatment step has been used to generate the epitope in CS glycosaminoglycans.

Immunochemical analysis of a large number of proteoglycans from many different animal species and tissues have indicated that the 3-B-3 (−) epitope is absent in native CS glycosaminoglycan chains of proteoglycans extracted from normal mature hyaline cartilages (14). However, expression of 3-B-3 (−) epitope is observed in cartilage proteoglycans from developing tissues (15) and in osteoarthritic cartilage (12; see below). Monoclonal antibody 3-D-5 recognizes an analogous 4-sulfated nonreducing terminal disaccharide on native CS glycosaminoglycans [3-D-5 (−)] and on mammalian hyaluronidase- or chondroitinase-generated CS fragments [3-D-5 (+)]. However, immunochemical studies have indicated that the 3-D-5 (−) epitope is present on proteoglycans from both normal and pathological tissues, indicating that CS chains terminating with hexuronate residues adjacent to N-acetylgalactosamine-4-sulfate are more common than those adjacent to N-acetylgalactosamine-6-sulfate, the 3-B-3 (−) epitope. The detailed biochemical characteristics of the epitopes recognized by the other native CS monoclonal antibodies (4-C-3, 4-D-3, 6-C-3 and 7-D-4) have yet to be determined. However, our preliminary analyses to date indicate that several of them recognize epitopes in oversulfated domains of CS glycosaminoglycans (13). In recent studies we have investigated the specificity of monoclonal antibody 7-D-4 (J. P. Griffin, C. E. Hughes, and B. Caterson, *unpublished observation*) and have identified a CS oligosaccharide containing 10–20 sugar residues that contain the optimal-size epitope recognized by this antibody. The oligosaccharide containing the 7-D-4 epitope most probably consists of a distinct sequence of sugar residues that contain several of the eight possible CS-isomer disaccharide combinations (13).

An example of the use of several of these anti-CS monoclonal antibodies to immunolocate different epitopes on the proteoglycans synthesized by monolayer cultures of bovine articular chondrocytes is shown in Fig. 2. Bovine articular cartilage chondrocytes were grown in high-cell-density monolayer cultures that maintain their chondrocyte phenotype for at least 10 days of culture. The proteoglycans were extracted from the cell layer matrix and subjected to composite

Chondroitinase ABC

Native

2-B-6(+) 3-B-3(+)   3-B-3(-) 7-D-4 4-C-3 6-C-3 4-D-3

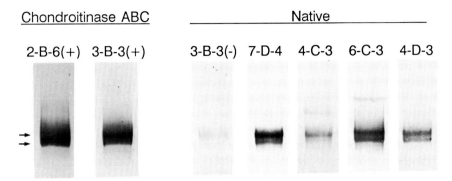

FIG. 2. Immunolocation analyses of proteoglycans isolated from monolayer cultures of bovine articular cartilage chondrocytes. Monolayer cultures were grown for 9 days with ascorbic acid (25 μg/ml) in the medium. The cell layer and associated matrix was extracted with 4 M guanidine HCl, and the extracts were processed prior to electrophoresis on composite agarose/polyacrylamide gels (12,22). Proteoglycans in these extracts were identified by immunolocation with a panel of monoclonal antibodies that recognize native and/or chondroitinase ABC-generated epitopes on CS glycosaminoglycans. The arrows denote the mobility of the two electrophoretic forms of the large proteoglycan subpopulations found in cartilage extracts; (+) and (−) denote whether or not the nitrocellulose sheet was pretreated with chondroitinase prior to immunolocation analysis.

agarose/polyacrylamide gel electrophoresis to separate the proteoglycans from other macromolecules in the extracts. The electrophoretically fractionated macromolecules were transferred to nitrocellulose and subjected to immunolocation analyses with our panel of anti-CS monoclonal antibodies. Some of the nitrocellulose sheets were digested with chondroitinase ABC prior to the immunolocation analyses with monoclonal antibodies that required this enzyme pretreatment in order to generate their respective epitopes, namely, 2-B-6 (+) and 3-B-3 (+). This study shows that different patterns of staining are observed with each of these anti-CS monoclonal antibodies. Staining with 3-B-3 (+) shows an immunolocation pattern that demonstrates the inherent heterogeneity of the two large aggregating proteoglycan subpopulations. Monoclonal antibody 2-B-6 (+) shows a less complicated pattern where immunostaining of the faster migrating large aggregating proteoglycan subpopulation predominates. Staining for native CS epitopes also shows differential staining patterns where different proportions of epitopes appear to be present in the two electrophoretically separated large proteoglycan subpopulations (compare 7-D-4 and 4-C-3 with 6-C-3 and 4-D-3). It is of interest to note that there are considerable differences in the 3-B-3 (−) and 3-B-3 (+) staining patterns. The 3-B-3 (−) epitope appears to be confined predominantly to the slower migrating large proteoglycan subpopulation and is also expressed on a considerably smaller number of the CS glycosaminoglycan chains. Monoclonal antibody 3-D-5 shows a similar pattern before (−) or after (+) chondroitinase pretreatment (results not shown). It thus appears that only the slower migrating large proteoglycan subpopulations contain the 3-B-3 (−) and 3-D-5 (−) epitopes in their CS glycosaminoglycan. The significance of this finding is presently not understood. These studies serve to illustrate the variable but distinctive distribution of different CS isomers within large aggregating proteoglycan subpopulations. The differential expression of some of these epitopes in proteoglycans from osteoarthritic cartilage is discussed below.

THE EXPRESSION OF ATYPICAL STRUCTURES IN CHONDROITIN SULFATE GLYCOSAMINOGLYCANS AS MARKERS OF OSTEOARTHRITIS

In several collaborative studies we have used these monoclonal antibodies against CS isomers to investigate cartilage proteoglycan metabolism in osteoarthritis. Of particular interest has been our discovery that subtle structural differences occur in the CS glycosaminoglycan chains of proteoglycans isolated from osteoarthritic cartilage that are not present in proteoglycans from normal articular cartilage (12). These atypical structures in the CS glycosaminoglycans are recognized by two monoclonal antibodies (3-B-3 and 7-D-4) that detect unique terminal and intrachain CS epitopes, respectively, in proteoglycans isolated from the osteoarthritic knees of animals from the Pond–Nuki dog model of osteoarthritis. These studies showed that the 3-B-3 (−) epitope was primarily expressed in the CS glycosaminoglycan chains of the slower migrating proteoglycan subpopulation whereas the 7-D-4 epitope was more generally expressed in the CS glycosaminoglycans in several of the osteoarthritic cartilage proteoglycan subpopulations (12). In other studies we performed immunohistochemical analyses investigating the focal expression of 3-B-3 (−) epitope (16) and 7-D-4 epitope in the Pond–Nuki and arthrotomy dog models of osteoarthritis. These studies showed that both epitopes preferentially stained superficial regions of the osteoarthritic cartilage where there was diminished proteoglycan in the extracellular matrix as determined by standard histochemical staining. Strong immunoreactivity was also observed in the territorial matrix surrounding chondrocyte clusters in areas where mechanically induced cartilage damage was evident.

We also investigated the differential expression of 3-B-3 (−) and 3-B-3 (+) epitope in the Hartley strain albino guinea-pig animal model that spontaneously develops osteoarthritis (17). Bendele and co-workers (18,19) first described the detailed histological analyses of articular cartilage obtained from the knee joints of Hartley strain guinea pigs. In this study they observed the time-dependent onset of degenerative changes in the cartilaginous tissue from knee joints of these guinea pigs that closely mimicked the development of osteoarthritis in humans. The earliest histological signs of cartilage fibrillation occurred in animals that were approximately 3 months old. The disease gradually progressed through to extensive cartilage degeneration, which was evident in most animals aged 12 months or older. There was no indication of any inflammation in the degenerative knee joints.

Figure 3 shows the differential expression of 3-B-3 (−) and 3-B-3 (+) epitope in proteoglycans extracted from articular cartilage obtained from the hip (H) and the medial (MK) and lateral (LK) tibial plateau of the knee joints of 3-month-old and retired breeder (>12 months) guinea pigs. The expression of 3-B-3 (+) epitope indicates that both large proteoglycan subpopulations were present in all three cartilage samples and that they were substituted with 6-sulfated CS glycosaminoglycan chains. However, replicate analyses for the presence of

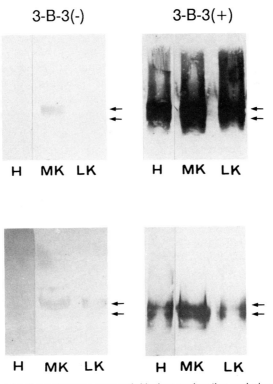

FIG. 3. Guinea-pig model of spontaneous osteoarthritis: Immunolocation analysis of proteoglycans extracted from articular cartilage obtained from the hip (H) and medial (MK) or lateral (LK) tibial plateau from 3-month-old (**top**) and >12-month-old (retired breeder) (**bottom**) Hartley strain guinea pigs. Proteoglycans were extracted from the cartilage and fractionated by composite agarose/polyacrylamide gel electrophoresis. Proteoglycan subpopulations were immunolocated with monoclonal antibody 3-B-3 with (+) or without (−) chondroitinase pretreatment. Positive immunostaining for 3-B-3 (−) epitope indicates the occurrence of atypical CS structures at the nonreducing termini of some glycosaminoglycans chains. The occurrence of this 3-B-3 (−) epitope is a biochemical marker for early changes in the development of osteoarthritis. Immunostaining for 3-B-3 (+) epitope shows the general occurrence of 6-sulfated proteoglycans in these immunolocation analyses. The arrows denote the electrophoretic mobility of the two large aggregating proteoglycans found in cartilage extracts.

3-B-3 (−) epitope in these proteoglycans indicated that CS glycosaminoglycans containing this epitope were only evident in proteoglycans extracted from the medial knee cartilage of the 3-month-old animal and both the lateral and medial tibial cartilage from the retired breeder. There was no expression of 3-B-3 (−) epitope in the hip articular cartilage from either of these animals (Fig. 3) or in any other animals that we have studied so far (ages 1–18 months old, results not shown). The weak expression of 3-B-3 (−) epitope in the medial compartment of the 3-month-old animal exactly parallels the histological findings of the earliest signs of cartilage degeneration in this model (18,19). This expression of epitope increases in all of the knee joint tissues as the disease progresses. The expression of the 3-B-3 (−) epitope is not an age-related phenomenon, because it is not expressed in other guinea-pig strains that do not develop osteoarthritis. This animal model provides yet another example of where the expression of 3-B-3 (−) epitope in the CS glycosaminoglycans can be used as an early marker that precedes cartilage destruction in the development of osteoarthritis. It is also of interest to note that the 3-B-3 (−) epitope is not expressed in the hip articular cartilage from the same leg of each animal even though these joints are subjected to similar weight-bearing experiences throughout the animal's life. This differential in the expression of 3-B-3 (−) epitope in the hip versus knee articular cartilage could be exploited as a suitable internal control for studies evaluating the efficacy of potential therapeutic agents in preventing the development of osteoarthritis.

We have also commenced some preliminary studies examining the expression of 3-B-3 (−) epitope in human osteoarthritic tissue (12). Figure 4 shows an example of the immunolocation analyses of proteoglycans extracted from normal knee articular cartilage and cartilage obtained from a patient with osteoarthritis who was undergoing total knee replacement. Once again, the expression of 3-

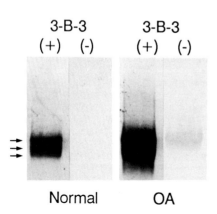

FIG. 4. Expression of 3-B-3 (−) epitope in proteoglycans isolated from human osteoarthritic cartilage. Proteoglycans extracted from normal and osteoarthritic (OA) articular cartilage samples were processed for composite agarose/polyacrylamide gel electrophoresis and immunolocation analysis as previously described (12). Nitrocellulose strips were immunolocated with monoclonal antibody 3-B-3 either before (−) or after (+) chondroitinase digestion of the proteoglycans immobilized on the nitrocellulose sheets. Immunoreactivity with 3-B-3 (+) shows the general staining pattern for 6-sulfated-CS-containing proteoglycans. 3-B-3 (−) reactivity is only observed in the proteoglycans from osteoarthritic cartilage samples. The arrows denote the electrophoretic mobility of the three major large aggregating proteoglycan subpopulations found in human articular cartilage.

B-3 (−) epitope is observed in the CS glycosaminoglycans of osteoarthritic cartilage proteoglycans, but it is not observed in similar proteoglycan samples obtained from normal human articular cartilage. These analyses indicate that expression of 3-B-3 (−) epitope can also be applied to studies of the pathogenesis of osteoarthritis in humans. Exploitation of these findings in future studies may also lead to the development of diagnostic assay procedures that can specifically monitor the progression of the disease in animal models and in humans who are predisposed to the development of osteoarthritis.

MONOCLONAL ANTIBODIES AGAINST PROTEOGLYCAN, LINK PROTEIN, AND ACTIVATED-METALLOPROTEINASE NEO-EPITOPES: THEIR POTENTIAL FOR MONITORING CARTILAGE MATRIX TURNOVER IN ARTHRITIS

In the past year we have begun studies that are directed toward producing monoclonal antibodies against proteoglycan and link protein neo-epitopes (new N- and C-terminal domains of proteins) that are produced on macromolecules as a result of post-translational modification or by the catabolic action of tissue proteinases (see Fig. 5; also see chapter by Roughley et al.). Our preliminary work on these studies has included the production of monoclonal antibodies against synthetic peptides that represent the "neo-epitope" N-terminal sequence of link protein 3 generated by the action of stromelysin on human articular cartilage proteoglycan aggregate (20). In addition, we have also raised a monoclonal antibody against the neo-epitope N-terminal sequence of stromelysin when it is activated from its proenzyme precursor. The N-terminal peptides (see Table

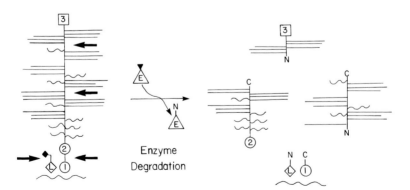

FIG. 5. Schematic representation of the neo-epitopes that are generated by the proteolytic action of tissue proteinases on cartilage proteoglycan aggregate. The arrows depict the hypothetical sites of a proteolytic enzyme (E) cleavage of the proteoglycan core protein and link protein (L); 1, 2, and 3 denote the G1, G2, and G3 domains of the proteoglycan monomer core protein, respectively; N and C depict the sites of new N- and C-terminal peptide domains ("neo-epitopes") created by the proteolytic action of the active enzyme. The generation of a N-terminal neo-epitope peptide on the activated form of the enzyme is also illustrated.

1) were prepared by solid phase peptide synthesis and then conjugated to a carrier protein before being used as antigens for monoclonal antibody production.

Specific screening strategies were developed to identify monoclonal antibodies against the different neo-epitope peptides. To date, three promising monoclonal antibodies have been identified: Two recognize the stromelysin-generated link protein 3 N-terminal peptide, and one recognizes the N-terminal peptide on activated stromelysin (66-B-3, 63-C-3, and 68-A-1, respectively). Screening procedures set up to determine the specificity of the antibodies showed that each antibody had strong reactivity against the immunizing antigen while showing no reactivity against other unrelated peptide conjugates (Table 1). More detailed characterization of the specificity of these antibodies still needs to be performed. Our recent preliminary analyses indicate that monoclonal antibodies 66-B-3 and 63-C-3 will preferentially recognize the new N-terminal sequence in link protein 3 that is produced after stromelysin cleavage of proteoglycan aggregates (21) isolated from a 21-year-old human articular cartilage sample. The lack of reactivity with link protein 1 or 2 strongly suggests that there is antibody specificity toward the N-terminal domains of this peptide. There was, however, additional reactivity with other non-link-protein components of this stromelysin digestion of human articular cartilage proteoglycan aggregates. At present we cannot explain this apparent cross-reactivity, but it could involve the low-affinity recognition of related neo-epitope sequences that occur in degradation products after stromelysin digestion of the proteoglycan monomer protein core.

Production of these and other neo-epitope antibodies have considerable potential for use in identifying the actions of specific enzymes responsible for normal matrix turnover and also matrix degradation products in arthritic diseases. Furthermore, the combined use of our structural, marker, and neo-epitope monoclonal antibodies may lead to the development of diagnostic procedures that can distinguish specific proteoglycan degradation patterns in patients with different pathological forms of arthritis.

TABLE 1. *Absorbance readings measured by direct enzyme-linked immunosorbent assay of monoclonal antibodies 63-C-3, 66-B-3 (raised against LP3), and 68-A-1 (raised against active stromelysin) using a panel of antigens[a]*

Peptide-conjugate	63-C-3	66-B-3	68-A-1
Link protein 3 (IQAENGPHLLC)	3.08[b]	3.16[b]	0.12
Active stromelysin (FRTFPGIPKWRC)	0.09	0.04	3.38[b]
Link proteins 1 and 2 (DHLSDNYTGGC)	0.13	0.04	0.09
Ovalbumin-cysteine (conjugate)	0.12	0.04	0.07

[a] Plates were coated with the peptide conjugates at 3 µg/ml. Sequences of the peptides conjugated to the carrier protein (ovalbumin) are shown in parentheses.
[b] Strong positive reactivity against the neo-epitope peptide.

SUMMARY AND CONCLUSIONS

The application of monoclonal antibody technology to the identification of immunological markers of cartilage proteoglycan metabolism in animal and human osteoarthritis shows considerable potential for development in the future. Our recent finding that the detection of subtle structural changes in CS glycosaminoglycans can be used as a biochemical marker for the development of osteoarthritis was a surprising one because many earlier studies had focused on looking for disease-specific changes related to the protein components of the cartilage proteoglycan aggregate. In our studies performed so far we have consistently observed the expression of 3-B-3 (–) epitope in proteoglycans isolated from osteoarthritic cartilage in several animal models and in human osteoarthritis. Similarly, the specific occurrence of 7-D-4 epitope in osteoarthritic proteoglycans has been observed in dog models of osteoarthritis and in humans but not in the guinea-pig animal model. The proteoglycan subpopulation containing the 3-B-3 epitope is generally the slower migrating electrophoretic species found after composite agarose/polyacrylamide gel electrophoresis. This subpopulation has an electrophoretic mobility that is similar to that of newly synthesized proteoglycans (22) before post-translational modifications that lead to increased proteoglycan heterogeneity have occurred. This observation suggests that at the early stages of the development of osteoarthritis, the newly synthesized proteoglycans contain some CS glycosaminoglycan side chains that have different non-reducing terminal disaccharide structures (i.e., different CS-chain termination mechanisms). Not all of the CS chains contain the 3-B-3 (−) epitope. Our preliminary findings suggest that those glycosaminoglycan chains that do are concentrated near the C-terminal (G3 domain) of the chondroitin sulfate attachment region (results not shown).

The biological function of the differential expression of these atypical structures within CS glycosaminoglycans is presently not known. However, our current working hypothesis is that they may be involved in regulating the local storage, binding, and/or activity of cytokines and growth factors within the extracellular matrix. It has also been of interest to us to note that the specific expression of 3-B-3 (−) and 7-D-4 epitopes occurs in the hypertrophic zone, but not in the resting or proliferative zones, of growth plate cartilage (12,23). This observation suggests that proteoglycans containing these epitopes in their CS glycosaminoglycans may be a marker for a change in the phenotypic expression of chondrocytes during normal growth and development (as in growth plate) and with the onset of cartilage pathology (as in osteoarthritis). Recent reports of the presence of type X collagen in osteoarthritic articular cartilage (24; also see chapter by von der Mark et al.) support this hypothesis, and this suggests that the development of osteoarthritis may involve changes in the phenotypic expression of the normally senescent articular cartilage chondrocyte when compared to that seen in the hypertrophic chondrocyte of the growth plate. Thus the osteoarthritic phenotype represents or mimics a progression of (normal) mature chondrocytes toward hypertrophic expression: a normal progression expressed in an abnormal setting.

ACKNOWLEDGMENTS

These studies were supported by grants from the NIH (AR32666 and AR40364), the Orthopaedic Research and Education Foundation (OREF), and Lilly Research Laboratories. The authors acknowledge the work of Dr. Robert Slater for his contributions to the OREF-supported component of this study, and we also would like to thank Ms. Janet Tilley for typing this chapter.

REFERENCES

1. Muir H. Current and future trends in articular cartilage research and osteoarthritis. In *Articular cartilage biochemistry.* Kuettner K, Hascall V, Schleyerback R, eds. New York: Raven Press, 1986;423–440.
2. Hardingham TE. Degenerative joint disease. In: Cohen RD, Alberti KGMM, et al., eds. *The metabolic and molecular basis of acquired disease.* London: Denman–Bel Aire–Tindel, 1990.
3. Maroudas A, Mizrahi J, Katz EP, Wachtel EJ, Soudry M. Physicochemical properties and functional behaviour of normal and osteoarthritic human cartilage. In: Kuettner K, Hascall V, Schleyerback R, eds. *Articular cartilage biochemistry.* New York: Raven Press, 1986;311–329.
4. Carney SL, Muir H. The structure and function of cartilage proteoglycans. *Physiol Rev* 1988;68: 858–910.
5. Mow V, Rosenwasser M. Articular cartilage: biomechanics. In: Woo SL, Buckwalter JA, eds. *Injury and repair of the musculoskeletal soft tissues.* American Academy of Orthopaedic Surgeons, Chicago. 1988;427–463.
6. Seno M, Anno K, Yaegashi Y, Okuyama T. Microheterogeneity of chondroitin sulfates from various cartilages. *Connect Tissue Res* 1975;3:87–96.
7. Michelacci Y, Dietrich C. Chondroitinase C from flavobacterium heparinum. *Biochim Biophys Acta* 1976;451:436–443.
8. Mankin HJ, Lipiello L. The glycosaminoglycans of normal and osteoarthritic cartilage. *J Clin Invest* 1970;50:1712–1720.
9. Wasterson A, Lindahl U. The distribution of sulphate residues in the chondroitin sulphate chain. *Biochem J* 1971;125:903–908.
10. Sorrell JM, Lintalla AM, Mahmoodian F, Caterson B. Indirect immunocytochemical localization of chondroitin sulfate proteoglycans in lymphopoietic and granulopoietic compartments of developing bursae of Fabricus. *J Immunol* 1988;140:4263–4270.
11. Sorrell JM, Mahmoodian F, Schafer IA, Davis B, Caterson B. Monoclonal antibodies that recognize novel epitopes in native chondroitin/dermatan sulfate glycosaminoglycan chains: their use in mapping functionally distinct domains of human skin. *J Histochem Cytochem* 1990;38:393–402.
12. Caterson B, Mahmoodian F, Sorrell JM, Hardingham TE, Bayliss MT, Carney SL, Ratcliffe A, Muir H. Modulation of native chondroitin sulfate structure in tissue development and in disease. *J Cell Sci* 1990;97:411–417.
13. Caterson B, Griffin J, Mahmoodian F, Sorrell JM. Monoclonal antibodies against chondroitin sulfate isomers: their use as probes for investigating proteoglycan metabolism. *Biochem Soc Trans* 1990;18:820–823.
14. Caterson B, Calabro T, Hampton A. Monoclonal antibodies as probes for elucidating proteoglycan structure and function. In: Wight T, Mecham R, eds. *Biology of the extracellular matrix: a series, "Biology of proteoglycans."* New York: Academic Press, 1987;1–26.
15. Sorrell JM, Mahmoodian F, Caterson B. Immunochemical and biochemical comparisons between embryonic chick bone marrow and epiphyseal cartilage chondroitin/dermatan sulfate proteoglycans. *J Cell Sci* 1988;91:81–90.

16. Visco DM, Johnstone B, Caterson B, O'Connor BL, Widmer WR, Jolly GA. Canine experimental osteoarthritis: a comparison of the Pond–Nuki and arthrotomy procedures; macroscopic, histochemical and immunolocalization results. *Trans Orthop Res Soc* 1991;16:328.
17. Caterson B, Blankenship-Paris T, Chandrasekhar S, Bendele A, Slater R. Biochemical characterization of guinea pig cartilage proteoglycans with the onset of "spontaneous" osteoarthritis. *Trans Orthop Res Soc* 1991;16:251.
18. Bendele A, Hulman JF. Spontaneous cartilage degeneration in guinea pigs. *Arthritis Rheum* 1988;31:561–565.
19. Bendele AM, White SL, Hulman JF. Osteoarthrosis in guinea pigs: histopathologic and scanning electron microscopic features. *Lab Anim Sci* 1989;39:115–121.
20. Nguyen Q, Murphy G, Roughley PJ, Mort JS. Degradation of proteoglycan aggregate by a cartilage metalloproteinase" *Biochem J* 1989;259:61–67.
21. Murphy G, Hembry RM, Hughes CE, Fosang AJ, Hardingham TE. Role and regulation of metalloproteinases in connective tissue turnover. *Biochem Soc Trans* 1990;18:812–815.
22. Carney SL, Bayliss MT, Collier JM, Muir H. Electrophoresis of ^{35}S-labeled proteoglycans on polyacrylamide–agarose composite gels and their visualization by fluorography. *Anal Biochem* 1986;156:38–44.
23. Byers S, Caterson B, Hopwood JJ, Foster BK. Immunolocation of glycosaminoglycans in the human growth plate. *J Histochem Cytochem* 1991; submitted.
24. Walker G, Fischer M, Thompson RC Jr, Oegema TR Jr. The expression of type X collagen in osteoarthritis. *Trans Orthop Res Soc* 1991;16:340.

DISCUSSION

Kresse: Have you done any quantitative studies with the 3-B-3 antibody to see what proportion of chondroitin sulfate chains bears that characteristic epitope? If all chondroitin sulfate chains had the same nonreducing end, this might help us understand the mechanisms of chain termination.

Caterson: There are about 100 chondroitin sulfate chains per proteoglycan monomer molecule, but only 10–20 of them appear to contain the epitopes. 3-B-3 tends to occur at a greater frequency on the slower migrating (larger) proteoglycan subpopulation. This suggests that the chains that contain the epitope are concentrated towards the G3 end of the molecule.

Sandy: Are molecules with these altered chondroitin sulfate epitopes released from cartilage into synovial fluid or serum?

Hardingham: We have developed in collaboration with Bruce Caterson ELISA methods for analyzing these chondroitin sulfate epitopes, and they can be detected easily in synovial fluid and in serum. We have not correlated their levels with patient history or disease progression.

Glant: Have you ever analyzed the proteoglycans detected by your antibody in the deepest layer of osteoarthritic cartilage? Are they new, are they the same molecules, or do they have the same core protein as aggrecan but with different glycosylation?

Caterson: In growth-plate cartilage the 3-B-3 epitope is concentrated in the hypertrophic zone where proteoglycans have longer chondroitin sulfate chains and appear to be larger in overall size. Biochemical changes in osteoarthritic proteoglycans are similar in that they have longer chondroitin sulfate chains. I guess that their protein cores are similar, if not identical, to aggrecan, but nobody has studied this in detail.

Glant: You discussed methods for developing monoclonals against "neo-epitopes" created by proteolytic cleavages in the proteoglycan core protein and link protein. My work suggests that such "neo-epitopes" may participate in the pathological process against cartilage.

Articular Cartilage and Osteoarthritis,
edited by K. Kuettner et al.
Raven Press, Ltd., New York © 1992.

30

Serum Keratan Sulfate: A Measure of Cartilage Proteoglycan Metabolism

Eugene J-M. A. Thonar,*·† Daniel H. Manicourt,‖
James M. Williams,*·†·‡ Kanji Fukuda,* Giles V. Campion,#
Barry M. E. Sweet,** Mary Ellen Lenz,*
Thomas J. Schnitzer,† and Klaus E. Kuettner*·§

*Departments of *Biochemistry, †Internal Medicine (Section of Rheumatology),
‡Anatomy, and §Orthopedic Surgery, Rush Medical College at Rush–Presbyterian–
St. Luke's Medical Center, Chicago, Illinois 60612; ‖Department of Internal Medicine
(Section of Rheumatology), Catholic University of Louvain, 1200 Brussels, Belgium;
#Department of Clinical Research (Section of Rheumatology), Hoechst
Aktiengesellschaft Werk Kalle-Albert, 6200 Wiesbaden 12, Germany;
and **Department of Orthopaedic Surgery, Medical School,
University of the Witwatersrand, Parktown, Johannesburg 2193, South Africa*

STUDIES OF THE RATE OF METABOLISM OF CARTILAGE AGGRECAN

The extracellular matrix of cartilage contains several populations of proteoglycans (PGs), viscoelastic molecules which enable the tissue to undergo rapid and reversible deformation. Aggrecan is, by far, the most abundant type of PG found in cartilage (1). It contains a core protein ($M_r = 2 \times 10^5$ daltons) to which numerous side chains of chondroitin sulfate (CS) and keratan sulfate (KS) are attached (1). Newly synthesized aggrecan molecules interact with hyaluronan and link proteins to form aggregates of large size which are entrapped very effectively within the abundant fibrous network made up of several types of collagen (2). When aggrecan molecules are degraded by proteolytic enzymes during normal turnover or as a result of abnormal disease-related processes, the resulting glycosaminoglycan-bearing fragments rapidly diffuse out of the tissue. The extrusion of these negatively charged fragments may be facilitated by repulsive forces exerted by the negative charges on PGs present at extremely high concentrations in the tissue (1). A large proportion of the fragments are eliminated by the lymphatic system, but some eventually reach the circulation before being cleared by the liver and kidneys (3).

Most KS-bearing peptidoglycans in human blood contain one or a few KS chains (3,4). They are considerably smaller than most of the PG fragments which diffuse out of the cartilage matrix. KS-bearing PG fragments injected intravenously in rabbits are eliminated from the blood at different rates, depending upon their size and composition (half-lives = 6–50 min) (1). Exposure of terminal galactose residues on KS chains and oligosaccharides causes a marked increase in the rate of elimination of fragments of all sizes, suggesting that binding of the fragments to galactose receptors on hepatocytes is an important, if not the major, pathway of elimination from the blood (1). Because KS-bearing molecules isolated from human blood have the longest half-life (approximately 50 min), they may not provide a true reflection of the structure and composition of all the KS-bearing fragments which enter the circulation (1). Future studies should help determine if the small KS-bearing fragments that predominate in blood are derived from the larger fragments which diffuse out of the cartilage matrix, and if they represent a major or, more likely, only a minor subpopulation of the KS-bearing molecules which enter the circulation.

Studies *in vitro* have provided important information about the mechanisms for turnover of PG molecules in cartilage. Cultures of articular cartilage explants have confirmed that when an aggrecan molecule is cleaved, greater than 90% of the fragment(s) containing the glycosaminoglycans is rapidly lost from the tissue (5). Measurement of the proportion of radiolabeled glycosaminoglycans appearing in medium daily can thus be used to obtain a measure of the rate of catabolism of PG molecules. When the cultures are maintained in steady state, the concentration of PGs in the explant remains constant; the rate of PG catabolism is equal to the rate of PG synthesis and thus also provides a measure of the rate of PG turnover (5). Measurements of the rate of catabolism or of turnover of cartilage PGs *in vitro* may not, however, always give an accurate representation of what is happening *in vivo*. For example, cartilage slices—or, as preferred by some, chondrocytes embedded in artificial matrices—are difficult to subject to physiological loading. Furthermore, the culture conditions often make use of factors that are not seen by the cells, and the oxygen tension may be quite different than that *in vivo*. In spite of these limitations, studies *in vitro* can be extremely useful in examining the response of chondrocytes to specific growth factors or drugs (5). However, they cannot be used to predict what will happen when the drug or factor is administered orally or by injection, because these agents may exert indirect effects (i.e., by promoting the production of molecules in noncartilagenous tissues which may, in turn, have a profound influence on PG metabolism in cartilage).

Recent developments have suggested that quantification of a highly sulfated epitope on KS chains (1) or of epitopes on the protein moiety (6) of aggrecan-derived fragments present in body fluids provides a useful measure of the catabolism of cartilage aggrecan *in vivo*. The level of such epitopes in synovial fluid can provide a measure of the degradation of aggrecan molecules within the cartilages in a single synovial joint. Because most of the KS in the mammalian body is present in cartilagenous tissues, a few years ago we proposed that the measurement of the blood level of a highly sulfated epitope present on KS chains in body fluids could provide useful information about the rate of catabolism of the PGs in these tissues (3). The serum or plasma level is much more difficult to interpret because the fragments on which the epitopes are present are derived from the many different cartilages (i.e., hyaline, elastic, and fibrous) which are rich in aggrecan. It should be noted that the concentration of the highly sulfated KS epitope varies not only from cartilage to cartilage, but also from region to region within a cartilage (7). For example, it is present at a much higher concentration in the deeper layers than in the most superficial layer of human articular cartilage from the femoral head (8).

In this chapter, we present a brief overview of recent studies of the highly sulfated KS epitope present in serum and discuss how they have contributed to a better understanding of the metabolism of KS-bearing PGs.

QUANTIFICATION OF THE HIGHLY SULFATED KS EPITOPE

The Competitive Indirect Enzyme-Linked Immunosorbent Assay (ELISA)

Most researchers who have quantified KS epitopes in body fluids have utilized a competitive indirect ELISA which uses the well-characterized 1/20/5-D-4 anti-KS monoclonal antibody (9). This antibody recognizes a highly sulfated sequence of several repeats of the disulfated disaccharide (6-sulfated N-acetylglucosamine-$\beta1,3$–6-sulfated galactose-$\beta1,4$) which is present in long KS chains distributed over the entire length of the polysaccharide-attachment region (1) (Fig. 1). Some of the longest KS chains have recently been shown to contain more than one epitope adjacent to each other (10).

KS-related epitopes are easier to quantify accurately than are some aggrecan-related protein epitopes. The hyaluronate-binding region, for example, must be denatured prior to quantification to prevent it from binding to hyaluronate (HA), link protein, or other HA-binding region molecules; such interactions have been shown to result in the masking or, in some cases, unmasking of epitopes (11). Although denaturation is easy to achieve, the need to remove the denaturing agent which can inactivate the antibody or suppress antigen–antibody interactions is a complicating factor.

The ELISA we developed to quantify the sulfated KS epitope (3) was recently modified after discovering that the anti-KS antibody bound to antigenic KS chains with greater avidity at pH 5.3 than at pH 7.0 (12). This modification yields steeper inhibition curves for both standards and unknowns and thus increases the ability to discriminate between concentrations of antigenic KS that are not markedly different (1). The ELISA gives a good measure of the epitope

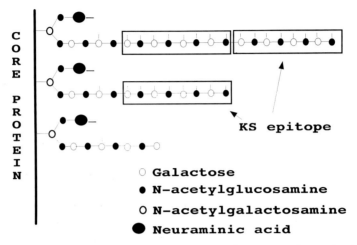

FIG. 1. Schematic representation of the tentative structure of antigenic and nonantigenic keratan sulfate (KS) chains. The longest KS chain is shown here as containing two contiguous epitopes on the basis of its ability to bind to at least two antibody molecules. The negatively charged sulfate groups on galactose and *N*-acetylglucosamine are represented as short vertical lines.

irrespective of the size of the molecule on which it is present (1). For example, pretreatment of aggrecan with keratanase (*Pseudomonas* species) and endo-B-galactosidase (*Escherichia freundii*), enzymes that cleave KS chains in nonantigenic regions, causes no detectable loss of KS epitope in the ELISA. On the other hand, similar treatment with keratanase II, a new KS-degrading enzyme (a kind gift from Seikagaku, Japan) which cleaves the β1-3 linkage between 6-sulfated *N*-acetylglucosamine and 6-sulfated galactose (13), causes total loss of antigenicity. It is important to note that not all anti-KS monoclonal antibodies can be used to quantify the KS epitope in serum by the competitive indirect ELISA; some of the antibodies bind with much lower affinity to KS epitope on soluble PG fragments than to the same fragments insolubilized on the plastic (1).

The ELISA is very sensitive. Quantification in duplicate requires less than 50 μl of serum or plasma. The epitope is extremely stable in serum. Samples stored at $-60°$C for several years, or frozen and thawed several times, show no detectable loss in antigenicity (1). Care should be taken to avoid hemolysis of red blood cells, because it may cause some loss in antigenicity when the hemolysis is very pronounced. Because the KS epitope recognized by the 1/20/5-D-4 antibody is not available in large quantities, the results in all of our studies are reported in terms of equivalents of an international standard of KS purified from human costal cartilage. One should avoid using undefined commercial standards of KS, because those we tested were not pure and had apparently lost much of their antigenicity during purification.

Significance of the Serum Level of KS Epitope

The serum level of KS epitope is surprisingly constant in normal individuals (14). It shows no apparent variation during the day or from day to day. It does not change significantly in naive runners following a 3-mile run or in experienced runners after a marathon (1). Likewise, bed rest is not usually accompanied by a detectable change in the serum level. However, if bed rest is maintained for several months, the level eventually shows a significant decrease (M. B. E. Sweet and E. J-M. A. Thonar, *unpublished observations*). Interestingly, the serum level returns to the pre-inactivity level following remobilization. These results suggest that measurement at a single time point provides a good indirect estimate of the rate of PG turnover in any individual. More importantly, they suggest that the rate of PG turnover is relatively constant over short periods of time.

The serum level of KS epitope shows a complex pattern of maturation-related changes in children (15). In adult life, levels are more stable but show a tendency to increase with age (3,16). Similar age-related changes have been detected in many different mammalian species (1). Within the adult population, levels vary, sometimes markedly, from individual to individual (1). We have postulated that the individual variations in the serum level of KS epitope within the adult population reflect differences in the rate of cartilage aggrecan catabolism/turnover (1). This contention that an adult who has an abnormally high serum level of KS epitope has an elevated rate of cartilage PG catabolism/turnover is based on several assumptions. First, we cannot rule out at this stage the possibility that a difference in the serum level of two adult individuals does not correspond, at least in part, to a difference in either (a) the proportion of cartilage-derived KS-bearing fragments that reaches the blood or (b) the rate of clearance of the fragments from the blood. Second, it is possible that adults with elevated serum levels of KS epitope have KS chains that are much more antigenic. A recent observation (17) that serum levels of KS epitope show a good correlation with the serum level of an epitope present on the core protein of aggrecan suggests that the level probably offers a good measure of total KS present. Studies are in progress to measure total KS (antigenic + nonantigenic) in serum to determine if, as hypothesized, the level of antigenic KS in serum provides an accurate measure of total KS present.

Abnormalities in the Metabolism of Corneal KS and Polylactosamines

The serum level of the KS epitope has been shown to provide important information about abnormalities or changes in the metabolism of KS-bearing PGs in a wide variety of conditions. Measurement of KS epitope in serum has proved useful not only in monitoring the catabolism of aggrecan molecules but also in shedding some light on the pathogenesis of macular corneal dystrophy

(MCD), an inherited blinding disease characterized by the accumulation of opaque deposits in the corneal stroma (18,19). Patients with type I MCD, the most prevalent form, appear to have an abnormality in the metabolism of one or both sulfotransferases which add sulfate residues onto galactose and *N*-acetylglucosamine in keratan chains (18,19). These patients, who are able to synthesize unsulfated keratan chains (19), have no detectable KS epitope in serum, cornea, or cartilage (20). Some individuals with clinical and histopathological evidence of MCD have detectable amounts of the highly sulfated KS epitope in serum and are now classified as having type II MCD (1,18). Some of the individuals belonging to this group have normal KS epitope levels, whereas others have levels that are unusually low. It is thus possible that additional groupings may be necessary to identify different abnormalities.

Because most of the KS epitope present in blood is derived from cartilage, the results suggested that in type I MCD, keratan chains in cartilage are also unsulfated, a contention that has since been corroborated by direct analysis of nasal cartilage from a patient (1,20). Since individuals with type I MCD do not appear to show an increased incidence of degenerative changes in cartilage, we have postulated that the sulfated groups on keratan chains are not essential for the functional properties of aggrecan molecules in this tissue (1,20).

Measurement of the level of KS epitope in serum has also proved useful in studying abnormalities in the metabolism of polylactosamines, which contain long segments of the repeat disaccharide *N*-acetylglucosamine–galactose (21). A patient with decreased amounts of membrane-bound galactosyltransferase in microsomal membranes from mononuclear cells was recently found to have an abnormally low serum level of KS epitope; this suggested that the chondrocytes were also affected by this galactosyltransferase defect (21).

Cartilage Tumors

The study of Kliner et al. (22) demonstrated that the serum level of KS epitope was elevated in patients with cartilage tumors, suggesting that some of the KS-bearing fragments in blood were derived from the degradation of PGs in the tumors. Levels dropped significantly in 9 out of 10 patients after removal of the tumor. Interestingly, the decrease was higher in patients with benign tumors containing relatively large amounts of KS and a well-differentiated cartilage matrix than in patients with lesser-differentiated matrix containing little KS. Although individual differences in the rates of metabolism of PGs in normal cartilage may make it difficult to use measurements of serum KS epitope to diagnose the presence of a tumor or ascertain tumor grade, sequential measurements in such patients may be very useful in monitoring secondary growth of cartilage tumors following primary excision. Alternatively, new monoclonal antibodies directed against other epitopes on the KS chains may allow more specific quantification of tumor-derived KS as opposed to normal cartilage-derived KS.

Abnormalities of Growth

Serum levels of KS epitope undergo marked age-related changes during growth (15). These reflect age-related changes in (i) the ratio of cartilage mass to body weight or to blood volume, (ii) the structure or concentration of KS in cartilage, (iii) the length of KS chains which may result in changes in the ratio of epitope to KS mass, (iv) the extent of cartilage replacement by bone, and (v) the rates of catabolism of PGs in the different cartilages that will not be replaced by bone (1). Interestingly, ossification of the cartilagenous backbone of the rapidly growing deer antler is accompanied by a rapid, but transient, rise in the serum level of KS epitope (23). This process, which occurs yearly, offers an excellent model for studying the relationship between changes in the serum level of KS epitope and replacement of growing cartilage by bone.

At any one age, the serum level of KS epitope shows a positive correlation with percentile height, supporting the contention that the rate of growth is a function of the activity of the chondrocytes (15). Children with constitutional delay of maturity (below the 5th percentile for height but not growth-hormone-deficient) and children who are growth-hormone-deficient have abnormally low levels (24). Administration of growth hormone to growth-hormone-deficient children resulted in a significant rise in the serum level of KS epitope, together with expected increases in annualized growth rate velocity and plasma levels of insulin-like growth factor 1 (24). A study is in progress to probe further the significance of these exciting findings.

Steroids and Nonsteroidal Anti-Inflammatory Drugs (NSAIDs)

In normal adults, the ratio of cartilage mass to blood volume, the concentration of KS in cartilage, and the size of the KS chains show only moderate changes with increasing age (1). The amount of cartilage PG catabolized during turnover is replaced via the synthesis and incorporation in the matrix of an equivalent amount of PG. It is worth noting that the mass of KS present in normal human blood at any one time has been calculated to be approximately 0.75 mg (3). This corresponds to about 38 mg of cartilage (i.e., less than 0.05% of the total mass of cartilage in the body). Because the serum level of KS epitope in normal adults does not fluctuate diurnally or from day to day (14), a single test result can be used as an indirect measure of the metabolic activity of chondrocytes.

Drugs which may either act as "chondroprotective" agents, help promote cartilage regeneration, or just simply increase the rate of PG synthesis are the subject of much debate. Studies of the effect of a particular drug on cartilage PG metabolism have had to limit themselves to examination of its effect on PG synthesis or turnover *in vitro* (25). A major advantage of the quantification of the KS epitope in serum is that it provides a measure of the effect of such drugs on the catabolism of cartilage aggrecan *in vivo*. Oral administration of piroxicam

(40 mg daily) or naproxen (1 g daily) for several weeks did not cause a significant change in the serum level of KS epitope, suggesting that these two NSAIDs have little, if any, effect on the rate of cartilage PG catabolism (26) (Fig. 2). In contrast, prednisone (40–60 mg daily) given orally for 3 days to patients attending an allergy clinic caused a rapid decrease in the serum level of KS epitope that was already evident after 24 hr and reached a maximum on day 4 (mean KS epitope level = 61% of pretreatment level) (26). Importantly, the effect of cortisone in these individuals who did not have joint problems appeared to be long-lasting; the serum level of KS epitope was still only 69% of pretreatment level 32 days after treatment was stopped (Fig. 2). More recently, Campion et al. (*this volume*) reported that a single intra-articular injection of corticosteroids in the knee joint of patients with osteoarthritis (OA) caused a similar decrease in the serum level of KS epitope (mean KS epitope level on day 7 after the injection = 68% of pretreatment level) (Fig. 2). Measurement of the serum level of KS epitope could

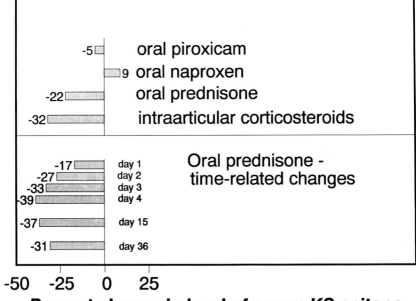

FIG. 2. Effects of drugs on the serum level of KS epitope. **Upper panel:** Summary of the findings in a study of patients with knee osteoarthritis who were tested after having taken piroxicam (40 mg/day, *N* = 40) or naproxen (1 g/day, *N* = 22) orally for several weeks and of patients with asthma (*N* = 7) who were tested immediately after a 4-day treatment with oral prednisone (40–60 mg/day) (26). A group of five patients with knee osteoarthritis who received a single intra-articular injection of corticosteroids were tested 1 week after the injection (Campion et al., *this volume*). The results for each of the four groups are reported as the mean percent change, using the mean level prior to treatment as the baseline value. **Lower panel:** Changes in the serum level of one of the asthma patients tested at various times after the initiation of the treatment with oral prednisone (26).

thus prove extremely useful in selecting the minimum dose needed to suppress the well-documented elevation in the rate of PG catabolism in OA joints. This approach could also help in reducing the risk of unduly suppressing PG synthesis.

Proteolytic Degradation of PGs in a Single Synovial Joint or Intervertebral Disc

Because KS epitope present in serum is derived from all cartilagenous structures in the body, a slight change in the rate of PG catabolism in a single synovial joint is unlikely to give rise to a measurable increase in the level of KS epitope in serum. However, recent studies have shown that massive and rapid degradation of the cartilage PGs in a single synovial joint causes a large transient rise in the serum level of KS epitope (12,27; also see chapter by Williams et al.). For example, the injection of as little as 20 μg chymopapain in one rabbit knee joint causes a severalfold increase in the serum level of KS epitope (See chapter by Williams et al.). Levels rise within 30 min and remain at a plateau for 24–48 hr before returning to preinjection values. In contrast, levels do not change in animals injected intra-articularly with saline or intramuscularly with the enzyme. The articular cartilage in the knee injected with chymopapain shows a marked loss in PG content at 24 or 48 hr after the injection. Importantly, articular cartilage in the contralateral knee is totally unaffected by this treatment. Replenishment of the PGs in the cartilage of the injected joint begins soon thereafter and is evident by day 9, when serum levels have returned to baseline. This observation that the level is not elevated during the repair phase supports the postulate that the KS-bearing molecules in blood are a marker of the degradation of aggrecan and not of its synthesis.

Similar large increases in serum levels of KS epitope have been observed in humans (14), dogs (28), and rabbits (29) following the injection of chymopapain or trypsin in intervertebral discs. The appearance of a rise in serum KS epitope following injection of chymopapain into the nucleus pulposus of a herniated human intervertebral disc provides the clinician with direct evidence that the enzyme was active and injected in the correct place and that the PGs in the tissue have been degraded. This approach was recently shown to be very effective in determining the minimum dose of chymopapain needed to degrade most of the aggrecan molecules in the nucleus pulposus of a single rabbit intervertebral disc (29) (Fig. 3). A similar study is in progress to determine the minimum dose needed to achieve a similar effect in humans; this will enable physicians to reduce the dose of chymopapain administered, thereby reducing the risk of anaphylactic shock.

Osteoarthritis

An elevation in the rate of degradation of PGs is widely believed to contribute to the progressive degeneration of articular cartilage in OA (1). This rise in the

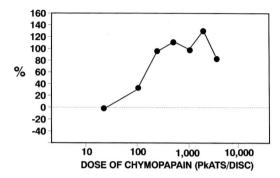

FIG. 3. Changes in the serum level of KS epitope following the injection of a single dose of chymopapain into a rabbit intervertebral disc (29). Individual adult rabbits received an injection of 20–4000 pKats of chymopapain into the L2–L3 intervertebral disc. Blood was drawn immediately before the injection and 24 hr later, and the serum was analyzed for content of KS epitope.

rate of PG catabolism which appears to begin while the condition is clinically silent is counterbalanced in its early stages by a corresponding increase in PG synthesis (30). We have suggested that this state of hypermetabolism, which interestingly appears to develop during middle age in some individuals without any evidence of joint disease, may predispose to OA (1,31,32). The rationale for this contention is based upon recent evidence that a proportion of the HA-binding regions which are generated during PG turnover may remain attached to HA, thereby reducing the number of sites which are accessible to newly synthesized PGs (1,33,34). These PG fragments which have been shown to accumulate in articular cartilage with age (33,34) contain no or few glycosaminoglycan chains and therefore contribute little to the functional properties of the tissue. With time, this probably weakens the ability of the articular surface to act as a unit in withstanding the high stresses that are placed upon it. In individuals who are turning over their cartilage PGs at accelerated rates, it is likely that the nonfunctional fragments do accumulate at a faster rate, thereby predisposing tissues to failure in regions that are heavily loaded (1).

Recent studies have shown that the mean levels of serum KS epitope are higher in populations of patients with generalized OA than in age-matched individuals without signs of joint disease (31,32,35,36). These results strongly support the widely held belief that aggrecan molecules in OA cartilages are being degraded at abnormally fast rates. It is worth noting that a proportion of patients with OA do not have elevated serum levels of KS epitope whereas a small percentage of adults without any clinical signs of OA do (31). Consequently, a single measurement of the serum level of KS epitope is not a useful marker of the articular cartilage destruction that is evident in patients who exhibit clinical symptoms. That point was made in an earlier paper published on the subject (32); in that study, the removal of a large joint exhibiting severe cartilage degeneration did not cause a significant, sustained decrease in the serum level of KS epitope in any one of the 31 patients studied.

Synovial joints contain only a small proportion of all cartilagenous structures containing KS (37). It is therefore probable that the excess KS present in the blood of some patients with OA is derived, in part, from other cartilages in the body as well. We have proposed that in individuals with generalized or polyarticular OA, the high serum level of KS epitope reflects a systemic state of PG hypermetabolism involving all the cartilagenous structures in the body (1,32). This raises the exciting possibility that the state of hypermetabolism may be under the control of a blood-borne factor.

Because OA is heterogeneous in regard to etiology, severity of degenerative changes, and number of joints involved (38), it is extremely difficult to correlate the serum level of KS epitope with one or more etiological or clinical aspects of the OA condition. If, as proposed above, the systemic state of hypermetabolism predisposes all cartilages in the body to failure, then one would expect individuals with sustained high levels of serum KS epitope to exhibit articular cartilage changes in many joints. Support for this hypothesis was recently obtained in studies of well-defined OA subpopulations: The serum levels of KS epitope were found to correlate positively with polyarticular joint involvement and other signs of generalized or polyarticular OA (32,35).

In a population of patients with knee OA, the serum level of KS epitope did not show a marked fluctuation from year to year (35). However, the results of a recent study of a patient exhibiting rapid articular destruction associated with avascular necrosis of the femoral head suggested that this may not always apply in all forms of OA. The rapid destruction of articular cartilage in one hip joint was accompanied by a marked rise in the serum level of KS epitope (Fig. 4). The level then returned to a more normal value following arthroplasty. Interestingly, the level rose again when the articular cartilage in the other hip joint began to show similar degenerative changes; the level again returned to a more normal value following arthroplasty and appeared to remain relatively stable for the next several months.

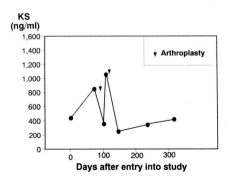

FIG. 4. Changes in the serum level of KS epitope in a patient with avascular necrosis of the femoral head (Fukuda et al., *unpublished observations*). Serum was obtained at entry into the study (day 0) and at various times thereafter. The two peaks correspond to times when articular cartilage in separate hips was undergoing rapid destruction; arthroplasty was performed at the times shown by the vertical arrow and was followed in each case by a marked drop in the serum level of KS epitope. Levels of KS epitope are reported in terms of equivalents of a standard of KS purified from dogfish cartilage.

Recent studies have suggested that quantification of KS epitope in synovial fluid and serum could prove most useful in assessing increases in the rate of PG catabolism during the early phase of OA. For example, Ratcliffe et al. (39), who studied patients with symptoms of pain and dysfunction of the temporomandibular joint which did not resolve with surgical treatment, found that the level of KS epitope in synovial fluid was nearly fourfold higher in individuals exhibiting signs of OA upon arthroscopic examination than in those who did not. In that study, clinical examination and diagnostic imaging had failed to reveal the presence of early OA changes in 14 out of 17 patients. Prospective studies have shown that the levels of epitopes on the peptide moiety of aggrecan-derived fragments or of KS epitope rise markedly during the first few weeks following ligament rupture or meniscal tear in the knee joint and, although they decrease thereafter, appear to remain elevated in some patients (6; also see chapter by Ongchi et al.). Another study showed that serum levels of KS epitope are elevated in individuals with severe acetabular hip dysplasia, a condition which predisposes to OA changes (K. Fukuda, *unpublished observations*). These prospective studies of patients at an increased risk of developing OA could prove useful in determining if individuals who exhibit long-lasting hypermetabolic states are more likely to develop OA. Current studies are in progress to measure the levels of KS epitope in the serum of these individuals in an attempt to obtain information concerning changes taking place in a synovial joint and systemically (level in serum).

Transection of the anterior cruciate ligament (ACLT) in the dog knee joint causes histological and biochemical changes (within a few months) similar to those observed in human OA (40). Although there was originally some concern that the changes were not progressive, a recent study has shown that with time the changes progress to full-blown destruction of the loaded cartilages in the operated joint (41). This model thus appears particularly useful to detect early changes in the metabolism of cartilage aggrecan in the knee and to shed some light on the significance of the subsequent development of the hypermetabolic state that develops systemically. Essentially all animals examined thus far have exhibited a significant rise in the serum level of KS epitope within a few weeks after ACLT (40,42). In contrast, levels in sham-operated dogs remained unchanged or showed a slight decrease (40). The cause of this rapid rise in the rate of catabolism of cartilage PGs in the transected ACL joint is not clear at the present time, nor is the relationship of this elevation to the subsequent development of the OA lesions. It is worth noting that because the PG content of the articular cartilages in the operated knee did not change during this time (40), the increase in the rate of degradation of PGs was almost surely accompanied by a corresponding increase in the rate of PG synthesis.

Manicourt et al. (40) have shown that the rise in the serum level of KS epitope can be detected as early as 7 days after ACLT in the dog (Pond–Nuki model). The level reaches a maximum by 2 weeks and remains elevated until sacrifice, 13 weeks after surgery (Fig. 5). At sacrifice, the level of KS epitope in serum

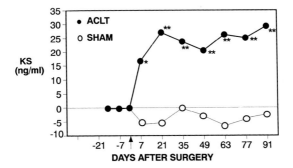

FIG. 5. Changes in the serum level of KS epitope in dogs at different times after anterior cruciate ligament transection (ACLT) or sham operation. In the ACLT ($N = 9$) and sham-operated ($N = 3$) groups, the result at each time point is expressed as the mean of the differences between the postoperative and preoperative levels.

from the operated joint was elevated and appeared to correlate with the magnitude of the rise observed in serum. However, the results of recent studies of humans with ACL injury (6; also see chapter by Ongchi et al.) suggest that an increase in PG catabolism in the operated dog joint was not the major contributor to the changes we observed in the serum of the operated animals. In those human studies, levels of PG fragments in synovial fluid are very high during the first 3–4 weeks after the injury but decline dramatically thereafter. Because levels of KS epitope in dog serum remain at a constant high between weeks 2 and 13 after ACLT, some of the KS appearing in serum must have been derived from other cartilagenous structures as well. Although the mechanisms involved in this stimulation of PG turnover are unclear, it is possible that factors which stimulate cartilage PG turnover systemically are released into the body fluids from articular cartilage, bone, or synovium of the unstable knee in this canine model of OA.

FUTURE PERSPECTIVES

Measurements of the serum level of KS epitope have enabled us to obtain answers to questions that otherwise could not have been asked. The results of studies performed thus far have clearly raised more questions than they have answered, but they have generated several exciting hypotheses.

This simple blood test should continue to be extremely useful in assessing changes in the metabolism of aggrecan in response to promising drugs and growth factors. Because the serum levels of KS epitope appear to correlate with the rate of growth in children, this approach may prove invaluable in studying the effects of such agents on the metabolism of growing cartilages. Rapid progress should also be made in determining the effect of mechanical forces on the turnover of this cartilage PG. The assay will clearly continue to be used as a tool to diagnose genetic abnormalities in the structure or metabolism of KS. These studies will also help improve our understanding of the function of KS chains on KS-bearing

PGs in cartilage and cornea as well as in tissues which have recently been found to contain small amounts of these molecules.

Because the serum levels of KS epitope vary markedly from individual to individual (or animal to animal), it is extremely important to relate levels to the pretreatment level, whenever possible. It is clear that the rise in the serum level of KS epitope, when calculated in this manner, can be used not only to identify the rapid depletion of aggrecan from a single cartilage but also to identify the slower, more progressive changes in the rate of turnover of cartilage aggrecan following experimentally induced joint injury. In patients who present themselves with degenerative cartilage changes and for whom a baseline value is not available, it is more difficult to assess the magnitude of the increase in the rate of aggrecan catabolism. Consequently, attempts to assess whether a change in the metabolism of aggrecan contributed to the initiation or progression of disease-related processes in articular cartilage are unlikely to generate simple answers. Such studies are further hampered by the fact that noninvasive techniques currently used by physicians to identify articular cartilage changes (i.e., x-rays and nuclear magnetic resonance imaging) are not very useful in identifying early changes or assessing disease progression.

Long-term prospective studies of well-defined subpopulations of patients at an increased risk of developing OA (i.e., individuals with joint injury, dysplasia, high levels of KS epitope, etc.) are currently in progress. When combined with arthroscopic examination of affected joints to identify early changes or assess the progression of the disease, these human studies and animal models seem to offer the best hope of unraveling the full potential of measurements of serum KS epitope in the assessment of articular cartilage degeneration.

ACKNOWLEDGMENTS

This work was supported, in part, by grants 1-P50-AR39239 and AG-04736 from the National Institutes of Health. We thank Dr. B. Caterson, the University of North Carolina at Chapel Hill, for his gift of the 1/20/5-D-4 monoclonal antibody; we also thank Drs. M. B. Mathews and A. L. Horwitz, the University of Chicago, for their gift of the international standard of keratan sulfate purified from human costal cartilage.

REFERENCES

1. Thonar EJ-MA, Williams JM, Maldonado BA, Lenz ME, Schnitzer TJ, Campion GV, Kuettner KE. Serum keratan sulfate concentration as a measure of the catabolism of cartilage proteoglycans. In: Kressina T, ed. *Monoclonal antibodies, cytokines, and arthritis. Mediators of inflammation and therapy.* New York: Marcel Dekker, 1991;373–398.
2. Mayne R, Irwin MH. Collagen types in cartilage. In: Kuettner KE, Schleyerbach R, Hascall VC, eds. *Articular cartilage biochemistry.* New York: Raven Press, 1986;23–35.
3. Thonar EJ-MA, Lenz ME, Klintworth GK, et al. Quantification of keratan sulfate in blood as a marker of cartilage catabolism. *Arthritis Rheum* 1984;28:1367–1376.

4. Thonar EJ-MA, Meyer RF, Dennis RF, et al. Absence of normal keratan sulfate in the blood of patients with macular corneal dystrophy. *Am J Ophthalmol* 1985;102:561–569.
5. Handley CJ, McQuillan DJ, Campbell MA, Bolis S. Steady-state metabolism in cartilage explants. In: Kuettner KE, Schleyerbach R, Hascall VC, eds. *Articular cartilage biochemistry.* New York: Raven Press, 1986;163–179.
6. Lohmander LS, Dahlberg L, Ryd L, Heinegard D. Increased levels of proteoglycan fragments in knee joint fluid after injury. *Arthritis Rheum* 1989;32:1434–1442.
7. Aydelotte MB, Thonar EJ-MA, Lenz ME, Schumacher BL, Kuettner KE. Differences in synthesis of keratan sulfate by subpopulations of cultured bovine articular chondrocytes. *Orthop Res Soc Trans* 1989;14:83.
8. Zanetti M, Ratcliffe A, Watt FMJ. Two subpopulations of differentiated chondrocytes identified with a monoclonal antibody to keratan sulfate. *Cell Biol* 1985;101:53–59.
9. Mehmet H, Scudder P, Tang PW, Hounsell EF, Caterson B, Feizi T. The antigenic determinants recognized by three monoclonal antibodies to keratan sulfate involve sulfated hepta- or larger oligosaccharides of the poly(N-acetyllactosamine) series. *Eur J Biochem* 1986;157:385–391.
10. Thonar EJ-MA, Manicourt DM, Williams J, et al. Circulating keratan sulfate: a marker of cartilage proteoglycan catabolism in osteoarthritis. *J Rheumatol* 1991;18(Suppl 27):24–26.
11. Thonar EJ-MA, Kimura JH, Hascall VC, Poole AR. Enzyme-linked immunosorbent assay analyses of the hyaluronate binding region and the link protein of proteoglycan aggregate. *J Biol Chem* 1982;257:14173–14180.
12. Williams JM, Downey C, Thonar EJ-MA. Increase in levels of serum keratan sulfate following cartilage proteoglycan degradation in the rabbit knee joint. *Arthr Rheum* 1988;31:557–560.
13. Nakazawa K, Ito M, Yamagata T, Suzuki S. Substrate specificity of keratan sulphate-degrading enzymes (endo-B-galactosidase, keratanase and keratanase II) from microorganisms. In: Greiling H, Scott JE, eds. *Keratan sulphate. Chemistry, biology, and chemical pathology.* London: The Biochemical Society, 1989;99–110.
14. Block JA, Schnitzer TJ, Andersson GBJ, Lenz ME, Jefferey R, McNeill TW, Thonar EJ-MA. The effect of chemonucleolysis on serum keratan sulfate levels in humans. *Arthritis Rheum* 1989;32:100–105.
15. Thonar EJ-MA, Pachman LM, Lenz ME, Hayford J, Lynch P, Kuettner KE. Age related changes in the concentration of serum keratan sulphate in children. *J Clin Chem Clin Biochem* 1988;26: 57–63.
16. Motoyoshi H, Tanaka S, Nagata Y, Yamasaki H, Fukuda K, Kita H. Age related alteration in levels of keratan sulfate in sera of orthopaedic patients. *J Jpn Orthop Assoc* 1989;63:1464–1468.
17. Saxne T, Hayford J, Heinegard D, Lenz ME, Thonar EJ-MA, Wollheim FA, Pachman L. Serum levels of the proteoglycan core protein and keratan sulfate correlate in juvenile rheumatoid arthritis. *Arthritis Rheum* 1989;32(4):S105.
18. Yang CJ, SundarRaj N, Thonar EJ-MA, Klintworth GK. Immunohistochemical evidence of heterogeneity in macular corneal dystrophy. *Am J Ophthalmol* 1988;106:65–71.
19. Hassell JR, Sundar Raj N, Cintron C, Midura R, Hascall VC. Alterations in the synthesis of keratan sulphate proteoglycan in corneal wound healing and in macular corneal dystrophy. In Greiling H, Scott JE, eds. *Keratan sulphate. Chemistry, biology, chemical pathology.* London: The Biochemical Society, 1989;215–225.
20. Edward DP, Thonar EJ-MA, Srinivasan M, Yue BJYT, Tso MOM. Macular dystrophy of the cornea: a systemic disorder of keratan sulfate metabolism. *Ophthalmology* 1990;97:1194–1200.
21. Fukuda MN, Masri KA, Dell A, Thonar EJ-MA, Klier G, Lowenthal RM. Defective glycosylation of erythrocyte membrane glycoconjugates in a variant of congenital dyserythropoietic anemia type II: association of low level of membrane-bound form of galactosyl transferase. *Blood* 1989;73: 1331–1339.
22. Kliner DJ, Gorski JP, Thonar EJ-MA. Keratan sulfate levels in sera of patients bearing cartilage tumors. *Cancer* 1987;59:1931–1935.
23. Dinsmore CE, Goss RJ, Lenz ME, Thonar EJ-MA. Correlations between phases of deer antler regeneration and levels of serum keratan sulfate. *Calcif Tiss Int* 1985;39:244–247.
24. Pachman LM, Green OC, Lenz ME, Hayford J, Thonar EJ-MA. Increase in serum concentration of keratan sulfate after treatment of growth hormone deficiency with growth hormone. *J Ped* 1990;116:400–403.
25. Brandt KD. A pessimistic view of serologic markers for diagnosis and management of osteoarthritis. Biochemical, immunologic and clinicopathologic barriers. *J Rheumatol* 1989;16(Suppl 18):39–42.

26. Campion G, Schnitzer T, Zeitz H, Lenz ME, Lindeman M, Thonar E. The effect of oral administration of prednisone and of the non-steroidal anti-inflammatory drug (NSAID) piroxicam on serum keratan sulfate (KS). *Orthop Res Soc Trans* 1990;15:334.
27. Williams JM, Moran M, Thonar EJ-MA, Salter RB. Continuous passive motion stimulates repair of rabbit knee articular cartilage following matrix proteoglycan loss. *Ortho Res Soc Trans* 1990;15: 127.
28. Oegema TR, Swedenburg SM, Bradford DS, Thonar EJ-MA. Levels of keratan sulfate-bearing fragments rise predictably following chemonucleolysis of dog intervertebral discs with chymopapain. *Spine* 1988;13:707–711.
29. Williams JM, Kiester D, Thonar EJ-MA, Andersson GB. The effect of intradiscal chymopapain on rabbit intervertebral discs. *Orthop Res Soc Trans* 1991;16(2):356.
30. Muir H. Current and future trends in articular cartilage research and osteoarthritis. In: Kuettner KE, Schleyerbach R, Hascall VC, eds. *Articular cartilage biochemistry.* New York: Raven Press, 1986;423–440.
31. Thonar EJ-MA, Schnitzer TJ, Kuettner KE. Quantification of keratan sulfate in blood as a marker of cartilage catabolism. *J Rheumatol* 1987;14(Suppl 14):23–24.
32. Sweet MBE, Coelho A, Schnitzler CM, et al. Serum keratan sulfate levels in osteoarthritis patients. *Arthritis Rheum* 1988;31:648–652.
33. Roughley PJ, Poole AR, Campbell IK, Mort JS. The proteolytic generation of hyaluronic acid-binding regions derived from the proteoglycans of human articular cartilage as a consequence of aging. *Orthop Res Soc Trans* 1986;11:209.
34. Bayliss MT, Holmes MWA, Muir H. Age-related changes in the stoichiometry of binding region, link protein and hyaluronic acid in human articular cartilage. *Orthop Res Soc Trans* 1989;14: 32.
35. Campion GV, McCrae F, Schnitzer TJ, Watt I, Dieppe PA, Thonar EJ-MA. Do serum levels of keratan sulfate help us with the heterogeneity of osteoarthritis? *Orthop Res Soc Trans* 1989;14: 162.
36. Kongtawelert P, Ghosh P. A new sandwich-ELISA method for the determination of keratan sulphate peptides in biological fluids employing a monoclonal antibody and labelled avidin biotin technique. *Clin Chim Acta* 1990;195:17–26.
37. Attencia LJ, McDevitt CA, Nile WB, Sokoloff L. Cartilage content of an immature dog. *Connect Tissue Res* 1989;18:235–242.
38. Sokoloff L, Hough AJ. Pathology of osteoarthritis. In: McCarthy DJ, ed. *Arthritis and related conditions.* Philadelphia: Lea & Febiger, 1985;1377–1399.
39. Ratcliffe A, Israel HA, Saed-Nejad F, Seibel MJ. Keratan sulfate epitope levels are elevated in synovial fluids from joints with arthroscopically diagnosed early osteoarthritis. *Orthop Res Soc Trans* 1991;16:228.
40. Manicourt DH, Lenz ME, Thonar EJ-MA. Levels of serum keratan sulfate rise rapidly and remain elevated following anterior cruciate ligament transection in the dog. *J Rheumatol* 1991 (in press).
41. Brandt KD, Braunstein EM, Visco DM, O'Connor B, Heck D, Albrecht M. Anterior (cranial) cruciate ligament transection in the dog: a bona fide model of osteoarthritis, not merely of cartilage injury and repair. *Orthop Res Soc Trans* 1991;16:331.
42. Brandt KD, Thonar EJ-MA. Lack of association between serum keratan sulfate concentrations and cartilage changes of osteoarthritis after transection of the anterior cruciate ligament in the dog. *Arthritis Rheum* 1989;32:647–651.

DISCUSSION

Levick: I think it is better to measure levels of markers in serum than in synovial fluids because the problems of interpretation are less severe. Nevertheless, there are some problems. The marker would depend on the volume of the plasma, but this can be assumed to be constant. The concentration also depends on the removal rate constant, which, in turn, depends on kidney and liver function, which change with time. For example, kidney function (glomerular filtration) deteriorates with age, as does liver function. This may not be a problem for short-term changes, as after an acute transection of cruciate ligaments. But in longer-term studies, changes in the input rate and changes in the time constants of removal by the liver and the kidney may be critical and would affect interpretation of changes in marker levels, with advancing age in the human population for example.

Thonar: We do not know too much about long-term changes taking place over a number of years. We have been surprised that the level of the keratan sulfate epitope is as constant as it is, because there are so many factors which could lead to a change with time. We were also amazed that levels were not affected by running a marathon. Our results suggest that the rates of input and removal of fragments remain quite constant in blood over a few months, at least in adults. Over a very long time you do see changes in individuals. At this stage we presume this is caused by a change in the rate of release of the fragments from the cartilage; however, we cannot rule out the possibility that in some individuals this is the result of a change in the rate of clearance of the fragments by the lymphatic system, liver, or kidneys. We hope to test this hypothesis in the future.

Dieppe: You showed that even short treatments with glucocorticoids cause a prolonged decrease in serum KS. What possible mechanisms might explain this? Secondly, how much variation is seen in different individual patients after a short course of steroid treatment? It may be a crazy idea, but one might be able to use a single shot of a steroid or a single growth factor to differentiate patient populations. You might detect people who have different metabolic responses in their connective tissue—in other words, invent a physiological test of joint integrity.

Thonar: There are a lot of relatively simple experiments that need to be done to answer some of the questions you have raised. Most individuals we have looked at have shown a decrease in the serum level of the keratan sulfate epitope in response to treatment with steroids. We do not know how little one would need to give to obtain an effect. This may vary from patient to patient and may depend upon the level of hypercatabolism in patients with osteoarthritis. Our assay is very helpful in determining how little one would need to administer to suppress the hypercatabolism that is observed in articular cartilage in osteoarthritis. This is well worth determining, because high doses of steroids are likely to result in a marked suppression of proteoglycan synthesis. We also hope to measure the serum level of keratan sulfate epitope to determine how long the suppression caused by a single injection lasts.

Glant: The monoclonal antibody 5-D-4 is a wonderful antibody with a very high avidity, but it requires a highly sulfated keratan sulfate segment with a given length. Do you think that the use of an anti-keratan sulfate antibody panel would increase the chance to differentiate between different diseases, which probably express variability of keratan sulfate sulfation?

Thonar: You are correct. In the coming years, we may well gain access to more useful antibodies. One of the problems with this type of keratan sulfate epitope is that it is found only in the longest keratan sulfate chains. In osteoarthritis, there appears to be a switchback to the synthesis of aggrecan molecules with shorter keratan sulfate chains. Consequently, it may be better to use an antibody which recognizes an epitope present in short keratan sulfate chains. No such antibody is currently available. It should be noted that even if such antibodies become available, they would need to have high affinity to be useful in immunoassays used to measure keratan sulfate epitopes present at low concentrations in serum.

Articular Cartilage and Osteoarthritis,
edited by K. Kuettner et al.
Raven Press, Ltd., New York © 1992.

31

Fibronectin in Osteoarthritis

Comparison of Animal and Human Diseases

George Lust and Nancy Burton-Wurster

James A. Baker Institute for Animal Health, College of Veterinary Medicine, Cornell University, Ithaca, New York 14853

Collagens and proteoglycans are the major organic constituents of articular cartilage, and they have been studied extensively. Their function is becoming well known for disease-free (normal) tissue. However, available information about their behavior in the degenerating cartilage of osteoarthritic joints is incomplete. These issues are being addressed in many laboratories and are discussed in this book. Attention is now also being given to noncollagenous and nonproteoglycan constituents of cartilage. It is reasonable to think that these minor components of cartilage have regulatory and/or organizational roles not yet understood.

A report based on data obtained from a canine hip dysplasia model of osteoarthritis initially suggested that a substantial increase in the glycoprotein fibronectin occurs in osteoarthritic cartilage (1). Similar increases in cartilage fibronectin were then reported for osteoarthritic canine knee and shoulder joints (2), surgically induced osteoarthritis in rabbit knee joints (3), and, recently, osteoarthritic joints of horses (Todhunter and Lust, *unpublished data*). Miller et al. (4) were the first to confirm that elevated levels of fibronectin in cartilage occurs in human osteoarthritic joints as well. Jones et al. (5) and Rees et al. (6) substantiated this. Thus it appears that increased fibronectin content in cartilage is a general feature of osteoarthritic joints.

The general subject of fibronectin has been well reviewed in a book by Hynes (7). Two other recent books have been written by Mosher (8) and Carsons (9). Some of the topics covered here have also been reviewed in ref. 9.

ANIMAL OSTEOARTHRITIS

Dogs

We previously reported (10) details of the osteoarthritis that develops in Labrador retrievers with hip dysplasia. The disease develops between 4 and 12 months of age, and at necropsy the hip joints have characteristic degenerative cartilage of one or both femoral heads. Occasionally, mild osteoarthritis also appears in the shoulder and knee joints (10). Mild synovitis usually is present, and osteophytes can also be identified. The fibronectin content in the deteriorating cartilage of dogs is increased, as much as 40-fold when compared to disease-free cartilage (Table 1). Up to 4 µg of fibronectin can be extracted from 1 mg of osteoarthritic cartilage, whereas values for normal cartilage are of the order of 100 ng/mg of wet cartilage. Cartilage from a region surrounding a focal lesion often also has elevated fibronectin content. As the disease advances, the areas of macroscopically "normal" cartilage from osteoarthritic joints can degenerate. Thus these regions may be thought of as an early stage of the disease process. In one report (11), fibronectin content was increased in cartilage in the early osteoarthritic stages whereas the glycosaminoglycan content remained in the normal range.

The source of the increased fibronectin in osteoarthritic cartilage is of interest. Two possibilities come to mind, namely, the chondrocytes and synovial fluid. The differences in structure between plasma and cartilage fibronectin make it unlikely that the plasma is the direct source of the accumulated cartilage fibronectin (12). Evidence that the chondrocytes are the source of at least some of the increased fibronectin in osteoarthritic cartilage includes the following observations: Cartilage explants can synthesize fibronectin; explants of damaged cartilage synthesized more fibronectin than normal and then retained more of this newly synthesized fibronectin within the matrix (13); fibronectin synthesized by cartilage explants had a molecular weight similar to that of the bulk of the fi-

TABLE 1. *Fibronectin of plasma, synovial fluid, and articular cartilage in four species*

| Species | Plasma (µg/ml) | Synovial fluid (µg/ml) | | Articular cartilage (µg/ml) | | References |
		Normal joints	Osteoarthritic joints	Normal joints	Osteoarthritic joints	
Dog	500–900	97	200	0.05–0.1	0.4–4.0	2,13
Horse	390–570	69	200	0.17	0.5	[a]
Rabbit	~300	30[b]	200[b]	0.05	4.5	3,20
Human	300–400	150	250	0.08	2.5	4,7

[a] The values were determined in the authors' laboratory or were taken from the listed references.
[b] Estimated from joint washes after injecting phosphate-buffered 0.9% NaCl into rabbit knee joints at necropsy.

bronectin which accumulated in degenerated cartilage (12). On the other hand, synovial fluid, which may contain a mixture of fibronectins from the synovium and the cartilage, cannot be ruled out as a source of cartilage fibronectin, especially in fibrillated cartilage. This was suggested by studies showing that purified plasma fibronectin labeled with biotin or iodine-125 was incorporated into cartilage explants. Degenerated cartilage from osteoarthritic joints accumulated nearly 10-fold more labeled fibronectin than did disease-free cartilage, although penetration occurred from the articular surface only (14). Disease-free cartilage excluded fibronectin from the articular surface. This was true even after the proteoglycan content was markedly reduced by incubation of the cartilage for several days with an extract of synovium (i.e., interleukin-1) or lipopolysaccharide (14).

We examined the relationship between fibronectin synthesis, cyclic adenosine monophosphate (cAMP), and cell shape in canine articular chondrocytes in monolayer cultures. Addition of dibutyryl cAMP to the cultures promoted retention of a rounded morphology and decreased fibronectin synthesis (15). The isotype of fibronectin synthesized in culture was also affected by the addition of dibutyryl cAMP to the culture medium. Untreated chondrocytes in culture had a polygonal morphology and expressed up to 25% of an isotype of fibronectin called ED-A-fibronectin. This isotype is prominent in fibroblasts, but was detected in cartilage fibronectin only at 1–2% (15). The percentage of fibronectin containing the ED-A sequence was reduced when chondrocytes were round in the presence of dibutyryl cAMP. The cultures treated with dibutyryl cAMP not only decreased fibronectin synthesis, but also increased production of keratan sulfate (16). It remains to be established whether that observation represents increased proteoglycan synthesis.

The fibronectin content of cartilage also was determined in two different experimentally induced canine models of joint degeneration. In the one model, osteoarthritis was induced in adult mongrel dogs by joint destabilization by anterior cruciate ligament transections (17). Animals were sacrificed after some 12 weeks, and articular cartilage was obtained from the habitually loaded areas of the femoral condyles. At an early stage, when macroscopic lesions were not observed, reduction in safranin-O staining was mild, and chondroitin sulfate levels were unchanged or increased, but some loosening of the fibrous subsurface network as well as chondrocyte cloning were seen. Small increases of fibronectin, up to 593 ng/mg wet weight of tissue, were observed in the cartilage taken from the operated joint. In the second model, proteoglycan depletion was induced by immobilization of one hind limb for 6 weeks. As described by Palmoski et al. (18), this model did not go on to develop osteoarthritis. Articular cartilage from the weight-bearing regions of the femoral condyles of the immobilized limb had reduced safranin-O staining, but there was no fissuring, fibrillation, or cloning. In one experiment, fibronectin levels in this proteoglycan-deficient cartilage were normal.

Rabbits

Osteoarthritis can be induced surgically in the rabbit knee as a result of joint destabilization as described by Colombo et al. (19). In this model, the collateral and sesamoid ligaments of the right knee are sectioned, and a slice of the anterior lateral meniscus is removed. This results in degenerated cartilage predominantly on the right lateral femoral condyle. Unoperated left knees, or a sham operation on the right knee of control animals, serve as controls. Moderate-to-severe cartilage lesions on the right lateral femoral condyle showed loss of safranin-O stain, loss of the superficial layer, fibrillation, loss of chondrocytes, and multicellular clusters, as observed on histochemical examination. This degenerated cartilage contained up to 20-fold more fibronectin than did normal cartilage from the contralateral or sham-operated knees as determined in an enzyme-linked immunosorbent assay on extracts of cartilage (Table 1). The synovial fluids of the affected joints had markedly elevated fibronectin concentrations (20).

Horses

The available information about the pathogenesis and pathology of osteoarthritis in horses has been reviewed by McIlwraith (21) and is consistent with osteoarthritis in other species in that the degenerating cartilage regions of diseased carpal joints contained a decreased quantity of proteoglycans and increased amounts of fibronectin. To date, the levels of fibronectin observed in the osteoarthritic joints have not been as high as for the other species, being below 1 μg/ mg of wet cartilage (see Table 1). An explanation for this difference must be sought in further studies. As in the case of diseased dogs and rabbits, the fibronectin concentration of equine osteoarthritic synovial fluids is increased about twofold (Todhunter and Lust, *unpublished data*).

HUMAN OSTEOARTHRITIS

The first independent confirmation that the fibronectin content was increased in osteoarthritic cartilage was made by Miller et al. (4). They presented data that fibronectin was increased in osteoarthritic cartilage of human femoral heads after surgical removal, and that explants of human osteoarthritic cartilage synthesized fibronectin. The authors estimated the fibronectin content of osteoarthritic samples to be about 2.5 μg/mg of wet cartilage, which is comparable to the values obtained for osteoarthritic cartilage from dogs and rabbits (see Table 1).

The presence of increased amounts of fibronectin in osteoarthritic cartilage subsequently also was confirmed in human femoral head samples by Jones et al. (5), who used immunoperoxidase localization. The fibronectin localized in a band in the matrix of the surface zone. The authors, and also Rees et al. (6), identified intracellular fibronectin in cells of the surface zone, as well as in deeper zones of cartilage, and they proposed that this indicated local synthesis of the protein *in vivo.* They postulated that the increased synthesis of fibronectin by osteoarthritic cartilage was a response by chondrocytes to change in the matrix. Brown and Jones (22) continued these studies and reported that there was a 10-fold increase of fibronectin in osteoarthritic human cartilage and presented data that fibronectin interacted strongly with proteoglycans, in that aggregation of cartilage proteoglycans by addition of hyaluronan also aggregated some of a fraction of the endogenous cartilage fibronectins. This latter observation also was made in a preliminary experiment by Burton-Wurster and Lust (*unpublished data*). Recent experiments to explain this finding by binding of cartilage fibronectin to large aggregating proteoglycan have been inconclusive, and research to explain this observation is continuing.

CONCLUSIONS AND SPECULATIONS

Mammalian diarthrodial joints are units, and all component parts are important. Articular cartilage is by necessity a resilient tissue, because it is subject to mechanical forces caused by weight-bearing and movement of the joint. Because mechanical factors are as much a part of the environment of cartilage as are biochemical factors, it is reasonable to expect that the chondrocyte, the cell responsible for maintaining the integrity of the cartilage matrix, will respond to mechanical stress. A goal in our laboratory is to maintain healthy cartilage in explant culture for an extended time and then to manipulate biochemical and mechanical parameters in such a way that we mimic, *in vitro,* the metabolic changes which we observe in tissue from osteoarthritic joints. Because it is well-documented that loss of proteoglycan and accumulation of fibronectin are characteristic features of degenerated cartilage, we have examined how the biosynthetic pattern of these macromolecules is altered in response to culture conditions, including culture under mechanical stress.

Results were published (23) showing that we can maintain and influence proteoglycan and fibronectin synthesis in cartilage explants cultured in a defined medium supplemented with insulin, calcium, and transforming growth factor β (TGF-β). The addition of TGF-β (2 ng/ml) to the defined medium not only maintained fibronectin synthesis but progressively increased the rate of synthesis until initial control levels were exceeded by fourfold. Nearly all of this newly made fibronectin was exported to the incubation medium. Yet as stated earlier in this chapter, fibronectin synthesis in osteoarthritic cartilage in explant culture also was markedly increased compared to normal cartilage; however, the osteoarthritic cartilage preferentially retained the newly synthesized fibronectin in the matrix.

We presented preliminary data (24) suggesting that cartilage responds to cyclic mechanical deformation by producing less fibronectin and decreasing the amount of proteoglycan released into the culture medium. In these two respects, the "loaded cartilage" appeared to behave like cartilage in a disease-free joint, and the data support the concept that cartilage requires mechanical forces to function normally.

Several investigators have made attempts to develop a blood test for osteo-arthritis that would enable them to detect cartilage degeneration early and follow its progression. In all cases the rationale has been that molecules normally found only in the articular cartilage are released into the bloodstream when cartilage degenerates. Although several cartilage-specific molecules have been studied, no effective diagnostic test is available.

Because fibronectin increases in osteoarthritic joints, we reasoned that some cartilage fibronectin may reach the blood. Detection of cartilage fibronectin in the blood, however, would be difficult unless a monoclonal antibody were available that recognizes specifically cartilage fibronectin in the presence of large amounts of plasma fibronectin. Generation of such an antibody has not been successful. This may be partly because the occurrence of a hybridoma producing a cartilage-specific antifibronectin antibody is expected to be rare. In preliminary work on this problem, we used a technique that involved labeling the hybridomas with fluorescent-labeled plasma or cartilage fibronectins and then using a fluo-rescence-activated cell sorter (FACS) to select those hybridomas that recognize only cartilage fibronectin-specific epitopes separately from those that recognize epitopes common to both plasma and cartilage fibronectin. Initial data suggest that this method has promise; if so, it may be useful to us and also to anyone faced with a similar selection problem.

A subject of interest to us and to many investigators in the field of osteoarthritis research is the metabolic activity of chondrocytes in healthy and diseased cartilage. It appears that in response to an as yet unknown perturbation to joint tissues, chondrocytes become hyperactive in fibronectin synthesis and fibronectin content of osteoarthritic cartilage increases; however, proteoglycan content becomes re-duced. As discussed above, in studies *in vitro,* TGF-β supplementation of explant cultures caused a dramatic stimulation of fibronectin production, whereas monolayer cultures of isolated chondrocytes in the absence of cAMP both in-creased the quantity and affected the type of fibronectin produced. In the canine cruciate ligament model, some workers have suggested that the natural early increase in metabolic activity involves synthesis of an "immature" proteoglycan. Thus it may be reasonable to propose that chondrocytes should be kept quiescent in order to favor cartilage matrix formation and maintenance. From our reading of the literature and also discussions with scientists on the subject of cartilage degeneration and regeneration in osteoarthritis, it appears that some investigators like the notion that stimulation of chondrocytes to increase their metabolic ac-tivity, and thus increase proteoglycan synthesis, is desirable for cartilage healing.

If this also results in increased fibronectin accumulation or in an inappropriate proteoglycan, the result may be counterproductive and would be undesirable. It just may be that drugs or other therapeutic procedures that selectively reduce, or that prevent increases, in metabolic activity of chondrocytes will be effective.

ACKNOWLEDGMENTS

The authors thank Margaret Vernier-Singer, Alma Williams, Raymond Recchia, Harry Leipold, Jürgen Steinmeyer, Rory Todhunter, and Dorothy Scorelle for assistance. Research was supported by NIH grant AR 35664 and by grants from the Ciba-Geigy Corporation.

REFERENCES

1. Wurster NB, Lust G. Fibronectin in osteoarthritic canine articular cartilage. *Biochem Biophys Res Commun* 1982;109:1094–1101.
2. Burton-Wurster N, Lust G. Fibronectin in cartilage. In: Carsons SE, ed. *Fibronectin in health and disease.* Boca Raton, FL: CRC Press, 1989;243–254.
3. Burton-Wurster N, Butler M, Harter S, et al. Presence of fibronectin in articular cartilage in two animal models of osteoarthritis. *J Rheumatol* 1986;13:175–182.
4. Miller DR, Mankin HJ, Shoji H, D'Ambrosia RD. Identification of fibronectin in preparations of osteoarthritic human cartilage. *Connect Tissue Res* 1984;12:267–275.
5. Jones KL, Brown M, Ali SY, Brown RA. An immunohistochemical study of fibronectin in human osteoarthritic and disease free articular cartilage. *Ann Rheum Dis* 1987;46:809–815.
6. Rees JA, Ali SY, Brown RA. Ultrastructural localisation of fibronectin in human osteoarthritic articular cartilage. *Ann Rheum Dis* 1987;46:816–822.
7. Hynes RO. *Fibronectins.* New York: Springer-Verlag, 1990.
8. Mosher DF, ed. *Fibronectin.* San Diego: Academic Press, 1989.
9. Carsons SE, ed. *Fibronectin in health and disease.* Boca Raton, FL: CRC Press, 1989.
10. Olsewski JM, Lust G, Rendano VT, Summers BA. Degenerative joint disease: multiple joint involvement in young and mature dogs. *Am J Vet Res* 1983;44(7):1300–1308.
11. Burton-Wurster N, Lust G. Fibronectin and water content of articular cartilage explants after partial depletion of proteoglycans. *J Orthop Res* 1986;4:437–445.
12. Burton-Wurster N, Lust G. Molecular and immunologic differences in canine fibronectins from articular cartilage and plasma. *Arch Biochem Biophys* 1989;269(1):32–45.
13. Wurster NB, Lust G. Synthesis of fibronectin in normal and osteoarthritic articular cartilage. *Biochim Biophys Acta* 1984;800:52–58.
14. Burton-Wurster N, Lust G. Incorporation of purified plasma fibronectin into explants of articular cartilage from disease-free and osteoarthritic canine joints. *J Orthop Res* 1986;4:409–419.
15. Burton-Wurster N, Leipold HR, Lust G. Dibutyryl cyclic AMP decreases expression of ED-A fibronectin by canine chondrocytes. *Biochem Biophys Res Commun* 1988;154:1088–1093.
16. Leipold HR, Burton-Wurster N, Steinmeyer J, Vernier-Singer M, Lust G. Fibronectin and keratan sulfate synthesis by canine articular chondrocytes in culture is modulated by dibutyryl cyclic AMP. *J Orthop Res* 1991; in press.
17. Palmoski MJ, Colyer RA, Brandt KD. Marked suppression by salicylate of the augmented proteoglycan synthesis in osteoarthritic cartilage. *Arthritis Rheum* 1980;23:83–91.
18. Palmoski M, Perricone E, Brandt KD. Development and reversal of a proteoglycan aggregation defect in normal canine knee cartilage after immobilization. *Arthritis Rheum* 1979;22:508–517.
19. Colombo C, Butler M, O'Byrne E, Steinetz BG. A new model of osteoarthritis in rabbits. I. Development of knee joint pathology following lateral meniscectomy and section of the fibular collateral and sesamoid ligaments. *Arthritis Rheum* 1983;26:875–886.

20. Lust G, Wurster NB, Harter SJ, et al. Fibronectin deposition in articular cartilage in spontaneous and surgically induced osteoarthritis. In: Otterness I, Lewis A, Capetola R, eds. *Therapeutic control of inflammatory diseases; new approaches to antirheumatic drugs.* Advances in Inflammation Research, vol. 11. New York: Raven Press, 1986;207–214.
21. McIlwraith CW. Diseases of joints, ligaments, tendons. In: Stashak TS, ed. *Adam's lameness in horses,* 4th ed. Philadelphia: Lea & Feabiger, 1987;339–485.
22. Brown RA, Jones KL. The synthesis and accumulation of fibronectin by human articular cartilage. *J Rheumatol* 1990;17(1):65–72.
23. Burton-Wurster N, Lust G. Fibronectin and proteoglycan synthesis in long term cultures of cartilage explants in Ham's F_{12} supplemented with insulin and calcium: effects of the addition of TGF-β. *Arch Biochem Biophys* 1990;283(1):27–33.
24. Steinmeyer J, Torzilli PA, Burton-Wurster N, Lust G. Effect of cyclic mechanical loading on fibronectin synthesis by articular cartilage explants. *Orthop Trans* 1990;15:129.

DISCUSSION

Rosenberg: Do you have any information about the immunohistochemical localization of fibronectin in relationship to the cellular events that are occurring in osteoarthritic cartilage?

Lust: Oh yes. Our immunohistochemical studies show that fibronectin is localized pericellularly and throughout the matrix. It is not preferentially localized near the surface or in the deep regions, nor with proliferating cells in the clusters in osteoarthritic cartilage.

Caterson: It is interesting that reducing the diet of the dogs lowers the incidence of hip dysplasia. Alison Bedele has shown similar effects in the guinea-pig model of osteoarthritis. The incidence of spontaneous osteoarthritis is significantly reduced if their diet is restricted.

Muir: Along the same lines, there is a widespread problem in the British pig industry, where intensive rearing of animals which are fed to excess leads to lameness, a condition known as *leg weakness.* We have shown that the articular cartilages of the lame animals were abnormal.

Howell: Have you studied turnover of fibronectin in osteoarthritis versus normal to see if it is degraded? Is it vulnerable to protease degradation?

Lust: Most of the fibronectin remains undegraded. Furthermore, it is turned over at the same rate in osteoarthritic as in normal cartilage, so differential rates of turnover cannot account for the accumulation of fibronectin in the osteoarthritic tissue. Its synthesis is increased in the osteoarthritic joints, more than overall protein synthesis.

Articular Cartilage and Osteoarthritis,
edited by K. Kuettner et al.
Raven Press, Ltd., New York © 1992.

32

Early Matrix Changes in Experimental Osteoarthritis and Joint Disuse Atrophy

Julio C. Pita,* Francisco J. Müller,* Daniel H. Manicourt,†
Joseph A. Buckwalter,‡ and Anthony Ratcliffe§

*Arthritis Division, Department of Medicine, University of Miami School of Medicine,
Miami, Florida 33101; †Department of Internal Medicine (Section of
Rheumatology), Catholic University of Louvain, 1200 Brussels, Belgium; ‡Department
of Orthopaedics, University of Iowa Hospital, Iowa City, Iowa, 52242; and
§Orthopaedic Research Laboratory, Department of Orthopaedic Surgery, Columbia
University College of Physicians and Surgeons, New York, New York 10032
Julio C. Pita is deceased*

Failure to repair damage affecting the surface of articular cartilage is a distinctive condition of osteoarthritis or osteoarthrosis (OA) which makes this disease very difficult to understand. Because of its human importance, this problem has attracted intense research efforts over a period of many years. Studies aimed at finding a therapeutic strategy to correct the inability of the injured articular cartilage to repair itself have led to numerous ingenious approaches that are discussed in recent reviews (1–3). Up to now, however, the failure of chondrocytes in injured articular cartilage to restore a functional matrix in spite of high metabolic activity remains a complex and challenging problem. Our research approach to the subject is based on studies comparing the irreversibility of OA progression with the reversibility of cartilage atrophy induced by short-term limb immobilization [disuse atrophy (DA)].

The initial outline of this project was presented in the Wiesbaden workshop of 1985 (4). Since then, some interesting progress has been made which identifies distinctive differences between the chemical composition of the matrix that results from limb disuse (DA) and that which results from cartilage abuse (OA). Our present study focuses on the proteoglycans (PGs) and their polymolecular aggregates in the articular cartilage extracellular matrix. This complements other studies that focus their attention more exclusively on chondrocytes and their metabolism or, alternatively, on the biochemical composition of other matrix components.

BACKGROUND

Healthy articular cartilage is characterized by large heterogeneity in the morphology of the cells and in the biochemical composition of the matrix. Chondrocyte size, shape, and cell density vary throughout the cartilage depth, as is clearly shown in the histological studies using light and electron microscopy (5). As a consequence of this morphological variation, chondrocyte metabolism can vary as demonstrated in the work of Aydelotte et al. (6), who studied chondrocytes recovered from different cartilage depths from the articular surface in agarose gel cultures. The variability of the chemical composition in normal cartilage matrix was illustrated by findings in our earlier publications (7,8) when PGs extracted from different depths of the knee joint articular cartilage of humans and dogs exhibited variable distributions with regard to (a) the PG content, (b) the sedimentation profiles of the purified PG preparations, (c) the proportion of the PG aggregates, and (d) the trimodal centrifugal populations of PG. These differences found between the upper and lower regions of articular cartilage and at various topological sites, such as low and high contact areas, are consistent with the distributions of the other aggregating components, namely, the hyaluronate (HA) and link glycoproteins (LPs) (9–11). Concerning the LP distribution, we have found more LPs in the PG aggregate preparations recovered from the middle and lower depths of the cartilage than in those extracted from the upper third. Characteristically, much of this heterogeneity is lost in the OA degradative process, resulting in a more homogeneous matrix composition with a substantial reduction in the proportion and sedimentation rates of the PG aggregates and a proportionate increase of PG monomers (7,12).

Significant differences in the molecular organization of normal and DA cartilage were also detected in canine knee joint articular cartilage. The major changes were those affecting the PG aggregates. In our model of mild joint disuse atrophy we found a reduction in the PG content and in the proportion of PG aggregates, confirming similar decreases observed in the earlier cast immobilization studies of Palmoski et al. (13,14) and in the recent work of Behrens et al. (15). In this study we hope to identify parameters which are characteristic of DA but absent in OA, and vice versa, particularly any which correlate with the reversibility of alterations provoked by DA.

A rather simple explanation of DA reversibility could be that the integrity of the collagen network is maintained whereas that in OA is not. But this cannot explain the loss of PGs and the change in their state of aggregation in DA, as described below. Moreover, it cannot explain why degradation is established, in the early stages of OA, before the collagen network has suffered any readily detectable breakdown. Other factors, then, are needed to distinguish OA from DA. As suggested in our previous study (4), the preservation of HA content in the DA tissue and its loss in OA might be one relevant factor.

METHODS AND SAMPLES

For this study, we have used our earlier developed methodologies for the nondissociative extraction of the PG molecules and their subsequent centrifugal

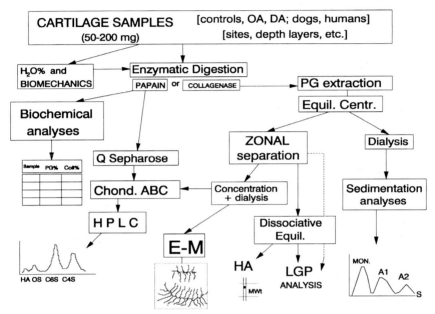

FIG. 1. Cartilage samples (about 50- to 200-mg-wet-weight slices, 200 μm thickness) from normal control, OA, or DA joints of dogs or humans, and from different topological sites and/or cartilage depth layers, were subjected to enzymatic digestion either with papain or with collagenase. Aliquots of papain-digested samples were analyzed for hydroxyproline (collagen percentage) and total hexuronate content (proteoglycan percentage). Other aliquots were separated from proteins through a Q-Sepharose column, digested with chondroitinase ABC, and analyzed using an HPLC system to determine HA (hyaluronate), OS (nonsulfated chondroitin), and chondroitin 6- and 4-sulfates (C6S and C4S, respectively). Collagenase-digested samples were nondissociatively extracted overnight and purified by equilibrium centrifugation (isopycnic flotation) for 72 hr. After equilibrium the PGs were located by hexuronate analyses. A small amount was dialyzed against 0.15 M sodium acetate buffer (pH 7), further diluted to about 0.3 mg/ml PG concentration, and analyzed by boundary velocity sedimentation. Usually, three well-defined "peaks" are observed: PG monomers and two PG aggregates, PGA-1 and PGA-2 (A1 and A2, respectively, in the diagram). The majority of the PGs obtained, however, are re-centrifuged by rate zonal centrifugation (triangular band method in an isovolumetric Cs₂SO₄ gradient), and the three PG populations are separated (sometimes even a fourth PG superaggregate reaching the bottom of the cell is also obtained). The zonally separated fractions are further concentrated by another equilibrium centrifugation (72 hr in Cs₂SO₄); after dialysis against an adequate medium, they can be subjected to any of the five following procedures: (i) Chondroitinase ABC digestion, for HPLC analyses; (ii) electron-microscopic (E-M) studies; (iii) HA molecular-weight determination using optoelectronic microviscosimetry; (iv) link glycoprotein (LGP) analyses; and (v) reaggregation experiments conducted as described earlier (8).

purification (Cs_2SO_4 equilibrium centrifugation), centrifugal analysis of polydispersity, and centrifugal zonal separation in isovolumetric density gradients of the PG populations (16,17). In addition, we have recently adapted a high-performance liquid chromatography (HPLC) technique originally designed for urine analysis (18) to determine the HA and chondroitin sulfate (CS) contents, either in papain-digested cartilage samples or in the polydisperse populations of PG molecules isolated by zonal centrifugation. We incorporated the use of Q-Sepharose (12), prior to the chondroitinase ABC digestion, to purify and separate HA and CS. This procedure ensures complete digestion of HA molecules, because the more abundant CS, the preferred substrate for the enzyme, might preclude the complete digestion of HA. The details and flow diagrams for these procedures are described in the legend of Fig. 1.

Samples were taken from the femoral condyles (FCs) and tibial plateaus (TPs) of the knee joint of healthy control young adult greyhound dogs and from comparable dogs subjected either to the experimental model of OA using the surgical procedure of Pond-Nuki (12) or to mild joint DA. In the latter animals, the right hind legs were restrained by strapping them around the thigh to the dog's body. This prevented the limb from bearing weight but did not limit a free 90° angle movement of the knee. The dogs immediately can ambulate on three legs, and while so doing they swing the constrained knee in a desirable way. In addition, for 1 hr every day the constrained legs were subjected to passive flexive movement.

Frozen cartilage samples weighing between 50 and 200 mg were cut in the microtome to slices about 200 μm in thickness. Samples used for the papain digestion were from the whole cartilage, whereas those used for the collagenase treatment and centrifugal studies corresponded to the lower two-thirds of the tissue thickness.

Our results are summarized under three main categories: (i) biochemical analyses of whole (nonextracted) cartilage samples; (ii) centrifugal purification and analyses of the PGs nondissociatively recovered from cartilage samples; and (iii) subsequent studies of the zonally isolated PG fractions and of their intrinsic components: PGA aggregation by electron microscopy; HA content by HPLC analysis; and LP by immunoassay as described in ref. 19.

BIOCHEMICAL STUDIES OF PAPAIN-DIGESTED SAMPLES

Overall Data (Tables 1 and 2)

The total PG content per dry weight was reduced by 15% in the DA dog joints, whereas it remained nearly constant in the OA cases. The opposite was true for the total collagen per dry weight: It remained constant for the DA cases, but decreased by 8% in the OA model. Water content increased 8% for the OA joints, but did not change for the DA cases. The HA (Table 2) decreased dramatically in OA joints (down to 19% of the control value), thus confirming our earlier

TABLE 1. *Overall biochemical analyses of canine articular cartilage*[a]

Group	H_2O %	PG %[b]	Collagen %[b]	PG/collagen
Control	76.9 ± 6.2	15.8 ± 2.6	59.0 ± 5.6	0.269 ± 0.5
(N = 76)	(100%)	(100%)	(100%)	
Disuse	77.0 ± 6.7	13.4[c] ± 2.4	59.8 ± 5.6	0.226[c] ± 0.05
(N = 80)	(100%)	(85%)	(101%)	
O.A.	82.7[c] ± 5.1	15.5 ± 3.2	54.3[c] ± 10.0	0.297[c] ± 0.09
(N = 82)	(108%)	(99%)	(92%)	

[a] Figures indicate averages ± SD. Taking the control values as 100% in each column results in the percentages shown in parentheses.

[b] Percentages are calculated on a dry weight basis. PG percentages were calculated by multiplying the hexuronate percentage by 4.55, and collagen percentages were calculated by multiplying hydroxyproline content by 8.3.

[c] These figures are statistically different from the respective control values in each case as calculated by analysis of variance followed by Newmann–Keuls multiple range tests ($p < 0.05$).

observations (20), but remained statistically unchanged in the DA cases. No statistically significant differences of the chondroitin 4- and 6-sulfates (C4S and C6S, respectively) were detected.

These figures reflect the average behavior of the three dog groups. When broken into more specific subgroups of samples, some interesting exceptions appear (see below). But the general trends did not change. They indicate a mild decrease of PG content in our disuse model coupled with no increase of water content. This clearly reflects the mildness of the semimobile strap immobilization procedure. In contrast, the OA cases revealed a dramatic loss of the HA matrix component.

Specific Data for Subgrouped Samples

Table 3 shows results for subgroups, namely, FC and TP after 4 and 8 weeks (DA) or 6 and 12 weeks (OA). The mild decrease of PG in the 4-week DA

TABLE 2. *HPLC analyses of normal, DA, and OA canine articular cartilage*[a]

Group	HA %	OS %	C6S %	C4S %	C6S/C4S
Control	3.0 ± 0.9	1.8 ± 0.9	52.5 ± 8.1	42.3 ± 8.2	1.31
(N = 7)	(100%)[b]				
Disuse	3.2 ± 0.3	2.1 ± 1.6	59.0 ± 9.2	35.8 ± 8.8	1.80
(N = 19)	(107%)				
O.A.	0.56[c] ± 0.3	10.3[c] ± 4.9	55.3 ± 6.3	33.8 ± 4.4	1.68
(N = 6)	(19%)				

[a] The figures express the hexuronate percentage in each component relative to the total hexuronate in the sample. HA, hyaluronate; OS, nonsulfated chondroitin; C6S and C4S, chondroitins 6- and 4-sulfate, respectively.

[b] Taking the control values as 100% in each column results in the percentages shown in parentheses.

[c] These values are statistically different from the respective control values in each case as calculated by analysis of variance followed by Newmann–Keuls multiple range tests ($p < 0.05$).

TABLE 3. *Biochemical analyses by weeks and sites of normal, DA, and OA canine articular cartilage*[a]

Group	N	Site	H$_2$O %	PG %	Collagen %	PG/collagen
Normal controls	37	FC[b]	76.3 ± 6.7	14.8 ± 2.7	58.8 ± 6.2	0.253
	39	TP	77.3 ± 5.9	16.7 ± 2.2	59.2 ± 5.0	0.283
4-week DA	24	FC	72.7 ± 5.3	12.0[c] ± 2.3	60.9 ± 5.8	0.200
	18	TP	76.3 ± 8.0	13.0[c] ± 1.4	58.5 ± 4.9	0.225
8-week DA	16	FC	76.9 ± 6.0	13.6 ± 1.8	60.5 ± 5.5	0.228
	12	TP	82.9[c] ± 3.4	15.1 ± 2.7	58.3 ± 7.2	0.260
6-week OA	22	FC	78.8 ± 4.7	14.2 ± 2.3	61.3 ± 7.8	0.235
	18	TP	82.6[c] ± 5.4	16.9 ± 3.0	53.5 ± 8.1[c]	0.326
12-week OA	25	FC	84.9[c] ± 6.2	14.5 ± 3.2	52.6 ± 8.8[c]	0.281
	17	TP	84.8[c] ± 3.8	17.2 ± 3.1	48.4 ± 11.3[c]	0.370

[a] Percentages are calculated on a dry weight basis. PG percentages were calculated by multiplying the hexuronate percentage by 4.55, and collagen percentages were calculated by multiplying hydroxyproline content by 8.3.

[b] FC, femoral condyle; TP, tibial plateau.

[c] These figures are statistically different from the respective control values in each case as calculated by analysis of variance followed by Newmann–Keuls multiple range tests ($p < 0.05$).

cartilage was 16% for FC and 19% for the TP samples. At 8 weeks of disuse, some spontaneous recovery of PG levels seems to be occurring (up to 92% of control values). The decrease of collagen percentage observed in OA (and not in DA) was more prominent in the TP than in the FC samples at 12 weeks, whereas the water increase was about the same for both.

CENTRIFUGAL ANALYSES OF THE NONDISSOCIATIVELY RECOVERED PROTEOGLYCANS

As indicated in the legend of Fig. 1, a mild collagenase digestion allows recovery of 65–70% of the PGs into a 0.4 M guanidine HCl nondissociative solution (21). The extracted PGs are further purified in a cesium sulfate isopycnic gradient for 72 hr at 39,000 rpm, with a loading density of 1.45 g/cm^3. The PG monomers band around 1.46–1.55 g/cm^3, and the proteoglycan aggregates (PGAs) band at around 1.38–1.46 g/cm^3. Both bands remained near the middle of the centrifugation cell. After recovery by aspiration from the top and subsequent dialysis against sodium acetate buffer (pH 7), the PGs were diluted to about 0.3 mg/ml for polydispersity analyses through velocity sedimentation (16).

A typical sedimentation profile, mathematically translated into a distribution function of sedimentation values, $g(S)$, is shown in Fig. 2 (*solid line*). Typical curves for DA and OA samples are shown by the long-dashed and short-dashed lines, respectively. The parameters of interest are the three "peak" S values and the three respective percentages (area under each peak) corresponding to each population of PG molecules. These data are summarized in Table 4. Row 4 gives the total percentage of aggregates. Interestingly, both DA and OA models have lost the same proportion of aggregates (down to 46%) when compared with

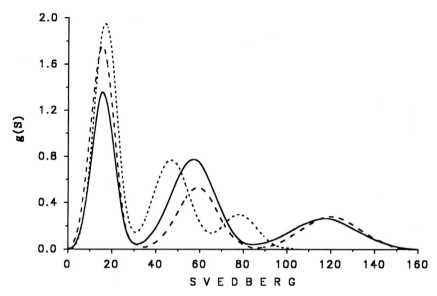

FIG. 2. Typical proteoglycan sedimentation profiles. Averaged polydispersity $g(S)$ functions are shown for PG preparations from normal (*solid line*), DA (*long-dashed line*), and OA (*short-dashed line*) canine articular cartilage. Each curve shows three peaks corresponding to the monomers (*leftmost peak*), PGA-1 (*center peak*), and PGA-2 (*right peak*) in each case. S values are in Svedberg units (x axis) and $g(S)$ in arbitrary units (y axis). For quantitative data on each peak S value and relative percentages, see Table 4.

the 63% aggregation in the control. The "quality" of aggregation, however (i.e., the size of the aggregates as reflected through their S values), was different as shown in row 5, where the (weighted) average S values are given. They indicate that the DA group ($S = 47$ S) is between the normal ($S = 54$ S) and OA ($S = 35$ S) values. This reflects higher overall sedimentation rates of the aggregates in

TABLE 4. *Centrifugal comparison of proteoglycan populations from normal, DA, and OA canine knee articular cartilage*

PG group or parameter	Normal		DA		OA	
	S^a	%	S	%	S	%
PG monomers	16	37	14	54[b]	17	54[b]
PGA-1	57	42	59	26	47	33
PGA-2	117	21	120	20	78[b]	13
Total % of aggregates		63		46[b]		46[b]
Average $\bar{S}_{wt}$	54 ± 15		47 ± 11		35 ± 3	
$S_2/S_1{}^c$	2.04 ± 0.1		2.02 ± 0.16		1.66[b] ± 0.09	

[a] S values are in Svedberg units.
[b] These figures are statistically different from the respective control values in each case as calculated by analysis of variance followed by Newmann–Keuls multiple range tests ($p < 0.05$).
[c] S_1 and S_2 refer to the peak S values of PGA-1 and PGA-2, respectively.

DA than in OA. For DA samples, the "quality" of the aggregates are unchanged from control (i.e., same $\bar{S}$ values for PGA-1 and PGA-2), with the major difference being a large decrease in the PGA-1 content. For OA samples, both aggregate populations decrease in average size and in content.

A direct appraisal of the PGA-2 versus PGA-1 behavior is presented by the ratio $S_2(\text{PGA-2})/S_1(\text{PGA-1})$ in row 6. The control and DA samples show the same ratio, 2, whereas the OA samples show a significant decrease in this parameter.

The fact that some aggregates still remain in the DA and OA samples is another indication of the mildness—and, hence, of the "earliness"—of the observed changes. A more drastic immobilization procedure as described in ref. 15, for example, eliminates practically all the aggregates from the matrix.

SUBSEQUENT STUDIES OF THE
ZONALLY SEPARATED PROTEOGLYCAN COMPONENTS
(COMPARISON OF THE TWO AGGREGATES)

PGs obtained from the purification equilibrium can be re-centrifuged in rate zonal gradients (17) to separate the PG components, especially the two aggregates. We modified this technique to improve analytical precision while retaining the preparative capability typical of zonal methods. "Triangular" zones of Britten and Roberts (22) were used instead of the commonly used rectangular zones. This provides clean separations of PG monomers, and of PGA-1 and PGA-2 aggregates. Occasionally, traces of a very fast sedimenting aggregate reached the bottom of the cell.

Electron-Microscopic Studies

Electron micrographs revealed ultrastructural features of PG monomers, and of the intermediate size and larger aggregates from normal cartilage. Typical examples for the two aggregates are shown in Fig. 3. Quantitative electron-microscopic (EM) average measurements of large populations of molecules are given in Table 5. The ratio of 2.9 for the relative HA length (HA_2/HA_1) harmonizes well with the ratio of 2 or more found for the corresponding peak S value ratios, S_2/S_1, described above. The spacing of the monomers along the HA filaments, however, was almost identical in both cases (26.6 and 26.8 monomers per nanometer, respectively). Thus, there is identical PG saturation of the HA in both cases, suggesting that the two aggregates consist of two different distributions of HA lengths ($\text{HA}_2 > \text{HA}_1$) having essentially the same monomers per unit HA length.

This interpretation, however, conflicts the observation that the two aggregate populations differ greatly in their S values. S_2 can only be much larger than S_1, as we observed previously (16,17), if the degree of monomer saturation in PGA-

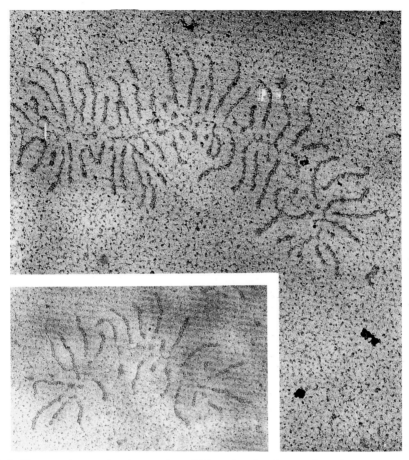

FIG. 3. Electron micrographs of a very large PGA (**top**) and an intermediate-sized one (**insert**). Both were obtained from zonal centrifugation as described in Fig. 1. The average data appearing in the "EM data" portion of Table 5 illustrate the ultrastructural features of molecules similar to those of this figure, although not exactly the same as the ones appearing here.

2 is greater than that of PGA-1. Otherwise the ratio of total mass to lateral slippage surface in both aggregates—and, hence, the S values—would be more nearly alike.

Two conflicting hypotheses seem to emerge, then, for explaining the existence of the two aggregates. Either (I) the two HA populations are unequal in length and have the same number, N, of monomers per unit length or (II) the two HA populations are equal and have a different N per unit length. This can be summarized symbolically as follows:

(I) $HA_2 > HA_1$,   with $N_2 = N_1$ (II) $HA_2 = HA_1$,   with $N_2 > N_1$

TABLE 5. *Comparative analyses of the PGAs from normal canine articular cartilage*

Parameter	Monomers[a]	PGA-1	PGA-2	PGA2/PGA1
EM data[b]				
HA length (nm)	—	400	1162	2.9
# Mon/Agg	—	15	44	2.9
HA nm/Mon	—	26.6	26.8	1.0
HPLC data[c,d]				
HA %	nd	4.1	2.4	
OS %	2.4	1.8	1.6	
Total CS %	97.6	94.1	96.0	
Total CS/HA	—	$R_1 = 23.0$	$R_2 = 40.0$	1.74
C6S/C4S	1.27	1.87	1.74	
LP data				
Conc (μg/ml)	nd	0.04	0.70	
LP/PG	nd	4.0	10.1	2.52

[a] Monomers are included for comparison when applicable.

[b] nm, nanometers; # Mon/Agg, number of PG monomers per aggregate; HA nm/Mon, nanometers of length observed between monomers along HA chain; nd, nondetectable.

[c] Percentages indicate hexuronate in component relative to total hexuronate in the sample.

[d] The PGAs used for HPLC and LP analyses had smaller S values than did those used for EM studies. The ratios S_2/S_1, however, were greater than 2 in all cases.

Other combinations of these parameters could also contribute, but the additional biochemical measurements described below seem to favor alternative II rather than I or any other combination.

HPLC Analyses and LP Content of the PG Components

The isolated PG components were analyzed after the standard digestion with chondroitinase ABC. Fractionation through Q-Sepharose cannot be used in this case, because of the extremely high molecular weights of the PGs. Thus enzyme concentration and the incubation time were increased to ensure complete hydrolysis of HA in the presence of the more competitive CS substrate.

The results of the HPLC analyses of the two aggregates (Table 5) show the ratios of total CS/HA to be $R_1 = 23$ and $R_2 = 40$ for PGA-1 and PGA-2, respectively. The ratio of these two ratios is, in turn, $R_2/R_1 = 1.74$, as shown in the last column. Similar R_2/R_1 ratios of 1.7 and 1.8 were found in other analyses using normal greyhound dogs. In addition, when articular cartilages from mongrel dogs with healthy knee joints were similarly examined, we found $R_2/R_1 = 43.5/24.4 = 1.78$. This provides strong evidence that there are about 1.8 more PG monomers in PGA-2 than in PGA-1 for the same HA content. This finding clearly favors hypothesis II, above. This result, however, although compatible with hypothesis II, does not unequivocally prove that the two HA chain lengths in both populations of aggregates are equal. To clarify the point, we isolated HA populations from the two aggregates by dissociating PGA-1 and PGA-2 in CsCl density gradients in the presence of 4 M guanidine HCl. Layers between the gradient densities of 1.4–1.5 g/cm^3 yielding positive hexuronate content were pooled, dialyzed against a highly diluted sodium phosphate buffer, and concentrated by evaporation to about 0.2 mg/ml as hyaluronate. The respective HA molecular weights, as estimated with an optoelectronic microviscometric technique (23), did not differ greatly (8).

Finally, LP determinations showed a significant increase of LP content in PGA-2 when compared with that in PGA-1. The ratio of LP/PG for the two aggregates was 2.52 (Table 5), harmonizing well with the general trend of the other ratios shown in the last column.

CONCLUSIONS

We have presented a comparison of DA and OA cartilage matrix components. The biochemical analyses (Tables 1–3) are mostly confirmatory of findings by others (24) for similar cartilages except that, because of the mildness of our immobilization method, the changes were less intense than those in other protocols. They also confirm our working hypothesis that HA is preserved in DA but not in OA, a factor that may be important to explain reversibility for DA but not for OA. Although both conditions lose PG aggregates (Table 4), DA readily reverts upon gradual remobilization of the limb. With enough HA still present in the tissue, an aggregate depleted matrix could recover when the normal PG synthetic rates are resumed. In contrast, OA degeneration seems to fail to populate the matrix with newly synthesized PG monomers for lack of HA filaments that would, via the aggregation process, bind the monomers and avoid their diffusion out of the tissue.

The content of LP should also play an important role in regulating the amount and stability of the PG monomers thus secured by aggregation with the HA. By controlling the relative amounts of LP, HA, and PG, the chondrocyte can orchestrate a wide variety of intermolecular interactions leading, at least, to two different kinds of PGAs as shown in this work. The EM evidence confirms the existence of the two aggregates isolated and analyzed by our centrifugation methods. At the same time, however, it appears to conflict with the detailed chemical description of each aggregate population. EM photography favors a model in which the two aggregates have different HA lengths with equal PG monomer spacing or saturation. On the other hand, the centrifugal (Table 4) and HPLC (Table 5) analyses and microviscosimetric measurements are compatible only with equal HA lengths and unequal PG monomer saturation.

An explanation to this interesting contradiction might hinge upon the fact that HA filament length deprived of monomers might not be entirely visible under the electron microscope. On the other hand, the amounts of link proteins interacting with the chain conferring stability to the aggregates (25) could regulate the unfolding (or apparent length) of the HA chain as well (26). The amount of link in the aggregates could vary from nothing (unstabilized aggregate) to saturation (maximally stabilized aggregates). With the smaller amount of link protein in the smaller aggregates, it is possible, then, that the HA might not be totally unfolded, whereas in the larger PGAs the HA chains with a higher proportion of LP could have acquired their maximum length and capacity for aggregation.

As reinforcement of the latter point, we recall from earlier studies using light-scattering that when the LP molecules bind to the HA chain, they induce a significant enlargement of its size (gyration radius), up to an increase of 50% (27). Also, when dynamic viscosity of highly concentrated solutions of PGs containing monomers and aggregates was determined at various rotating velocities, ω, the fluid seems to achieve superviscous values at high ω values. This behavior suggested that, somehow, the HA chains become unfolded beyond their non-saturated aggregation length, as a result of the rotation shearing forces (28). All these data seem to corroborate the suspicion that the apparently visible HA length in nonsaturated PG aggregates (typically, in the PGA-1) can be potentially unfolded and enlarged, thus bringing into harmony the detailed EM measurements with the rest of the centrifugal, biochemical, and viscometric data. A final decision, however, between hypothesis I or II, or any variation thereof, must be delayed until more detailed comparative studies can be completed.

Some interesting conclusions can be arrived at if we assume that the PG distribution profiles across different depth layers of canine cartilage are similar to those found for human cartilage (7). The latter type of cartilage showed more abundance of the PGA-2 toward the middle zones of the cartilage, with the PGA-1 being richer in the lowest and surface layers, especially in the latter zone, where the HA content is higher (9). Then one can infer that the shift observed in dogs from the normal distribution to the OA distribution depicted in Fig. 2 indicates that the middle zones of the cartilage have been involved in some disaggregation process of their PGA-2 components, with the whole OA cartilage becoming homogeneously similar to the surface and deepest layers. On the other hand, the immobilized cartilage tends to resemble more the PG centrifugal profiles of the middle zones, as if the surface and/or deepest layers had disappeared. These two contrasting pictures, reflected through PG aggregation patterns, point to a degradative involvement of the whole cartilage in the case of OA degeneration, whereas only a boundary or surface effect seems to be operative in disuse atrophy.

A complete substantiation of the preceding conclusions, however, must await for a detailed study of the two PGAs at different cartilage depth layers in DA and OA dogs by EM, HPLC, and LP analyses as done here for the normal cases. In addition, a study of the metabolic rates of HA in the various cases should throw much light on the interpretation of the equilibrium biochemical and centrifugal parameters reported in this chapter. Such a completed picture would bring us to a closer understanding of how the failure of OA to repair could be finally reverted by therapeutically induced changes in the matrix.

ACKNOWLEDGMENTS

This work was supported by NIH grants AR38733 and AR40032 and by research funds of the Veterans Administration Medical Center of Miami, Florida. We are grateful to Silvia S. Theye and Felix Soto for their technical help, and to Marta Ubals and Enrique Saez for their contribution in the HPLC analyses.

REFERENCES

1. Caterson B, Buckwalter JA. Articular cartilage repair and remodeling. In: Maroudas A, Kuettner K, eds. *Methods in cartilage research.* London: Academic Press, 1990;313–319.
2. Buckwalter JA, Mow VC. Articular cartilage repair after injury and during osteoarthritis. In: Howell DS, Mankin RW, Moskowitz RW, eds. *Osteoarthritis: diagnosis and management,* 2nd ed. Philadelphia: WB Saunders, 1991; in press.
3. Byers PD, Brown R. Reflections on the repair of articular cartilage. In: Maroudas A, Kuettner K, eds. *Methods in cartilage research.* London: Academic Press, 1990;319–321.
4. Pita JC, Manicourt DH, Müller FJ, Howell DS. Studies on the potential reversibility of osteoarthritis in some experimental animal models. In: Kuettner KE, Schleyerbach R, Hascall VC, eds. *Articular cartilage biochemistry.* New York: Raven Press, 1986;349–363.
5. Schenk RK, Eggli PS, Hunziker EB. Articular cartilage morphology. In: Kuettner KE, Schleyerbach R, Hascall VC, eds. *Articular cartilage biochemistry.* New York: Raven Press, 1986;3–20.
6. Aydelotte MB, Schleyerbach R, Zeck BJ, Kuettner KE. Articular chondrocytes cultured in agarose gel for study of chondrocytic chondrolysis. In: Kuettner KE, Schleyerbach R, Hascall VC, eds. *Articular cartilage biochemistry.* New York: Raven Press, 1986;235–254.
7. Muller FJ, Pita JC, Manicourt DH, Malinin TI, Schoonbeck JM, Mow VC. Centrifugal characterization of proteoglycans from various depth layers and weight-bearing areas of normal and abnormal human articular cartilage. *J Orthop Res* 1989;7:326–334.
8. Manicourt DH, Pita JC, McDevitt CA, Howell DS. Superficial and deeper layers of dog normal articular cartilage. *J Biol Chem* 1988;263:13121–13129.
9. Manicourt DH, Pita JC. Quantification and characterization of hyaluronic acid in different topographical areas of normal articular cartilage from dogs. *Coll Relat Res* 1988;1:39–47.
10. Poole AR, Pidoux A, Reiner L-HT, Choi M, Rosenberg L. The localization of proteoglycan subunit and link protein in the matrix of bovine articular cartilage: an immunohistochemical study. *J Histochem Cytochem* 1980;28:621–635.
11. Mort JS, Caterson B, Poole AR, Roughley PJ. The origin of human cartilage proteoglycan link-protein heterogeneity and fragmentation during aging. *Biochem J* 1985;805–812.
12. Manicourt DH, Thonar EJ-M, Pita JC, Howell DS. Changes in the sedimentation profile of proteoglycan aggregates in early experimental canine osteoarthritis. *Connect Tissue Res* 1989;23: 33–50.
13. Palmoski MJ, Perricone E, Brand KD. Development and reversal of proteoglycan aggregation defect in normal canine knee cartilage after immobilization. *Arthritis Rheum* 1979;22:508–517.
14. Palmoski MJ, Colver RA, Brand KD. Joint motion in the absence of normal loading does not maintain normal articular cartilage. *Arthritis Rheum* 1980;23:325–334.
15. Behrens F, Kraft EL, Oegema TR Jr. Biochemical changes in articular cartilage after joint immobilization by casting or external fixation. *J Orthop Res* 1989;7:335–343.
16. Pita JC, Müller FJ, Pezon CF. Centrifugal characterization of cartilage proteoglycans in isovolumetric density gradients. *Biochemistry* 1985;24:4250–4260.
17. Muller FJ, Pezon CF, Pita JC. Macro and micro rate zonal analytical centrifugation of polydisperse and slowly diffusing systems in isovolumetric density gradients. *Biochemistry* 1989;28:5276–5282.
18. Zebrower ME, Kieras FJ, Brown WT. Analysis by high-performance liquid chromatography of hyaluronic acid and chondroitin sulfates. *Anal Biochem* 1989;157:93–99.
19. Ratcliffe A, Hardingham TE. Cartilage proteoglycan binding region and link protein (radioimmunoassays and detection of masked determinants in aggregates). *Biochem J* 1983;213:371–378.

20. Manicourt DH, Pita JC. Progressive depletion of hyaluronic acid in early experimental osteo-arthritis in dogs. *Arthritis Rheum* 1988;31:538–544.
21. Manicourt DH, Pita JC, Pezon CF, Howell DS. Characterization of the proteoglycans recovered under non-dissociative conditions from normal articular cartilage of rabbits and dogs. *J Biol Chem* 1986;261:5426–5433.
22. Britten RJ, Roberts RP. High-resolution density gradient sedimentation analysis. *Science* 1960;131: 32.
23. Muller FJ, Pita JC. A simple electronic capillary microviscometer. *Anal Biochem* 1983;133:9–15.
24. Säämanen AM, Tammi M, Kiviranta I, Jurvelin J, Helminen HJ. Maturation of proteoglycan matrix in articular cartilage under increased and decreased joint loading. A study in young rabbits. *Connect Tissue Res* 1987;16:163–175.
25. Kimura JH, Hardingham TE, Hascall VC, Solursh M. Biosynthesis of proteoglycans and their assembly into aggregates in cultures of chondrocytes from swarm chondrosarcoma. *J Biol Chem* 1979;254:2600–2609.
26. Buckwalter JA, Rosenberg LC, Tang L-H. The effect of link protein on proteoglycan aggregate structure. *J Biol Chem* 1984;259:5361–5363.
27. Blanco LN, Pita JC. Light scattering study on the influence of the link glycoprotein and lysozyme on the hyaluronic acid molecules. *Arch Biochem Biophys* 1985;239:296–304.
28. Zhu WB, Mow VC. Viscometric properties of proteoglycan solutions. In: Mow VC, Ratcliffe A, Woo S-Y, eds. *Mechanics of diarthrodial joint,* vol 1. New York: Springer-Verlag, 1990;313.

DISCUSSION

Oegema: Have you tested the stability of the small and large aggregates with small hyaluronic acid oligomers to see if there really is not enough link protein to stabilize them, particularly the small aggregates?

Manicourt: We have not done that directly. We have studied the sedimentation of the two aggregate forms at different pH. The smaller aggregates were less stable to acid pH than were the larger aggregates. This is consistent with more functional link protein in the larger aggregates, because link-protein-stabilized aggregates are much more stable in lower pH solvents than are proteoglycan–hyaluronate complexes.

Rosenberg: Perhaps there is no discrepancy between the EM and the sedimentation velocity results. Proteoglycan monomers will only fill a proportion of a hyaluronate molecule until link protein is added, in which case the entire length of the hyaluronate can be filled to yield an aggregate of maximal size. Jody Buckwalter has studied the reassembly of aggregates with and without the link protein using electron microscopy.

Buckwalter: We have added variable concentrations of link protein to proteoglycan–hyaluronate complexes. As the proportion of link protein increases, the visible length of the HA filament in EM pictures also increases. There is a nice mathematical relationship between the concentration of link protein and the visible length of the HA filament.

Kuettner: The proportion of monomers increases in the disuse model. Can they interact with hyaluronic acid, and can they form aggregates?

Manicourt: They can interact with exogenous hyaluronic acid, but we did not investigate if they have lower affinity for hyaluronate than do monomers from normal articular cartilage.

Kuettner: Then why are these monomers not aggregated within the tissue? After all, hyaluronic acid does not decrease in that model. Could there be a change in the link proteins?

Manicourt: I do not think there is a decrease in link protein, since the faster sedimenting aggregates were preserved. It is possible that with disuse the monomers have a lower affinity for hyaluronate.

Heinegard: Matthias Mörgelein used associative extraction to isolate two types of aggregate from a chondrosarcoma and studied them by rotary shadowing. One had very closely spaced monomers, continuously distributed along the entire hyaluronate molecule. The other had clusters of monomers separated by an apparently "naked" filament of hyaluronate that had bound no link protein or monomer. I wonder if your two proteoglycan aggregates correspond to these structures?

Manicourt: This appears consistent with our hypothesis.

Pita (comment added in proof): I think that although many fine details are still missing, there is now strong evidence that the phenomenon of PG aggregation is more complex and variable than initially conceived. Questions of differential stability, monomer saturation, spacing, etc., within the two (or perhaps more) aggregates are still being investigated, and I hope that the physiological role of such heterogeneous aggregation states will eventually be understood.

Articular Cartilage and Osteoarthritis,
edited by K. Kuettner et al.
Raven Press, Ltd., New York © 1992.

Part IX: Experimental Osteoarthritis: Animal Models

Introduction

Ruth X. Raiss

*Department of Pharmacological Research, Hoechst AG Werk Kalle-Albert,
6200 Wiesbaden 1, Federal Republic of Germany*

Osteoarthritis (OA) is a disease of high incidence; however, it has poor predictability because of its multifactorial causes, the wide variation in its progression and severity, and the variety of the tissues and joints affected. For a disease of such heterogeneity in course and outcome and still of unknown pathogenesis, it is not surprising that a wealth of animal models have been described over the last few decades. Inherent in the term "model," however, is not only the comparability, but equally the limitations in its likeness to the original process. Depending on the purpose of each model, therefore, different emphasis and analogies have been sought. They can be assigned to two distinct approaches. The first focuses on certain parameters (or events) that are best (or least) understood, and, in a defined system, modifies them separately to learn more about their role in the complex pathology. This would represent an exploratory approach, mainly realized in induced models with definite onset and predictable course. The second approach aims to mimic the human pathology in its complexity and variability in order to interfere with it systemically. This would represent a modificatory approach, mainly focusing on genetically disposed models where OA occurs spontaneously. In the first chapter of this section (Pritzker), evolutionary closeness of the species to man is addressed using a primate model of a spontaneously occurring OA in macaques. The second chapter (Bayliss) defines some of the events that lead to OA after trauma or injury in the manifold models based on either joint instability, as obtained by meniscectomy or ligament dissection, or cartilage atrophy obtained by immobilization of the joint. This contribution highlights recent progress in experimental OA in a dog model, where the process of aging in mature cartilage, and its possible role in the development of the disease, is investigated. The role of weight-bearing and joint movement as in regular running, running stress, and overuse is not yet clear in its potential for inducing prearthrotic changes. The comparative study of running in Beagle dogs, and its effect upon articular cartilage, is presented in the third chapter (Helminen et al.). An important consideration in the sequence of cartilage degradation is the location of the "point of no return," when formerly reversible changes shift to irreversible ones. This question is addressed by the fourth chapter (Williams et al.), where chemically induced degradative changes in the joint can be modified by different protocols to give either mild, reversible changes or progressive, re-active changes. This helps define the boundary between attempts of repair and severe, irreversible progression to joint damage. Animal models of spontaneously occurring OA in a species with a conveniently short life span, such as in the STR ORT or the STR 1N mouse strains, seem promising for evaluation of therapeutic intervention. Further characterization of these strains is presented in the abstracts by Collins et al. and Raiss et al.

Articular Cartilage and Osteoarthritis,
edited by K. Kuettner et al.
Raven Press, Ltd., New York © 1992.

33

Cartilage Histopathology in Human and Rhesus Macaque Osteoarthritis

Kenneth P. H. Pritzker

Department of Pathology, Mount Sinai Hospital, University of Toronto, Toronto, Ontario M5G 1X5, Canada

Osteoarthritis is a disorder or group of disorders affecting synovial joints, characterized at the tissue level by degenerative, regenerative, and reparative structural changes in cartilage, synovium, and bone. Beyond this definition, which is too broad to be useful, lies controversy concerning four questions that relate structure to function. What precise structural features of cartilage can be associated with osteoarthritis? What are the characteristics of progression for each change and the temporal order of changes? What is the specificity of each feature for osteoarthritis? How do systemic or local factors contribute to the development of each structural feature? Lack of consensus on these questions has led to consideration of osteoarthritis as a general response of joint tissues to injury rather than as a specific set of diseases (1). Again, this alternative definition lacks operational utility.

Historically, degenerative changes in joints were long regarded as passive changes caused in part by "wear and tear" and in part by aging, without further defining either process. Since the demonstration by Collins and McElligott (2) in 1960 of ^{35}S uptake into chondrocytes and by Rothwell and Bentley (3) in 1971 of chondrocyte multiplication in osteoarthritic cartilage, articular cartilage has become recognized as an active tissue that is subject to structural modifications by systemic and local nutritional, endocrine, and metabolic factors, as well as by mechanical forces. The relationships of the structural features in osteoarthritis to the systemic and local factors that drive these changes are extremely complex. Understanding this complexity has been hampered by variable and inadequate access to human tissues early in the disease, lack of precise definitions for structural features, and lack of suitable animal models to study the systemic influences on osteoarthritis development and progression. Nonetheless, from clinical and radiologic studies, the traditional associations of osteoarthritis with aging, with excessive joint loading, and with structural changes such as osteophyte formation have been challenged (4).

HISTOPATHOLOGIC FEATURES OF
OSTEOARTHRITIC CARTILAGE

The ideal histopathologic understanding of osteoarthritis would associate precisely described structural features in joint tissues and would separate these features qualitatively, quantitatively, and temporally from changes in other degenerative joint diseases (Table 1). Unfortunately, unlike degenerative disorders such as calcium pyrophosphate dihydrate crystal arthropathy, no qualitative structural marker has yet been identified that is specific for osteoarthritis. Although synovial and bone tissues are as intimately involved in osteoarthritis as cartilage, this review is limited to structural alterations in hyaline articular cartilage. The currently accepted histopathologic classification of osteoarthritis is based on the grading systems established by Collins (5) in 1949 and by Mankin and co-workers (6,7) in 1970–1971. These semiquantitative classifications focused on cartilage structural features such as (a) disrupted surface integrity (fibrillation, erosion), (b) loss of proteoglycans as assessed by safranin-O histochemical staining, (c) reduplication of the calcified cartilage tidemark, and (d) an increase in chondrocyte density and clustering. Subsequent to these classifications, additional important structural features of osteoarthritic articular cartilage have been identified. In 1977, Venn and Maroudas (8) demonstrated edema in osteoarthritic cartilage and associated this component with early structural changes. More recently, Poole et al. (9), studying the role of articular chondrocytes and their territorial matrix, reestablished Benninghof's (10) concept of the chondron as the functional unit of articular cartilage. In retrospect, the Collins–Mankin histopathologic classification has several inadequacies. Although changes in cartilage and bone structure are noted, synovial structural features are ignored. There is omission of more recently identified features such as edema and chondrons, as well as neglect of changes in cartilage collagen distribution and orientation. Moreover, these classifications confuse and intermix *grading,* the appropriate histopathologic term for an index of disease activity, with *staging,* the term for an index of disease progression.

Even if only hyaline articular cartilage is considered, rearranging the structural features of osteoarthritis to segregate those features associated with disease activity (grading) from those associated with disease progression (staging) is a formidable, but urgently required, task. A preliminary list of recognized features, features under investigation, and features which may be desirable to assess is presented in Table 2.

TABLE 1. *Criteria for structural characteristics of osteoarthritic cartilage*

Precisely defined structural features
Specific qualitative or quantitative association with osteoarthritis
Specific temporal order and progression for each feature
Specific association with factor(s) that induce structural features

TABLE 2. *Osteoarthritic cartilage: structural features*

Cartilage component	Activity grading marker	Progression staging marker
Composite material	Edema	Fibrillation
		Delamination
		Decreased thickness
		Fibrocartilage
Proteoglycans	Depletion or excess	? Altered proteoglycan types
Collagen	? Collagen degradation products	Collagen distribution changes
		Collagen-type distributions
Mineral	Tetracycline uptake at tidemark	Tidemark reduplication
Chondrocytes	Increased cell density	Chondrocyte necrosis
	Increased clusters	

First, because the features are more familiar, criteria associated with staging of disease progression will be discussed. By definition, staging features are not reversible. These changes can affect either (a) the cartilage as a composite material or (b) specific structural components which contribute to cartilage architectural integrity (principally collagen distribution and orientation, as well as mineralization patterns and the tidemarks). Proteoglycans, while contributing to cartilage as a composite material, are not included here because these compounds are soluble and have high turnover relative to structural progression of the disease. Meachim and Emery (11) and Byers et al. (12) described extensively the fibrillation changes in osteoarthritic cartilage. We recognize that these changes now correspond to the processes of pitting and delamination in a synthetic composite material. Cycling tensile and compressive stresses acting tangent to the surface induce fibrillation in both high-density polyethylene and hyaline cartilage (13). Propagation of subsurface cracks appears associated with shear stresses (13). Therefore, fibrillation changes reflect the matrix as a composite of collagen and proteoglycan macromolecules, noncollagenous protein, and carbohydrates of intermediate molecular weight, solutes, ions, and water.

Erosion or decreased cartilage thickness reflects established degenerative structural alterations in cartilage that can result from delamination of superficial fragments and from structural changes within cartilage components, such as collagen rearrangement or loss and dehydration. In osteoarthritic cartilage, there are changes in the content of major and minor collagen types (14,15) and in biophysical properties of collagen (16). However, little is known about changes in collagen distribution and orientation, because the disease progresses before the replacement of the hyaline cartilage matrix by reparative fibrocartilage. Increased bound calcium has been associated with osteoarthritic cartilage in both humans and rhesus macaques (17,18). Both the histologic distribution of these ions within cartilage and the association of the changes with disease progression remain to be determined. A clear association exists between reduplication of the calcified cartilage tidemarks and tissue remodeling in osteoarthritis (5,6).

A cellular indicator of osteoarthritis progression in cartilage is chondrocyte necrosis. Distinguishing between necrosis of separate chondrocytes and necrosis of chondrocyte clusters (sites where chondrocytes previously proliferated) could assist in the histologic staging of osteoarthritis.

Recent advances in cartilage biology now enable us to compile a list of structural features associated with disease activity, thereby permitting grading of osteoarthritic cartilage. By definition, these features are transient structural changes or structural features which reflect cellular activities. Edema, a prominent early change in osteoarthritic cartilage (8), can now be recognized in injured intact cartilage by magnetic resonance imaging (19,20). The histochemical demonstration of proteoglycan depletion or excess (21), a feature of the Mankin classification (6,7), can be used as an indicator of disease activity, if it is understood that cartilage proteoglycans can reaccumulate rapidly after depletion (22) and that standard histochemical staining is insensitive to residual proteoglycan content where cartilage proteoglycan is partially depleted (23). The problem of proteoglycan histochemical quantitation can be addressed by omitting counterstain and by staining, in the same batch, a graded standard series of known proteoglycan composition.

Recently, Revell et al. (24) demonstrated patterns of tetracycline uptake in some calcified osteoarthritic cartilage tidemark zones. Thus, tidemark structure has emerged as a dynamic feature associated with osteoarthritis activity.

An entire literature has developed on how the chondrocyte modifies the structure of its surrounding matrix by secreting both degradative enzymes and structural macromolecule precursors (25,26). Many markers of chondrocyte activity can be assessed histochemically and immunohistochemically in small portions of cartilage. However, when evaluating osteoarthritic cartilage, it is often more practical to measure two indirect indices of chondrocyte activity, namely, cartilage cell density and chondrocyte cluster (chondrons) size and number (27). These features reflect previous chondrocyte proliferation and biosynthetic activity, respectively.

THE RHESUS MACAQUE AS A MODEL
FOR HUMAN OSTEOARTHRITIS

As a direct result of a systematic search for a spontaneous animal model for calcium pyrophosphate dihydrate (CPPD) crystal arthropathy (28), we found both CPPD crystal arthropathy and non-crystal-associated degenerative arthritis in the free-ranging rhesus macaque colony at the Caribbean Primate Research Center, Cayo Santiago and Sabana Seca, Puerto Rico (29). Furthermore, because of the colony size and the animal management protocol, it was feasible to use these animals as an experimental model for degenerative arthritis (Fig. 1). Even on preliminary examination of the joint tissues, both CPPD crystal arthropathy and a degenerative arthritis similar to osteoarthritis in humans were found in these animals (30). Most importantly, the degenerative arthritis could be observed in cartilage before osteological changes were evident (31). We described previously

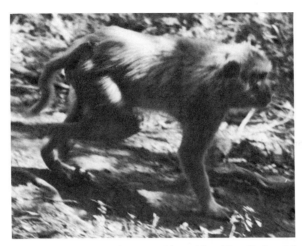

FIG. 1. Arthritic rhesus macaque, Cayo Santiago, Puerto Rico. Note flexion deformities of front and hind limb.

the advantages of this model for the study of osteoarthritis (29). There are abundant animals to study, and only a portion of the animals contract the disease. Much is known about constitutional factors such as matrilineage, social rank, and nutrition. Both degenerative arthritis and aging in these animals occur in an accelerated fashion compared to these factors in humans. The knee joints, which resemble human joints in both structure and function, are large enough to permit arthroscopy as well as biochemical and histologic study. If it were accepted that the degenerative arthritis in this model was identical to primary generalized osteoarthritis in humans, then the model could be utilized to study the systemic and local factors responsible for each structural change within osteoarthritic joints. Furthermore, any putative association of osteoarthritis with factors such as temperate climate, carnivorous diet, or locomotor adaptions peculiar to humans could be immediately discarded.

To characterize the histopathology of the disease and to describe its progression, we undertook a correlative biochemical and histomorphometic study of rhesus macaque knee joint tissues obtained at autopsy (17,27). As tissues became available because of acute fatal intercurrent conditions, principally trauma from fights and acute enteritis, it was possible to examine young and old as well as arthritic and nonarthritic animals. This enabled cross-sectional analysis of the natural history of the disease compared to age-matched controls. The biochemical and histomorphometric parameters were deliberately selected to be comparable to cartilage features that change in human osteoarthritis. We measured both biochemical and histomorphometric features within cartilage at standard sites on the femoral condyle. The femoral condyle was chosen because this side of the joint was afflicted less severely and had less secondary reparative changes. Independent of the morphometry, the degenerative arthritis was classified by experienced observers according to the Mankin grading system (6,7). The Mankin grade was applied after scoring sections of both the femoral condyle and tibia plateau cartilage. As with human osteoarthritis, we found the disease prevalent in adults before the onset of old age. Animals with degenerative arthritis had increased elemental concentrations of calcium, phosphorous, magnesium, and sulfur when compared to those in age-matched controls. Glycosaminoglycan content was increased primarily in younger animals with osteoarthritis, but was decreased in older animals affected with the disease. Collagen content as measured by hydroxyproline was decreased slightly in osteoarthritis when compared to that in controls. Many features present in the diseased cartilage, such as fibrillation and histochemical proteoglycan density, were initially excluded from morphometric analysis because the techniques available were not sufficiently rigorous to be adequately quantitative. The histomorphometric parameters chosen for study included the following: (a) indicators of disease progression, (b) articular cartilage depth (thickness), (c) subchondral bone depth, (d) tidemark number, and (e) indicators of disease activity such as cartilage cell density.

Important morphometric observations included a demonstration of increased cell density, particularly in the deepers zones of young osteoarthritic animals. This increased cell density persisted in the older diseased animals. As cartilage volume decreased with age in both diseased and controlled animals, the persistence of increased cell density could be identified as a structural marker for osteoarthritic activity in the presence of aging changes within cartilage (29).

THE RHESUS MACAQUE MODEL AND TISSUE ALTERATIONS IN OSTEOARTHRITIS: NEW INSIGHTS

We have established that the entire spectrum of degenerative arthritis in cartilage can be studied in the rhesus macaque model and that the model closely approximates, or is identical to, human osteoarthritis. Presently, we are investigating additional structural markers that undergo quantitative alteration with disease activity or progression. As demonstrated by Grushko et al. (32), tissue water undergoes both qualitative and quantitative changes within osteoarthritic cartilage. These changes appear critical to the biomechanical properties of cartilage. As recently discussed, accurate direct measurement of cartilage water content biochemically is extremely difficult (18). Fortunately, the techniques of magnetic resonance imaging are providing indices of water quantity, water quality, and spatial distribution within osteoarthritic cartilage while simultaneously measuring cartilage thickness. Proton-density (spin density) imaging, a modality which corresponds to the free water concentration in the tissues, offers particular promise. Thus, proton-density imaging provides an index of the physical binding of water to macromolecules and solutes. On average, the lower the proton-density signal, the more closely bound the water molecules will be to other constituents

(19,33). Thawed knee joints are analyzed in the 2-tesla, small-bore experimental magnetic resonance imaging facility at the Department of Radiology, Toronto Hospital, University of Toronto. In preliminary work, we have shown that the proton-density modality can image hyaline cartilage to a resolution of 0.1 mm (Fig. 2). Again, using the femoral condyle, the proton-density modality signal intensity is compared to cartilage thickness along 10 deciles of a parasagittal slice of cartilage volume. Preliminary data indicate that proton density decreases in osteoarthritic cartilage disproportionately and is unrelated to cartilage thickness (Fig. 3). The observed variation in proton density may reflect the variation in water interaction with macromolecules and other constituents of the cartilage matrix. Among other implications, these findings suggest that proton-density imaging at standardized local sites may provide a noninvasive indicator of osteoarthritic activity in cartilage.

In the search for an accurate morphometric marker for disease progression, we are studying the histochemical distribution of collagen. Collagen fibers in articular cartilage form an architectural framework (10). Although the changes in bulk collagen content determined by hydroxyproline assays are slight, the size, distribution, and orientation of collagen fibers are likely to be altered in osteoarthritis. To measure the collagen fiber distribution quantitatively, a reproducible method of collagen staining was found. Currently, we are pretreating

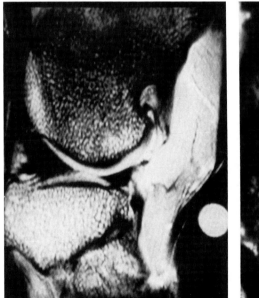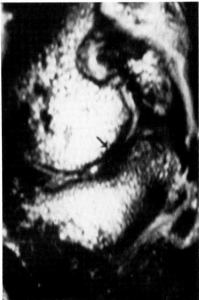

A   B

FIG. 2. Proton-density magnetic resonance imaging of rhesus macaque knee joint. **A:** Normal. **B:** Degenerative arthritis. Note loss of articular cartilage and increased thickness of articular bone plate in the arthritic joint (*arrow*).

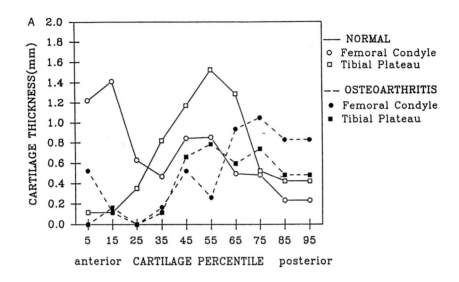

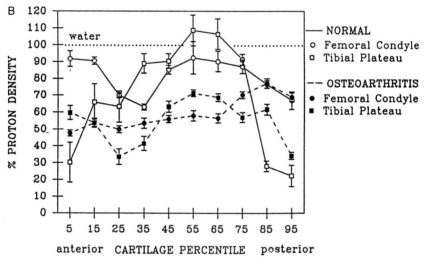

FIG. 3. Sample cartilage thickness (**A**) and proton-density (**B**) profiles of rhesus macaque articular cartilage. See text for details.

the sections with chondroitinase ABC for 5 hr to digest proteoglycans which may interfere with collagen staining or birefringence (34). The slides are subsequently stained with sirius red, a specific stain for collagen that also enhances the birefringence of collagen fibers viewed with polarized light microscopy (35). Our preliminary observations show increased sirius red staining in the matrix

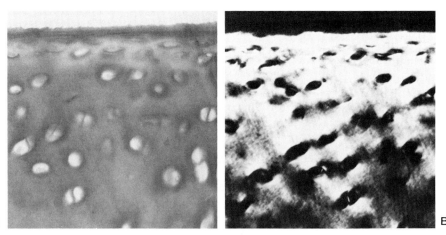

FIG. 4. Normal femoral condyle cartilage; sirius red stain. **A:** Light microscopy. **B:** Polarized light microscopy. Both the staining and birefringence are diffuse within the matrix. ×300.

surrounding osteoarthritic chondrons (4,5). With polarized light microscopy of the same sections there is less diffuse birefringence of collagen and increased perichondronal birefringence (Figs. 4 and 5). These findings suggest (a) a disruption of the interterritorial collagen organization and (b) increased organization of territorial collagen either by condensation of existing fibers or by new collagen formation. The validity of these histologic features as markers of osteoarthritis progression are being tested by histomorphometric analysis.

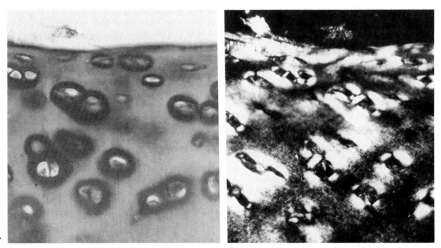

FIG. 5. Osteoarthritic femoral condyle; sirius red stain. **A:** Light microscopy. **B:** Polarized light microscopy. The cartilage thickness is decreased (erosion). Note the increase in the perichondronal staining and birefringence within the matrix. ×300.

DEGENERATIVE ARTHRITIS IN THE RHESUS MACAQUE: AN INTERIM APPRAISAL

Our studies have demonstrated many clinical, biochemical, and histological similarities between rhesus macaque degenerative arthritis and human osteoarthritis (36). Furthermore, we have shown that the rhesus macaque model can be used to gain understanding of the biochemical and histomorphometric characteristics of this disease. In the future, this model presents us with both problems and opportunities. As with human osteoarthritis, the problems are centered around understanding clusters of biologic events which change over time and for which there appear to be quantitative, but no specific qualitative, markers for the disease activity or progression. Moreover, the disease process does not occur in isolation, but instead proceeds with time, overlapping the aging process. The opportunities reside in the ability to study and eventually manipulate a model of generalized degenerative arthritis that is similar to the natural disease in humans. Study of this disease is enhanced by the presence of the disease in a population exposed to uniform environmental influences. Furthermore, this model of osteoarthritis is unencumbered by the variations in therapy offered to human patients prior to tissue sampling.

To date, the process of describing the model has demonstrated the value of quantitative measures in the histologic assessment of arthritis. Furthermore, it has raised questions concerning the values of the traditional histologic grading classification of osteoarthritis. This model provides us with the opportunity to define specific morphologic features quantitatively and to test their validity as markers of disease activity or disease progression. This, in turn, will enable the establishment of an accurate system for grading and staging osteoarthritis at the tissue level. Proton-density imaging and collagen distribution histochemistry must be considered as only two of several possible structural criteria. For example, could the histologic presence and distribution of collagen degradation products be a marker for disease activity? Could the histologic presence and distribution of abnormal proteoglycans or of collagen types prove to be a marker of disease progression? With suitable assays, we can assess questions of this kind in this model.

Once the structural markers are more precisely defined, other applications for this model of arthritis will emerge (34). Knowledge of genetics and social status, together with clinical assessment, may enable identification of clinical subsets with differing structural features and prognosis. Furthermore, the association of structural features with endocrine and environmental factors may lead to an understanding of how these factors drive the structural changes. Finally, with the availability of sufficient animals, it may be possible to develop treatment cohorts such that this model could be used to understand how chondroprotective agents and other therapeutic modalities alter beneficially the structural markers of osteoarthritis.

ACKNOWLEDGMENTS

This work was supported financially by the Arthritis Society. Dr. Matt Kessler, Dr. Tony Cruz, Dr. Marc Grynpas, Dr. Rita Kandel, and Ms. Joanne Chateauvert provided helpful discussions. Particular gratitude is expressed to Dr. Claude Lemaire for his expertise on magnetic resonance imaging and to Ms. Harpal Gahunia, who has worked extensively on both the current histomorphometric and magnetic resonance imaging studies. We thank the Division of Instructional Media, Mount Sinai Hospital, for photograph preparation. We also thank Ms. Lauretta Ross for typing the manuscript. The author assumes responsibility for any inaccuracies and all unsupported fanciful ideas in this chapter.

REFERENCES

1. Watt I, Dieppe P. Osteoarthritis revisited. *Skeletal Radiol* 1990;19:1–3.
2. Collins DH, McElligott TF. Sulphate ($^{35}SO_4$) uptake by chondrocytes in relation to histologic changes in osteoarthritic human articular cartilage. *Ann Rheum Dis* 1960;19:318–330.
3. Rothwell AG, Bentley G. Chondrocyte multiplication in osteoarthritic articular cartilage. *J Bone Joint Surg* 1973;55B:588–594.
4. Alexander CJ, Osteoarthritis: a review of old myths and current concepts. *Skeletal Radiol* 1990;19: 327–333.
5. Collins DH. Osteoarthritis. In: Collins DH, ed. *The pathology of articular and spinal diseases.* London: Edward Arnold, 1949;74–115.
6. Mankin HJ, Lippiello L. Biochemical and metabolic abnormalities in articular cartilage from osteoarthritic human hips. *J Bone Joint Surg* 1970;52A:424–434.
7. Mankin HJ, Dorfman H, Lippiello L, Zarins A. Biochemical and metabolic abnormalities in articular cartilage from osteoarthritic human hips II. Correlation of morphology with biochemical and metabolic data. *J Bone Joint Surg* 1971;53A:523–537.
8. Venn M, Maroudas A. Chemical composition and swelling of normal and osteoarthritic femoral head cartilage. *Ann Rheum Dis* 1977;36:121–129.
9. Poole CA, Flint MH, Beaumont BW. Chondrons in cartilage: ultrastructure analysis of the pericellular microenvironment in adult human articular cartilage. *J Orthop Res* 1987;5:509–522.
10. Benninghof A. Form unn bau der gelenkknorpel in ihren Beziehungen zur function II. Der aufbau nes gelenkknorpels in seinen Beziehungen zur function. *Z Zellforsch Mikrosk Anat* 1925;2: 783–862.
11. Meachim G, Emery IH. Quantative aspects of patello-femoral cartilage fibrillation in liverpool necropsies. *Ann Rheum Dis* 1974;33:39–47.
12. Byers PD, Contepomi CA, Farkas TA. Post-mortem study of the hip joint. *Ann Rheum Dis* 1976;35:114–121.
13. Bartel DL, Bicknell VL, Ithaca MS, Wright TM. The effect of conformity. Thickness and material on stresses in ultra-high molecular weight components for total joint replacement. *J Bone Joint Surg* 1986;68A:1041–1051.
14. Maynes RH. Cartilage collagen: What is their function and are they involved in articular disease? *Arthritis Rheum* 1989;31:241–246.
15. Yu LP, Smith GN, Brandt KD, Capello W. Type XI collagen-degrading activity in human osteoarthritic cartilage. *Arthritis Rheum* 1990;33:1621–1633.
16. Herbage D, Huc A, Chabrand D, Chapuy MC. Physicochemical study of articular cartilage from healthy and osteoarthritic human hips. Orientation and thermal stability of collagen fibres. *Biochim Biophys Acta* 1972;271:339–346.
17. Chateauvert JMD, Pritzker KPH, Kessler MJ, Grynpas MD. Spontaneous osteoarthritis in rhesus macaques. I. Chemical and biochemical studies. *J Rheumatol* 1989;16:1098–1104.

18. Pritzker KPH, Chateauvert JMD, Grynpas MD. Osteoarthritic cartilage contains increased calcium, magnesium and phosphorus. *J Rheumatol* 1987;14:806–810.
19. Pritzker KPH. Posttraumatic cartilage hypertrophy: edema or repair? *J Rheumatol* 1991;18:314–315.
20. Braunstein EM, Brandt KD, Albrecht M. MRI demonstration of hypertrophic articular cartilage repair in osteoarthritis. *Skeletal Radiol* 1990;19:335–339.
21. Christensen SB, Reimann I. Differential histochemical staining of glycosaminoglycans in the matrix of osteoarthritic cartilage. *Acta Pathol Microbiol Scand [A]* 1980;88:61–68.
22. Paul PK, O'Byrne E, Blancuzzi V, et al. Magnetic resonance imaging reflects cartilage proteoglycan degradation in the rabbit knee. *Skeletal Radiol* 1991;20:31–36.
23. Camplejohn KL, Allard SA. Limitations of safranin O staining in proteoglycan-depleted cartilage demonstrated with monoclonal antibodies. *Histochemistry* 1988;89:185–188.
24. Revell PA, Pirie C, Amir G, Rashad S, Walker F. Metabolic activity in the calcified zone of cartilage: observations on tetracycline labelled articular cartilage in human osteoarthritic hips. *Rheumatol Int* 1990;10:143–147.
25. Pelletier JP, ed. Osteoarthritis: update on diagnosis and therapy, *J Rheumatol* 18(Suppl27):63–117.
26. Fassbender HG. Role of chondrocytes in the development of osteoarthritis. *Am J Med* 1987;83:17–24.
27. Chateauvert JMD, Grynpas MD, Kessler MJ, Pritzker KPH. Spontaneous osteoarthritis in rhesus macaques. II. Characterization of disease and morphometric studies. *J Rheumatol* 1990;17:73–83.
28. Kandel RA, Renlund RC, Cheng P-T, Rapley WA, Mehren KG, Pritzker KPH. Calcium pyrophosphate dihydrate crystal deposition disease with concurrent vertebral hypertosis in a Barbary ape. *Arthritis Rheum* 1983;26:682–687.
29. Pritzker KPH, Chateauvert J, Grynpas MD, Renlund RC, Turnquist J, Kessler MJ. Rhesus macaques as an experimental model for degenerative arthritis. *Puerto Rico Health Sci J* 1989;8:99–102.
30. Renlund RC, Pritzker KPH, Kessler MJ. Rhesus monice (macaca mulatta) as a model for calcium pyrophosphate dihydrate crystal deposition disease. *J. Medical Primatology* 1986;15:11–16.
31. Pritzker KPH, Kessler MJ, Renlund RC, Turnquist J, Tepperman PF. Degenerative arthritis in aging rhesus macaques. *Am J Primatol* 1985;8:358.
32. Grushko G, Schneiderman R, Maroudas A. Some biochemical and biophysical parameters for the study of the pathogenesis of osteoarthritis: A comparison between the processes of ageing and degeneration in human hip cartilage. *Connect Tissue Res* 1989;19:149–176.
33. Konig H, Aicher K, Klose U, Saal J. Quantitative evaluation of hyaline cartilage disorders using flash sequence. *Acta Radiol* 1990;31:371–375.
34. De Campos Vidal B, Vilarta R. Articular cartilage: collagen II–proteoglycans interactions. Availability of reactive groups. Variation in birefringence and differences as compared to collagen I. *Acta Histochem* 1988;83:189–205.
35. Junqueira LCU, Bignolas G, Brentani RR. Picrosirius staining plus polarization microscopy, a specific method for collagen detection in tissue sections. *Histochem J* 1979;11:447–455.
36. Pritzker KPH, Chateauvert JM, Grynpas MD, Kessler MJ. Studies of naturally occurring degenerative arthritis in rhesus macaques as a model for degenerative arthritis in man. In: Maroudas A, Kuettner K, eds. *Methods in cartilage research.* London: Academic Press, 1990;341–342.

DISCUSSION

Thonar: You said that there was no change in MRI proton density in moderate osteoarthritis. Yet studies of animal models, like the Pond-Nuki model, show increases in water content in articular cartilage very early in the disease and before losses of proteoglycan.

Pritzker: This is resonating proton density, not total water content. So if the water is as free as the water in your glass, then the resonating proton density will be high. If all of the water is bound physically and is not resonating, then the density will be low, even if the total water content is the same.

Buckland-Wright: You referred to such features as fibrillation as indicators of disease progression in OA. Have you actually seen fibrillation in an MR image?

Pritzker: Our resolution is not sufficient to detect fibrillation.

Buckland-Wright: Surely there is synovial fluid lying over the articular surface and in between the actual fibrillation. I question whether MRI would ever detect such fibrillation.

Pritzker: There should be differences in the density of the water and that of the tissue, if there is in fact water between them. But there may not be much interstitial water. The joint is not sloshing around in synovial fluid. One surface is closely apposed to the other, with only a thin layer of fluid between the articular surfaces and within the fibrillation cleft.

Buckland-Wright: There is a fundamental problem in attempting to use MR images to measure joint space widths accurately. This relates to Pixel size and Pixel displacement due to the susceptibility artifact that occurs at boundaries of tissues with very different proton densities. In fact, Bill Martell and his colleagues showed that measurements of cartilage thickness from MR images are very unreliable, with coefficients of variation of about 35%.

Pritzker: Our apparatus is an experimental small bore machine with high resolution. Furthermore, we try to control the aspect ratio of the voxel which is kept relatively low. In this way we image just one plane which is relatively narrow in its depth.

van der Rest: Can you tell us more about the genetics in this population of monkeys? Is the OA dominant, and is it fully penetrant?

Pritzker: All of the animals come from about 500 monkeys that were placed on the island in 1938. About 50–60% of the animals have the disease. The matrilineages are known because it is easy to determine the mommies. Finding the daddies is more difficult. We are now using recombinant DNA techniques for precise genetic identification.

Articular Cartilage and Osteoarthritis,
edited by K. Kuettner et al.
Raven Press, Ltd., New York © 1992.

34

Metabolism of Animal and Human Osteoarthritic Cartilage

Michael T. Bayliss

Kennedy Institute of Rheumatology, Hammersmith, London W6 7DW, United Kingdom

Paul Dieppe's (1) concept that "osteoarthritis may be viewed as a multidimensional disease process depending on a variety of risk factors, and with variable outcome" is helpful, because it emphasizes the way in which the heterogeneous aspect of the disease complicates clinical and experimental investigations. While animal models and human studies *in vitro* independently provide useful insights, it is necessary to be cautious and try to draw together the disparate data currently available in order to develop a more complete understanding of the disease process.

Articular cartilage undergoes many changes in structure and organization during the development and progression of osteoarthritis. The extracellular matrix is very complex, and its composition and turnover vary in different joints (hip versus knee), topographically (anterior versus posterior), and through the depth of the tissue. The difficulty in identifying common events (other than the most general ones) when comparing biochemical changes observed in animal models of osteoarthritis and those in human osteoarthritic cartilage is therefore not surprising. Consideration must also be given to differences in the etiology and pathology of the disease. Joint diseases occur most frequently in the older age groups. It is therefore important that the changes associated with joint pathology are identified and distinguished from the age-related changes that occur in articular cartilage and chondrocytes. It is clear that the earliest changes in diseases, such as osteoarthritis, may well be symptom-free and occur long before pain, discomfort, or a loss of mobility bring the patient to the clinic. It is thus difficult to investigate the early, formative stages of the disease in patient groups. However, much can be learned of the early events by using experimental models where the way in which a joint responds to a single insult can be followed in some detail and the sequence of events determined. No single model can encompass all the features of human osteoarthritis, but studying joint responses to a range of experimental lesions will lead to a broader understanding of the way joints work and how they may fail. Indeed, this is the main advantage of animal models.

They enable dynamic events occurring at the earliest stages of an acute, rapidly progressing lesion to be studied. Thus, rather than considering them as models of a disease per se, they should be considered as a means of comparing and contrasting different processes of cartilage degeneration under controlled and reproducible conditions. The logic of this approach becomes apparent when comparisons are made with the main features of the human disease. Not only is it clinically ill-defined, its etiology is unknown but undoubtedly multifactorial, its rate of progression is much slower, and analysis of the available cartilage only reflects the state of the tissue at the end of the disease.

PROTEOGLYCAN METABOLISM

As identified experimentally, in osteoarthritis the cartilage may go through three main stages that lead to its destruction: (i) Increased matrix turnover and increased matrix synthesis occurs without matrix depletion; (ii) increased matrix turnover with net depletion of matrix components occurs, leading to major proteoglycan loss and tissue weakness; and (iii) mechanical damage and loss of the collagen network occur, resulting in cartilage destruction.

A decrease in the proteoglycan content of cartilage is the most consistent feature of all models of osteoarthritis and of the human disease. It is clear that this comes about via enzymatic damage (and possibly via free-radical damage) to these multimolecular complexes. Increased active proteoglycanase activity has been measured in both animal and human diseased cartilage. However, it is also clear that the chondrocyte can mount a concerted effort to counteract this degenerative spiral by increasing its biosynthetic activity, and it is this aspect of chondrocyte metabolism that illustrates one of the major problems encountered when trying to compare the biochemical changes in animal and human tissue. ·

Chondrocytes in cartilage from operated animal joints, when examined *ex vivo,* show an increased incorporation of [^{35}S]sulfate (2,3). In most cases, these changes are taking place in cartilage that would be graded as normal macroscopically because mechanical damage and surface fibrillation occur only after many weeks. In the case of the Pond-Nuki dog model, other areas of cartilage that do not become fibrillated also show these metabolic changes. Thus, the hypermetabolic activity in osteoarthritic animal cartilage is a very early event. However, it is important to appreciate that this is not a universal response and that there are animal models of osteoarthritis (defined by the loss of proteoglycan from cartilage matrix) that do not have increased rates of proteoglycan synthesis. For example, when the cruciate ligament of the dog was sectioned, but normal joint loading was prevented by immobilization of the knee in flexion, there was no stimulation of proteoglycan synthesis (4). In fact there was some decrease in rates of proteoglycan biosynthesis similar to that occurring following normal joint immobilization. Continued mechanical loading is thus the major driving force for the development and progression of this osteoarthritis-like lesion. This, of course, is no less than we should expect given the heterogeneous nature of the disease. The stages at which different extrinsic and intrinsic factors come into play will undoubtedly determine much of the metabolic response of the chondrocyte.

This may, to a certain extent, help to explain the variability in proteoglycan synthesis that is observed in all studies of cartilage from late-stage human osteoarthritic joints. Human joints usually have undergone 20–30 years of continuously changing mechanical and biochemical environments, and the disease has progressed at different rates in each individual before a patient comes to surgery. During that time, repair and remodeling processes must have been activated to a greater or lesser degree such that the remaining cartilage bears little resemblance biochemically to the changes that are presumed to have occurred in the earliest stages of the disease. The rate of synthesis is known to vary with the site from which cartilage is sampled from the normal hip and knee. When tissue is limited, as it is in surgical specimens, pooling of cartilage from different sites must influence the results. Finally, some of the most dramatic changes in chemistry and synthetic activity vary with cartilage depth. Most osteoarthritic joints, at least those removed under the auspices of the British National Health Service, have very small amounts of cartilage of variable thickness remaining on them. There can be little to gain from comparing the synthetic activity of partially thick diseased cartilage with full-thickness normal tissue. This latter feature could be one of the main reasons for the discordant results that have been obtained by different research groups. The studies of Mankin and co-workers (5,6) have consistently found a higher [^{35}S]sulfate incorporation by human osteoarthritic cartilage. When this was related to the severity of the lesion, as judged by a histochemical scale, there was a direct correlation: The higher the score, the higher the incorporation. However, the higher-scoring samples presumably consisted mainly of mid- and deep-zone cartilage, which, in normal tissue, contains cells that have a higher synthetic rate. Maroudas and co-workers (7), on the other hand, have equally consistently found no differences in proteoglycan synthesis between osteoarthritic specimens and normal age-matched cartilage, either in the knee or in the hip. Furthermore, Maroudas corrected for topographical and zonal changes by selecting tissue from the same region of the joint, slicing each specimen through the tissue depth, and only comparing equivalent slices.

In the late stages of the human disease, therefore, it is still unclear whether chondrocytes are metabolically hyperactive or if their presumed initial response has been inhibited by the multitude of mechanical and biochemical stimuli they experienced over the ensuing years. That human osteoarthritic chondrocytes do increase their rate of proteoglycan synthesis in the earliest stages of the disease is supported by a single specimen that I obtained from a femoral head after hind-quarter amputation for a tumor in the knee joint in a 38-year-old man. There was a well-delineated lesion (approximately 0.5 cm in diameter) on the superior surface of the joint, and although the cartilage had lost its smooth appearance, there was very little decrease in tissue thickness. Was this the early

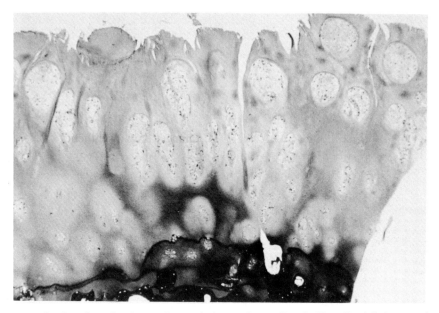

FIG. 1. Cartilage from the abnormal area of a human femoral head with an "early" degenerative lesion. Note the extensive cell clustering, fissuring of the tissue, and duplication of the tidemark. Masson's trichrome stain.

stages of osteoarthritis? It certainly had the classical histological signs of the disease, showing loss of metachromasia, profuse cell clustering, and duplication of the tidemark (Fig. 1). When analyzed subsequently for uronic acid, the lesion had a lower content than did the surrounding normal cartilage, but of greater significance was the higher rate of [^{35}S]sulfate incorporation (7.88 mmol/hr/g dry wt for the normal cartilage and 13.66 mmol/hr/g dry wt for the abnormal cartilage). Who knows? Serendipity may have provided the one and only specimen of preclinical human osteoarthritis!

PROTEOGLYCAN STRUCTURE

Glycosaminoglycan Changes

Numerous studies have examined changes in proteoglycan composition during the osteoarthritic process as an indication of the synthetic and degradative capacity of the chondrocyte. The predominant finding regarding glycosaminoglycan chains in human osteoarthritic cartilage is a decrease in the keratan sulfate content. This seems to be a real event and not one that is influenced by a decrease in cartilage thickness. Thus, the deeper layers of normal cartilage are richer in keratan sulfate than are the surface zones. The concomitant decrease in chondroitin 6-sulfate relative to chondroitin 4-sulfate gives an overall composition that is akin to immature cartilage. This has prompted the suggestion that the osteoarthritic chondrocyte reverts to a chondroblastic state and synthesizes a fetal-like or immature proteoglycan, one which may be unsuitable for the repair process. It has been suggested that the increased size of chondroitin sulfate chains in the Pond-Nuki dog model (3) could account for the increased molar ratio in $GalNH_2:GlcNH_2$. The higher ratio of (^3H)-$GalNH_2:(^3H)$-$GlcNH_2$ seen in cartilage in the rabbit menisectomy model (8) might also be similarly explained. There is, however, little evidence that these changes are biosynthetic in the late stages of human disease, and they could equally arise from catabolic events. For example, gel electrophoresis of normal and osteoarthritic human proteoglycans on agarose/polyacrylamide gels shows that in the diseased specimens it is the faster migrating, keratan sulfate-rich proteoglycan that is lost (Fig. 2).

Changes in the keratan sulfate/chondroitin sulfate and chondroitin 6-sulfate/chondroitin 4-sulfate ratios have not been a consistent finding in animal models, and it may be that these glycosaminoglycan changes occur late in pathogenesis. Specific modifications in the sulfation of chondroitin sulfate chains do, however, appear to be an early event (3 months) in the Pond-Nuki dog model and may be linked to the larger chain size that has been measured in this model. The proteoglycans isolated from cartilage of all regions of the operated joints in which the chondrocytes were activated reacted with a range of monoclonal antibodies to novel sequences of sulfation on chondroitin sulfate chains, and this finding was consistently present in all animals with experimental osteoarthritis (9) (see chapter by Caterson et al.). These epitopes were not present on proteoglycans purified from the contralateral joint cartilage. A similar, though less dramatic,

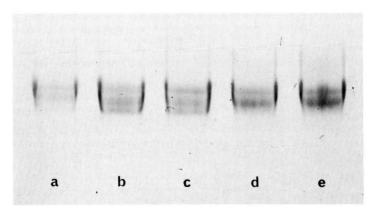

FIG. 2. Large-pore, agarose/polyacrylamide gel electrophoresis (dissociative gel in 4 M urea) of human articular cartilage proteoglycans. (**a**) Normal 9-year-old child; (**b**) normal 20-year-old adult; (**c**) normal 65-year-old adult; (**d**) osteoarthritic 58-year-old adult; and (**e**) osteoarthritic 63-year-old adult. Note the loss of the faster migrating band in the osteoarthritic specimens. Gel stained with toluidine blue.

immunoreactivity was observed on proteoglycans in extracts from human osteoarthritic cartilage (Bayliss, *unpublished data*) and from normal, immature cartilage, but not in extracts from normal, mature cartilage. It is worth noting that these epitopes were also present on the proteoglycans isolated from the "early osteoarthritic" specimen described above. The biological significance of these changes in chondroitin sulfate structure is unknown, but it is interesting to speculate that one function may be to increase the capacity of the matrix to bind growth factors, analogous to the known fibroblast growth factor (FGF)-binding properties of heparin and heparan sulfate chains which protect the growth factor from degradation, thereby increasing the local pool of these agents (10).

Proteoglycan–Hyaluronan Interactions

Abnormalities in aggregation, either from defects in link protein (or in the hyaluronan-binding region of proteoglycan) or from a deficiency in hyaluronan itself, have often been suggested as one route by which proteoglycans could be lost from the matrix. However, there is little evidence from either animal or human studies to support this hypothesis, although it is always possible to find some studies with divergent findings. Aggregation of the remaining endogenous proteoglycan pool is invariably normal, and although the hyaluronan content of osteoarthritic cartilage is reportedly lower than normal, there appears to be sufficient amounts to accommodate the reduced concentration of proteoglycan (7,11). Notable exceptions are (a) the natural and induced hip dysplasias in the dog and (b) models in which cartilage degeneration is induced by immobilization (12,13). In these models there is considerable impairment of aggregation. It is worthwhile remembering at this point that we are discussing reconstituted aggregates; how they are organized *in situ* may be very different, and possibly quite defective, compared to normal cartilage. Nevertheless, it appears that the hyaluronan-binding regions of the majority of proteoglycan monomers in osteoarthritic cartilage are fully functional. In most animal models this also applies to the newly synthesized proteoglycans, even though they are often larger than their normal counterpart, as in the Pond-Nuki model. However, those released from the osteoarthritic cartilage into the culture medium during culture *in vitro* cannot interact with hyaluronan and presumably have lost their hyaluronan-binding region (3). Whether these binding-region fragments are retained in the tissue and add to the existing pool that has accumulated during the aging process as a consequence of normal cartilage turnover, or whether they are lost from the matrix, is unknown. Corresponding studies of turnover of newly synthesized human osteoarthritic proteoglycans do not seem to have been carried out, but given the heterogeneous nature of the tissue and the variable nature of other biochemical parameters that have been measured, it is safe to assume that an equally diverse set of data would be obtained.

One aspect of adult human cartilage that does not seem to have been considered in relation to the animal models is the process by which newly synthesized proteoglycans are assembled into aggregates in the extracellular matrix; this may be due in part to the relative immaturity of many of the animals used. The rate of assembly in immature human cartilage is much faster than that in adults, where it can take up to 48 hr for the newly synthesized molecules to attain their full aggregating potential (14–18). Even then, many of the proteoglycans in the 4 M

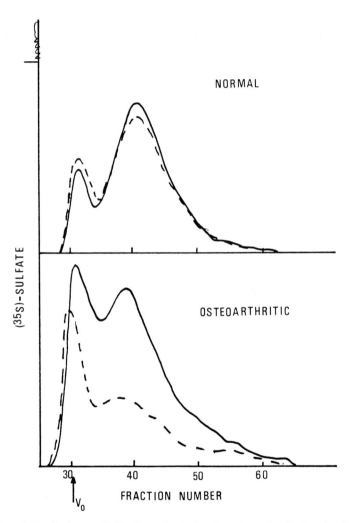

FIG. 3. Associative Sepharose Cl-2B chromatography of newly synthesized proteoglycans extracted with 4 M guanidine HCl from normal (84-year-old) and osteoarthritic (69-year-old) human articular cartilage. Cartilage was cultured for 4 hr in medium containing [³⁵S]sulfate (*solid curve*). Labeled samples were subsequently cultured for an additional 4 hr in isotope-free medium (*dashed curve*). A higher proportion of the proteoglycans extracted from the osteoarthritic cartilage were able to interact with hyaluronan after the initial 4 hr in culture, and aggregation was almost complete after an additional 4 hr in chase-culture. Acquisition of maximum hyaluronan-binding by the proteoglycans from normal adult cartilage was attained only after prolonged periods of chase-culture.

guanidine-extractable pool are not aggregated *in situ,* but are present in metastable states which are more or less easily extracted and which may represent different metabolic pools (19). Interestingly, the rate of aggregation was considerably faster than normal for many specimens of cartilage from late-stage human disease (Fig. 3). Paradoxically, however, the rate of aggregation in the "early" osteoarthritic sample described above was normal. Autoradiography of immature and mature cartilage after pulse and pulse-chase labeling with [^{35}S]sulfate also illustrates the effect of aging on the rate of extracellular transport and assembly of proteoglycans and highlights the heterogeneity of the proteoglycan pool in normal human cartilage (Fig. 4). This aspect of proteoglycan structure could profoundly affect

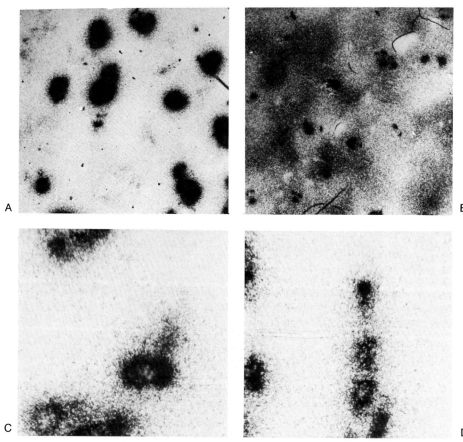

FIG. 4. Autoradiographs of the normal human articular cartilage. After 4 hr of labeling with [^{35}S]sulfate, the majority of proteoglycans synthesized by both specimens are localized in the pericellular regions [(**A**) 9-year-old child; (**C**) 60-year-old adult]. However, after culturing for an additional 20 hr in isotope-free medium, a much higher proportion of the proteoglycans are localized in the interterritorial regions of the immature cartilage; most of the newly synthesized proteoglycans remain in the pericellular regions of the adult cartilage [(**B**) 9-year-old child; (**D**) 60-year-old adult].

the turnover rates and could complicate further our understanding of the mechanisms of cartilage repair.

COLLAGEN METABOLISM

The dissolution of articular cartilage in osteoarthritis must eventually involve a loss of the collagenous component, and this probably involves proteolytic degradation of type II collagen and the "minor" collagens. Extrapolating from the studies on proteoglycan metabolism, it might also be expected that the chondrocyte would respond to this catabolic event by increasing collagen synthesis. It is not surprising, therefore, that alterations in collagen synthesis have been reported in spontaneously occurring osteoarthritis in the dog and that articular chondrocytes in the operated joints of the rabbit meniscectomy model and in the Pond-Nuki dog model of osteoarthritis have an increased rate of type II collagen synthesis (see chapter by von der Mark et al.). This stimulation occurs throughout the joint within 2 weeks of surgery and is maintained indefinitely at focal sites where lesions will develop (8,20). Investigation of collagen metabolism in human articular cartilage, however, has received far less attention than have the studies of proteoglycan turnover. This has stemmed mainly from the exceptionally long turnover time (500 years) that was measured in adult cartilage (21), suggesting that the mature chondrocyte would have little chance of even minimal repair of a defective collagen network. Nevertheless, an increase in collagen synthesis in human osteoarthritic cartilage was measured, as enhanced [^{3}H]proline incorporation, by Lippiello et al. (22) and is in keeping with the general concept of chondrocyte hypermetabolism in the disease. When type II collagen fibrils are formed in the extracellular matrix, the N- and C-propeptides are removed by specific proteases and are lost from the matrix. Using a radioimmunoassay for the C-propeptide (CP-II), Poole et al. (23) have recently demonstrated the synthesis of type II collagen in healthy human articular cartilage and have also shown that there is an increased content of CP-II in osteoarthritis, mainly in the lower mid- and deep zones around chondrocytes and not in the surface and upper mid-zone, where collagen degradation is more prevalent (24). These studies suggest that mechanisms are in place to attempt the repair of damaged cartilage, but in the case of type II collagen, this may be confined to cartilage in the deeper zones, where there is usually less pathological degradation of this molecule. How this zonal variation in collagen biosynthesis may compromise the conclusions of previously published studies, many of which (human and animal) will have used partial thickness tissue, awaits a detailed quantitative analysis of collagen synthesis through the cartilage depth.

The concept that the chondrocyte in mature cartilage is able to modify the type and concentration of collagen in the pericellular regions of the tissue as a potential repair mechanism, at least in the early stages of the disease, is appealing and is one for which there is a growing body of evidence. However, the effectiveness of this response in the later stages of cartilage degeneration, when major disruption of the collagen architecture has occurred in the intercellular matrix, seems less likely.

Little is known about the relative turnover rates of the various collagen types in normal adult or surgically modified joints. The finding that type IX collagen is covalently linked to the surface of type II collagen fibrils suggests that type IX turnover must be integral to the growth and remodeling of the fibrillar matrix (see chapter by Eyre et al.). It is significant, therefore, that in a recent study of rabbit joint cartilage after medial meniscectomy, the content of type IX collagen was consistently lower in the operated knee (25). Furthermore, although the synthesis of type II collagen was elevated, no consistent disturbance in the rate of type IX collagen synthesis was evident. The changes observed in human osteoarthritic cartilage are consistent with the animal model, but are much more pronounced, reflecting the advanced stages of the human disease (26). Type IX collagen, therefore, appears to be lost from the tissue at times when the cartilage is overhydrated and the collagen network is swollen. The latter is one of the earliest structural changes observed in both human and animal models of degenerative joint disease, and elucidation of the mechanisms controlling the coordinated synthesis of type II, IX, and XI collagens will be vital to our understanding of the chondrocyte's potential reparative activity.

Along with the degradative changes in matrix macromolecules that are so obvious in osteoarthritis, cartilage also undergoes major changes in mineralization, manifest mainly at the bone–cartilage interface. Type X collagen is regarded as a unique marker for hypertrophic chondrocytes, which are also rich in alkaline phosphatase activity, and one of the functions proposed for type X is that it plays a role in the mineralization scheme.

The chondrocytes in the deep zones of immature normal human cartilage are rich in alkaline phosphatase activity, consistent with the hypertrophic nature of these cells at this stage of development (27), and they also stain positively for type X collagen (28). In contrast, both activities are absent from mature normal cartilage, in keeping with the cessation of growth and the low rate of turnover of subchondral bone. In osteoarthritic cartilage, however, alkaline phosphatase activity is very high, often extending into the mid-zones of cartilage (Fig. 5), and type X collagen deposition is once again evident (29). It is of interest that Walker et al. (29) also observed type X collagen around chondrocyte clones near the surface of slightly fibrillated osteoarthritic cartilage, an area of tissue that does not normally calcify. That surface chondrocytes do have the potential to mineralize the matrix, given the appropriate stimuli, was illustrated by Archer et al. (28), who found that alkaline phosphatase and type X-negative cells, isolated from the surface of normal human cartilage, synthesized both components after 1 week in suspension culture over agarose. Investigations of mineralization of articular cartilage in osteoarthritis are scant compared with the extensive studies of collagen and proteoglycan metabolism relating directly to matrix structure and repair. However, it is clear that the structural macromolecules also play an important role in mineralization, and, given the potential for therapeutic intervention, a detailed analysis of the articular chondrocyte's metabolic activities

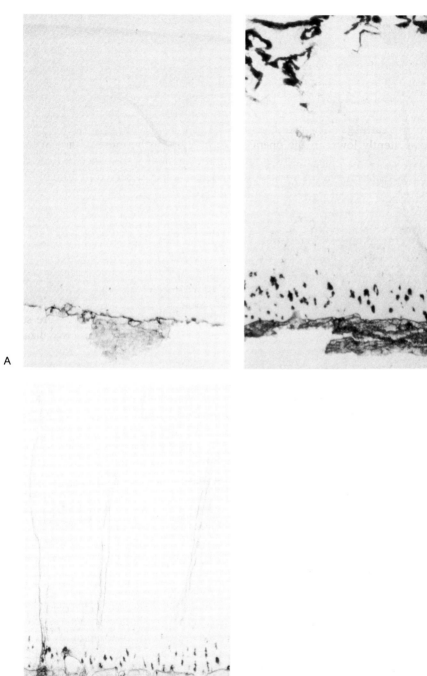

FIG. 5. Localization of alkaline phosphatase in normal 60-year-old (**A**), normal 10-year-old (**B**), and osteoarthritic 56-year-old (**C**) human articular cartilage.

relating to this process is long overdue; animal models of the disease will obviously have a vital role in establishing temporal events.

CONCLUDING REMARKS

Animal models may hold the key to our eventual understanding of the processes that lead to cartilage degeneration. Recent advances in chimeric and transgenic mice technology make it possible to introduce normal or mutated genes for cartilage macromolecules into the genetic complement. It has even been suggested that it may be feasible to develop the first authentic model of human osteoarthritis by this means (30). The fact that it has so far proved impossible to define human osteoarthritis clinically or biochemically must lead us to consider such a model with great caution. If we are ever to generate a model which can be accepted by clinicians and scientists, we are forced back to Paul Dieppe's (1) view of osteoarthritis. He suggests that clinical observations have to come first and that much current animal and human work *in vitro* is inappropriate because the right questions have not been formulated by the clinician. A more hopeful use of this technology may be to apply its undoubted possibilities to the processes of cartilage degeneration rather than striving to develop a model of the human disease, which in any case would be untestable.

ACKNOWLEDGMENT

This work was carried out with the major support of the Arthritis and Rheumatism Council of Great Britain.

REFERENCES

1. Dieppe P. Osteoarthritis: clinical and research perspective. *Br J Rheumatol* 1991;30 (Suppl 1):1–4.
2. Sandy JD, Adams ME, Billingham MEJ, Plaas A, Muir H. *In vivo* and *in vitro* stimulation of chondrocyte biosynthetic activity in early experimental osteoarthritis. *Arthritis Rheum* 1984;27: 388–397.
3. Carney SL, Billingham MEJ, Muir H, Sandy JD. Structure of newly synthesised (^{35}S)-proteoglycans and (^{35}S)-proteoglycan turnover products of cartilage explant cultures from dogs with experimental osteoarthritis. *J Orthop Res* 1985;3:140–147.
4. Palmoski M, Perricone E, Brandt KD. Development and reversal of a proteoglycan aggregation defect in normal canine knee cartilage after immobilization. *Arthritis Rheum* 1979;22:508–517.
5. Ryu J, Treadwell BV, Mankin HJ. Biochemical and metabolic abnormalities in normal and osteoarthritic human articular cartilage. *Arthritis Rheum* 1984;27:49–56.
6. Teshima R, Treadwell BV, Trahan CA, Mankin HJ. Comparative rates of proteoglycan synthesis and size of proteoglycans in normal and osteoarthritic chondrocytes. *Arthritis Rheum* 1983;26: 1225–1230.
7. Brocklehurst R, Bayliss MT, Maroudas A, Coysh HL, Freeman MAR, Revell PA, Ali SY. The composition of normal and osteoarthritic articular cartilage from human knee joints. *J Bone Joint Surg* 1984;66A:95–106.
8. Floman Y, Eyre DR, Glimcher MJ. Induction of osteoarthritis in the rabbit knee joint: biochemical studies on the articular cartilage. *Clin Orthop* 1980;147:278–286.

9. Caterson B, Mahmoodian F, Sorrell JM, et al. Modulation of native chondroitin sulphate structure in tissue development and in disease. *J Cell Sci* 1990;97:411–417.
10. Burgess WH, Maciag T. The heparin-binding (Fibroblast) growth factor family of proteins. *Annu Rev Biochem* 1989;58:575–606.
11. Bayliss MT, Venn M. Chemistry of human articular cartilage. In: Maroudas A, Holborow EJ, eds. *Studies in joint disease,* vol 1. London: Pitman Medical, 1980;2–58.
12. Eronen I, Vedeman T, Friman C, Michelsson J-E. Glycosaminoglycan metabolism in experimental osteoarthrosis caused by immobilization. *Acta Orthop Scand* 1978;49:329–334.
13. Inerot S, Heinegard D, Audell L, Olson S-E. Articular cartilage proteoglycans in ageing and osteoarthritis. *Biochem J* 1978;169:143–146.
14. Bayliss MT, Ridgeway GD, Ali SY. Differences in the rates of aggregation of proteoglycans from human articular cartilage and chondrosarcoma. *Biochem J* 1983;215:705–708.
15. Bayliss MT, Ridgeway GD, Ali SY. Delayed aggregation of proteoglycans in adult human articular cartilage. *Biosci Rep* 1984;4:827–833.
16. Melching LI, Roughley PJ. The role of link protein in mediating the interaction between hyaluronic acid and newly secreted proteoglycan subunits from adult human articular cartilage. *J Biol Chem* 1985;260:16279–16285.
17. Oegema TR. Delayed formation of proteoglycan aggregate structures in human articular cartilage disease states. *Nature* 1980;288:583–585.
18. Sandy JD, O'Neill S, Ratzlaff LC. Acquisition of hyaluronate-binding affinity *in vivo* by newly synthesised proteoglycans. *Biochem J* 1989;258:875–880.
19. Bayliss MT, Davidson C. Human articular cartilage: An investigation of *in situ* aggregation of proteoglycan. *Trans 37th Orthop Res Soc* 1991;16:5.
20. Eyre DR, McDevitt CA, Billingham MEJ, Muir H. Biosynthesis of collagen and other matrix proteins by articular cartilage in experimental osteoarthrosis. *Biochem J* 1980;188:823–837.
21. Maroudas A, and Urban JPG. Metabolism of cartilage. In: Maroudas A, Holborow, eds. *Studies in joint disease,* vol 1. London: Pitman Medical, 1980;87–116.
22. Lippiello L, Hall D, Mankin HJ. Collagen synthesis in normal and osteoarthritic human cartilage. *J Clin Invest* 1977;59:593–600.
23. Poole AR, Rizkalla G, Ionescu M, Rosenberg LC, Bogoch E. Increased content of the C-propeptide of type II collagen in osteoarthritic human articular cartilage. *Trans 37th Orthop Res Soc* 1991;16:343.
24. Dodge GR, Poole AR. Immunohistochemical detection and immunochemical analysis of type II collagen degradation in human normal, rheumatoid and osteoarthritic articular cartilages and in explants of bovine articular cartilage cultured with interleukin 1. *J Clin Invest* 1989;83:647–661.
25. Friedman JB, Winfield S, Robbins J, Lanzer WL, Sandell LJ, Eyre DR. Metabolic effects on collagen types II, IX and XI of articular cartilage in a rabbit meniscectomy model of osteoarthrosis. *Trans 37th Orthop Res Soc* 1991;16:63.
26. Ayad S, Brierley VH, Marriott A, Grant ME. Characterization of the collagens in normal and osteoarthrotic human articular cartilage. *Trans 37th Orthop Res Soc* 1991;16:249.
27. Bayliss MT. Biochemical changes in human osteoarthritic cartilage. In: Lott DJ, Jasani MK, Birdwood GFB, eds. *Studies in osteoarthrosis: pathogenesis, intervention, assessment.* Chichester: John Wiley & Sons, 1987;49–56.
28. Archer C, Stephens M, Kwan A, Bayliss MT. Human articular surface chondrocytes initiate alkaline phosphatase and type X collagen synthesis in suspension culture. *Trans 37th Orthop Res Soc* 1991;16:101.
29. Walker G, Fischer M, Thompson RC, Oegema TR. The expression of type collagen in osteoarthritis. *Trans 37th Orthop Res Soc* 1991;16:340.
30. Jimenez SA. Potential applications of molecular biology to osteoarthritis. In: Brandt KD, ed. *Cartilage changes in osteoarthritis.* Indianapolis, IN: Indiana School of Medicine, 1991;53–59.

DISCUSSION

Maroudas: I congratulate you on your iconoclastic statements. I think it was high time to bring out the differences between cartilage from human osteoarthritis and that from animal models of osteoarthritis. When you and I examined femoral condyle cartilage from joints removed for total joint replacement, we found that relatively large areas of cartilage, particularly in one of the compartments, were intact and had the same properties as cartilage from normal joints. Yet in animal models, the intact tissue usually shows changes. Can you comment on that?

Bayliss: In the Pond-Nuki model, before there is any surface change at all, chondrocyte metabolic activity changes. Conversely, the normal area of a human knee joint operated on for unicompartmental replacement has a normal metabolic activity and composition. To my mind, this tissue should also be considered abnormal, because it will degenerate when it has been put under conditions which will induce it to degrade.

Maroudas: I believe that a good proportion of osteotomies and unicompartmental prostheses have been successful. This implies that the residual cartilage must have been viable and functioning properly.

Kuettner: Jos van Kampen has identified two metabolic pools for proteoglycan turnover in adult rabbit articular cartilage. Do you think that the osteoarthritic disease process affects preferentially one of these pools?

Bayliss: The heterogeneity in proteoglycan metabolic pools is far greater in adult human cartilage than in animals. We have used a number of differential extraction procedures and have shown that proteoglycans in adult tissue are deposited in a variety of different pools that contain different sized monomers, aggregates, etc.

Kimura: You suggested proteoglycans made in osteoarthritic cartilage have some similarities to those made by embryonic cartilage. Embryonic cartilage proteoglycans have different ratios of 4- to 6-sulfate on chondroitin sulfate chains. Have you determined this ratio for proteoglycans synthesized in osteoarthritic cartilage?

Bayliss: The 4- to 6-sulfate ratios we have determined so far for newly synthesized proteoglycans in adult cartilage are very similar to those we see in immature cartilage.

Brandt: You referred to experiments using immobilization after cruciate ligament transection and noted that proteoglycan synthesis does not increase, in contrast to transected joints which are subjected to normal loading patterns. The immobilized joint does not develop osteoarthritis; rather, it undergoes cartilage atrophy, and that is quite different from osteoarthritis.

Bayliss: Right, exactly. That's the point that I was making. They are two different processes.

Brandt: In the animal models, for most parameters that are defined as abnormal, the reference is the contralateral joint which is always available. Because of the variation from dog to dog, comparative studies on the contralateral joint of the same animal are very important. Can you comment on how you define change or lack of change in human joint tissues when you do not have that advantage?

Bayliss: We do have the problems with controls in our human studies. Most of my specimens, certainly those for metabolic studies, have to be fresh tissues. I use mostly amputation specimens. I have collected some fresh postmortem samples of the same age, and they match up in chemistry and in metabolic activity. I feel quite happy that the normal tissues that I am using are suitable as controls for our studies of human osteoarthritic cartilage.

Articular Cartilage and Osteoarthritis,
edited by K. Kuettner et al.
Raven Press, Ltd., New York © 1992.

35

Effect of Motion and Load on Articular Cartilage in Animal Models

H. J. Helminen,* Ilkka Kiviranta,* Anna-Marja Säämänen,*
Jukka S. Jurvelin,* J. Arokoski,* R. Oettmeier,† K. Abendroth,‡
A. J. Roth,† and Markku I. Tammi*

**Department of Anatomy, University of Kuopio, SF-70211 Kuopio, Finland;
and Departments of †Orthopaedics and ‡Internal Medicine, University
of Jena, 0-6900 Jena, German Democratic Republic*

To what extent the development and maintenance of the delicate structure of articular cartilage is genetically determined, and which part is under extrinsic control, is unknown so far. Our long-term goal is to reveal the range of the alterations in articular cartilage exerted in response to one of the most important extrinsic factors, namely, the loading of the joint. The present chapter focuses on the models and results obtained from subjecting the animals *in vivo* to various intensities of joint loading.

There is evidence of hereditary defects that predispose to osteoarthritis, but it is also clear that work, sports, and lifestyle in general contribute to the development of the disease. By knowing more about the regulation of the articular cartilage matrix in response to joint loading, we may identify some avoidable risk factors of osteoarthritis.

EARLIER MODELS OF REDUCED LOADING

Splinting the knee, which restricts both movement and weight-bearing of the leg, has been used in several species, including rabbit, dog, guinea pig, rat, and mouse (for review see ref. 1). The "ankle" joint of sheep has been immobilized by plaster cast application on one foreleg (2). Sparing of a leg from weight-bearing without immobilization has been obtained by surgical operations on guinea-pig and canine limbs (1,3,4). Reduced joint loading—with or without immobilization—is more or less deleterious to the articular cartilage. Parameters such as position of the limb (extension/flexion), the possible induction of cartilage compression, the rigidity of the immobilization, and the species and age of the animals modify the response. The rabbit seems to be particularly susceptible to the adverse effects of immobilization, because cartilage matrix staining for proteoglycans is diminished after 2 days, and surface alterations are evident within 1 week after application of the splint. This is in contrast to canine articular cartilage, which does not show gross or microscopic deterioration after casting for up to 11 weeks (1).

REDUCED LOADING AND CARTILAGE MATRIX PROPERTIES

The biomechanical properties of articular cartilage are created by its extracellular matrix. The most important components of the matrix are the network of collagen fibrils and the proteoglycans that fill the network. It is the strongly hydrophilic nature of the glycosaminoglycan side chains of proteoglycans that provide the tissue with sufficient stiffness under normal compressive loads. Hence, any changes in glycosaminoglycan or proteoglycan content are expected to influence the biomechanical properties of articular cartilage.

Articular cartilage glycosaminoglycans decrease after reduced loading in all species studied so far (1). The reduction is at least partly reversible (5). The absence of cyclic compressive loading appears to be more important than restricted joint movement, because depletion of proteoglycans occurred also in amputated legs with full mobility but devoid of joint loading (4).

In contrast to the prominent changes in proteoglycan concentrations due to altered loading, collagen content remains unchanged. However, alterations in the structure and metabolic rate of collagen are possible (1).

Proteoglycan monomers from immobilized sheep (2) and dogs displayed a lower average molecular size compared with controls, and in some studies the ability of proteoglycans to aggregate was reduced, particularly if a rigid immobilization fixation was applied (5). The reduced content of proteoglycans was associated with a lower incorporation of [^{35}S]sulfate in cartilage slices taken from the unloaded animals (2,4,5). Lowered rates of proteoglycan synthesis in a grossly normal tissue suggested that the alteration should be classified as atrophy (4), although enhanced catabolic rate probably contributed to the proteoglycan loss (5).

In contrast to those occurring in sheep and dog, the alterations in articular cartilages of immobilized rabbits and rats cannot be regarded solely as atrophy, because the joints show inflammation, intra-articular adhesions, and extensive surface defects, sometimes with areas of complete cartilage loss. Rabbit knees immobilized in extension have been used as a model of osteoarthritis and do not represent the pure response to reduced loading (1).

MODELS OF INCREASED JOINT LOADING

Two different models have been used to study the effects of elevated joint loading. The first of these has utilized elevated weight-bearing, induced by experiments in which the use of one limb has been eliminated by operation (3), amputation (4), or casting (2). The contralateral limb, then, carries an increased load. A drawback in this model is that the gait is also slightly changed, shifting the loading pattern to different areas of the cartilage. The second model involves running, probably the most physiological way of enhancing articular cartilage load. Enhanced weight-bearing in the contralateral leg probably subjects the joint to more static loading compared to the intensified cyclic loading in the running programs.

ENHANCED WEIGHT-BEARING

Elevated weight-bearing, as it occurs in the contralateral leg to the splinted one, has not been reported to cause macroscopic damage to the articular cartilage (2–4), although in rabbits there were minor alterations in the cartilage surface as studied after 6 weeks' treatment (1).

The overall concentration of articular cartilage glycosaminoglycans is unchanged or slightly increased in the enhanced weight-bearing models of dogs and sheep (2,3,4), and the synthesis of proteoglycans is increased in the contralateral knee (5). In rabbits the proteoglycan content in articular cartilage is unchanged or slightly decreased (1,6). The structure of the proteoglycan matrix was altered in the rabbit by the enhanced weight-bearing, as suggested by the enlarged fraction of residual glycosaminoglycans not extracted with 4 M guanidinium chloride (1,6), an alteration opposite to that in reduced loading (6). Other proteoglycan alterations in the rabbit model of enhanced weight-bearing included elevated glucosamine/galactosamine ratios, suggestive of increased keratan sulfate content, and increased hyaluronan (6). The increase in keratan sulfate was observed also in the dog (3), but not in the sheep (2).

INFLUENCE OF RUNNING ON MATRIX

Experimental running exercise may injure articular cartilage, but there are also several examples of running exercise without adverse effects (1). A rapid beginning of a high-intensity training program in susceptible species (e.g., rabbit) is certainly deleterious. Also, articular cartilage which has atrophied due to preceding unloading suffers from running exercise (7). The relative intensity of the running is probably the most important factor that determines the response of the cartilage.

Gradually started, low-intensity training of young rabbits increases proteoglycan content in knee articular cartilages (1,8). In other studies, glycosaminoglycan content of articular cartilage has been reported to decrease after running training in dogs (9) and mice (10), and to remain unchanged in rabbits and guinea pigs (1). The variance between the results is probably accounted for by the initial and final intensities of the training, and possibly the age of the animals at the beginning of the experiment. Mature cartilage probably has a more limited capacity to cope with rapid shifts in the loading intensity or pattern than does the young cartilage.

As concerns the structural aspects of the proteoglycans in the running rabbits, nonstrenuous training of young animals induced more completely sulfated chondroitin sulfate chains, higher keratan sulfate/chondroitin sulfate ratios, and reduced extractability of proteoglycan—that is, alterations partly similar to those of elevated weight-bearing (6).

AIMS OF THE PRESENT STUDY AND EXPERIMENTAL APPROACH

We set out to investigate the biological responses of articular cartilage to varying degrees of mechanical stress. To reach this goal, we used a stable and reproducible animal model with beagle dogs to investigate the effects of joint loading and immobilization under physiological conditions. We utilized new, quantitative microscopic, biochemical, and biomechanical methods to assess the cartilage response. We paid primary attention to changes of articular cartilage following joint immobilization, remobilization following immobilization, and moderate as well as strenuous running training of the beagles. Measurements were also made to obtain quantitative microscopic data of the reactions of the subchondral bone.

IMMOBILIZATION AND REMOBILIZATION EFFECTS

Beagle stifle (knee) joint immobilization in flexion for 11 weeks in young, growing 6- to 7-month-old female beagles ($n = 6$) caused a decrease (mean 38%) of proteoglycans (PGs) in the articular cartilage. The depletion was greatest at the noncontact sites (i.e., at locations where joint surfaces did not carry load or stress) and least at the contact sites where cartilage was exposed to slight continuous or intermittent stress. The superficial zone of the articular cartilage was affected most severely, showing up to 58% loss of PGs. Chondroitin-6-sulfate (CS-6)/chondroitin-4-sulfate (CS-4) ratios showed a 14% reduction, suggesting either neosynthesis of new PGs (increase of CS-4-rich PGs) or enhanced catabolism of mature type, CS-6-rich PG molecules, or both. Immobilization made the articular cartilage softer, as indicated by the shear modulus, which decreased 17–25%. The effects of immobilization on articular cartilage are summarized in Table 1.

TABLE 1. *Beagles: immobilization (11 weeks)[a]*

- Decrease (mean 38%) of PGs in cartilage: Degree of depletion varies at different locations
- Superficial zone is affected most: Up to 58% of PGs are lost
- CS-6/CS-4 ratio shows 14% reduction
- Cartilage becomes softer: Shear moduli are decreased 17–25%

[a] Data from refs. 13–15.

TABLE 2. *Beagles: remobilization (15 weeks)[a]*

Incomplete restoration of parts of the cartilage on femoral condyles:
• PG content 18% less than in controls
• Larger PG monomer size
• CS-6/CS-4 ratio returned to control level
• Lateral femoral condyle cartilage remained softer than in the controls

[a] Data from refs. 15–17.

When a similar group of beagles ($n = 6$) were allowed to ambulate freely in their cages for 15 weeks after an 11-week immobilization period, many of the parameters mentioned above showed complete restoration. However, at some places (e.g., in femoral condyles), only partial restoration could be observed. PG content remained 18% less than in the controls, whereas at the same time the monomer size of PGs increased. CS-6/CS-4 ratios returned to the control level. The lateral femoral condyle cartilage remained softer than in the controls. The overall changes are summarized in Table 2.

Interestingly, in the knee joint contralateral to the splinted one, after the 11 weeks of immobilization, a localized anabolic reaction was observed as suggested by increases of PGs up to 54% in the condylar weight-bearing cartilage of femur (Table 3). This kind of response was not observed elsewhere in the femur, nor was it observed in the tibial plateaus. The increase was observed in the intermediate and deep zones of articular cartilage, not in the cartilage surface. There was no change in the CS-6/CS-4 ratio.

NONSTRENUOUS AND STRENUOUS RUNNING TRAINING

Nonstrenuous Running Training Effects (4 km/day)

When another group of beagles ($n = 6$) was trained on a treadmill with 15° uphill inclination [animals ran 4 km each working day for 15 weeks ("nonstrenuous" degree of stress on locomotor system)], general positive effects on articular cartilage properties were noted. The thickness of the uncalcified cartilage increased by 3–23%, and loaded cartilage areas showed up to 59% increase of PGs. Again, it was especially the intermediate, deep, and calcified zones, and not the superficial ones, which showed the response. We observed an increase of PGs unable to aggregate with hyaluronic acid, whereas the content of aggregating PGs did not change. The CS-6/CS-4 ratio increased in loaded areas. The cartilage was stiffer;

TABLE 3. *Beagles: limb contralateral to the splinted one[a]*

• Increase of PGs (up to 54%) in weight-bearing areas of femur, but not in more peripheral locations and tibial condyles; intermediate and deep zones, as well as the calcified cartilage, showed response
• No change of CS-6/CS-4 ratio

[a] Data from refs. 13 and 15.

TABLE 4. *Beagles: Nonstrenuous running training (4 km/day)*[a]

- Thickness of uncalcified cartilage increased 3–23%
- Increase of PGs (up to 59%) especially in loaded areas; intermediate and deep zones as well as the calcified cartilage showed response, not superficial zone
- Increase of PGs unable to aggregate with hyaluronan; no change in content of aggregating PGs
- CS-6/CS-4 ratio increased at loaded areas
- Cartilage becomes stiffer; shear moduli increased 10%

[a] Data from refs. 18–20.

the shear moduli showed a 10% average increase. The main observations are shown in Table 4.

Strenuous Running Training Effects on Cartilage (20 km/day or 40 km/day)

After more strenuous training, the articular cartilage showed (a) slightly increased thickness and PG content in the patella and the patellar surface of the femur, (b) nearly unaltered properties of the medial femoral and tibial cartilages, and (c) significantly reduced content and concentration of PGs in the lateral femoral and tibial condyles. The reduction was most marked in the superficial zone of the lateral tibial condyle, but the intermediate zone was also affected (Fig. 1). The cartilage stiffness showed an analogous trend as for the PG parameters; the cartilage became significantly softer at the lateral femoral and tibial condyles, showing a shear modulus decrease of 13–14% (Table 5).

Strenuous Running Training Effects on Subchondral Bone (40 km/day)

Estimated from the histological sections, the bone formation and remodeling rates, assessed from the area of osteoid and bone resorption surfaces, were significantly increased in the running beagles (Table 5). The trabecular bone volume was only increased in the femoropatellar area. On the other hand, the volume

TABLE 5. *Beagles: strenuous running (20 km/day and 40 km/day)*[a]

- PGs increased in femoropatellar area; this is because of an increase in cartilage thickness
- PGs in the superficial zone of cartilage: There is a decrease (up to 24–41%) on the summits of femoral and lateral tibial condyles
- Intermediate zones of lateral condyles lose PGs
- Stiffness of cartilage: There is a decrease at lateral femoral condyle; at lateral tibial condyle there is an increase of stiffness after 20 km/day but softening after 40 km/day
- CS-6/CS-4 ratio increased 52–72% at femoral patellar surface, but 10–25% decreased at femoral condyles, patella, and tibial medial condyle
- Subchondral bone remodeling clearly increased; osteoid and bone resorption surfaces are enlarged
- Trabecular bone volume increased only at femoropatellar area; here there is also subchondral plate thickening

[a] Data from refs. 15, 21, and 22.

of nonmineralized bone (osteoid) was increased in most locations investigated. The bone formation was sometimes four to five times more active than that in the control group.

JOINT-LOADING EXPERIMENTS AND KNOWLEDGE OF ARTICULAR CARTILAGE PHYSIOLOGY

To elucidate articular cartilage responses to loading, it is reasonable to adopt different types of research strategies. Experiments with animals is one approach, and we have used this strategy systematically (for a more comprehensive review see ref. 1). The conditions mimic in the best way the human physiological circumstances. Another strategy is to use controlled loading of cartilage fragments *in vitro* (11). This allows strict control of conditions of the chondrocytes, surrounded by the matrix, to respond to loading. The response can be investigated in the presence of suitable precursors, cytokines, growth factors, etc. The results obtained by these models complement, in a valuable fashion, our knowledge of articular cartilage properties.

It is most interesting that running training can cause PG depletion and softening of the articular cartilage. It is possible that these alterations are harmful for cartilage function. Many previous studies state unambiguously that physical exercise cannot cause untoward effects on articular cartilage (12). Our present observations open anew the discussion on this aspect. This line of investigation is therefore most justified and has to be continued.

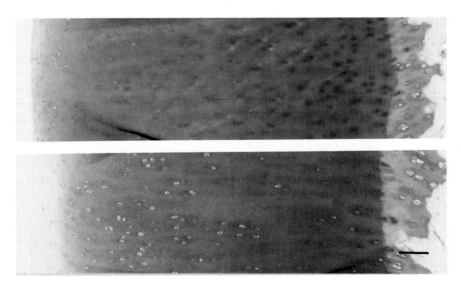

FIG. 1. Safranin-O-stained histological sections (3 μm thick) of beagle articular cartilage from lateral tibial condyle. **Top:** Control. **Bottom:** Specimen after running training (40 km/day). Lack of staining is evident in the superficial zone of the cartilage from the trained animal. Bar represents 100 μm.

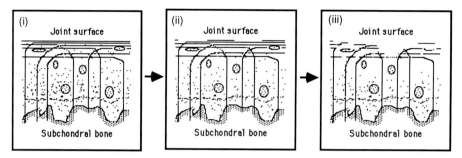

FIG. 2. Hypothesis of the etiopathogenesis of osteoarthrosis due to excessive joint loading. (i) Normal articular cartilage. Dots represent proteoglycans, curved lines represent collagens, and oval structures represent chondrocytes. (ii) Proteoglycan loss exposes the superficial collagen fibrils; condition is still reversible. (iii) Injury of collagen fibrils in the cartilage surface; additional loss of proteoglycans; "point of no return."

We put forward the hypothesis that the superficial zone depletion of PGs renders cartilage (especially its superficial collagen fibrils) prone to injury, leading gradually to osteoarthrosis (Figs. 1 and 2). This hypothesis appears very reasonable in light of our results, although we do not have direct experimental proof for the idea. So far we have not observed any injury in the superficial zone of articular cartilage, nor have we observed osteoarthrotic lesions of the tissue. It can also be argued that PG depletion and softening of the cartilage represent more or less normal physiological adaptation of the tissue to increased mechanical stress. We should continue the experiment to see whether true osteoarthrosis with typical pathological findings subsequently appears in response to increased mechanical loading, such as cartilage fibrillation, loss of cartilage fragments, formation of osteophytes, etc. Only this complete chain of observations would give us proof of the true role which mechanical factors play in the etiopathogenesis of osteoarthrosis.

REFERENCES

1. Tammi M, Paukkonen K, Kiviranta I, Jurvelin J, Säämänen A-M, Helminen HJ. Joint loading-induced alterations in articular cartilage. In: Helminen HJ, Kiviranta I, Tammi M, Säämänen A-M, Paukkonen K, Jurvelin J, eds. *Joint loading: biology and health of articular structures.* Bristol, England: John Wright (Butterworths), 1987;64–88.
2. Caterson B, Lowther DA. Changes in the metabolism of the proteoglycans from sheep articular cartilage in response to mechanical stress. *Biochim Biophys Acta* 1978;540:412–422.
3. Oláh EH, Kostenszky KS. Effect of altered functional demand on the glycosaminoglycan content of the articular cartilage of dogs. *Acta Biol Hung* 1972;23:195–200.
4. Palmoski MJ, Colyer RA, Brandt KD. Joint motion in the absence of normal loading does not maintain normal articular cartilage. *Arthritis Rheum* 1980;23:325–334.
5. Behrens F, Kraft EL, Oegema TR. Biochemical changes in articular cartilage after joint immobilization by casting or external fixation. *J Orthop Res* 1989;7:335–43.
6. Säämänen A-M, Tammi M, Kiviranta I, Jurvelin J, Helminen HJ. Maturation of proteoglycan matrix in articular cartilage under increased and decreased joint loading. A study in young rabbits. *Connect Tissue Res* 1987;16:163–175.
7. Palmoski MJ, Brandt KD. Running inhibits the reversal of atrophic changes in canine knee cartilage after removal of cast. *Arthritis Rheum* 1981;24:1329–1337.
8. Säämänen A-M, Tammi M, Kiviranta I, Jurvelin J, Helminen HJ. Running exercise as a modulator

of proteoglycan matrix in the articular cartilage of young rabbits. *Int J Sports Med* 1988;9:127–132.

9. Vasan N. Effects of physical stress on the synthesis and degradation of cartilage matrix. *Connect Tissue Res* 1983;12:49–58.

10. Krause, W-D. *Mikroskopische Untersuchungen am Gelenkknorpel extrem funktionell belasteter Mäuse—Ein Beitrag zur Aetiopathogenese degenerativer Gelenkveränderungen.* Dissertation. Köln: Gouder and Hansen, 1969.

11. Parkkinen JJ, Lammi MJ, Karjalainen S, et al. A mechanical apparatus with microprocessor controlled stress profile for cyclic compression of cultured articular cartilage explants. *J Biomech* 1989;22:1285–1291.

12. Stulberg SD, Keller CS. Exercise and osteoarthritis. In: Moskowitz RW, Howell DS, Goldberg VM, Mankin HJ, eds. *Osteoarthritis: diagnosis and management.* Philadelphia: WB Saunders, 1984;561–568.

13. Kiviranta I, Jurvelin J, Tammi M, Säämänen A-M, Helminen HJ. Weight-bearing controls glycosaminoglycan concentration and thickness of articular cartilage in the knee joint of young beagle dogs. *Arthritis Rheum* 1987;30:801–809.

14. Jurvelin J, Kiviranta I, Tammi M, Helminen HJ. Softening of canine articular cartilage after immobilization of the knee joint. *Clin Orthop* 1986;207:246–252.

15. Säämänen A-M, Tammi M, Jurvelin J, Kiviranta I, Helminen HJ. Proteoglycan alterations following immobilization and remobilization in the articular cartilage of young canine knee (stifle) joint. *J Orthop Res* 1990;8:863–873.

16. Kiviranta I. Joint loading influences on the articular cartilage of young dogs. Quantitative histochemical studies on matrix carbohydrates. Thesis. *Publ Univ Kuopio Med Orig Rep* 1987;14:1–91.

17. Jurvelin J, Kiviranta I, Säämänen A-M, Tammi M, Helminen HJ. Partial restoration of immobilization-induced softening of canine articular cartilage after remobilization of the knee (stifle) joint. *J Orthop Res* 1989;7:352–358.

18. Kiviranta I, Tammi M, Jurvelin J, Säämänen A-M, Helminen HJ. Moderate running exercise augments glycosaminoglycans and thickness of articular cartilage in the knee joint of young beagle dogs. *J Orthop Res* 1988;6:188–195.

19. Jurvelin J, Kiviranta I, Tammi M, Helminen HJ. Effect of physical exercise on indentation stiffness of articular cartilage in the canine knee. *Int J Sports Med* 1986;7:106–110.

20. Säämänen A-M, Tammi M, Kiviranta I, Jurvelin J, Helminen HJ. Levels of chondroitin-6-sulfate and nonaggregating proteoglycans at articular cartilage contact sites in the knees of young dogs subjected to moderate running exercise. *Arthr Rheumat* 1989;32:1282–1292.

21. Säämänen A-M. Articular cartilage proteoglycans and joint loading. A study in young rabbits and dogs. Thesis. *Publ Univ Kuopio Med Orig Rep* 1989;7:1–67.

22. Jurvelin J, Kiviranta I, Säämänen A-M, Tammi M, Helminen HJ. Indentation stiffness of canine knee articular cartilage—influence of strenuous joint loading. *J Biomech* 1990;23:1239–1246.

DISCUSSION

Handley: Do you have any metabolic data on cartilage from the exercised animals in order to get information about changes in the metabolism of cartilage as a consequence of the extent of exercise?

Tammi: Unfortunately we did not do this in the early experiments. We plan to repeat the immobilization experiment and study such metabolic parameters. We did sulfate labeling of cartilage slices from the femoral head in the 40 km/day exercise experiment. The hip cartilage is also actively mobilized and should show a response. But there was no difference really between control and runner groups.

Lust: Do you have any evidence of what happens in the hip joint of those dogs? Because quite often, when you immobilize or tie up one joint you get an abnormality in the hip joint.

Tammi: In the immobilization experiment, proteoglycans were also depleted in the hip joint, but no apparent change was observed in the running experiments.

Raiss: Have you considered an additional control in which dogs are exercised without load, such as swimming? Not 40 km, no!

Tammi: We have other animal models and hope to get some complementary data more readily in them, but I am afraid the experiments you suggest are not possible with the dog.

Okyayuz-Baklouti: Were any of the animals in the immobilization group subsequently exercised on the treadmill?

Tammi: No, we did not make the animals run after the immobilization. They were just allowed to resume normal physical activities.

Okyayuz-Baklouti: I want to point out that immobilization of the leg greatly affects muscle as well as the joint. After 11 weeks of immobilization, perhaps 50–60% of the muscle bulk will be lost at least in some muscle groups. This easily destabilizes the whole joint and changes the gait of the animal and alters the load on the cartilage. Thus, some of the consequences of immobilization on cartilage could derive from skeletal muscle atrophy.

Articular Cartilage and Osteoarthritis,
edited by K. Kuettner et al.
Raven Press, Ltd., New York © 1992.

36

Animal Models of Articular Cartilage Repair

James M. Williams,*·†·‡ Daniel Uebelhart,†·‡
Dennis R. Ongchi,‡ Klaus E. Kuettner,†·§
and Eugene J-M. A. Thonar†·‡

*Departments of *Anatomy, †Biochemistry, ‡Internal Medicine (Section of Rheumatology), and §Orthopedic Surgery, Rush Medical College at Rush–Presbyterian–St. Luke's Medical Center, Chicago, Illinois 60612*

Diseases of the synovial joint are a leading cause of disability worldwide. Osteoarthritis (OA) accounts for 60–70% of the various forms of joint disease. It is estimated that OA will be present in 67% of any population over 35 years of age (1). In the United States, OA is the second ranking cause of permanent incapacity in people over 50 years of age (1). This results in a significant social and economic burden. In joint diseases characterized by net loss of cartilage (e.g., OA), the deficiency of cartilage matrix is not attributable simply to wear and tear and may reflect an imbalance between the loss of matrix components and their replenishment/reorganization within the tissue. Articular cartilage contains a relatively small number of cells which elaborate an abundant extracellular matrix rich in proteoglycans (PGs), collagens, and other so-called "minor" components (2,3). Detailed descriptions of articular cartilage matrix are found elsewhere in this volume. Enzymes capable of degrading matrix components (4,5) and their inhibitors (6) are present in normal articular cartilage. Until the disease is far advanced, the loss of matrix in OA is associated with (a) increased synthesis of matrix constituents [i.e., protein (4), PGs (7,8), collagen (9,10), and DNA (7)] and (b) increased activity of degradative enzymes (5,11). These increases in metabolic activity reflect responses of the chondrocyte to alterations in its extracellular milieu and may be viewed as indications of an attempt by the chondrocyte to repair the cartilage damage.

REPAIR OF ARTICULAR CARTILAGE

The repair mechanisms of articular cartilage are poorly understood. They have important implications, however, with respect to the reversibility of articular cartilage injury. An understanding of the mechanisms responsible for cartilage destruction may shed light on the mechanisms involved in the successful (and unsuccessful) repair of articular cartilage. Reviews of articular cartilage repair have been published previously (12,13). It is important to note that the success of the repair process is dependent upon several factors such as age, size of the cartilage injury, location of the injury, and choice of therapeutic intervention. Articular cartilage injury may range from a loss of matrix components, which leaves the cells and collagen meshwork intact, to frank mechanical disruption of the cartilage and underlying subchondral bone. In the first case, Buckwalter et al. (12) note that if the source of matrix loss can be stopped and the demand on the chondrocyte is not excessive, repair of the articular cartilage injury can occur. However, if the damaging process continues or the demand is too great, irreversible damage occurs. The point where irreversible damage occurs is not clear.

Indications of putative attempts at repair by cartilage have been observed in naturally occurring and experimental OA. Such attempts include (a) increases in synthesis of DNA, protein, PGs, and collagen, (b) increases in ^{35}S, [^{3}H]-thymidine, and [^{3}H]proline incorporation by the cartilage, and (c) chondrocyte cloning (4–6), all of which suggest attempts by the chondrocytes to replenish lost matrix components. This increase in metabolic activity in OA cartilage may eventually fail, however, giving way ultimately to complete cartilage destruction. Thus, with progression of the disease in naturally occurring and experimental OA, repair attempts fail and severe joint destruction ensues. It is possible that chronic stress or excessive demand placed on the chondrocyte for repair may diminish the cell's ability to handle additional insults which will then result in loss of articular cartilage. Alternatively, it is possible that certain components of the extracellular matrix are selectively destroyed (or are not faithfully resynthesized by the chondrocytes) or that their replacement into the extracellular matrix is poorly coordinated. This implies a functional hierarchy of cartilage extracellular matrix components.

Other models of experimentally induced articular cartilage injury have been used to examine articular cartilage repair. Collagen synthesis and an increase in ^{35}S uptake by the chondrocytes have been noted following laceration of rabbit knee cartilage (14–16). Ghadially et al. (17,18) have described the ultrastructural features of repair of superficial and deep defects in rabbit articular cartilage and have noted that the most successful repair with hyaline-like cartilage occurs in young, skeletally mature rabbits. Importantly, full-thickness defects of articular cartilage which penetrate the subchondral bone are filled by repair tissue resembling either fibrocartilage or hyaline cartilage. In contrast, superficial lacerations which do not extend into subchondral bone fail to repair.

Immobilization of a synovial joint results in degenerative changes in the articular cartilage (19). Depending upon the experimental conditions, these changes are reversible or progressive. For example, compression of the articular surfaces, such as occurs with external fixation (irrespective of joint position) (20) or when the joint is placed in a position of extension (21), invariably results in irreversible injury to the articular cartilage. Immobilization of a synovial joint in flexion without compression of the articular surfaces also results in the loss of matrix PGs; however, these changes are reversed when the animals are permitted free activity during a period of remobilization (22,23). It is of interest to note that forced exercise on a treadmill following joint immobilization results in a failure of the cartilage to recover (24). It was suggested that loss of extracellular matrix caused by immobilization may have rendered the chondrocyte vulnerable to damage from increased loading during the exercise, thereby impairing its capacity for repair.

Therapeutic interventions aimed at redistributing the load on the articular surface may facilitate repair in OA cartilage. Factors such as age, size of the defect, and extent of the injury (i.e., extending through the thickness of the articular cartilage into the subchondral bone or not) and location of the injury (i.e., in habitually loaded or nonloaded regions) contribute to the repair outcome. These interventions have been reviewed thoroughly by Buckwalter et al. (12) A more recent technique used to facilitate repair of articular cartilage is the use of continuous passive motion (CPM). Salter et al. (25) have shown that CPM yields results superior to those of cast immobilization in the repair of small, full-thickness defects of articular cartilage which penetrate the underlying subchondral bone. Young rabbits show a greater ability to repair articular cartilage injury than do skeletally mature animals. Less successful results utilizing CPM occur with larger defects (i.e., >3 mm) (12). It is worth noting that CPM is in use in the clinical management of several joint-related conditions (i.e., open reduction and internal fixation of fractures; arthrotomy and arthrolysis for post-traumatic arthritis; synovectomy; release of joint contractures; osteotomies; arthroplasty; and ligamentous reconstruction) (26).

The experimental depletion of cartilage matrix components by application of matrix degrading enzymes *in vitro* has led to important observations regarding the interaction of the chondrocytes and their surrounding extracellular matrix. Papain, a proteolytic enzyme, has been used to demonstrate the reversible collapse of rabbit ear, tracheal, and costal cartilage after intravenous injection (27,28). These early studies suggested that the chondrocyte can replenish (repair) lost matrix components. Accordingly, Bosman (29) examined the effects of papain on growing chick tibias *in vitro*. Following a decrease in length and weight and a loss of cells, protein, and PGs, chondrocytes synthesized new PGs more rapidly than did control cartilage during a period marked by partial recovery of the lost extracellular matrix components. Similar results have been reported by Fitton-Jackson (30) using testicular hyaluronidase to remove most of the noncollagenous matrix. Hardingham et al. (31) later demonstrated that this rebound effect of chondrocytes resulted in the synthesis of PGs of much smaller size and lower chondroitin sulfate content. With time, these PGs became more like those from control samples. This chondrocyte rebound effect is also seen in enzymatically depleted human articular cartilage (32). Other parameters suggesting increased metabolic activity by chondrocytes following enzymatic perturbation of the matrix have been observed in rabbits; these changes include increases in glucose-6-phosphate dehydrogenase, glyceraldehyde-3-phosphate dehydrogenase, succinate dehydrogenase, and PG content as observed 9 days after a single intravenous injection of papain (33).

INTRA-ARTICULAR CHYMOPAPAIN AS A MODEL OF ARTICULAR CARTILAGE INJURY AND REPAIR

Injection of papain into a synovial joint has been used to induce degeneration and subsequent repair of articular cartilage in animal models (34–36). Following single or repeated intra-articular injections of papain into rabbit joints, PGs are lost from the cartilage matrix. This results in cell cluster formation, fibrillation of the articular surface, and chondrocyte loss which progresses with time to gross loss of cartilage and exposure of the underlying subchondral bone. Additionally, osteophyte formation at the joint margin has also been noted (36). Chondrocyte mitosis, thickening of fibrous tissue, and vascular invasion of the articular cartilage following intra-articular papain suggest attempts at cartilage repair which appeared to be more substantial in skeletally immature animals. It is important to note that in each of these above-mentioned models, which invariably result in articular cartilage destruction, single or repeated injections of relatively high concentrations of papain were used (i.e., a minimum of 9 mg per joint).

Our first use of intra-articular chymopapain involved testing the hypothesis that the concentration of keratan sulfate (KS) in serum reflects the extent and rate of cartilage PG catabolism (37). Adolescent male albino rabbits were injected with chymopapain (0.02 mg, 0.2 mg, or 2.0 mg in sterile water) into the left knee. These concentrations are, at most, one-fifth the concentrations used in the studies mentioned above. Prior to injection, serum samples were obtained on two or three occasions to determine baseline levels of serum KS. Serum was obtained at regular intervals (i.e., daily for 21 days and then monthly) thereafter until sacrifice. Other animals received intramuscular chymopapain or intra-articular water as controls. Serum KS epitope was quantified by an ELISA inhibition assay modified to permit quantification of rabbit serum KS. Changes in serum KS were determined by comparing each postinjection level to the preinjection baseline level. Samples of xiphoid cartilage and of articular cartilage from all knees of experimental and control rabbits were obtained at sacrifice for biochemical analysis [chondroitin sulfate (CS)/collagen ratios] and for histochemical staining with safranin O.

After injection of either 0.2 mg or 2.0 mg chymopapain into the left knee, serum KS levels rise above baseline within 5 hr, peak at 24 hr (Fig. 1), and remain elevated after 48 hr before returning to baseline after 9 days. Animals receiving only 0.02 mg chymopapain have peak serum KS values after 24 hr which are much lower than those obtained with the higher two doses and remain

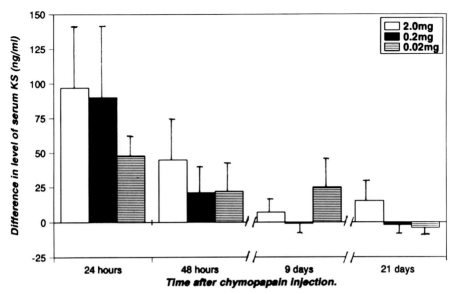

FIG. 1. Changes in the levels of keratan sulfate epitope following the injection of chymopapain into the rabbit knee. Levels are expressed in terms of equivalents of an international standard of keratan sulfate (KS) from human costal cartilage.

elevated above baseline after 9 days before returning to baseline. Serum KS values do not rise significantly above baseline in any animal afterward. Cartilage from all controls (i.e., contralateral noninjected knees, intra-articular sterile water, intramuscular chymopapain, xiphoid cartilage) are completely normal (Fig. 2A and 2B). In sharp contrast, stainable PGs are markedly reduced in animals receiving 0.2 mg or 2.0 mg chymopapain (Fig. 2C) after 2 days. Moderate loss of PG staining is seen at the same time in animals receiving only 0.02 mg chymopapain. Attempts by the chondrocytes to resynthesize matrix PGs after 9 days are noted in both 0.2- and 2.0-mg-injected animals (Fig. 2D). This reparative response continues for up to at least 6 months in animals receiving the lower dose of 0.2 mg (Fig. 2E and 2G), but fails in animals receiving the higher dose of 2.0 mg chymopapain (Fig. 2F and 2H). Virtually complete repair is noted in animals 6 months after receiving 0.02 mg chymopapain. A system for scoring the histologic changes [adapted from Mankin et al. (38)] has been applied to the femoral condyles, tibial plateaus, patellas, and patellar grooves of animals receiving 2.0 mg or 0.2 mg chymopapain (Table 1 and Fig. 3). Total joint scores for animals receiving 2.0 mg chymopapain are 22.4 ± 8.7 (after 2 days), 18.1 ± 9.2 (after 9 days) and 19.4 ± 9.7 (after 21 days). Total joint scores for animals receiving only 0.2 mg chymopapain are 18.2 ± 3.3 (after 2 days), 9.6 ± 7.4 (after 9 days), and 5.3 ± 5.4 (after 21 days). The ratio of chondroitin sulfate to collagen

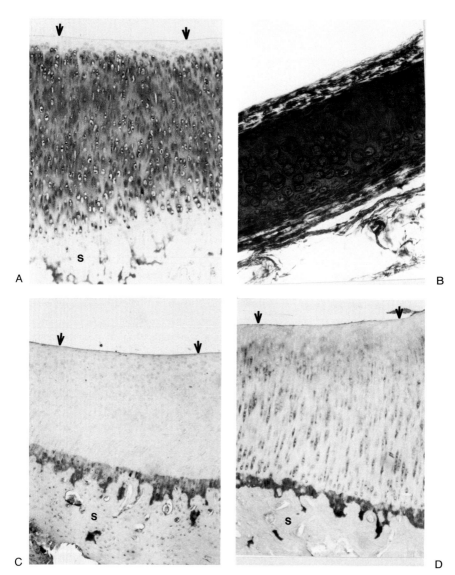

FIG. 2. Cross sections of rabbit knee articular cartilage (arrows identify articular surface) and underlying subchondral bone (s) isolated at various times following the injection of chymopapain. Safranin O, fast green stain. ×4. **A:** Normal control. **B:** Xiphoid cartilage. **C:** After 2 days. **D:** After 9 days. **E:** 0.2 mg after 21 days. **F:** 2.0 mg after 21 days. **G:** 0.2 mg after 6 months. **H:** 2.0 mg after 6 months.

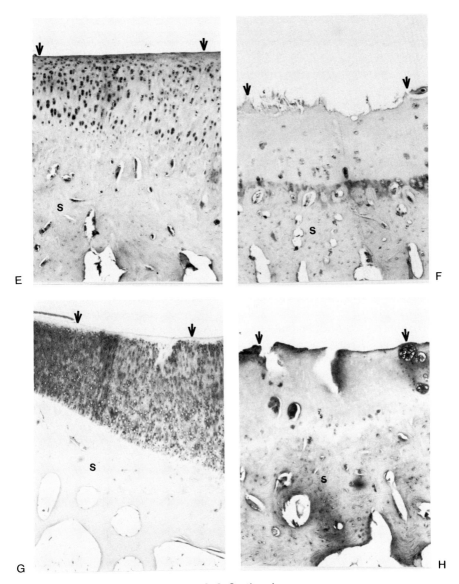

FIG. 2. *Continued.*

is reduced in all knees 2 days after receiving any of the chymopapain doses: 0.02 mg = 41 ± 9, 0.2 mg = 46 ± 12, and 2.0 mg = 46 ± 10 (Fig. 4). Elevated ratios suggesting resynthesis of PGs are noted after 9 days (2.0 mg = 70 ± 24, 0.2 mg = 59 ± 30). CS/collagen ratios are still elevated after 21 days (2.0 mg = 72 ± 22, 0.2 mg = 74 ± 26). After 6 months, CS/collagen ratios remain at 70 ± 9 in

TABLE 1. *Total histologic joint scores obtained at various times following the injection of chymopapain into the rabbit knee*

Time after injection (days)	Concentration of chymopapain (mg)	n	Total joint score
2	2.0	12	22.4 ± 8.7
	0.2	11	18.2 ± 3.3
	0.02	4	13.2 ± 1.9
9	2.0	12	18.1 ± 9.2
	0.2	12	9.6 ± 7.4
21	2.0	15	19.4 ± 9.7
	0.2	7	5.3 ± 5.4

animals receiving 2.0 mg, but rise to normal values in animals receiving 0.2 mg (116 ± 28) and 0.02 mg (115 ± 42). These results, with the exception of the high CS/collagen ratio seen in 2.0 mg animals after 21 days, are consistent with the histologic findings.

Numerous studies exist in the literature which support the notion that chondrocytes respond favorably to certain types of mechanical stimulation (39–42). In light of this and the apparent potential of CPM, we have performed a preliminary study to determine if CPM will affect the repair process following injection of chymopapain into the rabbit knee (43). Adolescent male albino rabbits were injected with chymopapain (0.2 mg or 2.0 mg in sterile water) into one knee. Blood was obtained to document the loss of PGs from the articular cartilage by measuring KS levels after the chymopapain injection. The results from this study

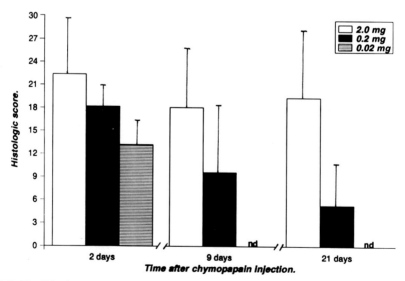

FIG. 3. Total histologic scores for femoral condyles, tibial plateaus, patellas, and patellar grooves obtained at various times following the injection of chymopapain into the rabbit knee.

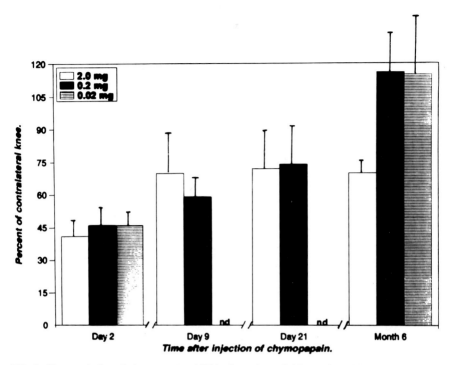

FIG. 4. Changes in the relative amounts of CS/collagen in medial femoral condyle articular cartilage at various times following injection of chymopapain in the rabbit knee. Results are expressed as percent of the ratios of CS/collagen in the contralateral noninjected knee. nd, no data available.

indicate that a period of cage rest followed by CPM of a chymopapain-injected knee may stimulate the spontaneous repair previously reported in rabbits injected with 0.2 mg chymopapain and may prevent the damage and stimulate resynthesis of matrix PGs following injection of 2.0 mg of chymopapain after 21 days (37). It is not known if this mechanically stimulated protection and repair will persist over a longer period of time (i.e., 6 months, 1 year).

In order to understand the mechanisms involved in the injury induced by intra-articular chymopapain injection, and the subsequent response, we have begun to examine other components of the extracellular matrix. Recently, we have measured urinary levels of two collagen cross-links, pyridinoline (Pyr) and deoxy-pyridinoline (D-Pyr), using a very sensitive high-performance liquid chromatography (HPLC) technique (44). The interassay variation of the whole assay in rabbit urine is 7.1% for Pyr and 13.1% for D-Pyr, and the recovery of Pyr and D-Pyr after spiking urine at the beginning of the processing was 97.2% and 71.6%, respectively (*unpublished data*). The age-related urinary excretion of Pyr and D-Pyr was measured in male New Zealand rabbits between 16 and 60 weeks of age and showed a steady state after 22 weeks of age (D. Uebelhart, *unpublished observation*). This is quite similar to the one described previously in humans (45). The effects of an intra-articular injection of a single dose of either 0.2 or 2.0 mg chymopapain in the rabbit has been followed over a 4-month period. Both low-dose and high-dose-injected rabbits show a very significant increase of Pyr as early as 24 hr after injection: 75% and 95% increase, respectively (Fig.

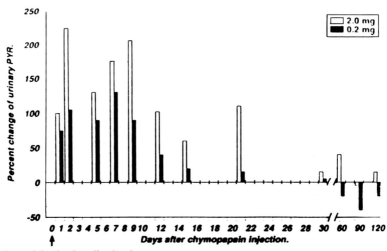

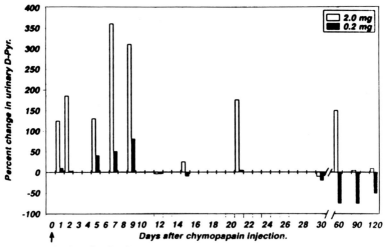

FIG. 5. Changes in urinary levels of Pyr (**A**) and D-Pyr (**B**) at various times following the injection of chymopapain into the rabbit knee. The arrow marks the time of injection. Pyr–2.0 mg chymopapain: n = 10. Pyr–0.2 mg chymopapain: n = 12. D-Pyr–2.0 mg chymopapain: n = 10. D-Pyr–0.2 mg chymopapain: n = 10.

5A). At day 2, Pyr was further increased in both low-dose (103%) and high-dose (220%) groups. A drop in urinary Pyr in both groups occurs at 5 and 7 days after injection, followed by a second peak for the low-dose group at day 7 (134%) and at day 9 for the high-dose group (208%). Pyr values for the low-dose group reach baseline after 1 month and are below baseline at 2, 3, and 4 months. Urinary Pyr values remain elevated for 21 days (115%) in the 2.0-mg group before returning to baseline at 30 days of evolution, but show novel increases at 2 months (37%) and 4 months (18%).

The urinary excretion of D-Pyr, the bone-specific cross-linking amino acid, is remarkably different for the low- and the high-dose-injected rabbits (Fig. 5B). D-Pyr is significantly increased in the high-dose group after 24 hr (127%) and 48 hr (179%) as compared with, respectively, 11% (24 hr) and 3% (48 hr) in the low-dose group which exhibit nearly no response. D-Pyr excretion reaches its maximum in the high-dose group at day 7 (309%). A slightly moderate rise in urinary D-Pyr is noted between days 5 and 9 in the low-dose group (60%). In both groups, D-Pyr reaches the baseline preinjection values at day 12. The low-dose group shows constantly negative values up to 4 months after the injection; however, the high-dose group shows further peaks at day 21 (163%) and at 2 months (145%), before returning to baseline at 3 and 4 months after the injection.

CONCLUDING REMARKS

It was stated previously that the repair mechanisms of articular cartilage are poorly understood. In naturally occurring OA, with progression of the disease, cartilage repair attempts fail and severe joint destruction ensues (7,8). What, then, is the key element (or combination of factors) which lead(s) to irreversible breakdown of articular cartilage? Several factors (e.g., age, extent, and location of the injury) have been discussed by Buckwalter et al. (12). It is possible that chronic stress or excessive demand placed on the chondrocyte for repair may diminish the cell's ability to handle additional insults. A second related possibility involves the loss of matrix PGs and a corresponding increase in water content, which is one of the earliest observed changes in articular cartilage injury (46). An increase in water content leads to a change in the mechanical properties of the articular cartilage, making it vulnerable to injury. However, it should be noted that the loss of PGs does not invariably lead to irreversible cartilage damage. A remarkable feature of articular cartilage injury is that over 50% of the matrix PGs can be lost and complete recovery can occur. This observation has been made previously through *in vivo* work following intravenous injection of crude papain which resulted in loss of matrix PGs and collapse of the ear cartilage which was rapidly reversible (27,28). Other work which has focused on the cellular response to enzymatic degradation of cartilage has revealed a rebound effect where metabolic activity of the chondrocytes is severalfold higher than normal (29–33). It is important to note, however, that markedly different outcomes can be achieved with a similar loss of PG from the cartilage. That is, intra-articular injection of 0.2 mg or 2.0 mg results in a similar loss of matrix PGs along with elevated serum KS, but different long-term outcomes. Accordingly, chondrocytes from joints receiving either concentration of chymopapain show elevated metabolic activity after 9 days. However, while this rebound response by the chondrocytes is sustained over the long term with the lower dose, it fails with the higher dose of chymopapain. This suggests that other factors may be involved, such as the selective destruction of other matrix components, the failure to resynthesize matrix components, poorly coordinated organization of newly synthesized matrix components, or concurrent damage to the underlying subchondral bone.

A third consideration in the repair of articular cartilage is the role of collagen. Collagen provides structural integrity for articular cartilage. In addition, it functions to constrain other matrix constituents, preventing their loss from the cartilage matrix. It has been long accepted that collagen is the main link in maintaining the integrity of the articular cartilage, because loss of integrity of the collagen meshwork almost invariably leads to tissue destruction. Studies by Broom and co-workers (47,48) have demonstrated the relationship between the collagen meshwork and matrix PGs and have shown how this contributes to the loading properties of articular cartilage. A role has been suggested for type IX collagen in structurally linking type II fibrils together, thus providing stability to the arcades of collagen fibrils in the matrix (49,50). Damage (or disorganization) to the collagen meshwork does not necessarily result in failure of the cartilage. Although the extent of damage/disorganization to the collagen meshwork is not known following intra-articular injection of chymopapain, complete recovery can occur.

A final consideration involves the physiologic coupling of articular cartilage and the underlying subchondral bone as set forth by Radin (51). In the chymopapain-induced articular cartilage injury model *in vivo,* depletion of matrix PGs was accompanied by the appearance of bone-specific collagen cross-links when there was a progressive degeneration of the articular cartilage. However, a similar depletion of matrix PGs which does not involve significant damage to the subchondral bone collagen cross-links results in spontaneous repair. Considering the distribution of both cross-links, D-Pyr is virtually only present in bone type I collagen and is absent from cartilage type II collagen (52). Even if a small fraction could be isolated and measured in cartilage type IX collagen (53), considering the magnitude of the urinary excretion of D-Pyr, it could clearly only originate from the subchondral bone compartment. These results, therefore, possibly demonstrate a dynamic coupling of articular cartilage with the underlying subchondral bone in an experimental animal model. The comparison between serum KS levels and urinary cross-link excretion suggests that chymopapain first degraded the PG fraction of articular cartilage as assessed by the raised serum KS levels, then cleaved the telopeptides of types IX and II collagen of cartilage (54), and later cleaved those of type I collagen in subchondral bone. These results serve to couple the articular cartilage and subchondral bone in an experimental animals model of the success or failure of cartilage repair.

What role, then, do other factors (e.g., mechanical forces, inflammation, cytokines) play in this model? The chymopapain effects are certainly associated with secondary mechanical events as well as with inflammatory factors and cytokine release. The greatest damage is seen histologically in the central weight-bearing regions. The increased mechanically related damage, combined with a longer stage of inflammation at the articular-cartilage–subchondral-bone level, could explain the absence of repair seen in the high-dose group as compared with the repair seen in the low-dose group. These interrelationships remain to be elucidated. As suggested by other work, the functional integrity of the extracellular matrix of articular cartilage is essential to allow the repair process to take place. Results from the chymopapain *in vivo* model are consistent with this notion. According to these data, the limiting factor for repair does not seem to be the PG content alone, but the degree of functional integrity of the collagenous meshwork. Disorganization and/or damage to the collagen meshwork occasionally can occur with complete repair. However, once it is too extensively disorganized and/or damaged, an effective repair process cannot be sustained and catabolism becomes the dominant feature.

REFERENCES

1. Peyron JG. The epidemiology of osteoarthritis. In: Moskowitz RW, et al., eds. *Osteoarthritis diagnosis and management.* Philadelphia: WB Saunders, 1984;9–27.
2. Mayne R, Irwin MH. Collagen types in cartilage. In: Kuettner KE, Schleyerbach R, Hascall VC, eds. *Articular cartilage biochemistry.* New York: Raven Press, 1986;23–35.
3. Heinegard D, Oldberg A. Structure and biology of cartilage and bone matrix noncollagenous macromolecules. *FASEB J* 1989;3:2042–2051.
4. Ali SY, Evans L. Enzymatic degradation of cartilage in osteoarthritis. *Fed Proc* 1973;32:1494–1498.
5. Sapolsky AI, Howel DS. Further characterization of a neutral metalloprotease isolated from human articular cartilage *Arthritis Rheum* 1982;25:581–588.
6. Kuettner KE, Harper E, Eisenstein R. Protease inhibitors in cartilage. *Arthritis Rheum* 1977;20:124–132.
7. Mankin HJ, Lippiello L. Biochemical and metabolic abnormalities in articular cartilage from osteo-arthritic human hips. *J Bone Joint Surg* 1970;52A:424.
8. Thompson RC, Oegema TR. Metabolic activity of articular cartilage in osteoarthritis. *J Bone Joint Surg* 1979;61A:407–416.
9. Lippiello L, Hall D, Mankin HJ. Collagen synthesis in normal and osteoarthritic human cartilage. *J Clin Invest* 1977;59:593–600.
10. Eyre DR, McDevitt CA, Muir IHM. Experimentally-induced osteoarthritis in the dog. Collagen biosynthesis in control and fibrillated cartilage. *Ann Rheum Dis* 1975;34(Suppl):137–140.
11. Ehrlich MG, Houle PA, Vigliani G, Mankin HJ. Correlation between articular cartilage collagenase activity and osteoarthritis. *Arthritis Rheum* 1973;21:761–766.
12. Buckwalter JA, Rosenberg L, Coutts R, Hunziker E, Reddi AH, Mow V. Articular cartilage: injury and repair. In: Woo SLY, Buckwalter JA, eds. *Injury and repair of the musculoskeletal soft tissues.* Illinois: American Academy of Orthopaedic Surgeons, 1987;465–482.
13. Sokoloff L. Cell biology and the repair of articular cartilage. *J Rheumatol* 1974;1:9–16.
14. Furukawa AT, Eyre DR, Koide S, Glimcher MJ. Biochemical studies on repair cartilage resurfacing experimental defects in the rabbit knee. *J Bone Joint Surg* 1980;62A:79–89.

15. Cheung HS, Cottrell WH, Stephenson K, Nimni E. *In vitro* collagen biosynthesis in healing and normal rabbit articular cartilage. *J Bone Joint Surg* 1978;60A:1076.
16. Meachim G. The effect of scarification of articular cartilage in the rabbit. *J Bone Joint Surg* 1963;45B:150–161.
17. Ghadially JA, Ghadially G, Ghadially FN. Long term results of deep defects in articular cartilage. A SEM study. *Virchows Arch [Cell Pathol]* 1977;25:125–136.
18. Ghadially FN, Ailsby RL, Oryschak AF. Scanning electron microscopy of superficial defects in articular cartilage. *Ann Rheum Dis* 1974;33:327–332.
19. Moskowitz, RW. Experimental models of osteoarthritis. In: Moskowitz RW, et al., eds. *Osteoarthritis: diagnosis and management.* Philadelphia: WB Saunders, 1984;109–128.
20. Hall MC. Articular cartilage changes in the knee of the adult rat after prolonged immobilization in extension. *Clin Orthop* 1964;34:184–195.
21. Telhag H, Lindberg H. A method for inducing osteoarthritic changes in rabbit knees. *Clin Orthop* 1972;86:214–223.
22. Palmoski MJ, Perricone E, Brandt KD. Development and reversal of a proteoglycan aggregation defect in normal canine articular cartilage after immobilization. *Arthritis Rheum* 1979;22:508–517.
23. Williams JM, Brandt KD. Temporary immobilization facilitates repair of chemically-induced articular injury. *J Anat* 1984;138:435–446.
24. Palmoski MJ, Brandt KD. Running inhibits the reversal of atrophic changes in canine knee cartilage after removal of a leg cast. *Arthritis Rheum* 1981;24:1329–1337.
25. Salter RB, Simmonds DF, Malcolm BW, Rumble EJ, MacMichael D, Clements ND. The biological effect of continuous passive motion on the healing of full thickness defects in articular cartilage. *J Bone Joint Surg* 1980;62A:1232–1251.
26. Salter RB, Hamilton HW, Wedge JH, Tile M, Torode IP, O'Driscoll SW, Murnaghan JJ, Saringer JH. The clinical application of basic research on continuous passive motion (CPM) for disorders and injuries of synovial joints. A preliminary report. *J Orthop Res* 1984;1:325–342.
27. Thomas L. Reversible collapse of rabbit ears after intravenous papain and prevention of recovery by cortisone. *J Exp Med* 1956;104:245–252.
28. McElligott TF, Potter JL. Increased fixation of sulfur 35 by cartilage *in vitro* following depletion of the matrix by intravenous papain. *J Exp Med* 1960;112:743–751.
29. Bosman HB. Cellular control of macromolecular synthesis: rates of synthesis of extracellular macromolecules during and after depletion by papain. *Proc R Soc [Biol]* 1968;169:399–425.
30. Fitton-Jackson S. Environmental control of macromolecular synthesis in cartilage and bone: morphogenetic response to hyaluronidase. *Proc R Soc Lond [Biol]* 1970;175:405–453.
31. Hardingham TE, Fitton-Jackson S, Muir IHM. Replacement of proteoglycans in embryonic chick cartilage in organ culture after treatment with testicular hyaluronidase. *Biochem J* 1972;129:101–112.
32. Verbruggen G, Luyten FP, Veys EM. Repair function in organ cultured human cartilage. Replacement of enzymatically removed proteoglycans during long term organ culture. *J Rheumatol* 1985;12:665–674.
33. Boussidan F, Nahir AM. Altered chondrocytic oxidative metabolism during the restoration of depleted intercellular matrix. *J Exp Pathol* 1990;71:395–402.
34. Murray DG. Experimentally induced arthritis using intra-articular papain. *Arthritis Rheum* 1964;7:211–219.
35. Bentley G. Papain-induced degenerative arthritis of the hip in rabbits. *J Bone Joint Surg* 1971;53B:324–337.
36. Inoue S, Glimcher MJ. The reaction of cartilage and osteophyte formation after the intra-articular injection of papain. *Seikeigeka Gakkai Zasshi* 1982;56:415–430.
37. Williams JM, Downey C, Thonar EJ-MA. Increase in the level of serum keratan sulfate following the degradation of cartilage proteoglycans in the rabbit knee joint. *Arthritis Rheum* 1988;31:557–560.
38. Mankin HJ, Dorfman H, Lippiello L, Zarins A. Biochemical and metabolic abnormalities in articular cartilage from osteo-arthritic human hips. II. Correlation of morphology with biochemical and metabolic data. *J Bone Joint Surg* 1971;53A:523–537.
39. Caterson B, Lowther DA. Changes in the metabolism of the proteoglycans from sheep articular cartilage in response to mechanical stress. *Biochim Biophys Acta* 1978;540:412–422.

40. DeWitt MT, Handley CJ, Oaks BW, Lowther DA. *In vitro* response of chondrocytes to mechanical loading: the effect of short term mechanical tension. *Connect Tissue Res* 1984;12:97–109.
41. Gray ML, Pizzanelli AM, Grodzinsky AJ, Lee RC. Mechanical and physicochemical determinants of the chondrocyte biosynthetic response. *J Orthop Res* 1988;6:777–792.
42. Sah RLY, Kim Y-J, Doong J-YH, Grodzinsky AJ, Plass AHK, Sandy JD. Biosynthetic response of cartilage explants to dynamic compression. *J Orthop Res* 1989;7:619–636.
43. Williams JM, Moran M, Thonar EJ-MA, Salter RB. Continuous passive motion stimulates repair of rabbit knee articular cartilage following matrix proteoglycan loss. *Orthop Trans* 1990;15:127.
44. Uebelhart D, Gineyts E, Chapuy MD, Delmas PD. Urinary excretion of pyridinium crosslinks: a new marker of bone resorption in metabolic bone disease. *Bone Miner* 1990;8:87–96.
45. Beardsworth LJ, Eyre DR, Dickson IR. Changes with age in the urinary excretion of lysyl- and hydroxylysylpyridinoline, two new markers of bone collagen turnover. *J Bone Miner Res* 1990;5:671–676.
46. Mankin HJ, Brandt KD. In: Moskowitz RW, et al., eds. *Osteoarthritis: diagnosis and management.* Philadelphia: WB Saunders, 1984;43–79.
47. Broom ND, Poole CA. Articular cartilage collagen and proteoglycans. Their functional interdependency. *Arthritis Rheum* 1983;26:1111–1119.
48. Broom ND, Marra DL. New structural concepts of articular cartilage demonstrated with a physical model. *Connect Tissue Res* 1985;14:1–8.
49. Broom ND. An enzymatically induced structural transformation in articular cartilage. *Arthritis Rheum* 1988;31:210–218.
50. Eyre DR, Apon S, Wu J-J, Ericsson LH, Walsh KS. Collagen type IX: evidence for covalent linkages to type II collagen in cartilage. *FEB* 1987;220:337–341.
51. Radin EL. Mechanical factors in the causation of osteoarthrosis. *Rheumatology* 1982;7:46–52.
52. Eyre DR. Collagen crosslinking amino-acids. In: Cunningham LW, ed. *Methods in enzymology,* vol 144. New York: Academic Press, 1987;115–139.
53. Wu J-J, Eyre DR. Cartilage type IX collagen is crosslinked by hydroxypyridinium residues. *Biochem Biophys Res Commun* 1984;123:1033–1039.
54. Strawich E, Nimni ME. Properties of a collagen molecule containing three identical components extracted from bovine articular cartilage. *Biochemistry* 1971;10:3905–3911.

DISCUSSION

Benya: When you observed some repair with regard to the hydroxypyridinoline crosslinks, I presume you are referring to decreased release with time. Do you know whether the cross-link content of the tissue also returns to its original level?

Williams: We are now in the process of correlating urinary levels of collagen crosslinks with the actual amount of cross-link in the tissue.

Pritzker: Richard Renlund and I developed a similar model by injecting hyaluronidase into rabbit joints. We observed some similar changes in terms of cartilage destruction and regeneration. We also observed very remarkable proliferative changes in the synovium, with the proliferation and establishment of hyperplasia of the synovial lining cells. Do you see this in your chymopapain model?

Williams: No, we do not see the same severity of change in the synovial lining. We see a mild inflammatory response which subsides after a few days.

Brune: Was continuous passive motion in your model beneficial for all doses?

Williams: It was beneficial at every dose. At the high dose in the absence of continuous passive motion, the cartilage degenerates. We therefore expected that this dose with continuous passive motion would erode the cartilage even faster and create a nice model for eburnation. We were wrong in that this treatment stimulated total repair.

Cooke: Where did the lesions develop in the joint?

Williams: We see the lesions in the central weight-bearing zone. At short distances away from the lesions, the cartilage appears histologically normal. It is important to note that when we remove cartilage samples for chemical analyses, some normal tissue from the more peripheral unloaded area may have been included.

Brandt: Your data showing enhanced release of bone-collagen-specific cross-links suggest that bone is damaged by the injection. That could occur by diffusion of chymopapain from the joint space, since these are younger animals with open epiphyses. The calcified cartilage retains intense safranin-O staining. How is bone metabolism activated?

Williams: Ted Oegema has examined patellas using this model, and the calcified cartilage does not appear to change. I don't think the mechanism of bone damage is as simple as the diffusion of chymopapain into bone compartments. Other systems, such as cytokine mediators or biomechanical changes, are more likely to be involved.

Heinegard: The decrease of staining for proteoglycans in your histological sections appeared to be much more pronounced than the loss of chondroitin sulfate measured chemically. Is there an explanation for that?

Williams: We need to be cautious in relating changes in histologic staining patterns with absolute measures of macromolecules. For example, 2 days following an intra-articular chymopapain injection, we can show a complete loss of stainable proteoglycans. However, biochemical analysis of cartilage samples taken at the same time show that 40–50% of the proteoglycans are still present.

Articular Cartilage and Osteoarthritis,
edited by K. Kuettner et al.
Raven Press, Ltd., New York © 1992.

Part X: Pharmacology in Osteoarthritis

Introduction

Rudolf Schleyerbach

*Department of Pharmacological Research, Hoechst Aktiengesellschaft Werk
Kalle-Albert, 6200 Wiesbaden 12, Federal Republic of Germany*

The dynamics of fluid flow in the synovium are very important in determining concentrations of markers for joint tissue metabolism or of pharmacological agents introduced during therapeutic intervention. The chapter by Levick describes the variety of parameters which influence volume and fluid flow measurements in the joint. The basic concepts described in his chapter form a framework for interpreting the data from synovial fluid samples which are central to many of the human and animal protocols currently under investigation. Inflammatory episodes within the joint are often a consequence of the progression of osteoarthritic diseases, and most therapeutic intervention is directed toward preventing inflammation and thereby reducing pain. The chapter by Lowther et al. describes a reliable rabbit model for carageenin-induced inflammation in knee joints, and it defines key roles for elastase and radicals derived from hydrogen peroxide generated by macrophages in the suppression of chondrocyte metabolism in the articular cartilage. This model is useful for testing efficacy of agents to intervene in this destructive process using protocols *in vivo* and on tissue *in vitro*. The clinician must struggle with the human consequences of the disease. The clinician-scientist has the additional burden of defining whether treatment protocols are beneficial or harmful. Although criteria for scientific proof are well defined, it is very difficult for the clinician-scientist to apply these criteria in well-controlled patient-based settings. The chapter by Brune evaluates this problem within the context of the nonsteroidal anti-inflammatory drugs (NSAIDs) and chondroprotective drugs that have been used clinically over the past few years. His assessment provides a cautionary note to investigators and clinicians in their worthy attempts to move promising leads in laboratory settings into clinical treatments to alleviate patient suffering.

Articular Cartilage and Osteoarthritis,
edited by K. Kuettner et al.
Raven Press, Ltd., New York © 1992.

37

Synovial Fluid

Determinants of Volume Turnover and Material Concentration

J. Rodney Levick

*Department of Physiology, St. George's Hospital Medical School,
London SW17 0RE, England*

Water, oxygen, nutrients, building materials, and drugs reach articular cartilage from blood by traversing the synovial capillary wall and overlying synovial tissue to reach the synovial fluid, which bathes the cartilage (Fig. 1). Conversely, cartilage metabolic end-products, extracellular matrix degradation products, and drugs leave the joint by permeating the intercellular spaces of the synovial lining. If they are highly diffusible (CO_2, urea, lactate, unbound drugs, small peptides) they then exit through the walls of synovial capillaries, but if they are larger and less diffusible (proteins, bound drugs, proteoglycan fragments, hyaluronan fragments) they exit via subsynovial lymphatics. In addition, synovial lining macrophages have the potential to take up and degrade macromolecules locally, but this probably contributes little to the removal of endogenous proteins from healthy joints, where the protein transit from joint cavity to bloodstream is known to be dominated by lymph flow. Foreign materials such as ferritin and glycogen, when injected into the synovial cavity, are taken up by synovial A cells, but the quantities involved are not clear.

DYNAMIC NATURE OF SYNOVIAL FLUID CONCENTRATION

Clinical interest in cartilage degradation products and protein-bound drugs in synovial fluid has highlighted the need for a better understanding of the factors governing intra-articular macromolecule concentration. These factors include: macromolecule input rate, the flow of water across the synovial lining, and probably also the properties of the synovial intercellular matrix (SIM). The first two factors will be assessed first.

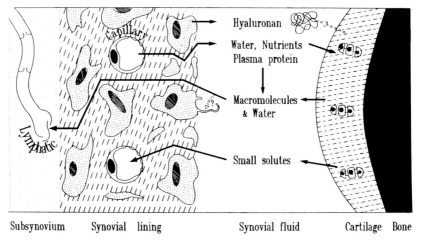

FIG. 1. Diagram depicting synovial transport pathways (not drawn to scale).

Synovial fluid is not stagnant but is constantly turning over (i.e., being replaced); this is because of capillary filtration and lymphatic absorption, which balance each other in the long term (Fig. 2). Macromolecule concentration is inversely related to the volume turnover rate because the input macromolecule is continually diluted in the stream of synovial fluid passing through the joint cavity. This is particularly important in arthritis, where fluid turnover rates are

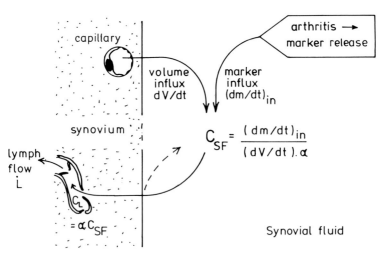

FIG. 2. Determinants of macromolecular concentration in a cavity where fluid is constantly being replaced by capillary filtration and lymphatic absorption. Dashed arrow indicates possible partial reflection of very large solutes by synovial interstitial matrix. For explanation of symbols, see text.

increased by 100–300% and where concentration values taken in isolation can be seriously misleading (1). The relationship between macromolecule concentration in synovial fluid (C_{SF}), the net input rate of the macromolecule ($\Delta m/\Delta t$; corrected for any local degradation), and synovial fluid turnover rate ($\Delta V/\Delta t$) follows directly from the definition of concentration (1):

$$C_{SF} = \frac{m}{V} = \frac{dm/dt}{dV/dt} = \frac{\text{marker net input rate}}{\text{fluid turnover rate}} \qquad [1]$$

provided that the macromolecule leaves the joint cavity at the same concentration that exists in the available water space within the synovial fluid (see later).

The synovial intercellular spaces are normally 1–2 μm wide and occupy 20–30% of the synovial surface (2) (Fig. 1). Small lipophobic solutes diffuse freely in such spaces. Hydraulic flow, however, experiences considerable resistance owing to the matrix of glycosaminoglycan (hyaluronan), proteoglycans, collagens (types I, III, IV, V, and VI), and glycoproteins (fibronectin, laminin) that occupy the synovial interstitium. Analogous polymer matrices in other tissues hamper macromolecular movement as well as water flow, and in many soft tissues the albumin diffusion coefficient is only ~25% of its normal value. Consequently, the question arises as to whether the synovial matrix also is sufficiently dense to retard macromolecular permeation. A pointer to the effective matrix density in synovium is provided by the studies of trans-synovial water flow described in the next section, and these also elucidate some factors controlling volume turnover.

FACTORS GOVERNING TRANS-SYNOVIAL FLOW

The rate at which water enters or leaves a joint cavity depends on the balance between intravascular and intra-articular hydrodynamic forces, the hydraulic permeability of the pathways, and subsynovial lymphatic function. Taking the intravascular factors first, studies in which synovial *microvascular blood pressure* and *plasma colloid osmotic pressure* (COP) were varied in rabbit knees showed that capillary pressure promotes filtration into the cavity and that plasma COP promotes absorption from it (3). They also showed that the hydraulic conductance of the blood-to-joint pathway increases as much as fourfold when pressure in the joint cavity is raised to pathological levels (>9 cm H_2O) by fluid infusion (4). At the same time, the synovial intercellular spaces become wider and the pathlength from the joint cavity to the microvasculature becomes shorter (2).

The influence of *intra-articular fluid pressure* (IAP) is illustrated in Fig. 3. A rise in IAP promotes the absorption of liquid from the joint cavity. The pressure–flow relationship steepens greatly above ~9 cm H_2O (yield point), which again indicates that synovial hydraulic conductance increases at high joint fluid pressures. IAP is determined by joint angle, fluid volume, periarticular tissue compliance, time, and muscle activity (4).

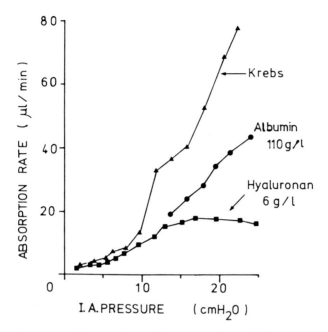

FIG. 3. Rate of trans-synovial absorption of fluid as a function of IAP in the normal rabbit knee (4,5).

When intra-articular plasma protein concentration is raised by adding albumin to the intra-articular fluid, absorption from the joint cavity is reduced (Fig. 3). This is partly because albumin modestly increases viscosity, and partly because it permeates the SIM to reach the pericapillary spaces, where it promotes capillary filtration by exerting a pericapillary osmotic pressure. An element of self-regulation arises here, because intra-articular protein both determines trans-synovial flow (Fig. 3) and depends on it (Eq. 1).

When intra-articular hyaluronan is added to intra-articular Krebs solution at physiological concentrations, not only is absorption rate greatly reduced but also the shape of the pressure–flow relationship is altered. The curve develops a plateau (5). At a certain trans-synovial fluid velocity, raising IAP fails to produce a maintained increase in trans-synovial flow. Indeed, flow 15–20 min after a pressure step sometimes even falls below that at the preceding lower pressure. The pressure required to drive unit trans-synovial flow is progressively raised, indicating that hyaluronan in the synovial cavity progressively increases the interstitial hydraulic resistance. This may be due to sieving of the synovial fluid hyaluronan molecules by SIM, causing a hyaluronan "filter-cake" to build up at, or within, the synovial surface. If this explanation is correct, SIM must be dense enough to retard (without necessarily totally blocking) the permeation of molecules as large as hyaluronan ($M_r \sim 800$ kD in these experiments).

TURNOVER RATES FOR LIQUID AND ENDOGENOUS MACROMOLECULES

The time-averaged volume turnover is estimated to be 2–4 μl/hr/cm^2 in normal human and rabbit knees (4), and this is equivalent to the cavity's water content turning over roughly once per hour. In human arthritis the average volume turnover rate *increases,* to ~1.8 ml/hr in the osteoarthritic knee and ~4.3 ml/hr in the rheumatoid knee (approximately four times normal) (6). *This is vital to bear in mind when interpreting intra-articular concentration data in arthritis* (see the denominator in Eq. 1). The volume turnover time, however (i.e. volume/volume turnover rate), is prolonged in arthritis because the effusion volume increases more than the volume turnover rate.

In contrast to the volume turnover time of an hour or so in normal joints, the turnover time for dissolved hyaluronan in synovial fluid, calculated as hyaluronan mass per joint cavity/mass turnover rate, is much longer, of the order of 24 hr (7). The half-life of intra-articularly injected, labeled hyaluronan is 14 hr (8). Evidently, therefore, hyaluronan experiences more difficulty in passing through SIM than does water, even though SIM is not an impenetrable obstacle for hyaluronan (8), and this implies that SIM is a relatively dense matrix. This view is supported by the high hydraulic resistance of synovium (see later). Before pursuing this, however, an important but often neglected biophysical effect of dissolved hyaluronan on macromolecule concentration in synovial fluid must be noted.

STERIC EXCLUSION BY DISSOLVED HYALURONAN: EFFECT ON APPARENT MACROMOLECULAR CONCENTRATION

The concentration C_{SF} in Eq. 1 is the concentration of a macromolecule in the *available* water space of synovial fluid (1), whereas the concentration measured analytically is solute mass divided by *total* volume. Hyaluronan excludes macromolecules from part of the total water space by creating pockets of fluid too tiny for macromolecules to enter (steric exclusion) (9,10). For example, at physiological concentrations, synovial fluid hyaluronan excludes albumin from 15–30% of the water space, and excludes α_2-macroglobulin from over 70% of the space (11).

When hyaluronan concentration falls, as in the arthritides, the available volume fraction increases, and this can be a large effect. For example, a fall in hyaluronan concentration from 3 g/liter (normal human knee) to 1 g/liter (rheumatoid knee) causes a 2.6-fold increase in the fractional available space for α_2-macroglobulin (M_r = 850 kD). As a result, the measured concentration of a macromolecule (namely, mass/volume of synovial fluid) can increase substantially in arthritis even without an increased input rate. This is especially so for large macromolecules, as can be seen from Ogsten's equation for the fraction of the water space available (K_{AV}) to a spherical macromolecule of radius a in a random assemblage of rigid molecular rods of radius r (9):

$$K_{AV} = \exp[-(z/r^2) \cdot (r + a)^2] \qquad [2]$$

where z is hyaluronan concentration, expressed as a volume fraction (concentration in g/ml $\times$ effective specific volume, 0.65 ml/g), and r is 0.35–0.6 nm for glycosaminoglycan chains. The validity of the above expression was proved experimentally by Laurent (10).

In the case of rod-shaped and other nonspherical convex solute molecules, analogous available-space expressions exist (12–14). There appears to be neither experimental nor theoretical work, however, on the fractional space available to nonaggregating proteoglycans within a hyaluronan solution, even though such information is needed to understand changes in the concentration of proteoglycan fragments in arthritic synovial fluid. The proteoglycan monomer is a bottle-brush-shaped molecule, and one might anticipate that K_{AV} for such a molecule will be greater than K_{AV} for a solid sphere of equivalent hydrodynamic radius (Eq. 2), but less than K_{AV} for dissociated chondroitin and keratan sulfate chains (12,13).

HYDRAULIC CONDUCTIVITY OF SIM AND ITS RELATIONSHIP TO COMPOSITION

Returning to the issue of the synovial matrix density, the hydraulic data provide a useful pointer in the absence of any analytical data. From the hydraulic data and morphometric measurements of pathway geometry in the rabbit knee, the interstitial hydraulic conductivity at low IAP is found to be 1.4–2.1×10^{-12} $cm^4 \cdot sec^{-1} \cdot dyn^{-1}$ for physiological saline at 37°C, which is similar to that of aortic interstitium and scleral stroma (14) and about 10 times that of femoral head cartilage.

Interstitial hydraulic conductivity is closely related to the concentration of polymer in a matrix (14,15). From the relations in (14) and allowing for a collagen content of 162 mg per milliliter of interstitium (estimated from data in ref. 17), the concentration of glycosaminoglycan (GAG) associated with the above value of conductivity is estimated to be 5–10 mg per milliliter of interstitium. Although this is only one-fifth to one-tenth of the GAG concentration in articular cartilage, it is sufficient to slow macromolecular transport markedly, because matrices of even lesser density have substantial effects on albumin transport (16).

MACROMOLECULE CONCENTRATION IN JOINT CAVITY WHEN EGRESS IS RETARDED

Although Eq. 1 is useful didactically, it derives from a specially simple case where macromolecules permeate synovium at the same rate as water, and thereby reach lymph at a thermodynamic concentration (mass/available volume) identical to that in synovial fluid (1). If, however, the matrix is sufficiently dense to impede macromolecular movement more than water, the lymph macromolecule concentration can be a variable fraction of that in synovial fluid (see Fig. 2). To allow for this we can write $C_L/C_{SF} = \alpha$. The requirements of conservation of mass now lead to a modified expression for steady-state concentration in synovial fluid available water (1), namely,

$$C_{SF} = \frac{dm/dt}{\alpha(dV/dt)} = \frac{\text{marker influx rate}}{\alpha \times \text{volume turnover rate}} \qquad [3]$$

This expression predicts raised concentrations of macromolecule in the joint cavity if α is less than 1.

SYNOVIAL REFLECTION COEFFICIENTS: CAN THEY BE ZERO FOR MACROMOLECULES?

When a solution is forced under pressure through a membrane that is less permeable to solute than to water, the solute undergoes partial molecular sieving or "reflection." The reflection coefficient σ is a measure of the proportion of solute molecules reflected at the limit of very high fluid velocities. Its value ranges from 0 to 1, and it depends on the solute partition coefficient Φ (15):

$$\sigma = (1 - \Phi)^2 \qquad [4]$$

Because the volume fraction z occupied by glycosaminoglycan is small, Φ is nearly equal to K_{AV} [$\Phi = K_{AV}/\exp(-z)$] (15). In many soft tissues the albumin partition coefficient is 0.5 or less, and in articular cartilage it is ~ 0.01 (18). In such cases the macromolecular reflection coefficient should be greater than zero. This has been confirmed in tissue excised from subcutaneous capsules, where the albumin and IgG reflection coefficients are 0.23 and 0.53, respectively, and the corresponding hydraulic permeability is 2.1×10^{-11} cm$^4 \cdot$ sec$^{-1} \cdot$ dyn^{-1} (16). The latter value indicates that subcutaneous tissue is actually more permeable than synovium, so it is unlikely that the macromolecular reflection coefficients of normal rabbit synovium[1] will be zero.

If interstitial matrix is represented as a uniformly random assemblage of rigid rods as in Ogsten's model, curves can be constructed that relate hydraulic conductivity and reflection coefficients, because both parameters depend on polymer concentration (14,15). Figure 4 illustrates such relationships for several proteins found in synovial fluid; the shaded zone indicates that synovial reflection coefficients are unlikely to be zero for molecules larger than albumin ($a = 3.55$ nm). Few data exist to test the theoretical curves, but the prediction for albumin at a conductivity within the articular cartilage range is close to that calculated via

---

[1] Not to be confused with endothelial barrier reflection coefficients cited in ref. 3.

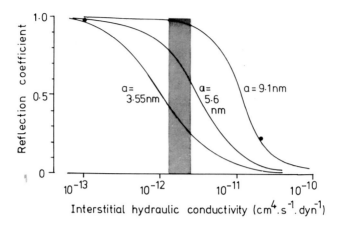

FIG. 4. Theoretical relationship between reflection coefficient for a rigid spherical solute of radius *a* (albumin, immunoglobulin G, α_2-macroglobulin) in a uniformly random network of rigid long rods (radius 0.6 nm; Eqs. 2 and 4) and interstitial hydraulic conductivity to saline at 35°C [based on glycosaminoglycan conductivity *in vitro* (14)]. Shaded zone covers range for normal synovial interstitial conductivity. Solid circles are data for albumin (*a* = 3.55 nm) in femoral cartilage [*left*, calculated from Maroudas's Φ value (18)] and in subcutaneous tissue (*right*, from ref. 16).

Eq. 4 from Maroudas's value for Φ in femoral articular cartilage (18). The reflection coefficients reported in ref. 16 actually exceed the predictions in Fig. 4.

The above model clearly has its limitations, because it implies virtual impermeability to particulate matter even though it is known that such matter can in fact slowly escape into the subsynovial lymphatics. The failure for very large particles could be due to the assumption of rigidity in the modeled rods. However, it seems unlikely that synovial matrix reflection coefficients to macromolecules will be zero, so how would this affect the intra-articular concentration of macromolecules?

THE "RACE" BETWEEN MACROMOLECULAR DIFFUSION AND REFLECTION

The reflection coefficient is a measure of the *greatest* separation of solute from solvent that a membrane can potentially achieve, but this is only achieved at high fluid velocities (15). This is because solute diffusion is continuously dissipating the concentration gradient set up by the process of reflection or "molecular sieving." At high flows, water velocity is high relative to solute velocity, and thus the downstream solution is dilute (Fig. 5). At low water velocities, however, the solute can more nearly "keep up" with the water, aided by diffusion, and the concentration gradient dissipates to some extent. In the limit of zero flow, downstream and upstream fluids equilibrate whenever σ is less than 1. Thus in a partially reflecting membrane, the transport of solute is a "race" between solute reflection, which tends to generate a concentration difference, and solute diffusion,

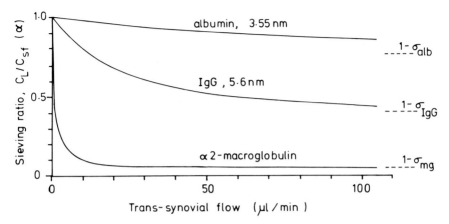

FIG. 5. Theoretical effect of steady trans-synovial absorption rate (Q) on macromolecular sieving [i.e., concentration in subsynovial lymph (C_L) relative to that in available space within synovial fluid (C_{SF})], for rabbit knee. σ is reflection coefficient. $C_L/C_{SF} = (1 - \sigma)/\{1 - \sigma[\exp(-\text{Pec})]\}$, where Pec $= Q(1 - \sigma)/PS$ (15). PS is diffusional permeability–surface-area product for interstitial path across whole synovial surface, calculated to be 128 μl/min (albumin), 53 μl/min (immunoglobulin G), 16.7 μl/min (α_2-macroglobulin). Mean turnover rate is approximately 0.5 μl/min in normal joint; flows at raised IAP are shown in Fig. 3.

which tends to dissipate it. As a result, the "sieving ratio" (filtrate concentration/ filtrand concentration; α in Eq. 3) varies between the limits $1 - \sigma$ (high fluid velocities) and 1 (very low fluid velocities), as shown in Fig. 5. Thus the concentration of a macromolecule in synovial fluid should be affected by fluid turnover rate for an additional reason besides that given in Eq. 1.

The mean trans-synovial flows in normal joints are very low (<1 μl/min in rabbit knees) in relation to diffusional capacity, so solutes of markedly different reflection coefficient (such as albumin and immunoglobulin G) may both have sieving ratios close to unity normally (see Fig. 5). For very large macromolecules at raised fluid velocities, however, sieving ratios may be less than 1, in keeping with the hyaluronan results in Fig. 3.

EXPERIMENTAL EVIDENCE CONCERNING MACROMOLECULAR SIEVING BY SYNOVIUM

Published data on the relative permeation rates of different macromolecules across synovium are very limited (Table 1), and most studies were conducted several decades ago, when the potential importance of trans-synovial fluid velocity was not fully recognized.

Several laboratories have reported that the half-life of radiolabeled albumin in joints is not significantly different from that of larger globulins (19–21). Two of these studies involved swollen, inflamed joints (human rheumatoid knees) (19,20), for which no estimates of SIM density exist. The paradoxical observations

TABLE 1. *Comparative studies of rates of macromolecular removal from joint cavity*

Species	Normal/ Synovitis[a]	Method	Intra-articular volume × normal[b]	Macromolecule[c]	Result[d]	Reference
Dog	Normal	Lymph analysis	6×; passive	Albumin Globulin	LMS	22
Human	RA	Half-life	40–250×	Albumin IgM	ND	19
Human	RA, OA	Half-life	Raised	Albumin IgG	ND	20
Human	Normal	Half-life	8×; bed rest	Albumin IgG	ND	21
Rabbit	Normal	Half-life	40×; mobile 4 hr	Albumin IgG	ND	21
Rabbit	Normal	Half-life	8×	Albumin Proteoglycan	LMS	23
Rabbit	Normal	Synovial resistance	~20×; immobile	Hyaluronan	LMS	5

[a] RA, rheumatoid knee; OA, osteoarthritic knee.
[b] Distension of synovial cavity given as multiple of normal volume. Comments in this column refer to passive motion, active mobility, etc.
[c] IgM, immunoglobulin M; IgG, immunoglobulin G.
[d] LMS, larger molecule slowed. ND, no difference between large and small macromolecular egress rates.

that the removal of heat-aggregated albumin was accelerated, as was that of macroalbumin particles of diameter 10–90 μm in one patient after 24 hr (20), raise the possibility of active degradation by synovial macrophages in rheumatoid arthritis. The third study involved normal rabbit knees injected with 1 ml of fluid (~40 times the normal synovial fluid volume); in these conscious animals, intermittent active flexion may have generated very high intra-articular pressures intermittently.

By contrast, three other studies have provided evidence for macromolecular selectivity in noninflamed synovium. In a classic direct attack on the problem, Bauer et al. (22) found that serum albumin escaped into thoracic duct lymph from normal dog knees (distended to 3–6 times normal) much faster than did a globulin fraction, during passive joint cycling or leg massage. However, the validity of their globulin immunoassay method has been questioned. More recently (23), a radiolabeled proteoglycan subunit of $M_r \sim 2.5 \times 10^6$ daltons was found to have a half-life of 12.4 hr in the rabbit knee, in contrast to 3.9 hr for albumin. In a study at defined trans-synovial flows, the effect of hyaluronan on fluid escape from noninflamed rabbit knees at raised fluid velocities indicated that the escape of hyaluronan of $M_r \sim 8 \times 10^5$ was severely slowed, relative to water, by normal rabbit synovium (4). Existing studies are thus in conflict regarding the ability of synovial interstitium to discriminate between various macromolecules, and further investigations are needed over a range of trans-synovial fluid velocities and a range of molecular sizes, shapes, and charges.

CONCLUSIONS

Although the basic principles underlying transport through matrices such as synovial interstitium are known, experimental studies in joints lag far behind and have not in general been formulated with these transport principles in mind. Important areas highlighted here are (a) the need to consider the dual effects of trans-synovial volume flow when assessing the concentration or half-life of a macromolecule in synovial fluid, (b) the need for studies of macromolecular sieving with attention to concomitant trans-synovial fluid velocities, and (c) the need for quantitative biochemical information about synovial interstitial composition analogous to that which has long been available for articular cartilage.

REFERENCES

1. Levick JR. The "clearance" of macromolecular substances such as cartilage markers from synovial fluid and serum. In: Maroudas A, Kuettner K, eds. *Methods in cartilage research.* London: Academic Press, 1990;352–357.
2. Levick JR, McDonald JN. Ultrastructure of transport pathways in stressed synovium of the knee in anaesthetized rabbits. *J Physiol* 1989;419:493–508.
3. Knight AD, Levick JR, McDonald JN. Relation between trans-synovial flow and plasma colloid osmotic pressure, with an estimation of the albumin reflection coefficient in the rabbit knee. *Q J Exp Physiol* 1988;73:47–66.
4. Levick JR. Synovial fluid and trans-synovial flow in stationary and moving joints. In: Helminen H, Kiviranta I, Tammi M, et al., eds. *Joint loading: biology and health of articular structures.* Bristol: Wright & Sons, 1987;149–186.
5. Levick JR, McDonald JN. Influence of intra-articular hyaluronan on flow across the synovial lining of knees in anaesthetized rabbits. *J Physiol* 1990;422:23P.
6. Wallis WJ, Simkin PA, Nelp WB. Protein traffic in human synovial effusions. *Arthritis Rheum* 1987;30:57–63.
7. Knox P, Levick JR, McDonald JN. Synovial fluid—its mass, macromolecular content and pressure in major limb joints of the rabbit. *Q J Exp Physiol* 1988;73:33–46.
8. Brown TJ, Laurent UBG, Fraser JRE. Turnover of hyaluronan in synovial joints: elimination of labelled hyaluronan from the knee joint of the rabbit. *Exp Physiol* 1991;76:125–134.
9. Ogsten AG. The spaces in a uniformly random suspension of fibres. *Trans Faraday Soc* 1958;54:1754–1757.
10. Laurent TC. The interaction between polysaccharides and other macromolecules. *Biochem J* 1964;93:106–112.
11. Levick JR. The permeability of rheumatoid and normal human synovium to specific plasma proteins. *Arthritis Rheum* 1981;24:1550–1560.
12. Ogston AG. On the interaction of solute molecules with porous networks. *J Phys Chem* 1970;74:668–669.
13. Jansons KM, Phillips CG. On the application of geometric probability theory to polymer networks and suspensions. *J Coll & Interface Sci* 1990;137:75–91.
14. Levick JR. Flow through interstitium and other fibrous matrices. *Q J Exp Physiol* 1987;72:409–438.
15. Curry FE. Mechanics and thermodynamics of transcapillary exchange. In: Renkin EM, Michel CC, eds. *Handbook of physiology, section 2: The cardiovascular system, vol IV—The microcirculation.* Bethesda: American Physiological Society, 1984;309–374.
16. Granger HJ, Taylor AE. Permeability of connective tissue linings isolated from implanted capsules. *Circ Res* 1975;36:222–228.

17. Eyre DR, Muir H. Type III collagen: a major constituent of rheumatoid and normal human synovial membrane. *Connect Tissue Res* 1975;4:11–16.
18. Maroudas A. Biophysical chemistry of cartilaginous tissues with special reference to solute and fluid transport. *Biorheology* 1975;12:233–248.
19. Brown DL, Cooper AG, Bluestone R. Exchange of IgM and albumin between plasma and synovial fluid in rheumatoid arthritis. *Ann Rheum Dis* 1969;20:644–651.
20. Sliwinski AJ, Zvaifler NJ. The removal of aggregated and nonaggregated autologous gamma globulin from rheumatoid joints. *Arthritis Rheum* 1969;12:504–514.
21. Rodnan GP, MacLachlan MJ. The absorption of serum albumin and gamma globulin from the knee joint of man and rabbit. *Arthritis Rheum* 1960;3:152–157.
22. Bauer W, Short CL, Bennett GA. The manner of removal of proteins from normal joints. *J Exp Med* 1933;57:419–432.
23. Page-Thomas DP, Bard D, King B, Dingle JT. Clearance of proteoglycan from joint cavities. *Ann Rheum Dis* 1987;46:934–937.

DISCUSSION

Campion: Your talk was somewhat disheartening for those of us who are used to getting up at meetings and presenting synovial fluid data. Do you have any ideas on how to make these measurements in patients without doing complicated turnover measurements?

Levick: I suppose the short answer is that you cannot have something for nothing! What is needed is not necessarily all that difficult. First, measure the hyaluronate concentration in the synovial fluid sample. You can then correct for the available volume space, which is small for big molecules. The second requirement is an estimate of fluid turnover using the method of Peter Simkin. Radiolabeled albumin is injected into the joint, and its clearance is followed for a few hours. Because albumin is removed via the lymph, this is an estimate of lymph flow and, thus, of fluid volume turnover.

van de Putte: You focused greatly on lymph as the efflux route from the joint. Are there other routes?

Levick: There are two others. One is by diffusion through the capillary wall into the bloodstream. That is where molecules much smaller than albumin go. The other route is local degradation by macrophages. There is no quantitative information about this, but Zvaifler and Sliwinsky looked at albumin clearance from the joint cavity and made a very strange observation. Heat-aggregated albumin particles, microns in size, were removed anomalously fast compared with undenatured albumin. One way to explain this is that the particles were being ingested and digested by macrophages.

Heinegard: One way to correct for the exclusion effects of hyaluronate and also for differences in volume flow is to use ratios between different marker molecules. The problem of permeability remains. In collaboration with Lindahl and Lindholm, we studied half-lives of a large proteoglycan fragment and a small proteoglycan fragment in horse joints. Other experiments used hyaluronate at several concentrations. In all experiments we obtained half-lives close to 10 hr whether the molecules were large or small or of high or low concentration. My impression, based on analyses of large numbers of synovial fluids, is that even if the effects you discuss are marked, their sum is rather constant.

Levick: Well that is very interesting.

Brune: You suggested that high concentrations of hyaluronate in the joint cavity can affect efflux of other molecules. Does that mean if physicians inject large quantities of hyaluronate into joints, this will interfere effectively with the traffic of other molecules in and out of the joint?

Levick: If my interpretation is right and if the accumulation of hyaluronate is sufficient to increase resistance to water movement, I would speculate that this might retard, but not prevent, the egress of other macromolecules.

Maroudas: When a labeling precursor is injected into a joint for metabolic experiments, the level of radioactivity that the chondrocytes see is dependent on the residence time of the tracer in the synovial fluid, which, in turn, is dependent on the factors you have been discussing. This may vary from one animal to the next and from one injected joint to another. Can you tell us how movement and exercise affect transport out of the joint cavity, because many people compare cartilage from mobile and immobile joints?

Levick: Well, moving a joint will generally cause the fluid to have a faster turnover, because it activates the lymphatic pump. Therefore I would imagine that movement would reduce the amount of time that a given molecule would spend in the joint cavity.

Dreher: Intra-articular pressures in rheumatoid patients with large effusions can be up to 400 cm water. Oxygen levels decreased, and we think that capillaries and lymphatics simply collapse under such high pressures. How does your absorption pressure hypothesis work with such high pressures?

Levick: Can I ask you? These extremely high pressures, I presume, were transient effects of flexing the joint. Am I right?

Dreher: You are right. When we moved the joints, pressure levels could increase 400 cm of water and more. If a leg is simply resting without being forced, pressures are around 100 cm water.

Levick: If the pressures are above 120 mm of mercury only transiently, I don't think there will be any great problem. Transient high pressures would promote a transient drainage of fluid out of the joint cavity, albeit at the expense of temporary hypoxia. As long as the high pressures are less than arterial pressure, which logically they have to be, they can be sustained. You could not sustain a pressure above a 120 mm of mercury without necrosis of the synovial layer, because there would be no blood flow.

Articular Cartilage and Osteoarthritis,
edited by K. Kuettner et al.
Raven Press, Ltd., New York © 1992.

38

Effect of Inflammation on Cartilage Metabolism

Dennis A. Lowther,* Absorn Sriratana,* and Mark S. Baker†

*Department of Biochemistry, Monash University, Clayton, 3168, Victoria, Australia;
and †Division of Clinical Sciences, John Curtin School of Medical Research,
Australian National University, Canberra, Australia*

In general, an inflammatory response is a natural physiological reaction for protection against a hostile environment and is focused on both the removal of the agent(s) producing the inflammation and the restoration of tissue damage. If the agent provoking the inflammation either cannot be removed or continuously returns, as, for example, in a rheumatoid joint, the resulting chronic inflammation leads to joint tissue damage. Several factors arising from cells involved in an inflammatory response are thought to contribute to joint tissue damage: lysosomal enzymes (1–3), toxic oxygen metabolites (4–6), prostaglandins (7), and cytokines (8). Lysosomal enzymes and toxic oxygen metabolites shed by inflammatory cells, such as polymorphonuclear (PMN) cells and macrophages, have been implicated in tissue damage during chronic arthritis (9). In recent years, *in vivo* models involving the production of a monoarticular acute inflammation in rabbit knee joints have been developed to examine the effect of PMN cells on the metabolism of articular cartilage (10,11).

PMN leukocytes are found in the inflammatory exudates in joint diseases (12–14) and in acute experimental arthritis where their appearance is accompanied by up to 40% loss of articular cartilage proteoglycan (10,15). PMN leukocyte proteinases have been suggested to play a central role in the degeneration of articular cartilage during inflammation of the joint (17–19). PMN elastase can degrade the core proteins of cartilage proteoglycans into fragments containing between one and five chondroitin sulfate chains and leaves the hyaluronate (HA) binding region bound to HA, thereby producing a chondroitin sulfate-free fragment (20). The proteoglycan fragments produced are too small to be entrapped by the collagen meshwork, and they diffuse out resulting in proteoglycan depletion. PMN elastase has been demonstrated in rheumatoid cartilage (21) and at the site of cartilage erosion (22), and it can be extracted from articular cartilage in experimental arthritis (16). A marked inhibition of proteoglycan synthesis also accompanies the appearance of PMN cells in inflamed joints (11,23–25). PMN cells readily produce super oxide and hydrogen peroxide (26,27), and there is some evidence that the oxidation of thiol groups detected in synovial fluid from inflamed joints could be generated by reactive oxygen intermediates (26,27). It has been shown that the hydrogen peroxide generated from oxygen by free radical generating enzyme systems causes inhibition of cartilage proteoglycan biosynthesis (28–30).

AIMS

The aim of this chapter is to describe mechanisms whereby the proteolytic enzyme elastase and the oxygen metabolite hydrogen peroxide, both of which can be produced by rabbit PMN cells, have a marked effect on articular cartilage *in vitro* and during inflammation *in vivo*.

MATERIALS

Radioisotopic [^{35}S] sulfate was obtained from Amersham International, Bucks, U.K. Glyceraldehyde-3-phosphate and glyceraldehyde-3-phosphate dehydrogenase from Boehringer, Mannheim. Dulbeco's modified Eagle's Medium (DMEM), fetal calf serum, and nonessential amino acids were from the Commonwealth Serum Laboratories, Melbourne, Australia. Adenosine triphosphate (ATP), 3-phosphoglyceric kinase, and firefly lantern extract (luciferase) came from Sigma Chemical Co., St. Louis, Missouri. The elastase inhibitor, nacetyl ala. ala. pro. val. chloromethyl ketone, was a gift from Dr. G. Powers, Georgia Institute of Technology, Atlanta, Georgia. Arteparon was a gift from Dr. P. Ghosh, Raymond Purves Laboratory, Royal North Shore Hospital, Sydney, Australia.

METHODS

1. *Production of an inflammatory response in rabbit joints.* Mature New Zealand white rabbits were injected with 3 mg of intraarticular lambda carrageenan dissolved in saline, and the articular cartilage was removed at varying times for the estimation of the proteoglycan, proteolytic enzyme content, and the rate of proteoglycan synthesis (10,16,23).

2. *Preparation of rabbit PMN cells and co-culture with rabbit or bovine cartilage.* Adult laboratory rabbits were injected intraperitoneally with 150 ml of 0.1% w/v glycogen dissolved in 0.15 M NaCl. After 18 hr, the rabbits were anesthetized and the peritoneal exudate was diluted with saline and collected by gravity drainage. The cell suspension was purified by centrifugation and lysis of

contaminating erythrocytes. A differential smear count gave an average viability of 97% and showed that PMN cells accounted for at least 94% of the total present. Normally each rabbit would yield approximately 5×10^8 cells per lavage.

Co-culture of rabbit PMN cells and slices of bovine or rabbit cartilage. Steer ankle joints or rabbit knee joints were opened under aseptic conditions and the cartilage was dissected off and placed in Dulbecco's modified Eagle's Medium. The tissue was diced into 0.5 mm slices and 50 to 100 mg wet wt was incubated with approximately 1×10^8 rabbit peritoneal PMN cells at 37° for 1 to 2 hr in air and with gentle shaking. The co-culture was stopped by chilling to 4° and aspirating off the PMN suspension and the cartilage was washed 2 to 3 times. Any PMN cells adhering to the cartilage surface were removed by brief sonication and again washed in Dulbecco's modified Eagle's Medium (41).

3. *Measurement of cartilage metabolism.* Proteoglycan content was estimated by papain digestions of cartilage and separation of the glycosaminoglycan (GAG) fraction on Sephadex G.25, and the proteoglycan content was calculated from determination of the hexuronate content (2,31). Proteoglycan synthesis was measured by the *in vitro* incorporation of [^{35}S] sulfate into cartilage explants as described previously (32). Proteolytic enzymes were extracted from inflamed and noninflamed cartilage with 4M guanidinium hydrochloride at 4°, and after dialysis were assayed by incubation with polyacrylamide discs containing ^{35}S-labeled proteoglycan as substrate. One unit of proteolytic activity is defined as that amount that results in the release of 1 μg of proteoglycan/min under the condition of assay (16).

The rate of degradation of proteoglycan was determined by incubating ^{35}S-labeled cartilage in Dulbecco's modified Eagle's Medium at 37° for varying periods of time. The ^{35}S fragments released into the medium were assayed, and the remaining intracellular cartilage proteoglycan in the tissue was extracted overnight with 0.1 N NaOH. ^{35}S-labeled cartilage was obtained following the intravenous injections at 0 and 24 hr of 0.75 mCi of [^{35}S] sulfate into rabbits. After an additional 24 hr, the rabbits received intraarticular injections of lambda carrageenan to induce inflammations, and the cartilage from the inflamed and normal joints was removed aseptically and incubated in Dulbecco's modified Eagle's Medium to determine proteoglycan degradation (41).

4. *Incubation of cartilage with a superoxide generating system or H_2O_2.* Eighty to 100 mg wet wt of cartilage slices were incubated for 120 min at 37° with 10 to 60 mU of xanthine oxidase and 2 mM hypoxanthine in 2 ml of Hanks' balanced salt medium supplemented with 5.8 mM glucose or with 0 to 10^{-4} M H_2O_2 (5,28). After incubation, the slices were washed three times in buffer and either incubated with [^{35}S]sulfate to measure proteoglycan biosynthesis or assayed for intracellular ATP and glyceraldehyde-3-phosphodehydrogenase (G-3-PDH) enzyme activity.

ATP. Cartilage ATP content was measured using the luciferin/luciferase system (35).

G-3-PDH. Activity in cartilage was extracted in 10 mM Tris/HCl pH 7.5, 1 mM ethylenediamine tetraacetic acid (EDTA), and 0.5% Nonidet P40 and measured by the consumption of NADH in the presence of substrate (35).

MEASUREMENT OF HYDROGEN PEROXIDE

Hydrogen peroxide was measured fluorimetrically in synovial fluid (34) or by titration with potassium permanganate.

RESULTS

Composition and Biosynthetic Activity of Rabbit Articular Cartilage at Various Times Following the Onset of Intraarticular Inflammation

The rates of proteoglycan synthesis and the proteoglycan contents of cartilage prepared from inflamed rabbit joints decreased markedly compared with the control joint from the same animal during the first 5 days (Fig. 1). Within 24 hr of inducing the inflammatory response, the rate of biosynthesis decreased by 30%, decreasing further to 60 to 70% of the control value by 5 days. Similarly, the proteoglycan content of the inflamed cartilage decreased by 15 to 20% at 24 hr and by approximately 40% by 7 days compared to the control. The proteoglycan contents of the articular cartilage eventually returned to normal. Proteoglycan synthesis in the inflamed joint recovered to a value comparable to the control joint by approximately 17 days, and then continued to increase to above normal for an additional 30 days, thus assisting the gradual restoration of the proteoglycan content of the tissue (Fig. 1). The rapid loss of proteoglycan from articular cartilage from the inflamed joint (Fig. 1) could be due to the rapid transient rise in the proteolytic enzyme activity shown in extracts from the inflamed cartilage between days 1 and 4 (Fig. 1). Evidence in Fig. 2 shows that an increased rate of degradation of proteoglycan also occurs when articular cartilage from inflamed joints is incubated *in vitro,* consistent with its being due at least in part to the increased proteolytic enzyme content (Fig. 1). No such changes occur in the noninflamed cartilage, and perhaps most significantly, the extracted proteolytic activity proved to be largely a serine proteinase not present in normal rabbit cartilage (16). Further evidence that serine proteinase in inflamed cartilage plays a role in the increased rate of degradation of proteoglycan is shown in Fig. 2.

The Effect of Inhibitors of Serine Protease on the Degradation of Proteoglycan in Cartilage Explants

The rate of loss of fragments of ^{35}S-labeled proteoglycan from cartilage explants into the medium was used as a measure of the enzymic degradation within the

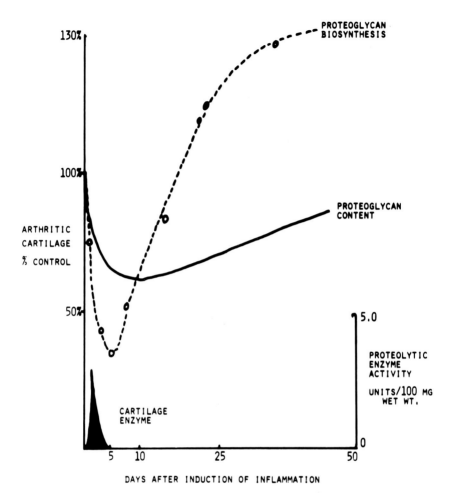

FIG. 1. Effect of a single intraarticular injection of carrageenan on the proteoglycan content and rate of proteoglycan biosynthesis in articular cartilage. Each point represents an average from three animals. The results are expressed either as the hexuronate content or rate of incorporation of $^{35}SO_4$ into GAG fraction from the inflamed joint as a percent of that in the control joint from the same animal. Proteolytic activity extracted with 4M GUCl is expressed as units/100 mg wet wt of cartilage. No proteolytic activity was found in extracts from control (noninflamed) joints. Proteoglycan biosynthesis (------); proteoglycan content (———).

tissue. As shown in Fig. 2B, arthritic cartilage shows considerably increased degradative activity, as indicated by the enhanced release of radioactive fragments of proteoglycan compared with that from a normal or control joint. Similarly, normal rabbit cartilage previously co-cultured for 1 hr with rabbit PMN cells and then sonicated and washed to remove adhering PMN cells also shows a significant increase in the rate of proteoglycan degradation compared with control cartilage not previously exposed to PMN cells (Fig. 2A).

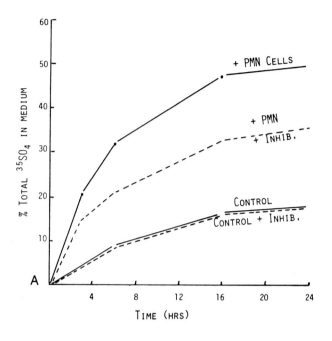

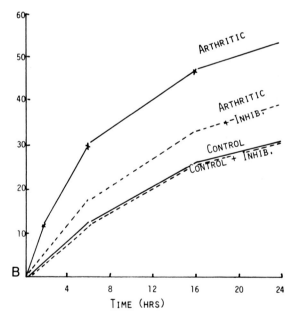

Thus, in both cases there is evidence for increased proteolytic activity which is significantly reduced if the specific elastase inhibitor AAAPVCK or a general serine proteinase inhibitor such as Arteparon is included in the culture. Neither inhibitor has any effect on the rate of degradation in normal articular cartilage, suggesting that the normal level of turnover of proteoglycan does not involve significant serine proteinase activity (Figs. 2A,B).

Evidence that Contact Between Rabbit PMN Cells and Cartilage is Essential for the Rapid Transport of Proteolytic Activity into the Articular Surface

Suspensions of rabbit peritoneal PMN cells were incubated in Hanks' balanced salt solution at 37° for 1 hr in the presence of slices of normal rabbit articular cartilage (8×10^7 PMN cells/100 mg wet wt cartilage). The PMN cells were removed by washing and the cartilage was briefly sonicated to disrupt adhering PMN cells, and was again washed thoroughly before the extraction of proteolytic enzyme with 4M guanidinium chloride as described in "Methods." It was assumed that the extracted enzyme was present within the cartilage matrix.

In a parallel experiment, the PMN cell population was incubated for 1 hr without the addition of cartilage slices. The PMN cells were removed by centrifugation and then cartilage slices were added to the supernatant and incubated for another hour at 37°C. After washing, the cartilage slices were again extracted with 4 M guanidinium chloride and the extracts were assayed for proteolytic activity. This was a measure of the ability of enzyme from PMN cells to penetrate cartilage in the absence of contact between PMN cells and cartilage. Finally, the experiment was repeated in the presence of synovial fluid which contains sufficient α-1-antiprotease to significantly inhibit the activity of any free secreted PMN elastase.

The results are shown diagrammatically in Fig. 3. Although the PMN suspension released 2.4 units of elastase activity into the medium, only 0.6 unit could be extracted from cartilage that was subsequently incubated in the cell-free medium. This was almost totally abolished if synovial fluid inhibitors were added with the cartilage. However, when the PMN suspension was co-cultured

←————————————————————————————————

FIG. 2. Serine proteinase activity and cartilage proteoglycan degradation (**A**) in cartilage from an inflamed joint and (**B**) induced by co-culture with PMN cells. **A:** 50 mg wet wt of ^{35}S-labeled cartilage were incubated in DMEM containing 10% serum and the rate of degradation of proteoglycan was measured by radioactivity appearing in the incubation medium. Arthritic cartilage from carrageenan-inflamed joint 24 hr after induction (■——■); cartilage from a saline noninflamed joint of the same animal (○——○); plus inhibitors 0.1 mM Nac AAAPVCK or 800 μg/ml Arteparon (○ ------ ○). **B:** 50–100 mg wet wt ^{35}S-labeled cartilage incubated for 2 hr with 2×10^7 PMN cells, cells were removed and tissue was sonicated and washed and then incubated in 2 ml DMEM for 0–24 hr at 37°, and the rate of ^{35}S-proteoglycan degradation was measured by release of radioactivity. Cartilage plus PMN cells (×——×); cartilage control (no PMN cells) (——); cartilage plus inhibitors 0.1 mM Nac AAAPVCK or 800 μg/ml Arteparon (------).

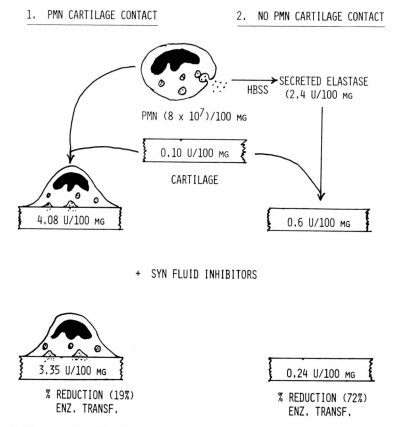

FIG. 3. The need for cell/cartilage contact to promote proteolytic enzyme transfer from PMN cells into cartilage matrix. Two ml suspensions of rabbit peritoneal PMN cells containing 8×10^7 cells were incubated in Hanks' balanced salt solution medium for 1 hr at 37° (incubation a) or in the presence of 100 mg wet wt of cartilage slices (incubation b). After incubation the PMN cells in (a) were removed by centrifugation before adding 100 mg of cartilage slices and incubating for a further 1 hr at 37° (incubation c). PMN cells were removed from (a) and (c) after chilling, slices were washed sonicated, and the proteolytic enzymes were extracted.

with slices of articular cartilage, the total amount of enzyme subsequently appearing in the cartilage was almost twice that secreted in the absence of cartilage; this suggests that cartilage can stimulate the release of PMN proteolytic enzyme. Moreover, the amount of enzyme transferred when PMN cells were in contact with cartilage was only slightly reduced in the presence of synovial fluid inhibitors. This suggests that the transfer mechanism involves the exclusion of soluble synovial inhibitors. This could occur if the enzyme transfer took place across the PMN/cartilage interface, and morphological evidence confirmed marked PMN adhesion to the cartilage surface. A similar mechanism of transfer has been suggested by Schalkwijk et al. 1986 (3).

The Effect of Oxygen Free Radical Scavengers on the Inhibitions of Proteoglycan Synthesis

Early studies showed the presence of a predominant PMN cell population in synovial fluid during the early phase of carrageenan-induced inflammation in rabbit joints (38). Such cells are known to generate superoxide and other free radicals (26). Thus, in order to examine whether oxygen free radicals or their derivatives might be responsible for the severe inhibition of articular cartilage proteoglycan biosynthesis in such joints, slices of normal articular cartilage, or suspensions of chondrocytes prepared from bovine cartilage, were exposed to a system generating as much superoxide as would be produced by a suspension of 10^8 PMN cells. This is the approximate cell population present in an inflamed rabbit joint after 24 hr (38).

By including scavengers for various free radical derivatives, it could be determined whether superoxide or a species derived from superoxide could be responsible for inhibition of proteoglycan synthesis. The results in Table 1 show that in the absence of scavengers, proteoglycan synthesis in cartilage slices is significantly inhibited. Suspensions of cartilage cells were much more sensitive as indicated by the much lower level of xanthine oxidase required to produce significant inhibition. This presumably reflects the scavenging effect of matrix components in cartilage slices, thereby requiring increased amounts of superoxide to produce an effect on chondrocyte biosynthesis. However, in both cases the only scavenger which significantly reduced the inhibition of proteoglycan synthesis was catalase. This indicates that the most effective species was the hydrogen peroxide derived from superoxide. The lack of effect of either superoxide dismutase or mannitol and detapac, an Fe^{2+} chelating agent, argues against either

TABLE 1. *Effect of oxygen free radical scavengers on the inhibition of proteoglycan synthesis by hypoxanthine/xanthine oxidase system*

| | % Inhibition proteoglycan synthesis | |
| | Cartilage slices (62.5 mU XO) | Chondrocyte suspensions (7.5 mU XO) |
Additions		
None	29%	79%
Superoxide dismutase	34%	66%
Catalase	8.5%	0%
Mannitol	34.4%	—
Detapac	—	78%

Superoxide dismutase and catalase were each used at 250 units/incubation.
Fifty to 100 mg wet wt of cartilage slices or 10^9 chondrocyte cells in 2 ml medium were incubated with 60 m units or 7.5 m units of purified xanthine oxidase, respectively, and 0.2 mM hypoxanthine for 2 hr at 37° in Hanks' balanced salt solution. Incubation was performed either in the absence or presence of free radical scavengers. After incubation and washing 3× in buffer proteoglycan, biosynthetic capacity of the scavenger-treated cartilage or chondrocyte suspension was estimated and expressed as a percentage of that produced in the absence of scavengers. Each incubation was repeated 3× and the results were expressed as a mean of those values.

superoxide itself or a derived hydroxyl radical as the critical species. Neither the xanthine oxidase nor its substrate hypoxanthine, when added in isolation, had any effect on proteoglycan synthesis (28).

Generation of Hydrogen Peroxide by PMN Cells from an Inflamed Joint

Inflammation was induced in rat joints by the injection of intraarticular carrageenan and at various times groups of 3 to 4 rats were killed. The hydrogen peroxide enzyme assay system was then injected intraarticularly and the synovial fluid and cells were washed from the joint and assayed for the production of hydrogen peroxide. The results shown in Fig. 4 indicate that provided catalase activity was blocked with sodium azide, measurable formation of hydrogen peroxide occurred. The amounts formed increased in parallel with increasing PMN cell population from the initiation of the inflammatory response (not shown).

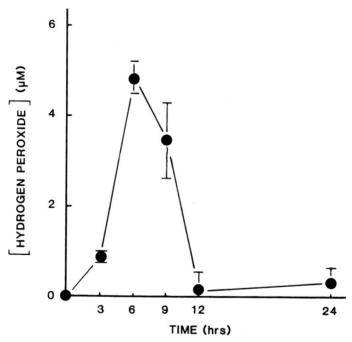

FIG. 4. Generation of H_2O_2 by synovial PMN cells from inflamed joints. Sprague-Dawley rats (250–500 gram) were given intraarticular injections of 50 μl of 3% λ carrageenan in physiological saline to induce a peak inflammatory response of synovial cells in 6–9 h. At various time points groups of three animals received intraarticular injection of the enzyme assay system used for the detection of hydrogen peroxide and the diluted synovial fluid was collected, cells were removed by centrifugation, and hydrogen peroxide was estimated in the total joint fluid. The results are plotted as μMol of H_2O_2/rat joint at the various time points postinduction of the carrageenan inflammatory response.

The maximum amount of hydrogen peroxide produced by the joint inflammatory cell population was 5 μM/rat joint (Fig. 4). This would indicate a concentration of H_2O_2 in the synovial fluid approaching the 10^{-4} M required to produce significant inhibition of proteoglycan biosynthesis (29).

Effect of H_2O_2 on Intrachondrocyte ATP Levels

When cartilage slices were exposed for 2 hr at 37°C to increasing concentrations of H_2O_2 ($0-10^3$ M H_2O_2), the intracellular levels of ATP decreased in a dose-dependent manner (Fig. 5). For example, control tissue was found to contain 9.0 ± 2.1 p mol ATP/mg tissue wet wt. After exposure to 10^{-4} M H_2O_2 for 2 hr, the ATP concentration fell to 5.2 ± 0.7 p mol ATP/mg tissue wet wt, a decrease of 42%. When explants from this same experiment were assessed for the level of proteoglycan synthesis by incorporation of [^{35}S] sulfate into proteoglycans (Fig. 5), the level of synthesis reflected the intrachondrocyte ATP concentrations. After exposure to 10^{-4} M H_2O_2, both intracellular ATP levels and

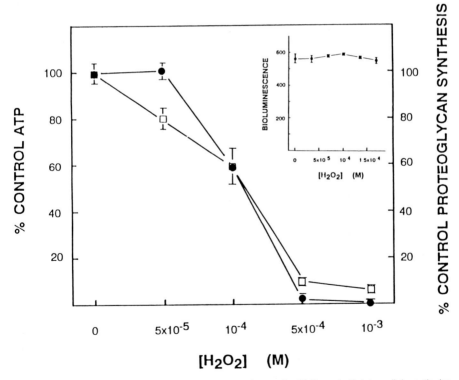

FIG. 5. The effect of exposing cartilage explants to increasing H_2O_2 on both intracellular articular cartilage ATP content (●) and proteoglycan synthesis (□) in cartilage explants and (*inset*) the inability of similar H_2O_2 to hydrolyze 300 μM ATP.

the rate of proteoglycan synthesis were decreased by 42% over the entire dose-response range $(0-10^3 \text{ M H}_2\text{O}_2)$; the greatest discrepancy between proteoglycan synthesis and ATP levels was 18% M. The depression of ATP levels by 10^{-4} M H_2O_2 was almost complete within 5 min of exposure (34), indicating that the lesion responsible for ATP depression occurred almost immediately. To determine if H_2O_2 hydrolyzed ATP directly, commercial ATP at levels similar to those found in cell extracts was exposed to H_2O_2 from 0 to 10^{-4} M for 2 hr at $37°$ (Fig. 5). There was no change in the observed bioluminescence, indicating that ATP is not directly hydrolyzed by H_2O_2. This result suggests that exposure of chondrocytes to H_2O_2 either inhibits ATP synthetic pathways or activates ATP consuming processes.

The Effect of H_2O_2 on G-3-PDH Activity

Articular cartilage depends largely on glycolysis for its ATP biosynthetic capacity (40). In addition, because G-3-PDH, a key enzyme in glycolysis, has been suggested to contain a critical, easily oxidizable-SH group (CYS 149) near the active center of the protein, the intrachondrocyte activity of this enzyme was measured as a function of exposure to H_2O_2. When cartilage was exposed to increasing concentrations of H_2O_2 $(0-10^{-3}$ M) (Fig. 6) and extracted without the addition of reducing agents, residual G-3-PDH activity was found to decrease immediately (<2 min) (data not shown) in a dose-dependent manner. Evidence has now been obtained that in either H_2O_2 treated cartilage or in cartilage from inflamed joints, the thiol groups of this enzyme are not available to react with $[^3\text{H}]$-IAA (34,36). These results suggest that decreased intracellular ATP levels in chondrocytes exposed to H_2O_2 both *in vitro* and *in vivo* may be due to inhibition of G-3-PDH activity.

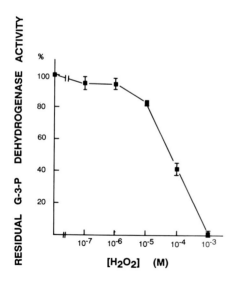

FIG. 6. The effect of increasing H_2O_2 for 2 hr at $37°$ on % residual cartilage G-3-PDH activity.

CONCLUDING REMARKS

The possible importance in arthritic disease of cartilage damage by PMN cells and their serine proteolytic enzymes have been emphasized by several reviewers (4,17). Immunological evidence for the presence of PMN elastase in human arthritic cartilage (22) has been complemented by the present and earlier studies (16). Within 4 days of inducing an inflammatory response with carrageenan, a serine proteinase appears in the articular cartilage which is absent from normal articular cartilage obtained from the same animal. The increased proteolytic activity in cartilage from the inflamed joint was only partly inhibited by specific serine proteinase inhibitors even though the enzyme extracted from such tissues with 4 M guanidinium chloride was completely inhibited. This would suggest that either some of the tissue serine proteinase is not accessible to the inhibitors, or that cartilage in response to inflammation and/or the presence of PMN cells may generate nonserine proteolytic enzymes such as mettallo proteinases. These have been demonstrated by exposure of cartilage to interleukin-1 (IL-1) (37). Proteoglycan degradation in noninflamed cartilage was not decreased in the presence of inhibitors of serine proteinases, which is consistent with current views that serine proteinases do not play a major role in normal cartilage proteoglycan degradation.

It seems likely that the rapid rate of proteoglycan degradation in the early phase of carrageenan-induced inflammation is due at least in part to the serine proteinase, elastase, secreted by invading PMN cells (16,21). The remainder would undoubtedly be due to cartilage metallo enzymes induced by IL-1 present in inflammatory exudates. The transient appearance of a serine proteolytic enzyme in cartilage from the inflamed joint parallels the rapid changes in the synovial cell population (38), indicating that PMN elastase transferred into cartilage is rapidly inactivated, either by chondrocyte endocytosis (38) or by specific serine proteinase inhibitor peptides. The need for PMN cells to be in contact with the cartilage surface for the efficient transfer of secreted elastase into the cartilage matrix has also been shown by Schalkwijk et al. (31). It seems likely that this mode of transfer protects secreted elastase from inactivation by proteinase inhibitors present in synovial fluid.

The inhibition of proteoglycan synthesis in cartilage exposed to oxygen free radicals (28) and hydrogen peroxide (5,33) has been well established. The question is whether the inhibition observed in cartilage from inflamed joints could also be due to hydrogen peroxide generated by activated PMN cells. The direct measurement of H_2O_2 production in inflamed rat joints indicates that at the peak of PMN infiltration, the concentration of H_2O_2 generated is at least half that shown in experiments *in vitro* to inhibit proteoglycan synthesis. Again it is likely that *in vivo,* some of the observed inhibition will be mediated by IL-1 (42). It seemed possible that an investigation of the mechanism of inhibition of proteoglycan biosynthesis by hydrogen peroxide using *in vitro* systems could be used to indicate whether this also occurs in an inflamed joint *in vivo.*

The immediate depletion of chondrocyte ATP after exposure *in vitro* to 10^{-4}

M H_2O_2 and the parallel decrease in biosynthetic pathways for DNA, protein, and hyaluronic acid (34,39) suggest that a decreased supply of ATP may occur because H_2O_2 blocks the glycolytic pathway. Chondrocytes in cartilage have an anaerobic pathway for ATP production (40), as indicated by the high lactate production to O_2 consumption. Thus the inhibition by H_2O_2 of 3-phosphoglyceraldehyde dehydrogenase, an enzyme occurring in the glycolytic pathway, may indicate the molecular site of H_2O_2 interaction and the reason for the subsequent inhibition of ATP production. Evidence for this in our experiments *in vitro* is shown by the nonavailability of SH groups near the active site of G-3-DPH for attachment of H^3-labeled iodoacetic acid in extracts from H_2O_2-treated cartilage compared to control untreated cartilage. Reduction by beta-mercaptoethanol restores this reactivity, indicating that exposure to hydrogen peroxide had oxidized the enzyme within the chondrocyte (34). Recent studies of extracts from inflamed cartilage have demonstrated the same inactivation of G-3-PDH, presumably due to H_2O_2 generated within the inflamed joint (36). Thus it seems likely that the PMN cell population in an inflamed joint may contribute to proteoglycan degradation and to the inhibition of proteoglycan biosynthesis by mechanisms other than those mediated by IL-1.

REFERENCES

1. Root RK, Metcalf J, Oshino H, Chance B. H_2O_2 release from human granulocytes during phagocytosis I. Documentation quantitation and some regulating factors. *J Clin Invest* 1975;55:945–955.
2. Bartholomew JS, Lowther DA, Handley CJ. Changes in proteoglycan synthesis following leucocyte elastase treatment of bovine articular cartilage in culture. *Arthritis Rheum* 1984;27:905–912.
3. Schalkwijk J, van den Berg WB, van den Putte LBA, Joosten LAB. Elastase secreted by activated polymorphonuclear leucocytes in vitro causes chondrocyte damage and matrix degradation in intact articular cartilage: escape from alpha 1 proteinase inhibitor and localisation in cartilage. *Br J Exp Pathol* 1987;68:81–88.
4. Weissman G. Lysosomal enzymes mechanisms of tissue injury in arthritis. *N Engl J Med* 1972;286:141–147.
5. Bates EJ, Johnson CL, Lowther DA. Inhibition of proteoglycan synthesis by hydrogen peroxide in cultured bovine articular cartilage. *Biochem Biophys Acta* 1985;838:221–228.
6. Schalkwijk J, van den Berg WB, van den Putte LBA, Joosten LAB. An experimental model for hydrogen peroxide-induced tissue damage. Effects of a single inflammatory mediator on periarticular tissues. *Arthritis Rheum* 1986;29:532–538.
7. Krane SM, Dayer JM, Goldring SR. Considerations of possible cellular events in the destructive synovial lesion in rheumatoid arthritis. In: Ziff M, Velo GP, Gorinis S, eds. *Adv Inflamm Res* 3: Rheumatoid arthritis. 1982;1–176.
8. Pettipher ER, Higgs GA, Henderson B. Interleukin-1 induces leucocyte infiltration and cartilage proteoglycan degradation in the synovial joint. *Proc Natl Acad Sci USA* 1986;83:8749–8753.
9. Cooke TDV, Sumia M, Maeda M. Deleterious interactions of immune complexes in cartilage of experimental immune arthritis. *Clin Orthop* 1985;183:235–245.
10. Lowther DA, Gillard GC. Carrageenin-induced arthritis. 1. The effect of intra articular carrageenan on the chemical composition of articular cartilage. *Arthritis Rheum* 1976;19:769–776.
11. Sandy JD, Lowther DA, Brown HLG. Antigen-induced arthritis studies on the inhibition of proteoglycan synthesis observed in articular cartilage during short-term joint inflammation. *Arthritis Rheum* 1980;23:433–447.
12. Ugai K, Ishikawa H, Hirohata K, Shirane H. Interaction of polymorphonuclear leucocytes with immune complexes trapped in rheumatoid articular cartilage. *Arthritis Rheum* 1983;26:1434–1441.

13. Pettipher ER, Henderson B, Moncada S, Higgs GA. Leucocyte infiltration and cartilage proteoglycan loss in immune arthritis in the rabbit. *Br J Pharmacol* 1988;95:169–176.
14. Mohr W, Pelster B, Wessinhage D. Polymorphonuclear granulocytes in rheumatic tissue destruction VI. The occurrence of PMN's in the menisci of patients with rheumatoid arthritis. *Rheum Int* 1984;5:39–44.
15. Lowther DA, Sandy JD, Santer VB, Brown HLG. Antigen-induced arthritis: decreased proteoglycan content and inhibition of proteoglycan synthesis in articular cartilage. *Arthritis Rheum* 1978;21:675–680.
16. Sandy JD, Sriratana A, Brown HLG, Lowther DA. Evidence for polymorphonuclear-derived proteinases in arthritic cartilage. *Biochem J* 1981;193:193–202.
17. Barrett AJ. The possible role of neutrophilic proteinases in damage to articular cartilage. *Agents Actions* 1978;8:11–18.
18. Keiser H, Greenwald K, Feinstein G, Janoff A. Degradation of cartilage proteoglycan by human leucocyte granule proteases. A model of joint injury. II. Degradation of isolated bovine nasal cartilage proteoglycan. *J Clin Invest* 1976;57:625–632.
19. Janoff A, Feisenstein G, Malemod CJ, Elias JM. Degradation of cartilage proteoglycan by human leucocyte granule neutral proteases—A model of joint injury. I. Penetration of enzyme into rabbit cartilage and release of $^{35}SO_4$-labelled material from the tissue. *J Clin Invest* 1976;57:615–624.
20. Roughley PJ. The degradation of cartilage proteoglycans by tissue proteinases: proteoglycan heterogeneity and the pathway of proteolytic degradation. *Biochem J* 1977;167:639–646.
21. Velvart M, Fehr K, Baici A, Sommermeyer G, Knopfel M, Cancer M, Salgam P, Boni A. Degradation in vivo of articular cartilage in rheumatoid arthritis by leucocyte elastase from polymorphonuclear leucocytes. *Rheum Int* 1981;1:121–130.
22. Menninger H, Burkhardt H, Roske W. Lysosomal elastase: effect on mechanical and biochemical properties of normal cartilage. *Rheum Int* 1981;1:73–78.
23. Gillard GC, Lowther DA. Carrageenan induced arthritis. II. The effect of intra articular injection of carrageenan on the synthesis of proteoglycan in articular cartilage. *Arthritis Rheum* 1976;19:918–922.
24. van den Berg WB, Kruysen MWM, van den Putte LBA, Beusekom HJ, van der Sluis-van der pol M, Zwartx WA. Antigen and zymosan induced arthritis in mice: studies on in vivo cartilage proteoglycan synthesis and chondrocyte death. *Br J Exp Pathol* 1981;62:308–317.
25. Sumi M, Maeda M, Cooke TDV. Deleterious interactions of immune complexes with tibial cartilage of antigen-induced arthritic rabbits. II: chondrocyte degradation. *Clin Orthop Rel Res* 1985;212:260–274.
26. Babior BM, Kipnes RS, Curnutte JT. Biological defense mechanisms. The production by leucocytes of superoxide a potential bactericidal agent. *J Clin Invest* 1973;52:741–744.
27. Root RK, Metcalf JA. H_2O_2 release from human granulocytes during phagocytosis: relationship to superoxide anion formation and cellular catabolism of H_2O_2: studies with normal and cytocholasin-B treated cells. *J Clin Invest* 1977;60:1266–1279.
28. Bates EJ, Lowther DA, Handley CJ. Oxygen free radicals mediate an inhibition of proteoglycan synthesis in cultured articular cartilage. *Ann Rheum Dis* 1984;43:462–469.
29. Bates EJ, Johnson LC, Lowther DA. Inhibition of proteoglycan synthesis by hydrogen peroxide in cultured bovine articular cartilage. *Biochim Biophys* 1985;838:221–228.
30. Schalkwijk J, van den Berg WB, van den Putte LBA. Hydrogen peroxide suppresses proteoglycan synthesis of intact articular cartilage. *J Rheum* 1985;12:205–210.
31. Bitter T, Muir H. A modified uronic acid carbazole reaction. *Anal Biochem* 1962;4:330–334.
32. Bartholomew JS, Lowther DA, Handley CJ. Changes in proteoglycan biosynthesis following leucocyte elastose treatment of bovine articular cartilage in culture. *Arthritis Rheum* 1984;27:905–910.
33. Hascall VC, Handley CJ, McQuillen DJ, Hascall GK, Robinson HC, Lowther DA. The effect of serum on biosynthesis of proteoglycans by bovine articular cartilage cells in culture. *Arch Biochem Biophys* 1983;224:206–223.
34. Ruch W, Cooper PH, Baggiolini M. Assay of H_2O_2 production by macrophages and neutrophils with homovanillic acid and horseradish peroxidase. *J Immunol Methods* 1983;63:347–357.
35. Baker MS, Feigan J, Lowther DA. The mechanism of chondrocyte hydrogen peroxide damage. Depletion of intracellular ATP due to suppression of glycolysis caused by oxidation of glyceraldehyde-3-phosphate dehydrogenase. *J Rheumatol* 1989;16:7–14.
36. Baker MS, Bolis S, Lowther DA. The oxidation of articular cartilage glyceraldehyde-3-phosphate dehydrogenase (G3-PDH) occurs in vivo during carrageenan induced arthritis. *Agents Actions* 1991;32:299–304.

37. Saklatvala J, Pilsworth LMC, Sarsfield SJ, Gavriloc J, Heath JK. Pig catabolin is a form of interleukin I. *Biochem J* 1984;224:461–466.
38. Santer V, Sriratana A, Lowther DA. Carrageenan-induced arthritis V. A morphologic study of the development of inflammation in acute arthritis. *Semin Arthritis Rheum* 1983;13:160–167.
39. Bates EJ, Lowther DA, Johnson CC. Hyaluronic acid synthesis in articular cartilage: an inhibition by hydrogen peroxide. *Biochem Biophys Res Comm* 1985;132:714–720.
40. Stockwell RA. *Biology of cartilage cells.* London: Cambridge University Press, 1979.
41. Lowther DA, Sriratana A, Bartholome JS. The role of serine proteinase in cartilage damage. *J Rheum* 1987 (Suppl. 14);14:49–51.
42. Tyler JA. Articular cartilage cultured with catabolin (Pig interleukin 1) synthesises a decreased number of normal proteoglycan molecules. *Biochem J* 1985;227:869–878.

DISCUSSION

Howell: In gonococcal arthritis there is evidence that the polymorph filopodia will actually break through the surface of the cartilage fibers and perhaps open up a way to allow enzymes in. Do the polymorphs in your experiments invade the surface after attaching?

Lowther: We have some scanning electron micrographs showing that polymorphs leave a disordered, roughened surface behind in places where they were attached, rather like the osteoclast does on bone. We also find evidence that polymorph filopodia can penetrate the cartilage surface.

Muir: There is a great deal of current interest in nitric oxide which may be generated by vascular endothelial cells and by other types of cells, including, perhaps, synovial cells. Nitric oxide reacts instantly with oxygen generated free radicals and deactivates them. Do you think that the synovial lining cells can help prevent damage to cartilage by neutralizing radicals produced by macrophages or the polymorphs?

Lowther: The only protective things I know of are catalase, superoxide dismutase, and many small molecules such as histidine which will mop up a variety of oxygen derived free radicals, including hydroxyl radicals. Whether the synovial membrane plays a specific role in producing such protective agents, I'm not sure.

Campion: Have you tried using animals rendered neutropenic?

Lowther: No, I have not. Animals rendered neutropenic still seem to show similar degenerative changes, at least to antigen derived arthritis. In other words, you don't need the polymorphs in order to get morphological changes of the sort that I have shown.

Hardingham: In the carrageenan-induced model, what is chemotactic for polymorphs?

Lowther: Complement appears to be activated, so the C5A and C3A are probably present. Such peptides and leukotriene B4 may attract the polymorphs.

Hirschelmann: Would catalase injection into the joint be an adequate therapy for this type of arthritis?

Lowther: We have shown that catalase is cleared from the joint extremely rapidly, and it must be present before the inflammation is induced to be effective. To reduce synovial clearance rates, we linked it to a large polymer in such a way that it still retained enzymatic activity. Similarly, the Dutch group at Nijmegen made catalase more cationic so that it really sticks to the cartilage surface. These modified catalases provided considerable protection from damage induced by inflammatory cells.

van den Berg: To clarify, we have shown that the charged modified catalase has mainly an effect on edema. There is only a slight protective effect on cartilage damage. If only the hydrogen peroxide is eliminated, other mediators will still induce significant damage.

Articular Cartilage and Osteoarthritis,
edited by K. Kuettner et al.
Raven Press, Ltd., New York © 1992.

39

Prophylactic and Therapeutic Use of Drugs in Joint Destruction

Kay Brune

Department of Pharmacology and Toxicology, The University of Erlangen-Nuernberg, D-8520 Erlangen, Germany

In all industrialized nations there is a constant increase in life expectancy. Consequently, an increasing number of the population is affected by chronic degenerative diseases, including osteoarthrosis. In Central Europe, approximately half of the people above the age of 50 show occasional signs of osteoarthrosis which interferes with their normal daily lives, causing impaired function, pain, and inability to perform work (1). It comes as no surprise that all types of remedies are offered to reduce the discomfort and impaired function of activated arthrosis. Numerous prophylactic treatments are on the market, supposedly to reduce the development of osteoarthritic joint damage. These remedies include not only so-called "natural medicines," but also homeopathic and other drugs of unproven activity (2,3). Typical examples are preparations or extracts of cartilage and joint tissues containing ground substances (3). They also comprise analgesics, particularly nonsteroidal antiinflammatory drugs (NSAIDs) which reduce pain (1). However, it is claimed that some of these drugs either accelerate joint decay or "protect" the joint from further damage (4,5). In this author's opinion, little proof of the prophylactic effect of so-called "chondroprotective" drugs is available. It also does not appear adequately supported to divide the group of NSAIDs into subdivisions which supposedly either accelerate cartilage damage or interfere with the progress of osteoarthrosis. The reasons are outlined as follows.

THE THERAPEUTIC USE OF DRUGS IN JOINT DESTRUCTION

In principle, joint damage leads to an inflammation of the joint tissues which may well result in mediator release and progressive joint destruction (5). In line with this reasoning, drugs which do interfere with inflammatory processes should reduce joint tissue damage, thus they may be regarded as being of prophylactic and therapeutic value. On the other hand, the main symptom of acute joint damage or acute phases of activated osteoarthrosis is pain, which is a physiological signal to protect the joint from intensive and excessive use. The application of analgesic NSAIDs reduces this pain symptom and may, therefore, allow an overriding of this physiological warning signal. Consequently, all NSAIDs, when taken in sufficient doses to guarantee pain relief, may also be regarded as damaging, or "chondrotoxic," because they facilitate overuse of an already damaged joint. Indeed, there is evidence that the latter mechanism is operating. Most physicians can name a variety of patients who take a NSAID before they engage in physical exercise like jogging, tennis, mountain climbing, etc. These patients know that this physical exercise will result in pain a few hours later, thus interfering with the night's sleep or the next day's well-being. It is obvious that this prophylactic use of NSAIDs cannot be regarded as directly interfering with joint destruction; rather, it accelerates this process.

Recently, similar evidence has been produced in animals. Hamsters are devoted tread mill walkers. If the joints of these animals are damaged, e.g., by trauma, the running performance per day is reduced to less than half (6). If these animals are fed sufficient quantities of NSAIDs, they make up their normal walking distance, regrettably at the expense of the joint healing process (6). These observations may be easily translated into the behavior of tennis players, joggers, or hikers who take the drug prophylactically. Under these conditions, the use of NSAIDs is obviously destructive for the joint, although it enhances physiological and psychological well-being. Moreover, data from Brandt (7) and others indicate that some NSAIDs cause joint damage in animals (dogs) suffering from traumatic joint destruction while others do not. The same authors show that the gait of the dogs is variable depending on the pain suffered. Consequently, the amount of joint damage appears to be negatively correlated with the analgesic effectiveness of the drug at a certain dosage level (7). These and other factors, such as the use of inadequate doses or concentrations, species differences, etc. (Table 1) have

TABLE 1. Effects of NSAIDs on joint tissue in vivo (Doses) or in vitro (Conc.) in different species

Species	Drug	Effect (+ or −)	Doses[a] mg/kg/d	Conc[a] µg/ml % (S)	ED_{50}[b] µg/kg/d	LD_{50}[b] µg/kg/d	D_{ther}[c] µg/ml	C_{ther}[c] µg/ml	Ref. no.
dog	aspirin	−	120	θ	70	400	50	30	8
	NA-salicylate	−	θ	160 (10)	70	400	50	30	9
	piroxicam	+	θ	3 (10)	5	300	0.3	5	9
rat	indomethacin	−	1	θ	0.25	10	2	1	10
	tiaprofenicacid	+	7	θ	10	200	10	10	10
chicken	phenylbutazone		30.0	θ	?	?	3	30	11
	diclofenac	+	1.5	θ	?	?	2	1	11
mouse	naproxen	−	50	θ	20	1,000	20	10	12
	diclofenac	+	3	θ	5	?	2	1	12
	Na-salicylate	−	θ	100 (0)	50	400	50	30	13
rabbit	indomethacin	−	θ	100 (10)	?	?	2	1	14
	diclofenac	+	θ	2 (10)	?	?	?	1	14

[a] Dosages or concentrations used by the authors.
[b] Effective (ED_{50}) and lethal (LD_{50}) doses defined in the species under investigation (from standard text books).
[c] Therapeutic dosages (D_{ther}) and concentrations (C_{ther}) of the NSAIDs in man.
S, serum concentration.
θ; not tested.

led to the contention that there are chondroprotective and chrondrotoxic NSAIDs. As indicated in Table 1, lack of comparability should argue against such claims. Sometimes the contentions of some investigators could not even be substantiated by later work of the same research group (see, e.g., refs. 12 and 15).

In conclusion, it may be stated that NSAIDs are of some therapeutic value when used to treat activated arthrosis and the pain resulting from it. However, this is true only if the patient continues to avoid use and overuse of the diseased joints. The contention that some NSAIDs may be analgesic *and* chondroprotective appears not well-supported by facts.

THE PROPHYLACTIC USE OF DRUGS

Aside from many medicines of dubious value (see, e.g., ref. 2), four types of so-called chondroprotective substances have been used in patients: Arumalone, Arteparone, *d*-glucosamine, and hyaluronic acid. The former two drugs are prescribed by brand names because they consist of (more-or-less) well-standardized mixtures of ingredients from calf cartilage and bone marrow (Arumalone: glycosaminoglycan-peptide complexes) or different esters of sulfated glycosaminoglycan(s) from connective tissue and cartilages (Arteparone) (16).

The first mention of the beneficial effect of bone marrow extracts in joint diseases is from the 17th century. In a collection of recipes gathered by the alchemist, Johann Joachin Becher (1635–1682), it is stated:

> *Der Mensch, das Ebenbild, welchs Gott ist angenehm, hat vier und zwanzig Stueck zur Arztney bequem. Vom Mark/wie auch vom Oel aus Beinen destilliert/Das schlimme Podagra heylsam vertrieben wird. Zerlassen Menschen-Fett ist gut vor lahme Glieder. So man sie darmit schmiert sie werden richtig wieder.*

Freely translated this means: "Man, the image that pleases God, has twenty-four remedies to offer: They are distilled from the marrow, as well as from the bones, cures severe gout. Melted human fat is very good when applied to the lame extremities, and makes them function again." Recent investigations have claimed (Table 2) that all the so-called chondroprotective substances are useful. Reviews of these studies are listed in Table 1. They have been discussed at length at several of the hearings of the German BGA in Berlin (BGA, Bundes Gesundheits Amt, the agency of the Federal Republic of Germany), an equivalent to the United States' Food and Drug Administration. The results of these investigations are that a *marginal* prophylactic or therapeutic effect of these compounds appears possible, but also that the administration, particularly the parenteral administration, of these compounds is accompanied by a sizeable incidence of unwanted side effects including bleedings, local allergic reactions, and systemic allergic reactions with acute glomerulonephritis and encephalitis (see Tables 1 and 2). Under these circumstances, in my personal opinion, the use of these remedies does not appear justified. Similar comments may be said of the different

TABLE 2. Evaluation of the use of three chondroprotective drugs

Composition	Brand name
D-glucosamine	Dona
glycosaminoglycan polysulfate	Arteparone
glycosaminoglycan-peptides (+ growth factors, etc.)	(A)Rumalone

Positive assessments (refs. 4, 16, 18):
Safe, but not very active; "protects" patients from NSAIDs use; use pays for research in osteoarthritis.
Negative assessments (refs. 3, 17, 18):
Report of many use-related side effects; very costly, thus ethically untenable; no outstanding clinical research on osteoarthritis patients in countries with wide use of chondroprotectives.

preparations of hyaluronic acids used as therapeutic and prophylactic means in the therapy of osteoarthrosis. Again, convincing clinical data are lacking but reports of side effects are available. Not even considered here are the additional costs to the community or the principal risk of intraarticular injections which accompanies any injection of such drugs in man.

REFERENCES

1. Wagenhauser FJ. Die medikamentöse Basisbehandlung der Arthrosen. 5th *Fortbildungskurs fuer Rheumatologie,* Basel. 1976;11:13–11.
2. De Smet PAGM. Drugs used in non-orthodox medicine. In: Dukes MNG, Beeley L, eds. *Side effects of drugs annual,* 13. Amsterdam, New York, Oxford: Elsevier, 1989;442–473.
3. De Smet PAGM. Drugs used in non-orthodox medicine. In: Dukes MNG, Beeley L, eds. *Side effects of drugs annual,* 14. Amsterdam, New York, Oxford: Elsevier, 1990;429–451.
4. Gosh P, Brooks P. Chondroprotection—exploring the concept. *J Rheumatol* 1991;18:161–166.
5. Calin A. Clinical aspects of the effect of NSAID on cartilage. *J Rheumatol* 1989;16(Suppl. 18): 43–44.
6. Ottterness I (in press).
7. Brandt KD. *Proceedings of the XVIIth Eular Congress of Rheumatology,* Rio de Janeiro, Brazil, 1989;368–372.
8. Palmoski MJ, Brandt KD. In vivo effect of aspirin on canine osteoarthritic cartilage. *Arthritis Rheum* 1983;26:994–1001.
9. Palmoski MJ, Brandt KD. Relationship between matrix proteoglycan content and the effects of salicylate and indomethacin on articular cartilage. *Arthritis Rheum* 1983;27:528–531.
10. Annefeld M, Raiss R, Cleres C. Einfluss steroidaler und nichtsteroidaler Antiphlogistika auf die Ultrastruktur von Chondrozyten der Ratte. *Arzneimittel-Forsch/Drug Research.* 1984;34:1763–1765.
11. Kalbhen DA. Biochemically induced osteoarthrosis in the chicken and rat. In: Munthe E, Bjelle A, eds. *Effects of drugs on osteoarthrosis.* Bern, Stuttgart, Vienna: Huber, 1983;48–68.
12. Maier R, Wilhelmi G. Preclinical investigations of drugs effects in models of osteoarthrosis. In: Munthe E, Bjelle A, eds. *Effects of drugs on osteoarthrosis.* Bern, Stuttgart, Vienna: Huber, 1983;90–96.
13. De Vries BJ, van den Berg WB, van de Putte LBA. Salicylate-induced depletion of endogenous inorganic sulfate. *Arthritis Rheum* 1985;28:922–929.
14. Mohr W, Kirkptrick CJ. In vitro experiments with chondrocytes. In: Munthe E, Bjelle A, eds. *Effects of drugs on osteoarthrosis.* Bern, Stuttgart, Vienna: Huber, 1983;75–89.
15. Pataki A, Riefe R, Witzemann E, Graf HP, Schweizer A. Spontaneous osteoarthritis of the knee-joint in C57BL mice receiving chronic oral treatment with NSAIDS or predisone. *Agents Actions* 1989;29:210–217.

16. Rejholec V. Long-term studies of anti-osteoarthritic drugs: an assessment. *Semin Arthritis Rheum* 1987;17(Suppl. 1):35–53.
17. Brune K. Stellungnahme zur Diskussion um Chondroprotektiva. *Akt Rheumatol* 1987;12:82–83.
18. Unpublished reports of the Deliberations of the German BGA (Bundes Gesundheits Amt), 1990.

DISCUSSION

Lust: I agree wholeheartedly with your assessment of chondroprotective drugs. In the United States, Arteparone is named Adequan when it is used to treat osteoarthritis in horses as approved by the FDA. Veterinarians that use it seem to think that it has some value. That is why I studied its effects on heriditary hip dysplasia in dogs. We studied 16 dogs with a high dose and repeated the study with a lower dose (2.5 mg/kg weight) with similar benefical results. Is there an explanation for this?

Brune: I know both your studies and those of David Howell. There were positive aspects in these animal studies but they have to be cautiously discussed. For example, did the control dogs receive an agent that also interferes with blood coagulation? Did the injection hurt? Was the drug given together with lidocaine, as is normally done in man? All these aspects may have effects, on the food intake of the dog, for example. Moreover, in your dogs the drug was given prophylactically, while in humans it is given therapeutically. Finally, the doses you used, while difficult to compare, were relatively high in comparison to human dosages. The human dose was reduced considerably a few years ago due to three lethal events in Switzerland. I do wholeheartedly agree that cautious investigations such as yours will give us hints as to what we should investigate.

Dieppe: It is quite easy to knock these trials, but one of the reasons is that they are extremely difficult to do. It is an almost overwhelming task to design a good clinical trial that will show that something is either chondroprotective or indeed deleterious to the joint. It is often forgotten that you need to design quite a different study to look for symptomatic benefit than to look for effects on structure or function of joints. These two aspects have been muddled up.

Brune: For a scientist, the statement which may be valid for a clinician, "it's very difficult to have better tests," docs not increase the quality of the proof available. I think that if there is no proof, there is no proof. The fact that it is difficult to do good research should make us think of better approaches. About 8 years ago, I suggested to the three producers of putative chondroprotective drugs to join in a controlled, prospective, double-blind trial without placebo. If the three drugs were compared against each other prospectively, the results would be meaningful. If all drugs show the same outcome, they are all either effective or ineffective. If there are significant differences, this would be meaningful, too.

Dieppe: I am skeptical as well. However, if there is anything impressive in chondroprotective agents, it is the hint coming from a number of studies, albeit not well controlled, which suggests that there may be some relatively early pain relief with some of them. This is unlikely to have anything to do with cartilage or indeed directly with osteoarthritis. Have you been impressed by that? What mechanisms could account for an effect on pain?

Brune: Indeed, one is sometimes impressed by pain relief early in treatment, but one should be cautious. Has the compound been injected intraarticularly or intramuscularly, with or without lidocaine, a local anesthetic? If you inject the drug into a hurting joint with lidocaine, immediate pain relief should occur. If given without lidocaine, my orthopedic colleagues tell me that injecting just plain sodium chloride into the joint helps for some time for no known reason. Early pain relief then, may have nothing to do with the drug *per se,* but is the result of intervention by the physician. Finally, the Yugoslavian study which exists only as a thesis shows that after short-term treatment, there was absolutely no difference between the placebo and the treatment groups.

Dieppe: The trial that needs to be done, then, is a proper placebo-controlled study of pain relief and not chondroprotection. We did, in fact, such a study with steroids in osteoarthritis and found the placebo injection was indeed a very effective treatment.

Hirschelmann: You used the term osteoarthrosis, while most others used osteoarthritis. Is it only terminology or do you mean a difference in pathology?

Brune: I think it is a typical game to argue about nomenclature. Some of my rheumatology and orthopedic colleagues love either one. If you prefer osteoarthritis, that is fine. If you prefer osteoarthrosis, that is also fine. We are facing a disease, which at different times is an "itis," that is inflammatory, and sometimes an "osis," that is degeneration without inflammation.

Articular Cartilage and Osteoarthritis,
edited by K. Kuettner et al.
Raven Press, Ltd., New York © 1992.

Part XI: Drug Evaluation in Osteoarthritis

Introduction

Roger M. Mason

*Department of Biochemistry, Charing Cross and Westminster Medical School,
London W6 8 RF, United Kingdom*

Laboratory evaluation of drugs for treating osteoarthritis should, ideally, test their ability to modify in a favorable way those cellular and molecular changes which are known to be involved in the initiation and development of the disorder. However, this logical approach poses problems for the investigator. First, our knowledge of such events is incomplete. Second, our ability to model osteoarthritis in the laboratory in order to test the effect of drugs on the disorder is limited. The aim of these introductory comments is to recall some of the biochemical processes which undergo change in osteoarthritis and to indicate the biological systems which are available for evaluating the action of drugs on such processes. The clinical evaluation of drugs for treating osteoarthritis is complementary to the laboratory evaluation but is outside the scope of this work. It should be mentioned, however, that recent advances in techniques such as magnetic resonance imaging and microfocal radiography provide new and sensitive methods to assess early osteoarthritic changes and, potentially, the impact of drug therapies on them.

One of the most striking changes in osteoarthritis is the depletion of proteoglycan from the extracellular matrix of the cartilage, the result of an increased rate of proteoglycan turnover, as measured in the Pond-Nuki canine model of osteoarthritis. There is also an increase in the rate of proteoglycan synthesis in both human and canine osteoarthritis, with matrix depletion occurring when this is exceeded by turnover. Qualitative changes in proteoglycan chemistry occur with a decrease in ratio of keratan sulfate to chondroitin sulfate in man and the expression of a new glycosaminoglycan epitope in the dog.

Most of the proteoglycan fragments released during turnover of the articular cartilage diffuse into the synovial fluid, and some eventually reach the blood. It seems likely, though not proven, that these fragments are generated by neutral metalloproteinase enzymes, and increased activity of two of these, collagenase and stromelysin, have been reported in both human and canine osteoarthritic cartilage. Metalloproteinases are synthesized as inactive proenzymes. After activation their proteolytic potential is limited by subsequent interaction with tissue inhibitor of metalloproteinases (TIMP). Increased metalloproteinase activity occurs in canine experimental osteoarthritis without any increase in TIMP, an imbalance which might promote enhanced matrix degradation.

Specific cytokines promote or inhibit the synthesis of proteoglycans in normal cartilage. IGF-1, TGFβ, IL-1, IL-6, and TNFα are made by various chondrocytes, suggesting that autocrine mechanisms may contribute to controlling the balance between proteoglycan synthesis and loss. Whether such controls are perturbed in the noninflammatory stages of osteoarthritis is unknown. However, the acquisition of drugs which, through an action on particular cytokines or their receptors, reestablish a balance between proteoglycan synthesis and turnover is a desirable therapeutic goal.

Since the cause of osteoarthritis is unknown, strategies for evaluating drugs to treat the disorder must relate to testing whether they are able to modulate one or more of the biochemical changes associated with the disorder. Methods are available for measuring rates of proteoglycan synthesis and turnover, for analyzing qualitative changes in proteoglycans, for the assay of fragments of proteoglycans or other matrix molecules in synovial fluid or blood, and for assessing the levels of mRNA, protein products, and activity of metalloproteinases, TIMP, and various cytokines and their receptors. A major problem for the investigator is the choice of a "biosystem" on which to test the effect of a drug on one or more of these biochemical parameters and how relevant that system is to human osteoarthritis. Broadly the choice lies between systems *in vitro* and *in vivo*. The former includes cell culture of articular chondrocytes under conditions which maintain their phenotype, and explant culture of whole cartilages (e.g., patella) from small animals or of pieces of articular cartilage from larger species. All three methods are represented in subsequent chapters or abstracts (Reiss *et al.*, van den Berg *et al.*, Mason and Goh). The advantage of *in vitro* systems is that they enable investigation of drug actions on specific biochemical pathways under rigorously controlled conditions. Large numbers of replicate cultures can be used relatively easily at a reasonable financial cost. However, the results must be interpreted with care since normal articular cartilage, usually of nonhuman origin, is invariably used in such experiments. Moreover, cells maintained *in vitro* are unlikely to be subjected to the same range and balance of effector molecules as they encounter *in vivo*.

The evaluation of drug actions on osteoarthritis *in vivo* poses further problems. Human osteoarthritic patients usually present at the clinic with advanced disease and are not necessarily suitable for such investigations. Moreover, ethical and financial considerations limit such investigation: for example, it is not usually acceptable to repeat arthroscopy and cartilage biopsy frequently. However, the recent introduction of sensitive immunoassays to monitor the concentration of cartilage matrix molecules, or their degradation products, in synovial fluid and blood may be applicable for studying drug action on human osteoarthritis joints as described here by Shinmei *et al.*

There are two main categories of animal models of osteoarthritis: those in which the disorder arises spontaneously and those in which it is induced experimentally. The former include murine models, for example, the osteoarthritis in the medial tibial plateau of the STR/ORT male mouse. Current investigations in our laboratory and elsewhere aim to describe the biochemical events accompanying the development of the disease, and when these are known, this model may prove useful for drug evaluation. The best studied experimentally induced osteoarthritis is the Pond-Nuki model in which articular cartilage changes similar to those of the human disorder are seen following section of the anterior cruciate ligament in the canine knee joint. Biochemical changes in the articular cartilage follow quickly, but a 2- or 3-year interval is required before matrix proteoglycans become depleted and cartilage fibrillation occurs. The disadvantages of this model for drug evaluation studies include the high cost of maintenance and provision of special animal facilities, together with the current unfavorable public attitude toward experiments involving dogs.

Articular Cartilage and Osteoarthritis,
edited by K. Kuettner et al.
Raven Press, Ltd., New York © 1992.

40

Drug Evaluation on Isolated Articular Chondrocytes

Ruth X. Raiss,* Monika Oestensen,†
and Margaret B. Aydelotte‡

*Pharmacological Research Hoechst AG Werk Kalle-Albert, Wiesbaden, Germany;
†Institute of Immunology and Rheumatology, University of Oslo, Oslo, Norway;
‡Department of Biochemistry, Rush-Presbyterian–St. Luke's Medical Center,
Chicago, Illinois 60612

In normal articular cartilage, chondrocytes control the morphological and functional integrity of the tissue by maintaining a well-balanced equilibrium between anabolism and catabolism of the matrix constituents. These cells synthesize not only the appropriate macromolecules, but also enzymes that degrade them and specific inhibitors, such as tissue inhibitor of metalloproteinases (TIMP). They also possess receptors for mediators considered to be involved in these processes, such as interleukin-1 (IL-1), insulin-like growth factor I (IGF-I), and transforming growth factor β (TGFβ). In rheumatic diseases involving cartilage deterioration, such as osteoarthritis (OA), the precise mechanism of cartilage matrix degradation is not yet fully understood, but there is strong evidence that the chondrocytes play a crucial role in their pathogenesis. In a process termed chondrocytic chondrolysis (1), chondrocytes can be stimulated *in vitro* to degrade their surrounding matrix in a manner similar to the cartilage destruction observed in osteoarthritis. Since this chondrolytic component in the joint diseases has not yet been prevented pharmacologically, methods for culturing chondrocytes *in vitro* have gained importance as assay systems to assess potential chondroprotective cartilage-restoring agents.

CONSIDERATIONS ABOUT ASSAY SYSTEMS OF CARTILAGE METABOLISM FOR DRUG TESTING

Chondrocytes differ in their metabolic activity according to the depth of the region in the cartilage from which they are derived (e.g., ref. 2). These initial differences disappear over time in monolayer culture, but are maintained in cultures over (3), or in (4) agarose gels. Most drug testing on isolated chondrocytes has been done with monolayer cultures which have the advantage of easy accessibility to the cells for agents dissolved in the nutrient medium. However, this is outweighed by the disadvantage of a limited time frame, after which these cells lose their chondrocytic characteristics (5). The agarose gel system, in contrast, combines the advantages of a homogeneous mixture of an otherwise heterogeneous cell population with the long-term stability of specific chondrocytic phenotype. In an agarose gel, many of the newly synthesized proteoglycan (PG) and collagen molecules are retained around the cells and incorporated into an extracellular matrix, whereas low-molecular PGs and matrix breakdown products, as well as low molecular weight drugs, diffuse freely between the gel and the liquid nutrient medium (6). Even after prior culture in monolayer, which favors mitogenesis and also "dedifferentiation," subsequent culture of chondrocytes in agarose gels leads to a reexpression of the chondrocyte phenotype (7). This redifferentiation within agarose gel is the more significant, as chondrocytic differentiation is considered to occur in multiple steps (8), and morphological modulation and loss of cartilage PG and collagen type II expression are not necessarily linked to each other during this process (9). Another promising culture system that preserves chondrocyte specificity is suspension within alginate beads (10,11), in which the density of the artificial matrix can be finely regulated and viable cells can be recovered by simple depolymerization. This system has not yet been used for drug testing, but with additional knowledge it will certainly provide a useful tool.

Important requirements for cell culture systems that are used to evaluate a broad spectrum of pharmacological agents are high levels of standardization and reproducibility. In articular cartilage, parameters such as cell density, PG turnover, and cellular response to mediators vary between species (12–15). Even within the same species, the size and composition of matrix PGs synthesized by chondrocytes can change considerably with age (16). The sensitivity to mediators also decreases with increasing age as, for example, 10- to 20-fold in human articular chondrocytes exposed to IL-1 (17). The data we present here are obtained with primary cultures of articular chondrocytes maintained in agarose gels. Articular chondrocytes obtained from human cartilage usually can not be collected sex- and age-matched because of the restricted availability of human tissue. Therefore, bovine cells derived from 18- to 20-month-old steers are used routinely for purposes of reproducibility and standardization. To evaluate drug effects upon various disease stages, however, human articular chondrocytes derived from donors of varying ages and health were selected. Proteoglycan metabolism, which is sensitive to early degradative stimuli, was selected as the main parameter, and was determined either histochemically as intensity of staining with alcian blue, or radiochemically via ^{35}[S]sulfate incorporation. To distinguish effects of cell proliferation from effects upon matrix metabolism, cell densities at the end of treatment protocols were recorded photometrically (Figs. 1A and 2A).

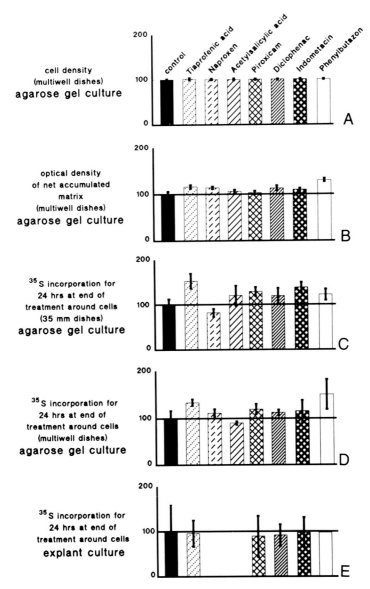

FIG. 1. Proteoglycan metabolism of bovine articular chondrocytes *in vitro* treated with NSAIDs over 8 days. The NSAIDs were administered in a concentration of 10^{-5} M anew with each change of medium every second day. Values of optical density for cell proliferation (A) and net matrix accumulation (B), and of [^{35}S]sulfate incorporation into matrix macromolecules (C,D,E) are expressed as percentage of untreated controls. The bars represent standard deviations of sextets (A,E) or quadruplets (B–D) per group. **A:** Cell density at the end of the experiment assessed by optical density measurement via inverted microscope, corrected for acellular agarose gel. **B:** Density of the net accumulated PGs retained in the agarose gel, assessed by optical density measurement via inverted microscope after staining with alcian blue. **C:** Proteoglycan (PG) synthesis of chondrocytes in agarose gel at the end of the treatment, assessed by [^{35}S]sulfate incorporation into PG macromolecules, in cultures of 35 mm diameter dishes. **D:** PG synthesis of chondrocytes in agarose gel at the end of the treatment, assessed by [^{35}S]sulfate incorporation into PG macromolecules, in 24 multiwell cultures. **E:** PG synthesis of cartilage explants per mg wet wt at the end of the treatment, assessed by [^{35}S]sulfate incorporation into PG macromolecules.

Compared to cultures of cartilage explants *in vitro,* where the chondrocytes remain embedded in their original matrix, isolated cells tend to respond to a greater extent to stimuli or drugs (Fig. 1C). They also react more reproducibly, and with less variation, than does tissue culture, based on the same cellularity (Fig. 1C,D) (18). Basically, these assay systems can serve two different purposes: to study the effects of agents upon normal physiological matrix metabolism as it presents itself under these conditions *in vitro,* or to investigate their effects upon chondrocytes in disease-related situations. We regard ascertaining potential effects upon the normal physiological matrix metabolism of chondrocytes as a first step in a screening profile for cartilage-supportive agents, and also as a prerequisite for drugs designed to combat other pathological events in the joint such as inflammation, pain, or autoimmune reactions. For instance, nonsteroidal antiinflammatory drugs (NSAIDs), used widely and successfully against joint inflammation, are prescribed frequently and often repeatedly in osteoarthritis, where cartilage is often already severely damaged. It is important that these drugs do not cause additional harm, and this is of high priority in the individual decision of which one to chose. The model can also be used to expose chondrocytes to disease-related conditions and study more specific interactions involved in the pathology. These conditions can be simulated in cultures by adding either synovial fluid (SF) obtained from rheumatic patients, or single mediators like IL-1, tumor necrosis factor (TNF), or retinol, all of which promote chondrocytic chondrolysis; or alternatively, by selecting human chondrocytes derived from diseased joints. We describe experiments using all three disease-related conditions: normal bovine and human chondrocytes cultured with IL-1, human chondrocytes cultured with SF from rheumatic patients, and human chondrocytes derived from diseased joints.

NSAID EFFECTS UPON BOVINE ARTICULAR CHONDROCYTES IN AGAROSE GEL CULTURE

We tested NSAIDs routinely used in basic treatment of inflammatory joint diseases—tiaprofenic acid, naproxen, acetylsalicylic acid, piroxicam, indomethacin, and phenylbutazone—on bovine articular chondrocytes cultured in agarose gels and on bovine articular cartilage explants. A concentration of 10^{-5} M was used for each over a period of 8 days. They had no effect upon cell proliferation in the chondrocyte cultures (Fig. 1A), but stimulated PG synthesis to a small, but not always significant degree (Fig. 1C,D), as well as the net accumulation of PGs (Fig. 1B). This slight stimulation, however, was not observed in cartilage explants, based on the same cellularity (Fig. 1E). When tested under conditions promoting chondrocytic chondrolysis (for methodological details, see ref. 19) induced by 0.05 ng/ml human recombinant IL-1 alpha (Fig. 2), none of the NSAIDs counteracted the IL-1–induced suppression of PG synthesis (Fig. 2B,C), or the enhanced PG degradation (data not shown). This agrees with results ob-

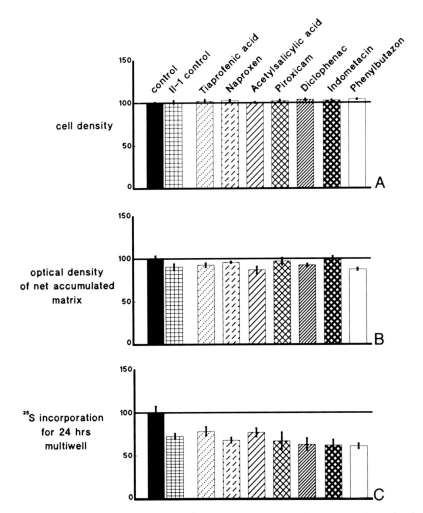

FIG. 2. Proteoglycan metabolism of bovine articular chondrocytes in agarose gels, under chondrocytic chondrolysis and treated with NSAIDs over 8 days. Chondrocytic chondrolysis was induced by 0.05 ng/ml interleukin-1, administered concomitantly with the NSAIDs at a concentration of 10^{-5} M and added anew with each change of medium every second day. Values of optical density for cell proliferation (A) and net matrix accumulation (B), and of [^{35}S]sulfate incorporation into matrix macromolecules (C) are expressed as a percentage of untreated controls. The bars represent standard deviations of sixtets (A) or quadruplets (B,C) per group. **A:** Cell density at the end of the experiment assessed by optical density measurement via inverted microscope, corrected for acellular agarose gel. **B:** Density of the net accumulated PGs retained in the agarose gel, assessed by optical density measurement via inverted microscope after staining with alcian blue. **C:** Proteoglycan (PG) synthesis of chondrocytes in agarose gel at the end of the treatment, assessed by [^{35}S]sulfate incorporation into PG macromolecules, in 24 multiwell cultures.

tained with calf chondrocytes grown in monolayer cultures and treated for 3 days with various NSAIDs (5). The stimulation of neutral proteinase synthesis by IL-1 also was not affected by NSAIDs in cultures of bovine and rabbit cartilage explants (13).

The final concentration of 10^{-5} M for a given drug is considered to be near that reached in the joint under physiological conditions. However, protein-binding characteristics of a drug, its transsynovial/transchondral kinetics, and higher synovial fluid turnover in diseased joints all may change the local concentration normally achieved. We therefore tested two NSAIDs over a broader range of concentrations for their potential effects upon chondrocytic chondrolysis. In the range of concentration from 10^{-7} M to 10^{-3} M, however, neither naproxen, nor tiaprofenic acid (TA) was effective in this model (Fig. 3). Despite a slight dose-dependent increase of ^{35}[S]-incorporation under TA, the IL-1–induced suppression was not reversed. The effect of naproxen was similar, although it actually further inhibited PG synthesis at the unphysiologically high concentration of 10^{-3} M. PG synthesis increased in cultures treated with TA in the absence of IL-1 over a broad range of drug concentration (Table 1), reaching significance at concentrations of 10^{-4} M and 10^{-3} M. The turnover, reflected in the amount retained in the matrix after prelabeling, also was unaffected at therapeutic concentrations, while at the two highest concentrations more matrix was retained than in the untreated control. Similarly, at therapeutically relevant doses, no

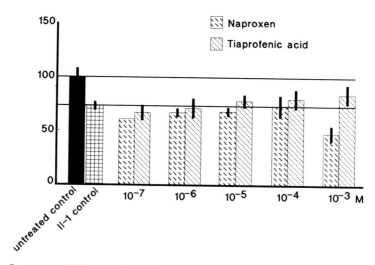

FIG. 3. Dose range of NSAIDs in their effect on proteoglycan synthesis under chondrocytic chondrolysis in bovine articular chondrocytes cultured for 8 days in agarose gel. Chondrocytic chondrolysis was induced by 0.05 ng/ml interleukin-1, administered concomitantly with the NSAIDs at concentrations of 10^{-7} to 10^{-3} M and added anew with each change of medium every second day. Values of [^{35}S]sulfate incorporation into matrix macromolecules at the end of the experiment are expressed as a percentage of untreated controls. The bars represent standard deviations of quadruplets per group.

TABLE 1. *Dose range of tiaprofenic acid in its effect upon proteoglycan metabolism in bovine articular chondrocytes cultured in agarose gels for 8 days*[a]

	Total incorporation	Retained matrix
Untreated control	100 ± 16%	54 ± 8%
Tiaprofenic acid 10^{-7} M	132 ± 19%	62 ± 9%
Tiaprofenic acid 10^{-6} M	112 ± 19%	56 ± 9%
Tiaprofenic acid 10^{-5} M	122 ± 6%	54 ± 3%
Tiaprofenic acid 10^{-4} M	157 ± 3%	67 ± 1%
Tiaprofenic acid 10^{-3} M	161 ± 10%	67 ± 4%

[a] Total incorporation: [^{35}S]sulfate incorporation after 24 hr labeling at day 8. Retained matrix: Remaining [^{35}S]sulfate incorporation around cells at day 8 after prelabeling at day 1.

change in PG turnover occurred in canine cartilage explants (20). Thus, TA does not markedly interfere with the PG metabolism of normal chondrocytes *in vitro* at physiological concentrations, and even at high concentrations, it stimulates PG synthesis and matrix retention rather than exerting harmful effects.

EFFECTS OF TIAPROFENIC ACID UPON HUMAN CHONDROCYTES IN AGAROSE GEL CULTURE

The effects of a drug demonstrated on cultured bovine chondrocytes provide an important indication for efficacy of the drug for human patients, but cannot be regarded as conclusive with respect to human pathology. Since the reactivity of articular chondrocytes varies between species (12), we also tested TA with cultures of human chondrocytes grown in agarose gels. Human articular cartilage was obtained from patients with rheumatoid arthritis (RA) and psoriatic arthritis during synovectomy of the wrist and elbow joints, and specimens from healthy controls were obtained from macroscopically intact femoral condyles and the patello-femoral joint of cadaveric knee joints within 12 hr after death. Cadaveric knee joints with visually detectable changes indicating degenerative joint disease were the source of OA cartilage which was macroscopically graded according to the four-scale grading system by Outerbridge (21).

Articular chondrocytes isolated from healthy cartilage were treated with TA in doses of 10^{-7} M reflecting a low dose concentration, 10^{-5} M reflecting a mean concentration reached in synovial fluid under therapeutic application, and 10^{-4} M reflecting the maximum concentration reached in plasma (22). At 10^{-5} M to 10^{-4} M, TA stimulated [^{35}S]sulfate incorporation in cultures after 1 week of incubation (Fig. 4A). After 2 weeks, this stimulatory effect disappeared at the concentrations relevant to synovial fluid, but it persisted to some degree at the 10^{-4} M dosage (Fig. 4B). These stimulations, then, may be interpreted as initial phenomena, not necessarily prevailing under chronic medication. DNA synthesis (^{3}H thymidine incorporation) in human chondrocytes after drug exposure showed no differences from untreated control at all TA concentrations tested. This indicates that the transient stimulation by TA was not related to an increase in

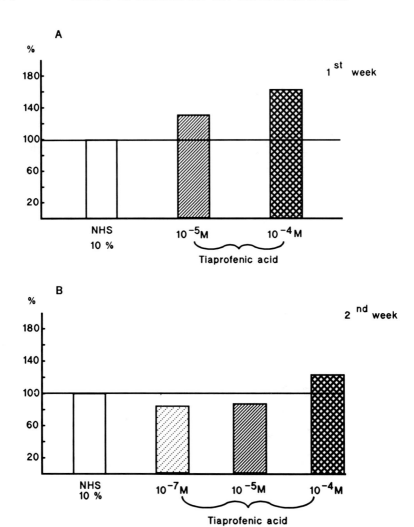

FIG. 4. Effect of tiaprofenic acid (TA) in different concentrations upon proteoglycan synthesis of normal human articular chondrocytes after 1 (**A**) or 2 (**B**) weeks in agarose gel culture. Values of [^{35}S]sulfate incorporation into matrix macromolecules at the end of the experiment are expressed as a percentage of untreated controls. They represent mean values of triplets per group. (NHS, Normal human serum.)

cell proliferation. The responsiveness of chondrocytes to a NSAID may be altered by inflammatory mediators which may be present in SF or serum from rheumatoid arthritis patients (RAS). Therefore the effect of TA under inflammatory conditions was investigated by supplementing the culture medium with 10% RAS or 10% SF instead of with 10% normal human serum (NHS). When healthy human chondrocytes were exposed to RAS, a stimulation of radiosulfate uptake around the cells was observed with most batches of RAS used (23). Addition of

TA adjusted the activity of the cells toward control levels (Fig. 5). Suppression of radiosulfate incorporation was consistently observed with 10% SF. In the experiment presented here, the suppression was to 50% of the control, but this was completely reversed by TA at both concentrations relevant to articular cartilage (Fig. 5). Thus, in both disease-related environments, TA exhibited a compensatory effect on human chondrocytes compared with the untreated controls and health-related culture conditions.

In short-term monolayer cultures, it has been shown that human chondrocytes differ in their reactivity to drugs according to the disease history of their donor

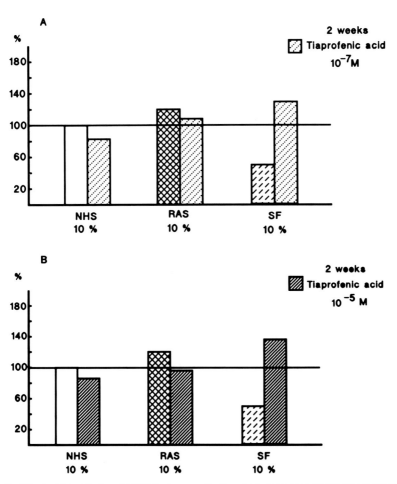

FIG. 5. Effect of tiaprofenic acid (TA) in therapeutically relevant concentrations on proteoglycan synthesis by normal human articular chondrocytes under normal human serum (NHS), serum from rheumatic patients (RAS), or synovial fluid from rheumatic patients (SF) after 2 weeks in agarose gel culture. Values of [^{35}S]sulfate incorporation into matrix macromolecules at the end of the experiment are expressed as a percentage of untreated controls. They represent mean values of triplets per group.

(24). We have found that the differences in metabolism and cell proliferation we observed between human chondrocytes derived from donors with varying disease severity were maintained in long-term agarose gel culture (23). For these reasons we studied the effect of TA on agarose cultures of articular chondrocytes from patients with rheumatic disease. As the samples obtained from rheumatic cartilages were generally small, we investigated drug effects upon PG metabolism exclusively by alcian blue staining which reflects the net amount of PG accu-

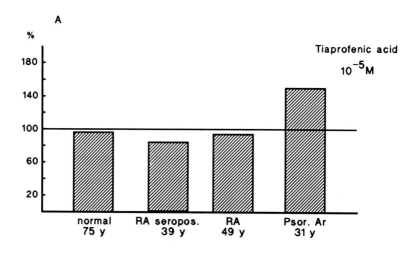

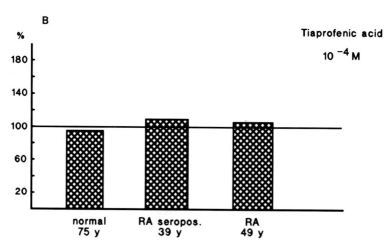

FIG. 6. Effect of tiaprofenic acid (TA) at two concentrations upon net accumulated proteoglycans of normal and rheumatic-patient–derived human articular chondrocytes under 10% normal human serum after 1 week in agarose gel culture. Values of optical density for net matrix accumulation are expressed as a percentage of untreated controls. They represent mean values of triplets per group. (RA, rheumatoid arthritis; Psor. Ar, psoriasis arthritis.)

TABLE 2. *Effect of serum of rheumatic patients (RAS), interleukin-1 (IL-1), and tiaprofenic acid upon proteoglycan synthesis in human articular chondrocytes derived from healthy and osteoarthritic cartilage, and cultured for 8 days in agarose gels[a]*

Treatment	43 y	OA 1.0 79 y	OA 1.5 71 y	OA 2.5 79 y	OA 3.0 87 y
10% NHS	100%	100%	100%	100%	100%
10% RAS	155%	154%	167%	286%	88%
IL-1 5 u/ml	24%	19%	23%	no incorp.	104%
Tiaprofenic acid 10^{-5} M	99%	131%	48%	112%	88%
Tiaprofenic acid 10^{-7} M	146%	143%	79%		
Tiaprofenic acid 10^{-5} M + IL-1	28%	23%	32%	28%	94%
Tiaprofenic acid 10^{-7} M + IL-1	23%	16%	25%	37%	

[a] The ages of the donors are indicated in years (y), and the severity of their osteoarthritis was macroscopically assessed along the 4-scale grading system of Outerbridge (21), with grade 1 indicating light, and grade 4 indicating most severe lesions.
Values of [^{35}S]sulfate incorporation are expressed as a percentage of untreated controls.

mulated over the culture period. In chondrocytes derived from three patients with inflammatory joint disease, incubation with therapeutic concentrations of TA neither altered cell proliferation (data not shown) nor impaired the accumulation of PGs over the culture period (Fig. 6). In the chondrocytes derived from a patient with psoriatic arthritis, TA even increased PG accumulation in comparison with the untreated control (Fig. 6).

Brandt and Slowman-Kovacs have shown that adverse effects of NSAID on cartilage are more marked or even expressed exclusively in OA cartilage (25). We therefore compared healthy chondrocytes with those from cartilage in various stages of OA in terms of their response to TA in the presence and absence of inflammatory mediators (Table 2). TA at therapeutic concentrations was mainly stimulatory, but in one case also suppressed PG synthesis. When administered concomitantly with IL-1, however, TA failed to compensate for the IL-1–induced suppression of PG synthesis in both healthy and diseased chondrocytes. RAS generally induced an increase in [^{35}S]sulfate incorporation, whereas IL-1 generally induced a severe suppression, down to 25% or less of the incorporation of the untreated control. Chondrocytes from the most severe stage of OA did not respond at all to RAS, IL-1, or TA (Table 2).

CONCLUDING REMARKS

We consider the agarose culture system for isolated articular chondrocytes as an appropriate and reproducible system for studying the direct effects of potential disease-modifying agents in the metabolism of these cells. The combination of densitometry and radiolabeling allows an easy distinction between effects on cell proliferation and those upon matrix metabolism, and furnishes additional information about the net accumulation of matrix over the time of incubation. Comparing the agarose gel culture system with explant cultures from the same source of cartilage, the variation is lower in agarose gel cultures. However, effects upon matrix metabolism are more marked in cell culture, probably because chondrocytes show an abnormally high rate of anabolism of matrix macromolecules following their isolation from normal cartilage matrix. While experience gained from experiments on animal cells may provide valuable insights, it may fail to reflect processes driving the human pathology. The data presented here suggest that bovine articular chondrocytes show reactions to mediators and drugs similar to those shown by healthy human chondrocytes, but may differ in respect to those shown by chondrocytes derived from human osteoarthritic cartilage.

NSAIDs, applied at concentrations reached under therapeutic administration, have no effect upon proliferation of cultured isolated chondrocytes. They exert a slightly stimulatory effect, in some cases significantly, upon PG synthesis. However, this was not observed in the explant system, and, at least in human chondrocytes, was not sustained over a longer period of exposure. These kinds of drugs do not overcome the IL-1–induced chondrocytic chondrolysis.

Tiaprofenic acid, a NSAID examined in more detail in this study, apparently exerts no adverse effects upon normal bovine or human chondrocytes, even at unphysiologically high concentrations at which some related drugs suppressed PG synthesis. TA also has no adverse or aggravating effects upon human chondrocytes derived from articular cartilage in various stages of disease. When PG metabolism is altered under disease-related culture conditions as shown by the addition of SF or RAS, no further aberrations were found with TA, and in part, even compensating changes were observed.

The culture of isolated articular chondrocytes within agarose gels is thus a system useful for evaluating mediators and drugs designed for pharmacological intervention of degenerative joint diseases. Although chondrocytes can be readily obtained from animal joints, it is also important to test human chondrocytes from both normal and diseased cartilage since these cells may differ in their sensitivity to the experimental agents. In culture, the chondrocytes can be exposed to concentrations of drugs higher than those which would be achieved clinically, in order to detect potential harmful effects. While it is not possible to simulate the complexity of the environment within the joint, the use of culture systems such as are described here can facilitate the study of multiple interactions between drugs such as NSAIDs and cytokines or growth factors.

ACKNOWLEDGMENTS

The authors wish to thank Irmgard Abt, Rolf Keiffer, Annlaug Oedegard, and Petra Schmidt for their skillful technical assistance, and Roland Röhrig and Hans Wedde for their expert help in preparing the figures.

REFERENCES

1. Aydelotte MB, Schleyerbach R, Zeck B, Kuettner KE. Articular chondrocytes cultured in agarose gel for study of chondrocytic chondrolysis. In: Kuettner KE, Schleyerbach R, Hascall VC, eds. *Articular cartilage biochemistry.* New York; Raven Press, 1985;235–256.

2. Zanetti M, Ratcliffe A, Watt F. Two subpopulations of differentiated chondrocytes identified with a monoclonal antibody to keratan sulfate. *J Cell Biology* 1985;101:53–59.

3. Archer CW, McDowell J, Bayliss MT, Stephens MD, Bentley G. Phenotypic modulation in subpopulations of human articular chondrocytes in vitro. *J Cell Science* 1990;97:361–371.

4a. Aydelotte MB, Kuettner KE. Differences between sub-populations of cultured bovine articular chondrocytes. I. Morphology and cartilage matrix production. *Connect Tissue Res* 1988;18:205–222.

4b. Aydelotte MB, Greenhill RR, Kuettner KE. Differences between sub-populations of cultured bovine articular chondrocytes. II. Proteoglycan metabolism. *Connect Tissue Res* 1988;18:223–234.

5. Kolibas LM, Goldberg RL. Effect of cytokines and anti-arthritic drugs on glycosaminoglycan synthesis by bovine articular chondrocytes. *Agents Actions* 1989;27:245–249.

6. Verbruggen GV, Veys EM, Wieme N, Malfait AM, Gijselbrecht L, Nimmegeers J, Almquist KF, Broddelez C. The synthesis and immobilisation of cartilage-specific proteoglycan by human chondrocytes in different concentrations of agarose. *Clin Exp Rheumatol* 1990;8:371–378.

7. Aulthouse AL, Beck M, Griffey E, Sanford J, Arden K, Machado MA, Horton WA. Expression of the human chondrocyte phenotype in vitro. *In vitro Cell Dev Biol* 1989;25:659–668.

8. Gerstenfeld LC, Kelly CM, von Deck M, Lian JB. Comparative morphological and biochemical analysis of hypertrophic, non-hypertrophic and 1,25(OH₂)D₃ treated non-hypertrophic chondrocytes. *Connect Tissue Res* 1990;24:29–39.

9. Mallein-Gerin F, Ruggiero F, Garrone R. Proteoglycan core protein and type II collagen gene expressions are not correlated with cellshape changes during low density chondrocyte cultures. *Differentiation* 1990;43:204–211.

10. Guo J, Jourdian GW, MacCallum DK. Culture and growth characteristics of chondrocytes encapsulated in alginate beads. *Connect Tissue Res* 1989;19:277–297.

11. Kuettner, Häuselmann, et al. (this volume).

12. Ismaiel S, Hollander AP, Atkins RM, Elson EJ. Differential responses of human and rat cartilage to degrading stimuli in-vitro. *J Pharm Pharmacol* 1991;43:207–209.

13. Arsenis C, McDonnel J. Effects of antirheumatic drugs on the interleukin-1 alpha induced synthesis and activation of proteinases in articular cartilage explants in culture. *Agents Actions* 1989;27:261–264.

14. Stockwell RA. *Biology of cartilage cells.* Cambridge: Cambridge University Press, 1979.

15. Sandell LJ, Daniel JC. Effects of ascorbic acid on collagen mRNA levels in short term chondrocyte cultures. *Connect Tissue Res* 1988;17:11–22.

16. Thonar EJMA, Bjornsson S, Kuettner KE. Age-related changes in cartilage proteoglycans. In: Kuettner KE, Schleyerbach R, Hascall VC, eds. *Articular cartilage biochemistry.* New York: Raven Press, 1985;273–288.

17. Bayliss MT, Hickery MS, Hardingham TE. Effects of IL-1 and TNF-alpha on human articular cartilage: differences in biosynthetic and degradative responses. *37th Annual Meeting, Orthopaedic Research Society,* March 4–7, 1991, Anaheim, California, p. 147.

18. Collier S, Ghosh P. Comparison of the effects of non-steroidal anti-inflammatory drugs (NSAIDs) on proteoglycan synthesis by articular cartilage explant and chondrocyte monolayer cultures. *Biochem Pharmacol* 1991;41:1375–1384.

19. Aydelotte MB, Raiss RX, Caterson B, Kuettner KE. Influence of interleukin-1 on the morphology and proteoglycan metabolism of cultured bovine articular chondrocytes. *Connect Tissue Res* (in press).

20. Muir H, Carney SL, Hall LG. Effects of tiaprofenic acid and other NSAIDs on proteoglycan metabolism in articular cartilage explants. *Drugs* 1988;35(Suppl. 1):15–23.

21. Outerbridge RE. The etiology of chondromalacia patellae. *J Bone Joint Surg* 1961;43B:752–757.

22. Nichol FE, Samanta A, Rose CM. Synovial fluid and plasma kinetics of repeated dose sustained action tiaprofenic acid in patients with rheumatoid arthritis. *Drugs* 1988;35(Suppl. 1):46–51.

23. Verbruggen G, Veys EM, Wieme N, Malfait AM, Gijselbrecht L, Nimmegeers J, Almquist KF,

Broddelez C. The synthesis and immobilization of cartilage-specific proteoglycan by human chondrocytes in different concentrations of agarose. *Clin Exp Rheumatol* 1990;8:371–378.

24. Oestensen M, Veiby OP, Raiss RX, Hagen A, Pahle J. Responses of normal and rheumatic human articular chondrocytes cultured under various culture conditions in agarose gel. *Scan J Rheumatol* 1991;20:172–182.

25. Brandt KD, Slowman-Kovacs S. Nonsteroidal antiinflammatory drugs in treatment of osteoarthritis. *Clin Orthop* 1986;213:84–91.

DISCUSSION

von der Mark: Your studies appeared to show that the NSAID tiaprofenic acid can stimulate proteoglycan synthesis somewhat above control levels in the agarose-chondrocyte cultures. Does this indicate improvement in terms of the physiological situation?

Raiss: I would not go that far. I think that these cells in this agarose system are more active and more prone to modification than they are in the explant system anyway. Thus, effects which we see in our cultures might be less marked in the explant system which may be closer to the actual physiological situation.

Lust: We studied the effect of Arteparone on chondrocyte monolayer cultures, which differ from your agarose-chondrocyte cultures. We saw an increase in the rate of fibronectin synthesis and in the content of fibronectin, an effect we did not see *in vivo*. It may be, however, that Arteparone does not get into the cartilage. It would be interesting to see if your cultures respond differently.

van den Berg: How does tiaprofenic acid affect proteoglycan degradation in your cultures?

Raiss: We tested this in pulse-chase experiments and saw no differences between normal and tiaprofenic acid-treated cultures. The drug did not prevent IL-1–induced degradation either.

Articular Cartilage and Osteoarthritis,
edited by K. Kuettner et al.
Raven Press, Ltd., New York © 1992.

41

Drug Evaluation on Normal and Arthritic Mouse Patellas

Wim B. van den Berg, Leo A. B. Joosten, Fons A. J. van de Loo,
Ben J. de Vries, Peter M. van der Kraan, and Elly L. Vitters

*Department of Rheumatology, University Hospital Nijmegen,
6525 GA Nijmegen, The Netherlands*

Cartilage destruction is a common feature in patients with rheumatoid arthritis (RA) or osteoarthritis (OA). In both diseases, depletion of the cartilage matrix is observed, and at later stages a total disruption of the matrix structure may occur, leading to irreversible joint damage. Enhanced degradation of cartilage proteoglycans is found in both rheumatoid arthritis and osteoarthritis. In contrast, proteoglycan (PG) synthesis is markedly inhibited during experimental joint inflammation (arthritis), whereas PG synthesis is stimulated in osteoarthritis, at least in the early stages of the disease. It is believed that the high amounts of proteoglycans synthesized are not properly incorporated in the matrix in the latter situation. Although the features of cartilage pathology are well characterized in both the human situation and experimental animal models, the exact mechanisms underlying cartilage destruction are still largely unknown. Treatment is therefore mainly symptomatic and may perhaps not even affect the underlying destructive process.

Nonsteroidal antiinflammatory drugs (NSAIDs) produce symptomatic improvement in terms of pain relief and better mobility. Steroids are clearly antiinflammatory, but their use in daily clinical practice is still controversial, mainly because of the fear of serious side effects on the articular cartilage. In recent years it has become clear that several NSAIDs may also have harmful side effects on cartilage. Initial studies by Palmoski and Brandt (1,2) showed that salicylates and some other NSAIDs suppress cartilage proteoglycan synthesis. Furthermore, this effect appeared much greater on OA cartilage compared to normal cartilage. It is still unclear whether the deterioration of cartilage damage in OA models by certain NSAIDs is due to the higher susceptibility of OA cartilage or to overuse of damaged joints after pain relief.

In RA the effect of antiinflammatory drugs on the articular cartilage may be two-fold: suppression of inflammation, with concomitant relief of inflammation-mediated damage to the cartilage, and direct side effects on the cartilage, which may potentially be higher on arthritic versus normal cartilage.

In this chapter we review the impact of NSAIDs and steroids on articular cartilage under various experimental conditions. When cartilage is studied under conditions of experimental joint inflammation, it is referred to here as arthritic cartilage. Cartilage taken from (models of) osteoarthritis is termed osteoarthritic (OA) cartilage throughout. Discussion of disease modifiers, used in the treatment of RA, is beyond the scope of this review.

INFLUENCE OF NSAIDs ON ARTICULAR CARTILAGE *IN VITRO*

Plain organ cultures of slices of canine articular cartilage were used to show that several NSAIDs (e.g., salicylates, fenoprofen, and isoxicam) inhibited net proteoglycan (PG) synthesis. In contrast, drugs like indomethacin, piroxicam, and diclofenac appeared to have no effect. The augmented synthesis of PG in cartilage slices from OA dogs was suppressed by salicylate to a much greater extent, and suppressive effects were then also noted with indomethacin (1,2). Using intact murine patellas, we confirmed the suppressive effect of salicylate (3,4), but this was blocked when high amounts of serum were used in the culture medium. The latter finding questions the relevance *in vivo* of data from culture systems in which low amounts of serum were used. Recent studies with the new drug Tenidap showed a similar trend: significant suppression of PG synthesis *in vitro* at therapeutic concentrations, which was abolished with 30 to 100% serum. Thorough screening *in vivo* did not show any disturbance of chondrocyte synthetic function when Tenidap was applied at therapeutic concentrations for several weeks (unpublished observations).

Apart from plain cartilage cultures, numerous studies have been performed in cocultures of cartilage with inflamed synovium, or with passively added destructive inflammatory mediators such as interleukin-1 (IL-1α,β). NSAIDs do not block IL-1 biosynthesis or IL-1 action on the articular cartilage (5–7), with the potential exception of Tiaprofenic acid. It has been claimed that this drug suppresses IL-1–mediated cartilage degradation (8). Steroids do not interfere with IL-1 action, but are potent inhibitors of IL-1 production.

INFLUENCE OF NSAIDS ON CARTILAGE
PG SYNTHESIS *IN VIVO*

Apart from direct effects on the chondrocyte, drugs may exert effects on systemic factors *in vivo*, e.g., the sulfate concentration, and this may have a direct impact on cartilage metabolism. It will be clear that such effects will be overlooked when only drug screening *in vitro* is performed. We have shown that the suppressive effect of salicylate on PG synthesis in the mouse is mainly due to its potential ability to deplete sulfate (9). Similar observations have been done for paracetamol in the rat. The latter drug has no direct effect on cartilage metabolism *in vitro*. However, PG synthesis was markedly suppressed *in vivo*, and this was related to the degree of sulfate depletion. The mechanism of sulfate depletion is linked to sulfate conjugation of paracetamol by liver enzymes. Prolonged paracetamol treatment resulted in significant PG depletion in the articular cartilage (10).

We investigated the sulfate-depleting potential of a series of drugs (11), and also examined the threshold levels that result in either suppression of PG synthesis or undersulfation of PGs. The latter appeared to occur only under extreme sulfate depletion (12,13), and is therefore not physiologically relevant after drug treatment. Inhibition of synthesis of normal PGs consistently occurs after 50% reduction of normal sulfate levels. This was found for patellar cartilage from different species and slices from human cartilage, cultured at increasing sulfate concentrations ranging from 0 to 1 mM. Interestingly, only the rate of sulfated glycosaminoglycan (GAG) synthesis in human cartilage appeared rather sensitive to *small* deviations from the physiological sulfate concentration. Sulfate dependence appeared to be similar for normal, arthritic, and osteoarthritic cartilage (14).

In contrast to the studies with isolated cartilage *in vitro*, the studies *in vivo* are always a mix of direct and indirect effects, e.g., on systemic factors or on the inflammatory process in the joint. To avoid this complexity and to clarify conclusions, many researchers do favor studies *in vitro*. However, when drug effects are screened *in vitro* on a piece of cartilage taken from a diseased joint, part of the control of chondrocyte metabolism occurs in an autocrine fashion, and the experiments are complicated anyway by cytokines, growth factors, and enzymes, which are produced/activated within the cartilage matrix.

SUSCEPTIBILITY OF ARTHRITIC CARTILAGE

As noted above, salicylate had a more pronounced suppressive effect on proteoglycan synthesis in osteoarthritic compared to normal cartilage. This could be related to changes in the matrix resulting in a different penetration of the drugs, or to a changed susceptibility of osteoarthritic chondrocytes. A recent study using isolated chondrocytes from osteoarthritic cartilage did not provide evidence for the latter possibility (15), but it can not be excluded that specific properties have been lost during isolation and subsequent culture. In addition, experiments related to the diminished proteoglycan content of the matrix were performed. Greater drug effects were noted in cartilage from unloaded compared to loaded regions, and in enzymatically PG-depleted cartilage (16). However, partition measurements did not yield conclusive data on enhanced drug uptake. It seems unlikely that the uptake of low molecular weight drugs is heavily influenced by the matrix unless serum proteins function as drug carriers within the matrix.

Using arthritic patellar cartilage taken from zymosan-induced joint inflammation, we could not find enhanced susceptibility to NSAIDs in short-term culture studies (17). In contrast to the situation in osteoarthritic cartilage, proteoglycan synthesis is already markedly suppressed (50%) shortly after induction of joint inflammation. Salicylate had no greater impact on chondrocyte synthetic function in this cartilage. Tiaprofenic acid and piroxicam remained without effect. Prednisolone, without effect on normal cartilage, significantly enhanced PG synthesis in arthritic cartilage, probably due to its potent antiinflammatory action and therefore relief of inflammation-mediated suppression.

In patellar cartilage taken several weeks after induction of zymosan arthritis, PG synthesis had increased to 150% in an attempt to restore the depleted matrix, but enhanced susceptibility to adverse drug effects was not found in this cartilage.

EFFECTS ON PG DEGRADATION

Most studies on adverse drug effects have been done on PG synthesis, probably related to the fact that synthesis can be measured easily by radiolabel uptake. Moreover, the first claims of adverse effects of NSAIDs were on synthesis and not on degradation. Salicylate, for example, had a clear-cut suppressive effect on PG synthesis, but the rate of catabolism of PG in normal canine cartilage was unaffected (16). It should be emphasized that the maintenance of an intact matrix depends on the delicate balance of both synthesis and breakdown (17,18). As a parameter of proteoglycan turnover, we measured the loss of ^{35}[S]sulfate from prelabeled murine patellae *in vivo* under normal and inflamed conditions. Turnover is high in young mice (30–40% loss of ^{35}[S]PG in 2 days), and degradation is markedly enhanced (20–40%) after induction of zymosan arthritis. This provides a sensitive screening system to measure potential protective action of drugs on both basal and stimulated breakdown. Of the NSAIDs tested, only tiaprofenic acid significantly suppressed loss of prelabeled PG (Table 1). In addition, prednisolone significantly inhibited the enhanced degradation in the arthritic joint.

A similar potential was noted by Pelletier et al. (8), who showed that both Tiaprofenic acid and hydrocortisone suppressed proteoglycan catabolism in human OA cartilage *in vitro*. They claimed that the mechanism could be related to reduction in synthesis of neutral metalloproteases. Recent data from our laboratory indicate that proteoglycan turnover in our murine patella *in vitro* is under stringent control of insulin-like growth factor (IGF-1). In line with earlier observations in bovine explants, IGF-1 appeared to be the main anabolic factor controlling PG synthesis in murine patellas, but it is also a very potent inhibitor of PG loss (19–21). In the absence of IGF-1, steroids seem to mimic IGF effects on catabolism. However, this observation should be considered tentative since

TABLE 1. *Degradation of [35S]prelabeled PG in vivo*

Drug twice daily	Dose mg/kg	[35S]content in patellar cartilage (%)	
		Normal	Arthritic
—	—	71 + 14	48 + 12
Salicylate	200	70 + 7	45 + 7
Tiaprofenic acid	16	90 + 21[a]	69 + 22[a]
Piroxicam	10	73 + 21	45 + 12
Prednisolone	1	86 + 26	58 + 13*

[a] Significantly different from the control group ($p < 0.01$).
Data represent the mean + SD of patellae obtained from at least 10 mice with unilateral zymosan arthritis. Mice were prelabeled by i.p. injection of [35S]sulfate (2 uCi/g) at day −1, arthritis was induced in one knee joint, and patellae were isolated 2 days later. Drugs were given twice a day, starting at −8 hr. [35S]content is expressed as a percentage from the amount present at day 0.

the mechanism is unknown. It is a given that proteoglycan catabolism requires metabolically active chondrocytes, and any nonspecific inhibitor may well reduce catabolism.

EFFECT OF NSAIDs ON CARTILAGE DESTRUCTION IN ANTIGEN-INDUCED ARTHRITIS

The best net effect of NSAIDs on normal and arthritic cartilage can be obtained after prolonged treatment in an animal model. We induced unilateral murine antigen-induced arthritis (AIA) by intraarticular antigen injection into the knee joint of preimmunized animals. This is a model of allergic arthritis and it has many features in common with RA. Cartilage destruction is characterized by enhanced degradation of PG and inhibited PG synthesis. NSAIDs were given twice a day from the onset of arthritis. All drugs tested significantly suppressed edema formation, and slight effects were also noted on cellular infiltration (22,23). However, cartilage damage was unchanged. Inhibition of chondrocyte PG synthesis was similar in the control and drug-treated animals, and no change in the degree of proteoglycan loss was noted (Fig. 1). Either the NSAIDs lack a specific influence on a particular destructive process in this model, or the overall effect is a balance between inhibition of inflammation-mediated cartilage damage and direct adverse drug effects on the chondrocyte. We did not observe any adverse drug actions on the cartilage of the contralateral normal joint in these experiments, and other studies (see above) could not provide evidence for enhanced susceptibility of arthritic chondrocytes. This suggests that NSAIDs have an impact on some parameters of the inflammatory process, but apparently leave the underlying cartilage destructive process untouched.

In a separate series of experiments, we investigated further the mechanism and possible mediators involved in cartilage destruction in AIA. Granulocytes

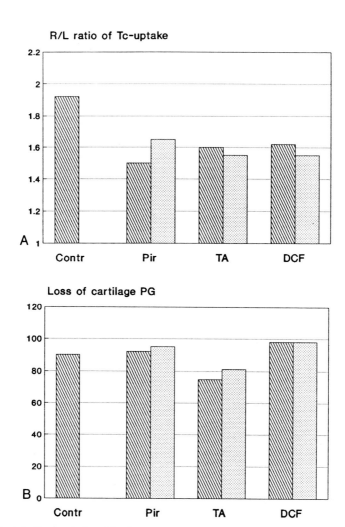

FIG. 1. A: Arthritis was induced in the right knee joint by intraarticular injection of mBSA in preimmunized mice. Groups of at least seven mice were treated twice daily with NSAIDs: piroxicam (2.5 and 7.5 mg/kg); tiaprofenic acid (10 and 30 mg/kg); diclofenac (2.5 and 7.5 mg/kg). Edema was measured at day 4 by 99mTechnetium uptake, and proteoglycan loss was scored at day 7 by loss of staining in the patellar cartilage (joint sections). **B:** Significant suppression of edema was found for all drug doses (*dotted bars* represent the highest dose), but significant changes in PG depletion were not seen.

appeared of minor importance and evidence has recently been obtained suggesting that IL-1 is a key mediator. Inhibition of chondrocyte proteoglycan synthesis could be abolished by treatment with neutralizing anti-IL-1ab antibodies (Fig. 2), and cartilage proteoglycan depletion was markedly reduced (24–26). The latter is a combination of enhanced proteoglycan breakdown and inhibited synthesis. Although a key role of IL-1 in degradation is not proven, the restoration

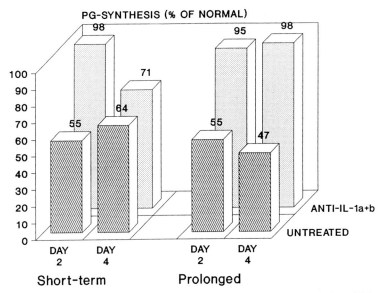

PG-SYNTHESIS (% OF NORMAL)

FIG. 2. Arthritis was induced in the right knee joint by intraarticular injection of mBSA in preimmunized mice. Treatment with anti–IL-1ab serum was given at day −2 (short-term) or again at day 0 and day 2 (prolonged protocol). The control group received nonrelevant antiserum. Patellae were isolated, and PG synthesis in the arthritic patella was expressed relative to the contralateral control. Anti–IL-1 treatment markedly abolished PG synthesis inhibition at day 2, and suppression was evident on day 4 in the short term protocol (lack of neutralizing capacity), but could be totally prevented upon prolonged antiserum treatment.

of PG synthesis appeared to be of major importance in the high turnover cartilage matrix of the murine patella.

As discussed above, common NSAIDs have no direct effect on IL-1–mediated cartilage damage, and this seems to explain the lack of protection within AIA. As an exception, tiaprofenic acid was noted to suppress PG degradation, but was essentially neutral in action on cartilage destruction in AIA, which seems contradictory. However, many NSAIDs are potent inhibitors of prostaglandin production, and prostaglandin E2 is known to suppress the production of IL-1 by mononuclear cells. In fact, it has been claimed that indomethacin aggravates cartilage destruction in AIA (27), and this could well be related to enhanced generation of IL-1. Moreover, NSAIDs may interfere with IL-1 inhibitor production (28,29), which further complicates the expected overall impact on articular cartilage.

EFFECT OF STEROIDS ON CARTILAGE DESTRUCTION IN AIA

Claims have been made that corticosteroids may cause severe cartilage degeneration in normal joints. Marked suppression of proteoglycan synthesis by chondrocytes was noted and oral or intraarticular steroid treatments may worsen OA cartilage lesions (30). However, many of the early studies used very high doses of oral steroids or repeated local injections and the clinical relevance of these observations is questionable. More recent studies using careful experimental conditions and therapeutic dose regimens revealed efficacy of steroid injections in relieving OA symptoms as well as cartilage damage (31).

We examined the effect of local depot preparations (prolonged steroid release) on chondrocyte function in normal and arthritic murine joints, using therapeutic antiinflammatory dosages. Single injections of rimexolone or triamcinolone hexacetonide (THA) markedly suppressed proteoglycan synthesis in normal patellas (up to 40%), and this effect may last several weeks (32). However, when THA was given in arthritic joints, e.g., at day 3 after arthritis induction, the inflammation-mediated suppression of PG synthesis was readily abolished (Fig. 3). The fact that chondrocyte synthetic function returns to normal values may reflect that the chondrocytes in the arthritic cartilage, which is markedly depleted at that time point, are in essence prone to shift to highly enhanced synthesis (overshoot) at the moment that the suppressive inflammatory mediators are blocked by the steroid. In combination with the adverse effect of steroids on PG synthesis, the net effect will go down from the expected overshoot to normal values. Another intriguing possibility would be that arthritic chondrocytes are rather insensitive to the adverse effect of steroids, related to reduced receptor expression.

Recent observations in OA cartilage have demonstrated markedly reduced numbers of steroid receptors (33), and we are actually looking at steroid receptors

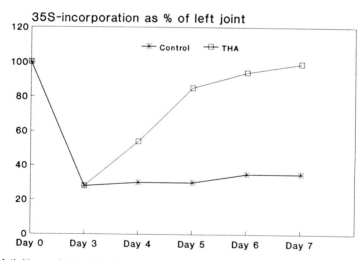

FIG. 3. Arthritis was induced in the right knee joint by intraarticular injection of mBSA in preimmunized mice. At day 3 triamcinolone hexacetonide (THA, 25 μg) was injected into the right arthritic knee. The control group received saline. Patellae were isolated at various days and chondrocyte proteoglycan synthesis was assessed by a 3 hr pulse with ^{35}[S]sulfate *ex vivo*. Incorporation is expressed as percentage of the left patella.

in chondrocytes from arthritic cartilage. In conclusion, the net effect of steroid treatment seems beneficial to the arthritic cartilage, and this urges a reappraisal of careful steroid regimes in the treatment of both RA and OA.

To further examine whether chondrocyte synthetic function in arthritic cartilage is really normalized after steroid treatment, we screened the responsiveness to IGF-1 and the chromatographic pattern of newly synthesized, radiolabeled PG. Figure 4 shows the well-known IGF nonresponsiveness in arthritic cartilage upon 24 hr culture *ex vivo* (34,35). PG synthesis in normal patellar cartilage is markedly reduced within 24 hr in the absence of IGF-1, but can easily be stimulated above the original synthetic rate by IGF-1. Arthritic cartilage lacks this latter responsiveness. The THA-treated cartilage shows a normal reaction pattern to IGF-1.

Chromatography was performed of radiolabeled PG which was extracted from cartilage, incubated for 3 hr with ^{35}[S]sulfate, followed by a 24 hr chase. In the absence of IGF-1, around 40% of the labeled PG is lost from the cartilage during a 24 hr chase, compared to 10% in the presence of IGF-1. The latter value is in agreement with the rate of loss of radiolabeled PG. *in vivo.* Fig. 5A verifies that IGF-1 is highly essential in this chase period to maintain both a normal rate of loss of PGs and a normal structure of retained PG. Proteoglycans from the arthritic cartilage, treated with THA *in vivo,* show a nearly identical pattern compared to control cartilage processed in the presence of IGF-1. This illustrates

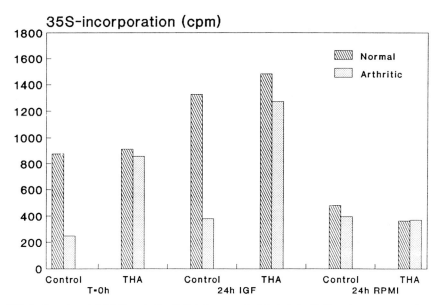

FIG. 4. Experimental details as in Fig. 3. Patellae were isolated at day 7. Chondrocyte proteoglycan synthesis was assessed by a 3 hr pulse with ^{35}[S]sulfate *ex vivo,* either directly after isolation (t = 0 hr) or after a 24-hr culture period in the presence or absence of IGF-1.

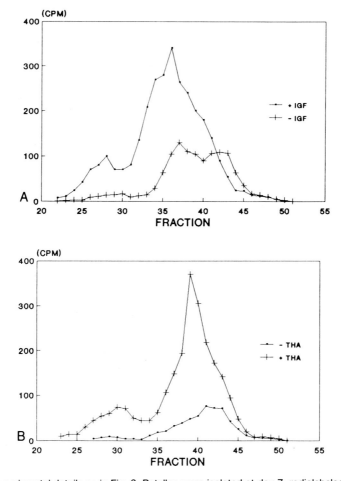

FIG. 5. Experimental details as in Fig. 3. Patellae were isolated at day 7, radiolabeled by a 4 hr pulse with [35][S]sulfate and chased for 24 hr in the presence or absence of IGF-1. Thereafter proteoglycans were extracted and applied on a Sephacryl S-1000 column under associative conditions. **A:** Normal cartilage. **B:** Arthritic cartilage treated at day 3 with or without THA (processing with IGF-1). Bovine proteoglycans were added as a carrier and showed consistent patterns after each run.

recovery of IGF-1 responsiveness not only with regard to PG synthesis, but also with regard to degradation. The pattern in the arthritic control cartilage points to severe degradation, and this may perhaps also reflect the IGF-1 nonresponsiveness. For logistic reasons, chromatography with murine articular cartilage PG has received little attention up to now, and good reference material is lacking. Profiles after various chase periods are presently under study.

CONCLUSION

Common NSAIDs like piroxicam, diclofenac, and tiaprofenic acid lack the adverse effect as noted for salicylate on chondrocyte proteoglycan synthesis. It seems obvious that newer drugs will be routinely screened for this potential and become more attractive if this side effect on cartilage is absent. A first screen can be done on slices or even isolated chondrocytes, but it must be clear from this review that potential drug actions on systemic factors can be easily overlooked, that it is essential to determine the impact on both synthesis and degradation, and that the most relevant information still has to come from the net effect in an animal model. In fact, as demonstrated for corticosteroids, a drug with marked side effects on chondrocytes can still be of great value in arthritic conditions, and it would be a pity if newer drugs do not even stand the chance to be screened *in vivo* because they show an adverse effect at an early stage on one aspect of chondrocyte metabolism. If NSAIDs are given just as analgesics, it should be clear that any side effect on cartilage is unwanted.

Apart from NSAIDs, much interest has recently been focused on so-called chondroprotective drugs like Rumalon or Arteparone, or the therapeutic potential of growth factors. It remains to be seen whether there is a place for the latter therapy. In arthritis we found IGF-1 nonresponsiveness, making mere addition of IGF-1 senseless. Another likely candidate, TGFb, is now under study in many laboratories. An important breakthrough in chondroprotective therapy must await a more detailed understanding of the exact mechanism of cartilage destruction in the various arthritic conditions.

It has been claimed that IL-1 is a key mediator in both OA and RA, but some contradictory findings make it unlikely that chondroprotective therapy should be similar in both diseases. IL-1 inhibits proteoglycan synthesis in articular cartilage, whereas synthesis is enhanced in early OA. Moreover, Tiaprofenic acid shows efficacy in OA models, but is essentially without effect on cartilage destruction in allergic arthritis. Studies with selective drugs/inhibitors in the various models are warranted to yield further insight into the underlying destructive processes.

REFERENCES

1. Palmoski MJ, Brandt KD. Effect of some nonsteroidal antiinflammatory drugs on proteoglycan metabolism and organization in canine articular cartilage. *Arthritis Rheum* 1980;23:1010–1020.
2. Palmoski MJ, Colyer R, Brandt KD. Marked suppression by salicylate of the augmented proteoglycan synthesis in osteoarthritis cartilage. *Arthritis Rheum* 1980;23:83–91.
3. van den Berg WB, Kruysen MWM, van de Putte LBA. The mouse patella assay. An easy method of quantifying articular cartilage chondrocyte function in vivo and in vitro. *Rheumatol Int* 1982;1: 165–169.
4. de Vries BJ, van den Berg WB, Vitters E, van de Putte LBA. The effect of salicylate on anatomically intact articular cartilage is influenced by sulfate and serum in the culture medium. *J Rheumatol* 1986;13:686–693.

5. Rainsford KD. Effects of antiinflammatory drugs on IL-1 induced cartilage proteoglycan resorption in vitro. *J Pharm Pharmacol* 1989;41:112–117.

6. Arner EC, Pratta MA. Independent effects of IL-1 on proteoglycan breakdown, proteoglycan synthesis and prostaglandin E2 release from cartilage in organ culture. *Arthritis Rheum* 1989;32: 288–297.

7. Arsenis C, McDonnell J. Effects of antirheumatic drugs on the IL-1α-induced synthesis and activation of proteinases in articular cartilage explants in culture. *Agents Actions* 1989;27:261–264.

8. Pelletier JP, Cloutier JM, Martel-Pelletier J. In vitro effects of Tiaprofenic acid, sodium salicylate and hydrocortisone on the proteoglycan metabolism of human osteoarthritic cartilage. *J Rheumatol* 1989;16:646–655.

9. de Vries BJ, van den Berg WB, van de Putte LBA. Salicylate induced depletion of endogenous inorganic sulfate. Potential role in the suppression of sulfated glycosaminoglycan synthesis in murine articular cartilage. *Arthritis Rheum* 1985;28:922–929.

10. van der Kraan PM, Vitters E, de Vries BJ, van den Berg WB, van de Putte LBA. The effect of chronic paracetamol administration to rats on the glycosaminoglycan content of patellar cartilage. *Agents Actions* 1990;29:218–223.

11. de Vries BJ, van der Kraan PM, van den Berg WB. Decrease of inorganic blood sulfate following treatment with selected antirheumatic drugs: potential consequence for articular cartilage. *Agents Actions* 1990;29:224–231.

12. van der Kraan PM, de Vries BJ, Vitters EL, van den Berg WB, van de Putte LBA. The effect of low sulfate concentrations on the glycosaminoglycan synthesis in anatomically intact cartilage of the mouse. *J Orthop Res* 1989;7:645–653.

13. Sobue M, Takeuchi J, Ito K, Kimata K, Suzuki S. Effect of environmental sulfate concentration on the synthesis of low and high sulfated chondroitin sulfates by chick embryo cartilage. *J Biol Chem* 1978;253:6190–6196.

14. van der Kraan PM, Vitters EL, de Vries BJ, van den Berg WB. High susceptibility of human articular cartilage glycosaminoglycan synthesis to changes in inorganic sulfate availability. *J Orthop Res* 1990;8:565–571.

15. Slowman-Kovacs SD, Albrecht ME, Brandt KD. Effects of salicylate on chondrocytes from osteoarthritic and contralateral knees of dogs with unilateral anterior cruciate ligament transection. *Arthritis Rheum* 1989;32:486–490.

16. Brandt KD. Effects of nonsteroidal anti-inflammatory drugs on chondrocyte metabolism in vitro and in vivo. *Am J Med* 1987;83(Suppl. 5A):29–34.

17. de Vries BJ, van den Berg WB, Vitters E, van de Putte LBA. Effects of NSAIDs on the metabolism of sulfated glycosaminoglycans in healthy and (post)arthritic murine articular cartilage. *Drugs* 1988;35(Suppl. 1):24–32.

18. Ghosh P. Therapeutic modulation of cartilage catabolism by nonsteroidal antiinflammatory drugs in arthritis. *Semin Arthritis Rheum* 1989;18(Suppl. 1):2–6.

19. McQuillan DJ, Handley CJ, Campbell MA, Bolis S, Milway VE, Herington AC. Stimulation of proteoglycan biosynthesis by serum and IGF-1 in cultured bovine articular cartilage. *Biochem J* 1986;240:423–430.

20. Luyten FP, Hascall VC, Nissley SP, Morales TI, Reddi AH. Insuline like growth factors maintain steady-state metabolism of proteoglycans in bovine articular cartilage explants. *Arch Biochem Biophys* 1988;267:416–425.

21. Schalkwijk J, Joosten LAB, van den Berg WB, van Wijk JJ, van de Putte LBA. Insuline like growth factor stimulation of chondrocyte proteoglycan synthesis by human synovial fluid. *Arthritis Rheum* 1989;32:66–71.

22. de Vries BJ, van den Berg WB. Impact of NSAIDs on murine antigen induced arthritis. I. An investigation of antiinflammatory and chondroprotective effects. *J Rheumatol* 1989;16(Suppl. 18):10–18.

23. de Vries BJ, van den Berg WB. Impact of NSAIDs on murine antigen induced arthritis. II. A light microscopic investigation of antiinflammatory and bone protective effects. *J Rheumatol* 1990;17:295–303.

24. van de Loo AAJ, van den Berg WB. Effects of murine recombinant IL-1 on synovial joints in mice: quantification of patellar cartilage metabolism and joint inflammation. *Ann Rheum Dis* 1990;49:238–245.

25. van den Berg WB. Impact of NSAIDs and steroids on cartilage destruction in murine antigen induced arthritis. *J Rheumatol* 1991;18(Suppl. 27):122–123.
26. van de Loo AAJ, Arntz OJ, Otterness IG, van den Berg WB. Protection against cartilage proteoglycan synthesis inhibition by anti-IL-1 antibodies in experimental arthritis. *J Rheumatol,* (in press).
27. Pettipher ER, Henderson B, Edwards JCW, Higgs GA. Effect of indomethacin on swelling, lymphocyte influx, and cartilage proteoglycan depletion in experimental arthritis. *Ann Rheum Dis* 1989;48:623–627.
28. Herman JH, Appel AM, Khosla RC, Hess EV. In vitro effect of select nonsteroidal antiinflammatory drugs on the synthesis and activity of anabolic regulatory factors produced by osteoarthritic and rheumatoid synovial tissue. *J Rheumatol* 1989;16:75–81.
29. Herman JH, Sowder WG, Hess EV. NSAID induction of IL-1/catabolin inhibitor production by OA synovial tissue. *J Rheumatol* 1991;18(Suppl. 27):124–126.
30. Pelletier JP, Martel-Pelletier J. The therapeutic effects of NSAID and corticosteroids in OA: to be or not to be (Editorial). *J Rheumatol* 1989;16:266–269.
31. Pelletier JP, Martel-Pelletier J. Protective effects of corticosteroids on cartilage lesions and osteophyte formation in the Pond-Nuki dog model of OA. *Arthritis Rheum* 1989;32:181–193.
32. Joosten LAB, Helsen MMA, van den Berg WB. Protective effect of Rimexolone on cartilage damage in arthritic mice: a comparative study with Triamcinolone Hexacetonide. *Agents Actions* 1990;31:135–142.
33. DiBattista JA, Martel-Pelletier J, Cloutier JM, Pelletier JP. Modulation of glucocorticoid receptor expression in human articular chondrocytes by cAMP and prostaglandins. *J Rheumatol* 1991;18(Suppl. 27):102–105.
34. Schalkwijk J, Joosten LAB, van den Berg WB, van de Putte LBA. Chondrocyte nonresponsiveness to IGF-1 in experimental arthritis. *Arthritis Rheum* 1989;32:894–900.
35. van den Berg WB, Joosten LAB, Schalkwijk J, van de Loo AAJ, van Beuningen HM. Mechanisms of cartilage destruction in experimental arthritis: lack of IGF-1 responsiveness. In: Lewis AJ, Doherty NS, Ackerman NR, eds. *Therapeutic approaches to inflammatory diseases,* New York: Elsevier Science, 1989:47–54.

DISCUSSION

Brune: Steroids are less catabolic in rodents. It is possible that the beneficial effects of steroids you observe in your mouse system may not be easily transferred to the human situation.

van den Berg: I hope you are not correct. Although steroids clearly inhibit proteoglycan synthesis in normal mouse cartilage, they also block normal degradation. When the total balance of degradation and synthesis is taken into account, there is only a slight overall negative effect. As for a potential beneficial role in human, work by Pelletier with human OA cartilage explants also showed some positive effects of steroids.

Benya: In your antigen-induced arthritis, why do the mice respond to the steroids but not to IGF-1?

van den Berg: The steroids probably block the inflammatory process by interfering with all kind of mediators including the ones causing IGF-1 nonresponsiveness. The latter phenomenon is not simply related to IL-1. If IL-1 is injected into a joint, proteoglycan synthesis is inhibited, but normal responsiveness to IGF-1 is maintained. In the antigen-induced arthritis, enzymes released from either granulocytes or macrophages may degrade IGF-1 receptors on chondrocytes.

Tyler: You observed a lack of response to IGF-1 when you put the antigen-induced arthritic patellae into culture. Do they recover responsiveness if you leave them in culture?

van den Berg: No, they do not, at least not within 2 days. Initial experiments with

TGF-beta have not stimulated recovery of IGF responsiveness either. So the culture system seems to lack specific factors needed for full recovery.

Dreher: Your model is a nonerosive one. The cartilage is not destroyed and will recover within 2 or 3 weeks. How can you equate results in this acute inflammation model with osteoarthritis or rheumatoid arthritis?

van den Berg: I agree that it is not a model for osteoarthritis, and that we should be careful extrapolating findings in these models to human diseases. This model can be chronic if the right antigens are used. When we use cationic antigens in hyperimmune animals, a T-cell–driven process is elicited which causes chronic progression of the disease and irreversible damage to chondrocytes and cartilage.

Articular Cartilage and Osteoarthritis,
edited by K. Kuettner et al.
Raven Press, Ltd., New York © 1992.

42

The Potential of Cartilage Markers in Joint Fluid for Drug Evaluation

Masayuki Shinmei,* Yasuaki Inamori,* Yasuo Yoshihara,*
Toshiyuki Kikuchi,* and Taro Hayakawa†

*Department of Orthopedic Surgery, National Defense Medical College,
Tokorozawa, Saitama, 359, Japan; †Department of Biochemistry, School of Dentistry,
Aichi-Gakuin University, Chigusa-ku, Nagoya, Aichi, 464, Japan*

The destruction of articular cartilage and loss of joint function is a common and most crucial terminal pathway in any kind of arthritides. In spite of recent rapid progress in technologies for diagnosing and treating the arthritides, it is very hard to recognize subtle changes in either disease progression or improvement without using invasive methods, arthrotomy, or arthroscopy. Of the noninvasive procedures, only high resolution magnetic resonance imaging (MRI) can be expected to detect variations in cartilage thickness and focal defects of the order of 1 mm (1). However, MRI instrumentation is very expensive, and the number of patients which can be assessed in a day is limited. Under such circumstances, the attempt to discover macromolecules which are specific and sensitive markers for degeneration and repair processes of cartilage and to develop reliable assay kits for these molecules is a most challenging problem. In addition, the quantification of these marker molecules in body fluids has much greater advantages for multiple assessments in patients and may be less expensive. What kinds of macromolecules may be candidates for joint disease markers? Recent rapid progress in molecular biology of articular cartilage is offering many possibilities in this respect. All components which are unique to or enriched in cartilage may be possibilities.

Proteoglycans, which represent about 20% of the dry weight of cartilage, were the first target to be evaluated. Cartilage proteoglycan structures released into synovial fluid in an experimental osteoarthritis developed in dogs were assayed with immunoassays using polyclonal rabbit antisera raised against bovine or canine proteoglycans. The concentration of chondroitin sulfate-rich proteoglycan antigens was higher in operated knees (2).

The proteoglycan concentrations in knee joint exudates of human arthritic patients have also been measured, and an inverse relation between the extent of cartilage destruction and proteoglycan concentration was observed (3). Further, it was suggested that proteoglycan concentration could serve as a marker correlating with cartilage destruction and therefore could be used to monitor the effects of intraarticular injection of glucocorticoid (4) or the systemic administration of various drugs to the patients with rheumatoid arthritis (5). Proteoglycan levels in joint fluids increased greatly shortly after trauma and decreased thereafter. However, higher than normal levels were maintained during a period of years (6). Mean values of the concentration and the total amount of the hyaluronic acid binding region of proteoglycans (radioimmunoassay) and sulfated glycosaminoglycans (dimethylmethylene blue assay) in joint fluid were higher in Reiter's syndrome and gout than in osteoarthritis and rheumatoid arthritis (7). However, another study suggested that the concentration of glycosaminoglycans in joint fluid was higher in rheumatoid arthritis and osteoarthritis compared to normal (8). Similarly, keratan sulfate levels in joint fluid from patients with various acute and chronic arthritis were higher than normal, probably reflecting the rapid depletion or greatly increased turnover of proteoglycan in the articular cartilage during acute inflammation in the joint (9).

Joint disease has three different aspects independent of the cause: cartilage destruction, repair processes, and synovial inflammation. Consequently, the attempts to discover new markers should be expanded to cover all of these different aspects of joint disease. If this can be done, we will be able to understand the degree and extent of the pathology of cartilage more precisely. For this reason, we began to investigate three different molecules as potential markers to reflect different aspects of joint disease: type II procollagen C-peptide, chondroitin sulfate isomers (chondroitin 4-sulfate and 6-sulfate), and tissue inhibitor of metalloproteinases.

TYPE II PROCOLLAGEN C-PEPTIDE AS TYPE II COLLAGEN SYNTHETIC MARKER

Type II collagen accounts for about 90% of the total cartilage collagen and is synthesized by chondrocytes as a procollagen molecule with noncollagenous aminopropeptide and carboxypropeptide extensions. These extensions are removed by specific procollagen peptidases before type II collagen is incorporated into fibrils. Type II procollagen C-peptide (pColl-II-C) remains in the tissue for a time, associated with or incorporated into newly formed fibrils. pColl-II-C was extracted and purified from growth cartilage of fetal bovine, and was initially thought to be a new molecule and was named chondrocalcin (10). After it was identified (11), it was shown to be present in all embryonic and immature cartilaginous tissues where synthetic activity of type II collagen is high (12). Immunolocalization showed that it is present mainly in the calcified zone of growth plate cartilage and adult articular cartilage (13). The biological role of pColl-II-C is still unknown, however, although important roles in calcification processes and fibrillogenesis have been suggested (14).

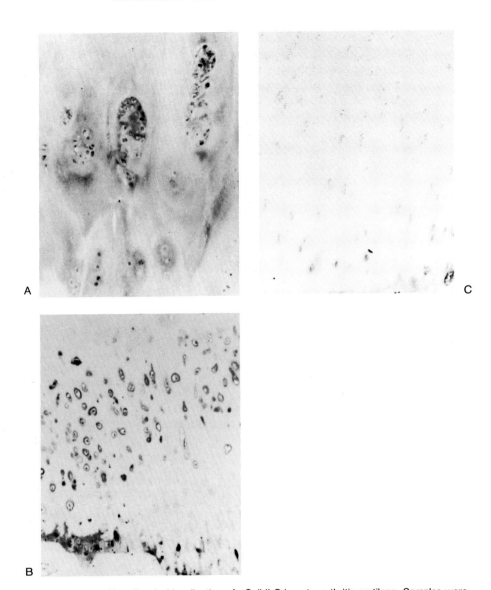

FIG. 1. Immunohistochemical localization of pColl-II-C in osteoarthritic cartilage. Samples were fixed with 4% formaldehyde. Sections of 3 μm thick were preincubated with chondroitinase ABC. Rabbit polyclonal antibody against bovine pColl-II-C extracted was used to immunostain tissue with an avidin-biotin method. Sections show positive staining of matrix in clusters of cells in osteoarthritic cartilage (**A**) and in the matrix of the superficial and calcified zones and the cytoplasm of chondrocytes of middle zones in a chondro-osseous spur from a osteoarthritic joint (**B**). Normal cartilage shows occasionally positive stain in calcified zones (**C**).

Type II collagen is present in human osteoarthritic cartilage and chondro-osseous spurs (15). It is also synthesized in degenerated cartilage *in vivo* and *in vitro* as shown by studies in human osteoarthritic tissue (16) or in animal models of osteoarthritis (17). On the other hand, others have reported a reduced deposition of collagen in the matrix (18) with an accumulation of procollagen in degenerative cartilage (19). This would suggest the existence of a partial defect in conversion of procollagen to collagen (19). Indeed, the deposition of pColl-II-C has been observed in the cartilage of osteoarthritic joints with high frequency compared to normal or rheumatoid joints (20) (Fig. 1). From these facts, it is conceivable that in an osteoarthritic joint, synthesis and accumulation of type II procollagen increases, with a concomitant increased release of pColl-II-C into the joint fluid.

Therefore, we determined pColl-II-C concentration in joint fluid as a potential marker reflecting synthetic activity of type II collagen in diseased joints. Rabbit antibodies were raised against bovine pColl-II-C and immobilized on polystyrene

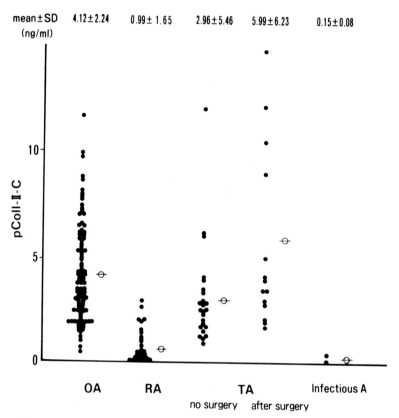

FIG. 2. Concentration of pColl-II-C in joint fluid samples for patients with different joint diseases. pColl-II-C levels were measured by enzyme immunoassay. Concentration refers to equivalent ng of pColl-II-C for fetal bovine growth plate cartilage. OA, osteoarthritis; RA, rheumatoid arthritis; TA, traumatic arthritis.

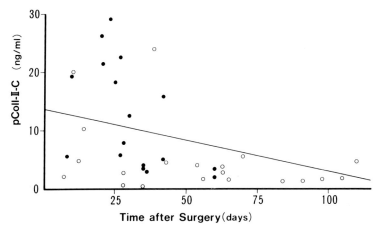

FIG. 3. Time-concentration relationship in traumatic arthritis group after surgery. *Open circles* denote arthroscopic meniscectomy patients and *closed circles* denote patients with reconstructive surgery of anterior cruciate ligament by arthrotomy.

balls for use in an ELISA (21,22). The detection limit of the method is 0.2 ng/ml. Joint fluid pColl-II-C concentrations varied widely among patients in all groups tested (Fig. 2). There were no significant differences between the pColl-II-C levels with respect to age and sex in adults. Highly significant differences were observed between the patient groups of osteoarthritis and rheumatoid arthritis, and between patient groups of traumatic arthritis and rheumatoid arthritis. Levels of pColl-II-C over 2 ng/ml were observed in only 11% of rheumatoid patients, but in more than 88% of osteoarthritis patients. The pColl-II-C levels were higher in the patients with moderate osteoarthritis than in advanced ones when the mean values were compared for each group previously classified according to the severity of radiological changes.

Traumatic arthritis means the joint effusion which occurred due to the joint derangement, the causes of which are mostly meniscal tear and ligament rupture. Some of these patients are treated surgically. Thus, patients of traumatic arthritis were further subdivided into two groups; those with or without surgery. A higher mean value was obtained in the patient subgroup that received surgery. Moreover, pColl-II-C levels were high after the surgery and decreased with time (Fig. 3). The reasons for such high concentrations of pColl-II-C in joint fluids of patients with traumatic arthritis are not clear, but it is feasible that in this case the chondrocytes have much higher metabolic activities because the mean age of the patient group was only 35 ± 9 years.

CHONDROITIN SULFATE ISOMERS AS CATABOLIC MARKERS OF PROTEOGLYCANS

The presence of galactosamine in joint fluid was noted more than 35 years ago, and this was subsequently attributed primarily to chondroitin sulfate (CS) apparently released from cartilage. As keratan sulfate (KS) does not have significant amounts of galactosamine and DS is not a major constituent of cartilage proteoglycans (PGs). However, correlations were not found between the concentrations of the acidic glycosaminoglycans, as calculated from the galactosamine, and the degree of articular changes in early stages of rheumatoid arthritis, even though galactosamine concentrations were high in joint fluids from patients with advanced stages of rheumatoid arthritis in which osteoarthritic change was complicated (23).

In human articular cartilage, chondroitin 6-sulfate (C-6-S) is the predominant isomer of CS. In fact, almost all the CS in adult articular cartilage is C-6-S (24). The biological meaning of this is not understood, but it suggests that C-6-S may be related to the integrity of matrix structure. Indeed, C-6-S increases in cartilage at the contact area in animals subjected to strenuous exercise (25).

Based on these observations, we measured CS isomers in joint fluid as possible indicators of proteoglycan metabolism. Unsaturated disaccharide isomers formed by chondroitinase ABC digestion of joint fluid samples were analyzed by high-performance liquid chromatography using an amine-bound silica column (26,27). The method was linear from 5 nmol to 2 pmol. The total amounts of C-6-S and C-4-S were higher in the following order: traumatic arthritis, osteoarthritis, and rheumatoid arthritis. Differences were significant between each group.

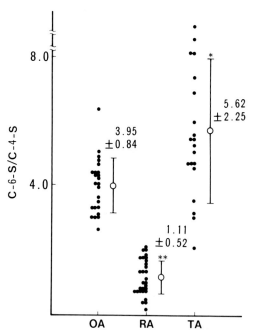

FIG. 4. The ratios of C-6-S/C-4-S in joint fluid samples from patients with OA (osteoarthritis), RA (rheumatoid arthritis) and TA (traumatic arthritis). The concentrations of C-6-S and C-4-S were determined by high-performance liquid chromatography as unsaturated disaccharide isomers formed after chondroitinase ABC digestion of joint fluids. *$p < 0.05$; **$p < 0.001$.

The ratios of C-6-S to C-4-S were also calculated. The mean values in the joint fluids of osteoarthritis, rheumatoid arthritis, and traumatic arthritis were 3.95 ± 0.84, 1.11 ± 0.52, and 5.62 ± 2.25, respectively (Fig. 4). These results demonstrated that the distribution of CS isomers is characteristic of the disease and could be a good diagnostic marker. The ratio also decreased with the progress of osteoarthritis (unpublished data). Since these results appear to be very similar to the changes of proteoglycan levels in joint fluids (3,6), we suggest that the CS levels and C-6-S/C-4-S ratios reflect catabolism rather than anabolism of proteoglycans of cartilage.

TISSUE INHIBITOR OF METALLOPROTEINASES AS A MARKER OF JOINT INFLAMMATION

A family of matrix metalloproteinases produced by chondrocytes, synovial cells, and a variety of inflammatory cells are thought to be involved in joint destruction. Most of these cells can also produce specific inhibitors of matrix metalloproteinases such as tissue inhibitor of metalloproteinases (TIMP) (28). Accordingly, the balance between the enzymes and TIMP may be crucial for the maintenance of cartilage matrix integrity. Inhibitors isolated from the numerous connective tissue cells and explants appear to be identical to or closely related to TIMP (29). The immunological identity of TIMP from various human sources, including plasma, amniotic fluid, and synovial fluid, has also been reported (29).

Collagenase inhibitor activities were first detected in rheumatoid synovial fluids (30), and the purified enzyme inhibitor was able to block the activities of collagenase, gelatinase, and proteoglycanase properties similar to those of TIMP. TIMP values in paired serum and joint fluid samples from rheumatoid arthritic patients were measured using a radioimmunoassay. TIMP levels were always higher in joint fluid compared to serum, indicating local synthesis of TIMP within the joint (31). Excess TIMP in joint fluids could inhibit cartilage degradation, perhaps cooperating with α_2-macroglobulin infiltrated from serum. This idea has been supported by recent studies on septic arthritis. No biologically active collagenase inhibitor activity could be demonstrated in joint fluid even though high molecular weight proteinase-TIMP complexes were identified (32).

We measured TIMP levels in joint fluid samples with an immunoassay (33). The detection limit of this method is 1.5 pg/well for human TIMP. The mean value of joint fluid TIMP was significantly higher in a patient group with rheumatoid arthritis than in one with osteoarthritis (Fig. 5). Joint fluid TIMP levels did not correlate with either erythrocyte sedimentation rates or C-reactive protein levels in serum from rheumatoid arthritic patients. It is noteworthy that TIMP levels in joint fluids from patients with traumatic arthritis were in the same range as those with rheumatoid arthritis (Fig. 5). In addition, TIMP levels were high after the surgery and reduced with time (Fig. 6). Therefore, we suggest that TIMP

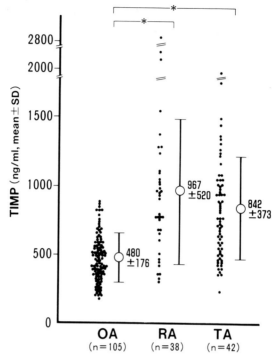

FIG. 5. Concentration of TIMP in joint fluid samples from patients with OA (osteoarthritis), RA (rheumatoid arthritis), and TA (traumatic arthritis). TIMP was measured by a one-step sandwich EIA. *$p < 0.001$.

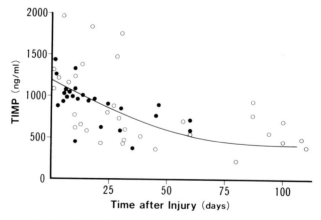

FIG. 6. Time-concentration relationship in the TA group after surgery. *Open circles* denote patients after arthroscopic meniscectomy and *closed circles* denote patients after reconstructive surgery of the anterior cruciate ligament by arthrotomy.

levels in joint fluids reflect the activity of inflammation in the joint irrespective of whether the patient has acute or chronic arthritis.

THE ROLE OF JOINT MARKERS IN DRUG EVALUATION

There have been no widely used methods to evaluate the therapeutic and/or adverse effects on cartilage of drugs administered to patients to suppress joint inflammation. In addition, the efficacy of various surgical treatments designed to protect degenerated cartilage or to accelerate repair processes has been evaluated only by radiography and clinical assessment. Therefore, there is a great need to develop biochemical markers enabling us to assess the metabolism of cartilage both qualitatively and quantitatively.

Intraarticular injection of glucocorticoid reduces proteoglycan concentrations in joint fluids of rheumatoid patients (4). Further, decreases in proteoglycan levels were observed in two patients whose arthritis spontaneously subsided. Conversely, higher concentrations of proteoglycan epitopes were observed in both joint fluids and sera of rheumatoid patients after oral administration of low doses of prednisolone compared to the patients given nonsteroidal antiinflammatory drugs or slow-acting antirheumatic drugs (5).

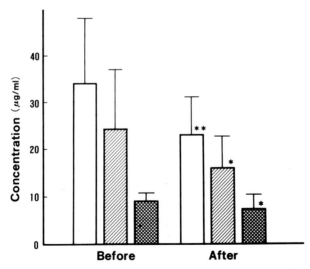

FIG. 7. Concentrations of chondroitin sulfate isomers in joint fluid samples from patients with osteoarthritis either before or after intraarticular injections of 2.5 ml of 1% superpurified hyaluronan (Arz®). The injections were repeated every week and mean injection times of nine patients were 4.3. The significant decrease of each mean value was observed when the changes were compared with between before and after the injection. Chondroitin 6S + 4S (□); Chondroitin 6S (▨); Chondroitin 4S (▩); $^*p < 0.05$; $^{**}p < 0.01$.

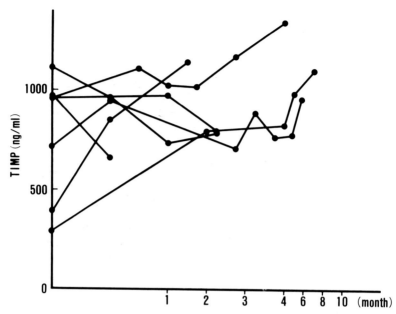

FIG. 8. Change of TIMP levels during and after intraarticular injections of glucocorticoid in the patients of rheumatoid arthritis. The injections were repeated every 2 to 4 weeks up to a maximum of six times. Three cases out of six have shown increased tendency of TIMP levels in joint fluids.

The changes of pColl-II-C and CS isomer concentrations were monitored after intraarticular injection of purified hyaluronan in the knee joints of osteoarthritis. Levels of pColl-II-C increased and levels of both C-6-S and C-4-S decreased (Fig. 7). A similar study was undertaken with the patients of rheumatoid arthritis in whom glucocorticoid was injected intraarticularly. In this case, the concentrations of pColl-II-C and TIMP were measured before and after 5 to 6 injections. Although there was no change in pColl-II-C levels, TIMP increased significantly in three out of six cases (Fig. 8).

CONCLUDING REMARKS

The basic events of cartilage destruction appear to be rather common for many types of joint diseases. The participating cells and the degree of response may differ with each disease state, but the differences should be quantitative rather than qualitative. Humoral factors which act as catabolic or anabolic effectors on chondrocytes are now thought to be produced by almost all mesenchymal and inflammatory cells. Thus, cross-talk between the cells in abnormal conditions might play a fundamental role in the pathogenesis of cartilage destruction.

The attempts to identify molecules related to cartilage metabolism and to develop simple and accurate assay methods which are applicable to clinical studies should be encouraged (34). Assays of proteoglycan, keratan sulfate (35), and hyaluronic acid (36) have been forerunners in this field. The pColl-II-C, chondroitin sulfate isomers, and TIMP assays described here will expand our understanding of different aspects of cartilage metabolism in diseased joint states.

ACKNOWLEDGMENT

This research was supported in part by a Silver Science Grant from the Ministry of Health and Welfare in the Japanese Government.

REFERENCES

1. Karvonen RL, Negendank WG, Franser SM, Mayes MD, An T, Fernandez-Madrid F. Articular cartilage defects of the knee: correlation between magnetic resonance imaging and gross pathology. *Ann Rheum Dis* 1990;49:672–675.
2. Heinegård D, Inerot S, Wieslander J, Lindblad G. A method for the quantification of cartilage proteoglycan structures liberated to the synovial fluid during developing degenerative joint disease. *Scand J Clin Lab Invest* 1985;45:421–427.
3. Saxne T, Wollheim FA, Pettersson H, Heinegård D. Proteoglycan concentration in synovial fluid: predictor of future cartilage destruction in rheumatoid arthritis? *Br Med J* 1987;295:1447–1448.
4. Saxne T, Heinegård D, Wollheim FA. Therapeutic effects on cartilage metabolism in arthritis as measured by release of proteoglycan structures into the synovial fluid. *Ann Rheum Dis* 1986;45:491–497.
5. Saxne T, Heinegård D, Wollheim FA. Cartilage proteoglycans in synovial fluid and serum in patients with inflammatory joint disease. Relation to systemic treatment. *Arthritis Rheum* 1987;30:972–979.
6. Lohmander LS, Dahlberg L, Ryd L, Heinegård D. Increased levels of proteoglycan fragments in knee joint fluid after injury. *Arthritis Rheum* 1989;32:1434–1442.
7. Carroll G. Measurement of sulfated glycosaminoglycans and proteoglycan fragments in arthritic synovial fluid. *Ann Rheum Dis* 1989;48:17–24.
8. Bensouyad A, Hollander AP, Dularay B, Bedwell AE, Cooper RA, Hutton CW, Dieppe PA, Elson CJ. Concentrations of glycosaminoglycans in synovial fluids and inflammatory mediators in rheumatoid arthritis. *Ann Rheum Dis* 1990;49:301–307.
9. Ratcliffe A, Doherty M, Maini RN, Hardingham TE. Increased concentrations of proteoglycan components in the synovial fluids of patients with acute but not chronic joint disease. *Ann Rheum Dis* 1988;47:826–832.
10. Choi HU, Tang LH, Johnson TL, Pal S, Rosenberg LC, Reiner A, Poole AR. Isolation and characterization of a 35,000 molecular weight subunit fetal cartilage matrix protein. *J Biol Chem* 1983;258:655–661.
11. van der Rest M, Rosenberg LC, Olsen BR, Poole AR. Chondrocalcin is identical with the C-propeptide of type II procollagen. *Biochem J* 1986;237:923–925.
12. Niyibizi C, Wu J-J, Eyre DR. The carboxypropeptide trimer of type II collagen is a prominent component of immature cartilages and intervertebral-disc tissue. *Biochem Biophys Acta* 1987;916:493–499.
13. Poole AR, Rosenberg LC. Chondrocalcin and calcification of cartilage. *Clin Orthop* 1986;208:114–117.
14. Kujawa MJ, Weitzhandler M, Poole AR, Rosenberg L, Caplan AI. Association of the C-propeptide of type II collagen with mineralization of embryonic chick long bone and sternal development. *Connect Tissue Res* 1989;23:179–199.
15. Goldwasser M, Astley T, van der Rest M, Glorieux FH. Analysis of the type of collagen present in osteoarthritic human cartilage. *Clin Orthop* 1982;167:296–302.

16. Lippiello L, Hall D, Mankin HJ. Collagen synthesis in normal and osteoarthritic human cartilage. *Clin Invest* 1977;59:593–600.
17. Eyre DH, McDevitt CA, Muir H. Experimentally induced osteoarthrosis in the dog. *Ann Rheum Dis* 1975;34(Suppl.):138–140.
18. Burton-Wurster N, Hui-Chou CS, Greisen HA, Lust G. Reduced deposition of collagen in the degenerated articular cartilage of dogs with degenerative joint disease. *Biochem Biophys Acta* 1982;718:74–84.
19. Miller DR, Lust G. Accumulation of procollagen in the degenerative articular cartilage of dogs with osteoarthritis. *Biochem Biophys Acta* 1979;583:218–231.
20. Shinmei M, Naramatsu Y, Tanaka O, Inamori Y, Kikuchi T, Shimomura Y, Matsuyama S, Matsuzawa Y. Increased levels of chondrocalcin (type II collagen C-propeptide) in osteoarthritic synovial fluid. *Arthritis Rheum* 1989;32(Suppl.):S108.
21. Shimmei M, Inamori Y, Yoshihara Y, Hayakawa T, Shimomura Y. Molecular markers of joint disease: significance of the level of type II collagen C-propeptide, chondroitin sulfate and TIMP in joint fluid. Transactions of the 37th annual meeting, Orthopaedic Research Society, 1991;16: 230.
22. Shinmei M, Ito K, Matsuyama S, Inamori Y, Matsuzawa K, Shimomura Y. Carboxy-terminal type II procollagen peptide levels in joint fluids as a marker of collagen biosynthesis of cartilage in joint diseases. *Ann Rheum Dis* (submitted).
23. Seppala PO, Karkkainen J, Lehtonen A, Makisara P. Chondroitin sulfate in the normal and rheumatoid synovial fluid. *Clin Chim Acta* 1971;36:549–553.
24. Mourao PAS. Distribution of chondroitin 4-sulfate and chondroitin 6-sulfate in human articular and growth cartilage. *Arthritis Rheum* 1988;31:1028–1033.
25. Saamanen A-M, Tammi M, Kiviranta I, Jurvelin J, Helminen HJ. Levels of chondroitin-6-sulfate and nonaggregating proteoglycans at articular cartilage contact sites in the knees of young dogs subjected to moderate running exercise. *Arthritis Rheum* 1989;32:1282–1292.
26. Toyoda H, Shinomiya K, Yamanashi S, Koshiishi I, Imanari T. Microdetermination of unsaturated disaccharides produced from chondroitin sulfates in rabbit plasma by high performance liquid chromatography with fluorometric detection. *Anal Sciences* 1989;4:381–384.
27. Yoshida K, Miyauchi S, Kikuchi H, Tawada A, Tokuyasu K. Analysis of unsaturated disaccharides from glycosaminoglycuronan by high-performance liquid chromatography. *Anal Biochem* 1989;177:327–332.
28. Docherty AJP, Murphy G. The tissue metalloproteinase family and the inhibitor TIMP: a study using cDNAs and recombinant proteins. *Ann Rheum Dis* 1990;49:469–479.
29. Murphy G, Docherty JP. Molecular studies on the connective tissue metalloproteinases and their inhibitor TIMP. In: Glauert AM, ed. *The control of tissue damage.* Amsterdam: Elsevier, 1988;223–241.
30. Cawston TE, Mercer E, De Silva M, Hazleman BL. Metalloproteinases and collagenase inhibitors in rheumatoid synovial fluid. *Arthritis Rheum* 1984;27:285–290.
31. Cawston TE, McLaughlin P, Hazleman BL. Paired serum and synovial values of α_2-macroglobulin and TIMP in rheumatoid arthritis. *Br J Rheumatol* 1987;26:354–358.
32. Cawston TE, McLaughlin P, Coughlan R, Kyle V, Hazleman B. Synovial fluids from infected joints contain metalloproteinase—tissue inhibitor of metalloproteinase (TIMP) complexes. *Biochem Biophys Acta* 1990;1033:96–102.
33. Kodama S, Iwata K, Iwata H, Yamashita K, Hayakawa T. Rapid one-step sandwich enzyme immunoassay for tissue inhibitor of metalloproteinases. An application for rheumatoid arthritis serum and plasma. *J Immunol Methods* 1990;127:103–108.
34. Lohmander LS. Therapy evaluation in joint disease: the role of cartilage markers in joint fluid and serum. In: Raspe HH, ed. *Therapeutic approaches to joint disease.* Munchen: Zuckschwerdt Verlag, 1990;28–36.
35. Thonar EJ-MA, Lenz ME, Klintworth GK, Caterson B, Pachman LM, Glickman P, Katz R. Quantification of keratan sulfate in blood as a marker of cartilage catabolism. *Arthritis Rheum* 1985;28:1367–1376.
36. Engstrom-Laurent A, Hallgren R. Circulating hyaluronic acid levels vary with physical activity in healthy subjects and in rheumatoid arthritis patients. *Arthritis Rheum* 1987;30:1333–1337.

DISCUSSION

Dieppe: We have preliminary data that may agree with some of your findings. In collaboration with Robin Poole we studied synovial fluid from a small group of patients before and after single injections of yttrium into the joint to cause synovial ablation. In each case there was a marked and inverse change in keratan sulfate which decreases and the Col(II) propeptide which increases. It is tempting to suggest that this reflects beneficial responses on the joint.

Shinmei: We have not yet studied the relationship between keratan sulfate and the Col(II) propeptide in joint fluids. However, our preliminary data suggest an inverse correlation between Col(II) propeptide and chondroitin-6 sulfate in osteoarthritis joint fluids.

Mason: Can you speculate on the dramatic reduction in the chondroitin 6-sulfate in the synovial fluid after treatment with hyaluronate?

Shinmei: Hyaluronate may have some coating effect on the degenerated cartilage, resulting in the reduction of proteoglycan release from the cartilage matrix.

Lohmander: Can you provide some details about your hyaluronate treatment protocols?

Shinmei: Intraarticular injection of hyaluronate has been approved in the treatment of osteoarthritis of the knee joint in Japan since 1987. Hyaluronate solution (1%, 2.5 ml) was injected every 1 or 2 weeks and repeated 5 or 10 times with an improvement of the symptoms.

Caterson: I was intrigued by your observation that chondroitin-4-sulfate increased relative to chondroitin-6-sulfate in rheumatic patients. In normal older adults most chondroitin sulfate in cartilage is 6-sulfated. Is the 4-sulfated form coming from somewhere else?

Shinmei: Reduction of chondroitin 6-sulfate in the joint fluids from rheumatoid arthritis patients seems to reflect the loss of cartilage mass in the joint. Further, it is well known that in the rheumatoid arthritis joint the synthetic activity of cartilage proteoglycan is very low. Therefore, I suppose that a relative increase reflects release of chondroitin 4-sulfate from inflamed synovial membrane and infusion from the serum.

Articular Cartilage and Osteoarthritis,
edited by K. Kuettner et al.
Raven Press, Ltd., New York © 1992.

43

General Discussion for Chapters 37–42

Schleyerbach: New collagen types, their genes, and aspects of their promoters are now known, but it is hard to define their physiological and pathological functions. Can transgenic animals be developed with collagen gene modifications which will help determine these functions?

Olsen: The answer is yes, and several laboratories are trying to make them. We are trying to knock out type IX to make a transgenic mouse that hopefully will survive without making type IX collagen. We have knocked out the gene alpha-1(IX) in embryonic stem cells in collaboration with Rudolf Jaenisch, and the results so far are promising. Time will show whether we can obtain transgenics and breed them to homozygosity. We have tried to produce a transdominant negative mutation by making a gene that would code for the amino terminal globular domain of type IX collagen without the rest of the molecule. This could produce a transgenic mouse which expresses an excess of this globular domain in cartilage where it might compete with the endogenous domain on type IX collagen molecules for binding sites in the matrix and alter its organization. Since this mutation may be lethal, we are transfecting the gene into stem cells in culture which will be injected into blastocysts to produce chimeric mice that carry the transdominant mutation.

Hascall: Dr. Shinmei, are the markers you study in synovial fluid present in detectable amounts in serum? If so, do they correlate with the synovial fluid volumes? Can cohorts of such markers be used to increase the significant differences between a patient set and a normal set?

Shinmei: We can measure serum levels of Col(II) propeptide and TIMP. The serum concentrations of Col(II) propeptide and of TIMP are approximately a tenth and a fifth of their concentrations in synovial fluid. Thus, serum levels can be correlated with synovial fluid levels, but they are less reliable. Concerning arthritic patients, then, analyses of synovial fluid are better indicators of the cartilage condition. Measurements of these markers in serum have much greater value in more systemic diseases such as growth retardation, osteoporosis, or chondrodysplasia.

Heinegård: Comparing marker levels in serum and synovial fluids will add complications. The range of values in serum will be much greater, because some patients have disease activity in one joint and others in several joints. Furthermore, the background will be high due to contributions from tracheal, nasal, and other cartilages. Therefore, analysis of synovial fluids has its merits as well as problems and analysis of serum has its problems as well as merits.

Hascall: If markers are to be used eventually to define populations at risk, I think that serum must be the place to look. Can marker cohorts be developed, independent of which joints might be involved, that can narrow down the standard deviations in these assays enough to address this particular question?

Lohmander: In general, I think that the markers should only be used in a diagnostic or prognostic way. You can also use them to learn more about disease mechanisms, and if that is one of your goals, then synovial fluid markers should be investigated, because many of them will disappear between the synovial fluid and serum.

Heinegård: I think that neoepitopes created by the disease process have a great potential for becoming very useful markers in terms of making both prognostic and perhaps diagnostic assays. Assays based on such epitopes may well be suitable for serum samples.

Campion: I think Dr. Lohmander is right about the usefulness of synovial fluid for learning about disease progression of a distinct joint site pragmatically, though the final aim has to be to develop serum markers as they are the only ones useful for population studies. Moreover, compartmentalization is a real problem in synovial fluids. There are compartments that are probably not reached by dilution markers such as radiolabeled albumin. Serum markers are good for prospective and long-term studies where the patients are their own controls and marker stability with time can be shown. Such variables as changes in hepatic and liver function can also be assessed. In sum, I think relevant data can be obtained about changes in connective tissue metabolism with serum markers.

Levick: To support what Dr. Campion just said, to interpret serum levels of markers, one must know the time constants of removal and whether they change with time. The latter probably is not a real problem. Conversely, there are at least five uncertainties in interpreting the synovial fluid concentrations that I outline in my chapter. Thus on general principles, serum levels are safer to interpret than synovial fluid levels. To be fair, if you do measure synovial fluid markers, the kind of problems I am talking about probably cause concentrations to vary by less than an order of magnitude. If the marker concentration changes by two or three orders of magnitude, then I think worries about excluded volumes and turnover rates can be disregarded. However, if the changes are merely within one order of magnitude, then you have to worry about them. The general point is that serum levels are safer to interpret than synovial fluid levels.

Articular Cartilage and Osteoarthritis,
edited by K. Kuettner et al.
Raven Press, Ltd., New York © 1992.

Part XII: Clinical Aspects of Osteoarthritis

Introduction

Giles V. Campion

*Section of Rheumatology, Clinical Research, Hoechst Werk Kalle-Albert,
6200 Wiesbaden 12, Germany*

In many ways, this section marks both the climax and the nadir of the workshop. It is the climax in that it is to the patient with osteoarthritis (OA) that this workshop must be dedicated. It is to be hoped that a better understanding of the processes of the joint in health and disease will enable us to contribute more to helping the patient with osteoarthritis than has been the case until now. It is the nadir in that of all the sections, this is the one where our understanding proves to be at its most primitive. Our pens hesitate over the first pages of the protocols as we still struggle with definitions, methodology, and finding the proper reagents.

IF WE HAD A PROMISING DRUG, HOW WOULD WE APPLY IT TO THE CLINICAL SITUATION? HOW WOULD WE STUDY IT?

The first approach would be to identify the subject at risk. The second would be to pick a homogenous group to study. Population studies tell us that OA is a common disease, but that it is a heterogeneous and, in the final analysis, a very poorly understood disease. We know that OA of the hip is a different disease from OA of the knee and that some procedures such as meniscectomy increase the subsequent risk of developing OA (see Dieppe et al.). We also know that OA progresses in different patients at different rates, that in the majority the process may stabilize with resolution of symptoms, but that in others, rapid joint failure and destruction occur. As yet we are unable to distinguish between such people in the early stages of their disease.

But population studies tell us that our ability to identify clinically significant OA is poor. The extensive Health Examination Survey conducted on 6,672 US adults between 1960 and 1962 tells us that 85% of patients between 75 and 85 years of age have OA as defined by radiological criteria. What does this mean? Does it mean anything?

Certainly not all individuals would be suitable candidates for a trial with our promising drug. The dichotomy between radiological and clinical findings is a real problem for the clinical scientist. An attempt is being made to set diagnostic criteria for OA at different sites. A laudable aim, but given the length of the disease process, the important patient to study is precisely the one who has yet to fulfill these same criteria. More recently, mutations have been described in the Type II collagen gene in familial OA. The relevance of this finding to OA in the population as a whole has yet to be determined, but it may well provide a means of subsetting some types of OA.

The advent of magnetic resonance imaging (MRI) has revolutionized our ability to image the joint and we are perhaps only beginning to discover the potential of this technique. For the first time the possibility of directly imaging the soft tissues of the joint is available (see Hodgson et al.). With the best scanning techniques and with the use of contrast enhancement, it is possible to show osteochondral lesions as small as 1 mm. Calculation of the T1 and T2 relaxation times in normal articular cartilage enables the detection of increased hydration of the superficial layers and vascular invasion of the deeper layers. Unappreciated intraarticular pathology such as meniscal derangements can become evident and this may account for some of the symptoms previously attributed to the OA process. Moreover, using techniques such as diffusion and spectroscopy, it may be possible to come to grips with the pathophysiology of the joint *in vivo.*

One of the outstanding breakthroughs in the history of medicine has been the introduction of the prosthetic joint. This advance has transformed the lives of many OA patients, relieving them from pain and disability and enabling the resumption of functional, pain-free movement of a failed joint. Another surgical procedure, osteotomy, gives us the unusual possibility of studying the process of repair afforded through joint realignment. Arthroscopy gives us the opportunity to visualize the joint directly and may provide valuable information about the early stages of osteoarthritis as well as tell us something about its heterogeneity (see Puhl). Moreover, with the miniaturization of equipment and the development of sophisticated technology, arthroscopy may become a consulting room procedure, with the possibilities of directly recording parameters such as synovial blood flow and cartilage softening.

However, despite the possibilities offered to us by the modalities discussed above for identifying early disease or for following the results of therapeutic intervention, each has its disadvantage in terms of cost or practicality. And so much hope for the future must rest in the subject of the final contribution of this section (see chapter by Lohmander). The increased understanding of joint biochemistry together with the advent of techniques such as monoclonal antibodies have vastly improved our ability to measure connective tissue components in body fluids that can reflect events occurring in the matrix of the joint tissues. However, a note of caution is advisable. The significance of these measurements in tissue fluids, especially in serum, can only be made in relation to a thorough understanding of the epitope that is being recognized, its stability in relation to sample collection and handling, and to knowledge of the circulation and clearance of the molecule. A wide biological variation in levels of components is often evident, which underlines the need for comprehensive patient assessment, preferably as part of large prospective studies. With this caveat apart, a panel of assays measuring different matrix products may be available in the future to give us dynamic information about the health of the joint and its response to therapy.

With the developments enumerated above, we hope that it will become much easier to study a putative, disease-modifying agent in osteoarthritis after identification of a homogenous, at-risk group with early disease. Superior monitoring of the effects of therapy will be available with the aim of obtaining a result comparable if not superior to arthroplasty. So although the current state of knowledge is poor in many ways, the outlook for real progress during the next 6 years is very bright.

Articular Cartilage and Osteoarthritis,
edited by K. Kuettner et al.
Raven Press, Ltd., New York © 1992.

44

Epidemiology, Clinical Course, and Outcome of Knee Osteoarthritis

Paul Dieppe, Janet Cushnaghan, and Tim McAlindon

Rheumatology Unit, Bristol Royal Infirmary, Bristol BS2 8HW, United Kingdom

Osteoarthritis (OA) is characterized by specific *pathological* changes in synovial joints. When severe, these changes are reflected by *radiographic* abnormalities which are used to diagnose the presence of OA in epidemiological and clinical practice. *Clinical* manifestations are less specific and cannot be accurately predicted from pathological and radiographic changes.

Several large surveys of the pathological and radiographic abnormalities have been reported. As a result, much information is available on the prevalence of advanced OA. Several risk factors or associations have also been delineated. However, very little is known about the incidence of the condition, and almost nothing is known about its natural history and outcome.

Improved understanding of the biology and biomechanics of synovial joints is leading to the introduction of new therapeutic options. It is going to be essential to have accurate information on the natural history of the disease, and on the factors that control outcome, before any new therapy can be used rationally.

THE IMPORTANCE OF JOINT SITE

The main joint sites affected by OA include the apophyseal joints of the spine, the knee, the hip, and certain small joints of the hands and feet. Of these, the spinal, knee, and hip joints cause the major problems in terms of consequent pain and disability.

The risk factors of knee, hip, and spinal OA are different. For example, they have different age and sex prevalence, and whereas knee OA is strongly associated with obesity, hip OA is not (1). In a recently reported study of 500 patients with peripheral joint OA, knee and hand disease were found to be related to each other, but hip and knee OA had no significant association (2). Hip and knee OA should be regarded as quite different conditions.

Our own studies are concentrating on knee OA. Even then, problems of joint site arise, as OA has a focal distribution within, as well as between, joints. There are three major compartments in the knee: the patello-femoral articulation, and the medial and lateral tibio-femoral joints; OA of each of these three compartments may have different associations.

ESTABLISHED DATA AND CURRENT GAPS IN OUR KNOWLEDGE OF THE EPIDEMIOLOGY, CLINICAL COURSE, AND OUTCOME OF KNEE OA

Definitions

Large studies of knee OA have relied on radiographic definitions of the condition. The "gold standard" was produced by Kellgren and Lawrence in the late 1950s (3). They described five grades of knee OA using a combination of signs, including osteophytes, joint space narrowing, and subchondral bone changes. There are many problems with this approach. Linearity and a constant association between each of the different features seen on the x-ray are assumed. In fact, osteophytes alone are common, and perhaps unrelated to OA; and severe joint space narrowing can occur with few other changes (4). Furthermore, the system only involves the antero-posterior view of the knee joint alone, so that no assessment can be made of the patello-femoral joint.

Clinical definitions present even greater difficulties. The American College of Rheumatology has recently attempted to provide a framework for the clinical description of knee OA (5), but this has been severely criticized (6). In a large survey of clinical and radiographic changes at the knee joint, the relative lack of correlation between x-rays, clinical signs, and symptoms was confirmed, and clinical changes proved very poor predictors of radiographic OA (7).

Prevalence, Incidence, and Impact

All data on the prevalence and incidence of knee OA must be interpreted in the light of the problems discussed above, i.e., the difficulty in defining the condition. However, advanced OA of the tibio-femoral joint is easily recognized radiographically, and data are available on the prevalence of this condition. Figures from Europe and North America are similar, and suggest a prevalence of less than 1% among people aged 25 to 34, rising to about 30% in those aged 75 and above (1,8). In those under 45, knee OA is more common in men than in women. There is then a steep rise in the prevalence in women between ages 45 and 65, and the condition is about three times more frequent in women overall. Only one study on incidence has been reported (9). An overall incidence of around 200/100,000 person-years for hip and knee OA was estimated.

Data on the impact of the condition are sketchy and indirect. Knee pain appears to be extremely common in older members of the community, with a recorded prevalence in one study of 33% in women and 16% in men aged 70 (10). Physical disability, particularly lack of mobility, is also extremely common in the elderly, and much of the problem has been attributed to OA. However, little direct evidence on the impact of knee OA or on the relationships between knee pain, radiographic evidence of OA, and disability is available.

Risk Factors

Individual risk factors for knee OA can be divided into two categories: those that relate to a generalized systemic predisposition to the condition, and those that relate to abnormal biomechanical loading of the joint.

Apart from age and sex, the most obvious systemic risk factor is obesity. The association is strong, marked obesity conferring up to a 7× increased risk of knee OA. Other interesting associations that have been described include reproductive variables in women (e.g., hysterectomy and menopause), hypermobility, cigarette smoking (which may be protective), diabetes, hypertension, and hyperuricemia (11).

Mechanical factors include previous surgery or trauma, abnormalities of joint shape, and the use and abuse of the knee joint. Cruciate ligament rupture and total meniscectomy are both well-known factors which predispose to knee OA. However, the interval is often very long, and local factors may interact with systemic predisposition, and the majority of those who have had a meniscectomy still have a good knee joint some 25 years later (12). Joint shape has proved difficult to study *in vivo,* but Cooke and his colleagues have suggested that minor abnormalities in the angulation of the femoral condyles ("knee dysplasia") may be a major factor in the pathogenesis of knee OA (13). Moderate, normal exercise appears to be unrelated to OA, but recent data suggest that there may be an association with activities that involve knee bending (11).

Any strategy for the prevention of knee OA will depend on a better understanding of the risk factors and associations, and in particular, of the interaction between systemic and localized factors.

Course and Outcome

Surprisingly, there are almost no data about the course and outcome of the condition. It is generally described as a slowly progressive disorder, but clinical studies emphasize the heterogeneity of knee OA (2). Hernborg and Nilson reviewed 71 patients between 10 and 18 years after a knee x-ray first showed evidence of OA. Symptoms were reported to have worsened in 56% and improved in 17%. The majority of the radiographs showed deterioration even if symptoms had improved (14). Massardo and colleagues reported an 8 year follow-up of 31 patients. The majority worsened clinically, with increased pain and disability, but two of the patients showed a striking improvement in their conditions. The x-rays changed little (15). Data from large epidemiological studies in the United States also indicate that the majority of cases, but not all, progressively worsen. However, there are few data on the risk factors or determinants of the progression and outcome of the disease. Risk factors for progression could be different from those that predispose to contracting OA, and need to be studied separately.

Conclusions

Knee OA is a common disorder, with a major impact through consequent pain and disability. It is strongly related to age, sex, and obesity, and a variety of other systemic and local risk factors are likely to be important in its pathogenesis. Very little is known about its incidence, natural history, or outcome, and almost nothing is known about the factors that control the variable expression of the disease. The causes of both pain and disability remain obscure. Little is known about the relative importance of the three different compartments of the knee joint; most epidemiological surveys have paid little or no attention to the patello-femoral joint.

SOME CURRENT INVESTIGATIONS ON THE EPIDEMIOLOGY, CLINICAL COURSE, AND OUTCOME OF KNEE OA

Methodology: Establishing Appropriate Clinical, Imaging, and Biochemical Techniques for Studying Knee OA

Clinical Methodology

Unlike basic scientists, clinicians rarely test the validity of their bedside techniques. However, if clinical criteria are going to be used for the classification and assessment of OA (5–7) it is vital to know if the recording of signs is reproducible.

We have recently completed a study of the within- and the between-observer variations of common signs used in the clinical assessment of knee OA (16). Some signs showed reasonable reproducibility, including bony swelling and tibio-femoral crepitus (with kappa statistics of >0.6, indicating a high level of agreement between observations), but others, particularly evidence of instability and signs of patello-femoral disease, were poor. This has implications in the design and interpretation of clinical studies.

The Plain Radiograph

Various new approaches to the production and interpretation of x-rays in OA are currently being investigated, including the use of macroradiography and computerized assessment of the interbone volume in the tibio-femoral joint (17).

We assess each of the main signs of OA at the knee joint separately, rather than using a composite score. Thus joint space narrowing, osteophytes, subchondral bone sclerosis, cysts, and any evidence of bony destruction are each scored on a 0–2 scale for each of the three compartments of the knee joint. As for clinical signs, we have examined the validity of this methodology and found that the reproducibility of our scoring system is again better for the tibio-femoral than for the patello-femoral joint (18). Tibio-femoral joint space narrowing performed well (kappa 0.66, 95% CI 0.58–0.74), suggesting that the use of complex methods of measuring interbone distance is unnecessary. The method also allows us to assess changes in bone and cartilage separately, and to follow their progression and associations longitudinally in each of the three joint compartments.

Other Imaging Techniques

The x-ray has the advantages of being simple, cheap, and well understood. However, it can only provide a static, unidimensional picture of historical changes in the anatomy of the joint, and principally reflects the bony component of OA. Other imaging techniques can provide dynamic, physiological information, as well as better anatomical data that include the soft tissues (17).

In conjunction with Fiona McCrae, Iain Watt and colleagues, we have investigated the value of *scintigraphy* (bone scans) in knee OA. Several different scan patterns have been delineated that appear to reflect different aspects of the OA process (19). We are particularly interested in McCrae's recent data which suggest that certain scintigraphic features may predict radiographic and clinical changes at the knee joint (20). It may be that the technique can be used to aid prognosis, although we need to collect more data over a longer time interval. We have also compared x-ray and scintigraphic findings with magnetic resonance images (MRI). *MRI* proved to be a sensitive technique for detection of both soft tissue and bony changes, and correlated with some scintigraphic patterns, indicating, for example, that activity within growing osteophytes and changing subchondral bone can be imaged (21).

It would appear that the pathophysiology of OA, as well as a wide range of anatomical changes, can be assessed with these techniques. MRI may prove particularly useful in following disease progression in individual patients and in monitoring the effects of any experimental treatment.

Biochemical Methods

The development of biochemical markers for the assessment of OA is discussed in other chapters. We have begun to use some of these assays in our ongoing studies of patients with knee OA.

Although it seemed less likely that serum biochemistry would be of value than examination of synovial fluids, we have recently correlated assays of serum keratan sufate (KS) performed by Eugene Thonar and hyaluronate (HA) performed by Giles Campion and Warren Knudson and their colleagues with clinical and x-ray changes in a large population of patients with knee OA (22,23). KS epitope levels showed some correlation with the number of involved joints in women, and were higher in men with knee OA than in women with similar degrees of OA (22). Our early data with the HA assay suggest that serum levels are much higher in OA than in controls, and correlate quite strongly with the severity of the radiographic changes at the knee joint (Table 1) (23). This provocative finding is currently being tested in another population of patients.

Levels of KS epitope in the synovial fluid are much higher than those in the serum (22) by a factor of about 10 times. They are also inversely related to the degree of joint space narrowing on the radiograph. We are currently investigating the use of other markers in synovial fluids obtained from patients with knee OA, including products of collagen turnover, as well as proteoglycans.

Pain, Disability, and Knee OA in the Community: A Study of People Over the Age of 55

Validated techniques for assessing disability, such as the Health Assessment Questionnaire (HAQ), have recently been developed, allowing large surveys of the relationships between pain, disability, and OA to be performed.

We have undertaken a postal survey of 2,102 people over the age of 55, inquiring about knee pain (using validated questions) and disability using the HAQ (24). Replies were received from 677 men and 1,017 women, a response rate of over 80%. Knee pain was common, age-related, and more frequent in women than in men. Disability was also age-related, and showed a strong statistical association with the presence of knee pain at all ages ($p < 0.05$).

A proportion of those surveyed, some with and some without knee pain, have been interviewed, examined, and had their knees radiographed. The data are being examined for risk factors as well as associations between pain, disability, and knee OA. Radiographic evidence of OA of the knee was found in 53% of 273 people with knee pain, and in 17% of 240 controls without knee symptoms. In men, medial compartment disease predominated, whereas in women patello-

---

TABLE 1. *Correlations between knee OA and serum hyaluronan*

Patient group: N = 83 (61F, 22M), with established knee OA	
Average age 64.9 years (±10.8)	
Disease duration 16.1 years (±jkl 3.4)	
Correlations with radiographic and scintigraphic changes:	
Total knee x-ray score:	$r_s = 0.49$
Joint space narrowing:	$r_s = 0.42$
Osteophytosis:	$r_s = 0.43$
Total scintigraphic score:	$r_s = 0.33$
Generalized pattern:	$r_s = 0.36$

All correlations are significant at 0.01 degree or more.
See Campion et al., ref. no. 23.

femoral joint OA was the most common finding. The highest disability scores (HAQ) were found in those with patello-femoral OA (Table 2).

These data suggest that men and women have quite different patterns of knee OA, and that the patello-femoral joint, which has been largely ignored in previous community-based studies, may be a more important cause of disability than tibio-femoral joint OA.

Natural History, Response to Therapy, and Outcome: Longitudinal Studies of Groups of Patients with Knee OA

Hospital-based studies are less representative than community-based surveys, but much can still be learned from a careful follow-up of well-characterized patients. In addition to patient groups already referred to (19,22,24), we are engaged in long-term prospective studies of two other cohorts.

500 Patients with Peripheral Joint OA

The demographic data of this group at entry to the study have already been published (2). The 500 patients all presented with symptomatic OA of nonspinal joints. The group comprises 342 women (mean age, 65.3 years) and 158 men (mean age, 59.7 years). The condition was confined to one or two joint sites in 83.4% of cases, only involving three or more sites in 16.6%. Three patterns of disease stood out: (a) isolated hip disease in younger men; (b) knee and hand disease in obese, middle-aged women; (c) polyarticular disease in older women, often associated with joint (bone/cartilage) destruction and/or crystal deposition. These patterns overlap and are not mutually exclusive.

The group has been reviewed 3 years after entry, and the data are currently being analyzed. It is already apparent that many of these patients have changed little over 3 years, although a minority have had a rapid evolution of OA in one

TABLE 2. *The relationship between disability and OA of different compartments of the knee joint*

	No disability	HAQ > 0	HAQ ≥ 2
Controls	82.5	17.5	4.8
Medial TF			
Compartment OA	54.0	46.0	12.7
Controls	75.0	25.0	3.6
PF joint OA	35.7	64.3	16.1

The figures show the percentages of controls and cases with radiographic evidence of lone OA of either the medial tibio-femoral (TF) or patello-femoral (PF) compartments of the knee joint who report lower limb disability. Disability, scored by the Health Assessment Questionnaire (HAQ), is divided into three categories: none (HAQ = 0), some disability (lower limb HAQ 0–1.9), severe disability (HAQ ≥ 2). Controls are age-sex matched people with no radiographic changes of OA. All differences are significant at 95% level.

or more joints; symptoms have resolved in a few cases. There is obviously scope in this study to uncover risk factors for improvement as well as progression, but we may have to wait several more years to observe enough change in sufficient numbers to obtain meaningful data. One of our major conclusions from the study so far is that "generalized OA" is not a distinct entity. Hand and knee disease are associated with each other, and the presence of hand disease is often used loosely to indicate polyarticular, nodal, or generalized OA. However, involvement of several sites seems to be age-related and arises from a gradual acquisition of new joints being involved as patients with a susceptibility to OA get older.

A 2-Year Therapeutic Trial

Patients with painful knee OA are often treated with nonsteroidal antiinflammatory drugs (NSAIDs). They may continue to take these agents for years. Short-term trials over a period of a few weeks have demonstrated that they provide better pain relief than a placebo, but long-term trials have not been conducted. We undertook this study to establish the feasibility of long-term, placebo-controlled studies in knee OA, and to assess the changes observed in patients studied carefully over a 2-year period (25).

Eighty-nine patients with established knee joint OA (65 women and 24 men;

TABLE 3. *Change over 2 years in a group of 51 patients with osteoarthritis of the knee joints, treated with either placebo or diclofenac[a]*

	Total no. completing study (N = 51)		Placebo group (N = 20)		Diclofenac group (N = 31)	
	Entry	2 Years	Entry	2 Years	Entry	2 Years
Number with rest pain (%)	23 (45)	21 (41)	8 (40)	6 (30)	15 (48)	15 (48)
Number with instability (%)	3 (6)	8 (16)	1 (5)	3 (15)	2 (6)	5 (16)
Mean range knee flexion	112°	111°	112°	111°	111°	112°
Number with functional difficulty:						
Walking (%)	8 (16)	15 (29)	2 (10)	8 (40)	6 (19)	7 (23)
Stairs (%)	44 (86)	37 (72)	18 (90)	16 (80)	26 (84)	21 (68)
Patient opinion:						
Better		25		9		16
Same		10		5		5
Worse		16		6		10
X-ray change						
No change (%)		31 (62)		13 (68)		18 (58)
Change (%)		19 (38)		6 (32)		13 (42)

[a] The data indicate little change over 2 years, irrespective of treatment.

mean age, 63 years) entered a randomized, double-blind, placebo-controlled trial of 100 mg diclofenac daily. Forty-four were randomized to placebo and 45 to diclofenac treatment. The patients were assessed at 6-month intervals for 2 years. Fifty-one (57%) completed the study, 20 of whom were on placebo and 31 on diclofenac. Most dropouts occurred early and were mainly due to lack of efficacy (3 active, 12 placebo, $p < 0.01$) or side effects (6 active, 5 placebo). At completion of the study there were few group differences, and 25 of the 51 (49%, 9 on placebo and 16 on diclofenac) reported improvement in their symptoms over the 2-year period (Table 3).

This study emphasizes the fact that once established, knee OA is often static over long periods of time. It also shows that many patients improve symptomatically, irrespective of tablet treatment used. Unfortunately, no variables correlating with a good or bad outcome, other than increasing age being associated with lack of tolerance to NSAIDs, have emerged from the study. However, it is clearly possible to carry out long-term, placebo-controlled studies in knee OA, and they should be sources of valuable data on the natural history and effects of any treatment on the disease.

CONCLUSIONS

1. Joint site is important in OA. Hip and knee disease should be regarded as quite different conditions, which may have a different etiopathogenesis, treatment response, and outcome.
2. Existing knowledge on knee OA in the community is limited because of the relatively crude methods which have been used to study the condition, and the tendency to ignore the patello-femoral joint. The patello-femoral joint may be a more important source of symptoms and disability than tibiofemoral disease, especially in women. Better methods for investigating this site are needed for population-based studies.
3. Risk factors for the development of knee OA need better definition, as they provide clues to the etiology of the condition. Rapid progression and a poor outcome occurs in a minority of cases. Determinants of outcome, which may be different from disease associations, also need to be defined.
4. New imaging and biochemical methods, along with better use and validation of existing clinical and x-ray techniques, are dramatically increasing the power and sensitivity of patient-based studies.
5. Long-term prospective studies of knee OA are feasible and underway. Placebo-controlled trials can be carried out over a period of years rather than weeks. Data so far indicate that once established, OA often remains stable for many years.

ACKNOWLEDGMENTS

This work is generously supported by the Arthritis and Rheumatism Council for Research (ARC). We would also like to acknowledge the generous help of numerous colleagues, especially those in Bristol and those at Rush University, Chicago.

REFERENCES

1. Felson DT. Epidemiology of hip and knee osteoarthritis. *Epidemiol Rev* 1988;10:1–28.
2. Cushnaghan J, Dieppe P. Study of 500 patients with limb joint osteoarthritis. 1. Analysis by age, sex, and distribution of symptomatic joint sites. *Ann Rheum Dis* 1991;50:8–13.
3. Kellgren JH, Lawrence JS. Radiological assessment of osteoarthrosis. *Ann Rheum Dis* 1957;16: 494–501.
4. Ahlbäck S. Osteoarthritis of the knee: a radiographic investigation. *Acta Radiol* 1968;(Suppl.): 277.
5. Altman R, Bloch D, Bole GJ, et al. Development of clinical criteria for osteoarthritis. *J Rheumatol* 1987;14(Suppl. 14):3–6.
6. McAlindon T, Dieppe PA. Osteoarthritis: definitions and criteria. *Ann Rheum Dis* 1989;48:531–532.
7. Claessens AAMC, Schouten JSAG, van den Ouweland FA, Valkenburg HA. Do clinical findings associate with clinical osteoarthritis of the knee? *Ann Rheum Dis* 1990;49:771–774.
8. van Saase JLCM, van Romunde LKJ, Cats A, et al. Epidemiology of osteoarthritis: Zoetermeer survey. *Ann Rheum Dis* 1989;48:271–280.
9. Wilson MG, Michet CJ, Ilstrup DM, Melton LJ. Idiopathic symptomatic osteoarthritis of the hip and knee: a population-based incidence study. *Mayo Clin Proc* 1990;65:1214–1221.
10. Bergstrom G, Bjelle A, Sundh V, Svanborg A. Joint disorders at ages 70, 75 and 79 years—a cross-sectional comparison. *Br J Rheum* 1986;25:333–341.
11. Spector TD, Campion GD. Generalised osteoarthritis: a hormonally mediated disease. *Ann Rheum Dis* 1989;48:523–527.
12. Doherty M, Watt I, Dieppe P. Influence of primary generalised osteoarthritis on development of secondary osteoarthritis. *Lancet* 1983;2:8–11.
13. Cooke TDV. Pathogenetic mechanism in polyarticular osteoarthritis. *Clin Rheum Dis* 1985;11(2): 203–238.
14. Hernborg JS, Nilson BE. The natural course of untreated osteoarthritis of the knee. *Clin Orthop Rel Res* 1977;123:130–137.
15. Massardo L, Watt I, Cushnaghan J, Dieppe P. An eight year prospective study of osteoarthritis of the knee joint. *Ann Rheum Dis* 1989;48:893–897.
16. Cushnaghan J, Cooper C, Dieppe P, Kirwan J, McAlindon T, McCrae F. Clinical assessment of osteoarthritis of the knee. *Ann Rheum Dis* 1990;49:768–770.
17. Cobby M, Watt I, Dieppe P. Imaging in osteoarthritis. In: Russell RGG, Dieppe PA, eds. *Osteoarthritis: research and prospects for pharmacological intervention.* London: IBC Ltd, 1991;34–50.
18. Cooper C, Cushnaghan J, Kirwan J, Rogers J, McAlindon T, McCrae F, Dieppe P. Radiographic assessment of the knee joint in osteoarthritis. *Ann Rheum Dis* (in press).
19. McCrae F, Shouls J, Dieppe P, Watt I. The scintigraphic assessment of osteoarthritis of the knee joint. *Ann Rheum Dis* 1991 (in press).
20. Dieppe P. Osteoarthritis: clinical and research perspective. *Br J Rheumatol* 1991;30(Suppl. 1): 1–4.
21. McAlindon TEM, Watt I, McCrae F, Goddard P, Dieppe PA. Magnetic resonance imaging in osteoarthritis of the knee: correlation with radiographic and scintigraphic findings. *Ann Rheum Dis* 1991;50:14–19.
22. Campion G, McCrae F, Schnitzer TJ, Lenz ME, Dieppe PA, Thonar J-MA. Levels of keratan sulfate in the serum and synovial fluid of patients with osteoarthritis of the knee. *Arthritis Rheum* 1991 (in press).
23. Campion G, McCrae F, Dieppe P, Watt I, Thonar J-MA, Schnitzer TJ, Knudson W. Serum hyaluronan levels in osteoarthritis. *Trans Orth Res Soc* 1991 (abstract in press).
24. McAlindon TE, Cooper C, Kirwan JR, Dieppe PA. Knee pain and disability in the community. *Ann Rheum Dis* 1991 (in press).
25. Dieppe PA, Cushnaghan J, Jasani K, McCrae F, Watt I. A two-year, placebo-controlled trial of

a non-steroidal anti-inflammatory (NSAID) in knee osteoarthritis (OA). *Br J Rheumatol* 1990;29(Suppl. 2):129 (abstract).

DISCUSSION

Brand: How many patients were in the subsets you examined in your postal survey?

Dieppe: The initial survey was 2,000 with a response of 80%. From that we have picked about 200 OA cases that were pain positive and x-ray positive, and 400 controls that were pain negative and x-ray negative for a risk factor analysis of osteoarthritis. The data on the risk factors are not yet available. Two other groups of about 100 each were also selected: first the pain negative and x-ray positive group and second the pain positive and x-ray negative group. We intend to study these as a separate issue to better understand pain.

Cooke: How do you define patello-femoral joint space and alignment? Are standing x-rays of the knees analyzed?

Dieppe: In the community-based study we are not able to study alignment fully with long-leg x-rays. We always do standing x-rays and have some data on standing versus lying x-rays. We assess the joints by a visual scoring system where we score osteophyte, joint space narrowing, and subchondral bone change separately. Evaluation of patello-femoral joint space narrowing is often an impossibility. So we depend more on subchondral bone changes and osteophytes. We do not include people unless they have subchondral bone changes as well as an osteophyte. Osteophyte alone does not indicate osteoarthritis.

Zborovsky: How many patients with osteoarthritis do you have altogether?

Deippe: Altogether we have cohorts numbering something like 1,000 people that we are following longitudinally. Two hundred are from the community, the rest is a hospital-based population. Therefore we can study differences between hospital and community-based OA populations.

Khaltaev: Have you looked at central obesity among your patients?

Dieppe: We have height, weight, and girth measurements so that we can look at central versus peripheral obesity, but have not done so yet. We are also hoping to obtain data on the time progression of obesity, including childhood weight.

Articular Cartilage and Osteoarthritis,
edited by K. Kuettner et al.
Raven Press, Ltd., New York © 1992.

45

Magnetic Resonance Imaging of Osteoarthritis

R. J. Hodgson, T. A. Carpenter, and Laurance D. Hall

*University of Cambridge, School of Clinical Medicine,
Cambridge, CB2 2PZ, United Kingdom*

Magnetic resonance imaging (MRI) provides a unique opportunity for visualizing and inspecting the soft tissues of joints. Its completely noninvasive nature makes it suitable for long-term serial studies, while its spatial localization allows images to be made of single slices, multiple parallel slices, or even of an entire three-dimensional region of interest. The protocol used to acquire the image is infinitely variable, and basic physical constants lead to a complex interplay between the image contrast, the image resolution, and the time required to acquire it. The main objective of this chapter is to give some insight into how these variables and constraints determine the uses and limitations of MRI in the investigation of joint structure, state, and function, concentrating largely on the articular cartilage, and extending this to osteoarthritis (OA) in particular.

Starting in the clinic with the large joints of the hip and knee, the question of articular cartilage visualization in terms of both spatial resolution and differentiation from adjacent tissue is addressed, together with what changes may be seen in the cartilage. MRI manifestations of OA are reviewed together with their use in differential diagnosis and staging of the disease. Moving away from the clinic to the laboratory, the feasibility of imaging the more technically demanding subjects of laboratory animals and human finger joints is examined, as are developments in these areas to date. Information is also drawn from *in vitro* studies. Finally, because the investigation of OA by MRI is still in its infancy, the prospects for the future are assessed, particularly the extension of *in vitro* and animal studies to man, effects of improved technical performance, and some practical applications.

THE POTENTIAL OF MRI FOR CLINICAL ASSESSMENT OF CARTILAGE

Typically, an MR image of a human joint may be obtained from a series of 3 to 5 mm thick, parallel, nearly adjacent slices through the knee with a resolution of 0.5 to 1 mm (1–8); similar images may be obtained from a 3 to 5 mm slice in the hip with in-plane resolution of 0.6 to 1 mm (5,7). Imaging time may vary from 2 to 17 min (1–3), depending on the nature of the protocol used, but this will affect the contrast. A typical normal knee image is shown in Fig. 1. The cortical bone appears very dark, as is true on all MR images. The marrow in the bone appears bright, although this may appear darker depending on the experiment, almost down to the level of cortical bone (Figs. 2, 3, 4). Clearly, good contrast between compact bone and marrow is useful for observing bone restructuring (Fig. 5). Similarly, the menisci are always dark (unless damaged). The articular cartilage varies from intermediate (Fig. 1) to high (Figs. 2, 3, 4) intensity (3,9); thus the hyaline cartilage is well distinguished from either, although in fact it is only the upper layers of cartilage that are seen, the calcified basal layer being of very low intensity, similar to cortical bone. Adjacent layers of articular cartilage may often be delineated by a thin, dark line which has been reported in the knee both *in vitro* (10,11) and *in vivo* (12,13), where it was seen in most of 28 cases (12) and in the proximal and distal (Figs. 2, 3) interphalangeal joints *in vivo* (11,14). This has been attributed to the superficial zone of cartilage with tangentially oriented collagen fibers (13).

There is clear potential for observing cartilage abnormalities with MRI; indeed, many have been reported including softening, swelling, surface irregularity, focal

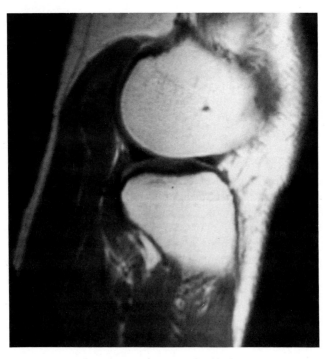

FIG. 1. Image of a normal healthy knee.

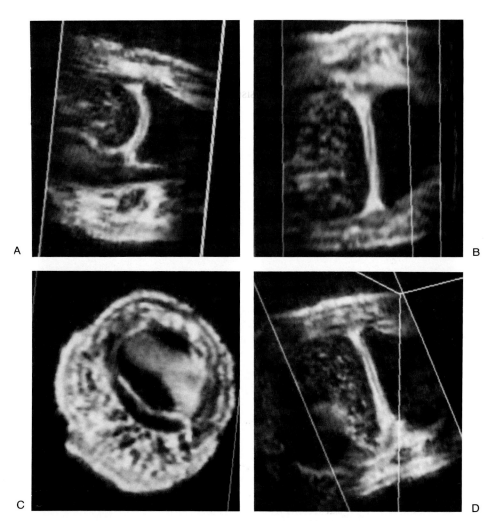

FIG. 2. Sections through three dimensional images of a normal, healthy, distal interphalangeal joint: **(A)** saggital, **(B)** coronal, **(C)** transverse, and **(D)** oblique.

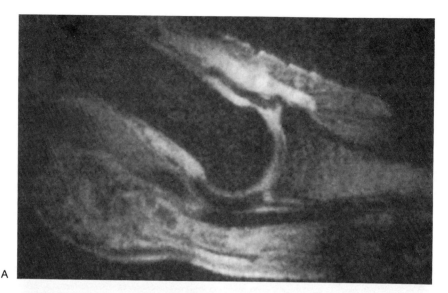

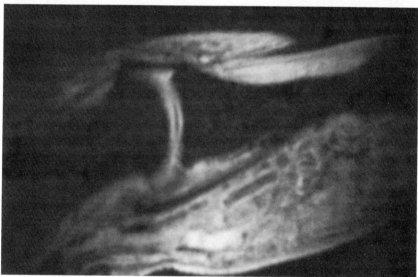

FIG. 3. Images of a normal, healthy, distal interphalangeal joint in flexion: (**A**) bent backwards, (**B**) almost straight, and (**C**) bent forwards.

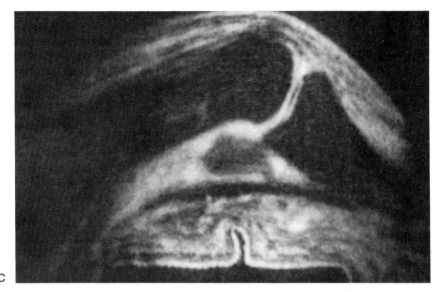

C

FIG. 3. *Continued.*

and diffuse thinning, cartilage loss, and joint space narrowing (Fig. 6). Softening has been observed in the knee as inhomogeneities in intensity within an otherwise normal layer of cartilage, in patello-femoral chondromalacia (2,12). Swelling has been observed *in vitro* (10) and in *in vivo* cases demonstrated by arthroscopy (2), and is associated with decreased intensity on MRI. Focal thinning has been reported in the hip in avascular necrosis (15) and in the knee in chondromalacia patellae (2). Focal lesions appear as localized regions of intensity which may be higher or lower in intensity than the articular cartilage depending on the experiment; with an inappropriate protocol they may not be discernible. Cadaveric studies suggest that lesions can be detected down to about 3 mm in size (6,10), although intraarticular injection of contrast media may reduce this to about 2 mm and also reduce the imaging time (6,10). Contrast media may not be necessary in the presence of joint effusion (9).

Diffuse effects include loss of the dark line between articulating cartilage layers, attributed to fibrillation, which may also be associated with decreased signal intensity extending to the cartilage surface (10). Diffuse thinning has been widely reported, and is seen as a decrease in the thickness of the high intensity band of cartilage in the knee (1,16) and in the hip (17) in rheumatoid arthritis (5) and in avascular necrosis *in vitro* (13). *In vitro* studies of the knee suggest errors in the measurement of cartilage thickness between MRI and sectioning to be about 0.7 mm, of the order of the MR image resolution (0.6 mm), without a consistent

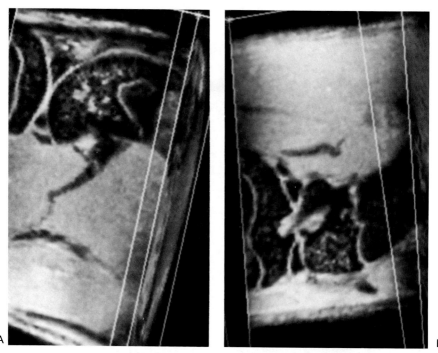

FIG. 4. Sections through a three-dimensional image of a normal, healthy rat knee: **(A)** saggital, **(B)** coronal, **(C)** transverse, and **(D)** multiply sliced.

over- or underestimation (18). In more extreme cases, cartilage loss may extend down to the cortical bone (1,2,4,5,12,17). The joint space between the cortical bone surface may be observed to decrease (1,18); again, good correlation is observed between values measured from MRI images and from sections (18).

These features allow the staging of cartilage degeneration with good correlation with arthroscopic findings, with the possible exception of early cartilage softening (2,10,12).

In addition to articular cartilage changes, bone lesions can also be demonstrated (1,5). In a study of subjects with rheumatoid arthritis, more bone erosions were detected on MRI images than on x-rays in 11 out of 19 cases, a finding attributed to the ability of MRI to look at thin slices (5). Joint effusions may also be observed in appropriate experiments as regions of relatively high intensity in the joint space (4,5,7,16,17). MRI, then, has been demonstrated not only to have the capability for imaging cartilage, but the contrast and resolution reveal degenerative features which allow disease staging.

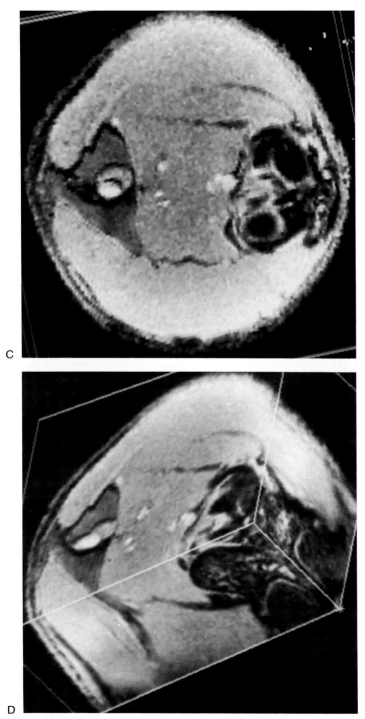

FIG. 4. *Continued.*

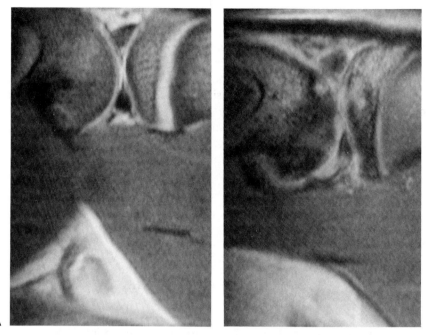

A   B

FIG. 5. Images through rat knees: **(A)** normal and **(B)** after experimentally induced arthritis.

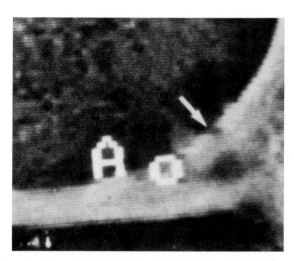

FIG. 6. Image through a knee with osteoarthritis, demonstrating localized cartilage defects (*arrow*). (From Konig et al., ref. 8, with permission.)

CLINICAL STUDIES OF OSTEOARTHRITIS

Having demonstrated the potential for MRI in the investigation of OA, three studies involving osteoarthritis are reviewed.

In a comparison of different imaging techniques for studying cartilage, Konig et al. studied various patients, including six with osteoarthritis, (three of the knee and three of the hip) (7). Plain x-rays revealed abnormalities in only two subjects, while histology showed a slight reduction in the proteoglycan and chondrocyte concentration in two and a distinct reduction in four. MR showed a significant decrease in signal intensity in the hyaline cartilage of all six joints. Good correlation between histologic reductions in proteoglycan was seen on MR images. MR, then, is of use not only because it allows earlier detection of OA than does plain x-ray, but also because it reveals information about the stage of proteoglycan loss.

Konig et al. studied a group of 24 normal volunteers and 106 patients with osteoarthritis, acute arthritis, rheumatoid arthritis, and activated osteoarthritis (8). Based on two MR intensity parameters of cartilage and joint effusion (19), they attempted to discriminate between the diseases. They were able to split the patients into five classes: (a) early/late OA, (b) activated OA/rheumatoid arthritis, (c) joint effusion, (d) acute arthritis, and (e) normal cartilage. Out of 144 cases, 78% were diagnosed correctly and 7% placed on the borderline between two classes. One of the most interesting findings of the study was a strong correlation between one of the MR parameters of cartilage measured and the age of normal volunteers. This has been attributed to the biochemically recognized structural changes which occur with aging, with no associated changes in water content. Thus MR is useful not only for differentially diagnosing osteoarthritis, but images can yield parameters that chart the proteoglycan structural changes, as well as being sensitive to water content change.

In an approach to OA investigation with MR based not solely on cartilage signal, Li et al. investigated 10 patients with late stage OA of the hips (20). Although their equipment allowed images of a resolution down to only 1.7 mm from 10 mm slices, they were able to classify joints into five grades based on their MR appearance: 0. normal; 1. inhomogeneity of articular cartilage; 2. inhomogeneity and discontinuity of articular cartilage and loss of intensity and blurring of the trabecular pattern in the femoral head and neck; 3. loss of articular cartilage, irregular cortical bone outline, blurring of trabecular pattern, loss of intensity in femoral head and neck, and regions of intermediate intensity with dark rims in the femoral head; 4. as 3. but with less intensity from marrow and more deformity in femoral head. These gradings were compared with functional capacity, as were plain x-ray gradings. In distinguishing between some and almost complete incapacity, plain x-rays were superior to MRI images, but for distinguishing between discomfort or limited mobility and severe incapacity, MR was more successful than x-ray. Clearly this study concentrated on the later stages of OA, but even so it demonstrated the superiority of MR over plain x-ray for staging in the less severe cases. Clearly the higher resolution typically available would enhance ability to further graduate the earlier grades.

Clinical studies of OA by MR have potential for diagnosis and staging. They also reveal and chart proteoglycan structural changes as well as changes in water content.

LABORATORY STUDIES OF JOINTS

One factor which is of particular importance to imaging small joints in both animals and in man is that it becomes more difficult to attain the same resolution relative to the joint size as the joint size decreases. Nevertheless, high resolution images are attainable. Figures 3 and 4 show images of the distal interphalangeal joint, where resolution of 0.1 to 0.2 mm from slices 1.8 to 2.5 mm thick is attainable (11,14; Fig. 3). This allows measurement of the cartilage thickness to a precision of about 0.1 mm and, while this is likely to be less than the true value (11), it should be consistent to this level of accuracy if the experimental protocol remains unchanged. Measurement of thickness is a potentially useful guide to cartilage state, and can be extended to area and volume. Figure 2 shows sections through a three-dimensional image of the distal interphalangeal joint with resolution of $0.2 \times 0.2 \times 0.4$ mm. The dark line between cartilage layers is clearly visible (Fig. 2) and appears more pronounced than on larger joints. This may be due in part to the different experimental conditions (11), but it might be expected if it does indeed correspond to the superficial layer of tangentially oriented collagen (13). Figure 3 demonstrates the appearance of the joint at different angles of flexion; such studies are useful for investigating joint physiology and have also been performed in the knee, where a series of the images showed sliding of the articular cartilage layers at the patello-femoral joint (21).

Imaging of animals is of particular interest for the testing of pharmaceuticals and both the rabbit and the rat are commonly used for model arthritis. Figure 4 shows a three-dimensional image of a normal rat knee at a resolution of 0.2 mm; the articular cartilage is clearly visible throughout the joint. Figure 5 shows two-dimensional images of the knee of two rats from a 0.8 mm slice with 0.15×0.08 mm resolution; (**A**) is a normal rat and (**B**) is a rat some time after experimental model arthritis has run its course. Extensive joint alterations have occurred in the latter, including cartilage restructuring, resulting in a thickened layer of high intensity cartilage of nonuniform thickness and bone remodeling, leading to localized loss of intensity from marrow in trabecular bone in the bone heads. Rats with this arthritis have had their knees imaged at different stages in the disease, and changes in cartilage signal, cartilage thinning, cartilage loss, and bone edema have also been detected.

In the rabbit knee, a resolution of 0.2 to 0.6 mm from 2 to 3 mm slices may be obtained. Bone changes and remodeling have been demonstrated in model arthritis (22). In an interesting series of experiments by Paul et al. (23), a rabbit knee was imaged before and after the injection of papain, which resulted in a decrease in the proteoglycan by a factor of about 19; the intensity of the cartilage thickness decreased significantly. That study demonstrates the feasibility of following by MR proteoglycan changes in the rabbit knee, suggesting it might be useful for following experimentally induced arthritis.

Studies of MR parameters on arthritis induced in pig knees by Konig et al. (19) used six different experimental forms of arthritis, including osteoarthritis from surgically induced incongruence and consecutive abnormal loading, and compared the results to biopsy findings and x-rays. Subchondral bone marrow lesions were seen earlier with MR than with x-ray. Although the type of induced arthritis could not be detected from the MR data, the matching in these parameters was well correlated with the maximum histological change, suggesting MR can accurately follow the time course of proteoglycan change in arthritis.

MR has also been used to study experimentally induced arthritis in the dog (24). Osteoarthritis was induced by transection of the anterior cruciate ligament, and MR images were acquired 3 years later. Gross thickening of regions of the articular cartilage of up to 350% compared to control knees was observed. Cartilage margins on the control knees were sharply defined, while on the osteoarthritic knee they were indistinct.

MR of animals has attained technical levels where even down to the size of a rat, articular cartilage can be clearly seen and changes in it during arthritis can be demonstrated. The ability to perform many serial studies on the same animal allows disease courses to be followed without the biological variation introduced by using many animals or the invasive use of biopsies.

In vitro investigations of bovine cartilage by Lehner et al. have revealed internal structure not appreciated *in vivo* (25). MR experiments were performed on articular cartilage from bovine patellae. Although many MR experiments showed the cartilage to be homogeneous, certain protocols revealed two layers, superficial and deep, of slightly different intensity, and of similar thickness, which were attributed to different zones. When normal cartilage samples were subject to low compression, an impression appeared in the image of the superficial lamina with lateral fluid flow while the deep lamina was unchanged. After increased or prolonged pressure, the intensity of the image of the deep layer increased, which is behavior attributed to fluid loss. Normal cartilage took about 20 min for the image to return to normal after cartilage was subjected to compression, but on the cartilage samples showing fibrillation, the cartilage images had not reverted to their previous appearance in this time.

All the images described so far have been obtained from the hydrogen atoms in the sample, in common with almost all MR images. Images can, however, be obtained with other nuclei, although they will be of poorer quality. In particular, sodium imaging of joints has revealed images in which intense regions have been tentatively assigned to cartilage and joint fluid (26). Unfortunately, the resolution is very low (3–4 mm from a 10 mm slice).

FUTURE PROSPECTS

The study of osteoarthritis by MR imaging clearly has a long way to go before it reaches maturity, but already much has emerged and the direction for future work is taking shape. Already anatomic changes in articular cartilage can be seen at a level useful for staging arthritis.

In the early stages with little or no gross anatomical change in the cartilage, variations in contrast have been demonstrated which clearly relate not only to water content but also to the proteoglycan state. While there is much work to be done in understanding the behavior of MR images in terms of these biochemical changes, the data available from MR images will clearly give qualitative information and it may well be possible to quantify this to some degree.

The ability to distinguish specific points in the early progression of OA has been demonstrated, as has MR's capability for staging the later effects. Earlier and more accurate staging should be possible based on the spatial appearance of the cartilage images, and the ability to identify early points in the disease which has been seen should lead to very early staging based on proteoglycan and small water changes. Since MR allows similar images to be obtained from animals and from man, it will provide a useful tool in determining how closely animal models of OA correspond to human OA. The noninvasive nature of MRI, permitting the arthritis in a single animal to be followed over its complete time course, will allow the assessment of efficacy of pharmaceutical intervention. The data, unlike histologic examination, will benefit from different time points having been obtained from a single animal; also, fewer animals will be required for the study.

In humans, the early staging of OA will allow the assessment of treatment success, which is potentially useful not only for individual therapeutic planning, but also for investigating the success of different therapeutic regimes. In particular, the use of the finger joints may allow testing that would otherwise produce unacceptable discomfort.

Finally, it might be hoped that the accurate following of the early stage of OA with MRI might produce insights into the basic processes at work.

ACKNOWLEDGMENTS

The authors thank Dr. Herchel Smith for the endowment which made this work possible (L. D. Hall and T. A. Carpenter) and for a studentship (R. J. Hodgson).

REFERENCES

1. Yulish BS, Lieberman JM, Strandjord SE, Bryan PJ, Mulopulos GP, Modic MT. Hemophilic arthropathy: assessment with MR imaging. *Radiology* 1987;164:759–762.
2. Yulish BS, Montanez J, Goodfellow DB, Bryan PJ, Mulopulos GP, Modic MT. Chondromalacia patellae: assessment with MR imaging. *Radiology* 1987;164:763–766.

3. Stoller DW. Fast MR improves imaging of musculoskeletal system. *Diagn Im Int* 1988;Apr:44–51.
4. Hartzman S, Reicher MA, Bassett LW, Duckwiler GR, Mandelbaum B, Gold RH. MR imaging of the knee. Part II. Chronic disorders. *Radiology* 1987;162:553–557.
5. Beltran J, Caudill JL, Herman LA, Kantor SM, Hudson PN, Noto AM, Baran AS. Rheumatoid arthritis: MR imaging manifestations. *Radiology* 1987;165:153–157.
6. Gylys Morin VM, Hajek PC, Sartoris DJ, Resnick D. Articular cartilage defects: detectability in cadaver knees with MR. *Am J Roentgenol* 1987;148:1153–1157.
7. Konig H, Sauter R, Deimling M, Vogt M. Cartilage disorders: comparison of spin-echo, CHESS, and FLASH sequence MR images. *Radiology* 1987;164:753–758.
8. Konig H, Aicher K, Klose U, Saal J. Quantitative evaluation of hyaline cartilage disorders using FLASH sequence. II. Clinical applications. *Acta Radiol* 1990;31:377–381.
9. Hajek PC, Sartoris DJ, Neumann CH, Resnick D. Potential contrast agents for MR arthrography: in vitro evaluation and practical observations. *Am J Roentgenol* 1987;149:97–104.
10. Hayes CW, Sawyer RW, Conway WF. Patellar cartilage lesions: in vitro detection and staging with MR imaging and pathologic correlation. *Radiology* 1990;176:479–483.
11. Cole PR, Jasani MK, Wood B, Freemont AJ, Morris GA. High resolution high field magnetic resonance imaging of joints: unexpected features inproton images of cartilage. *Br J Radiol* 1990;63:907–909.
12. Reiser MF, Bongartz G, Erlemann R, et al. Magnetic resonance in cartilaginous lesions of the knee joint with three-dimensional gradient-echo imaging. *Skeletal Radiol* 1988;17:465–471.
13. Harms SE, Muschler G. Three-dimensional MR imaging of the knee using surface coils. *JCAT* 1986;10:773–777.
14. Carpenter TA, Hall LD, Hodgson RJ. Investigation of the distal interphalangeal joint under flexion. *Magn Reson Imaging* 1990;8(Suppl. 1):79.
15. Mitchell DG, Joseph PM, Fallon M, et al. Chemical-shift MR imaging of the femoral head: an in vitro study of normal hips and hips with avascular necrosis. *Am J Roentgenol* 1987;148:1159–1164.
16. Beltran J, Noto AM, Mosure JC, Weiss KL, Zuelzer W, Christoforidis AJ. TI: the knee: surface coil MR imaging at 1.5T. *Radiology* 1986;159:747–751.
17. Brower AC, Kransdorf MJ. Imaging of hip disorders. *Radiol Clin North Am* 1990;28:955–974.
18. Chandnani VP, Ho C, Chu P, Trudell D, Resnick D. Knee hyaline cartilage evaluated with MR imaging: a cadaveric study involving multiple imaging sequences and intraarticular injection of gadolinium and saline solution. *Radiology* 1991;178:557–561.
19. Konig H, Aicher K, Klose U, Saal J. Quantitative evaluation of hyaline cartilage disorders using flash sequence. I. Method and animal experiments. *Acta Radiol* 1990;31:371–375.
20. Li KC, Higgs J, Aisen AM, Buckwalter KA, Martel W, McCune WJ. MRI in osteoarthritis of the hip: gradations of severity. *Magn Reson Imaging* 1988;6:229–236.
21. Niitsu M, Akisada M, Anno I, Miyakawa S. Moving knee joint: technique for kinematic MR imaging. *Radiology* 1990;174:569–570.
22. Checkley D, Johnstone D, Taylor K, Waterton JC. High-resolution NMR imaging of an antigen-induced arthritis in the rabbit knee. *Magn Reson Med* 1989;11:221–235.
23. Paul PK, OByrne E, Blancuzzi V, et al. Magnetic resonance imaging reflects cartilage proteoglycan degradation in the rabbit knee. *Skeletal Radiol* 1991;20:31–36.
24. Braunstein EM, Brandt KD, Albrecht M. MRI demonstration of hypertrophic articular cartilage repair in osteoarthritis. *Skeletal Radiol* 1990;19:335–339.
25. Lehner KB, Rechl HP, Gmeinwieser JK, Heuck AF, Lukas HP, Kohl HP. Structure, function, and degeneration of bovine hyaline cartilage: assessment with MR imaging in vitro. *Radiology* 1989;170:495–499.
26. Granot J. Sodium imaging of human body organs and extremities in vivo. *Radiology* 1988;167:547–550.

DISCUSSION

Okyayuz-Baklouti: Is it possible to perform volume-selective phosphorous or proton spectroscopy in cartilage of the knee joint?

Hall: Phosphorous spectroscopy of joints is very, very hard. Proton spectroscopy is just about achievable, but it will probably not yield much important information currently because the water in cartilage gives very broad resonances as do other small molecules. The shape of cartilage is very awkward. Existing techniques sample cubes of tissue and unfortunately cartilage does not come in convenient cubes. We are developing methods to obtain proton resonances from arbitrary shaped volumes, but it's very hard.

Okyayuz-Baklouti: There is a new field, NMR microscopy, which is very hard to use in tissues which have movement artifacts. Maybe more rigid systems like cartilage or joints might be a target for NMR microscopy.

Hall: I agree. The family of NMR-imaging experiments which we refer to as chemical NMR microscopy are meant to produce very high-resolution images from small volumes of tissue. However, there are physical limitations; for a 1-mm sample, you can achieve resolution of about 5 microns. Eventually 1 micron resolution will be possible, but that is about the limit. So this is not really microscopy; it is just high-resolution imaging.

Thonar: Can you comment on the potential of MRI to measure very small changes in water content in articular cartilage, distinguishing 70% water content from 72%, for example?

Hall: Yes, in principle, but in practice this is very difficult. We have funds from oil industry to see if we can quantitate brine and oil in lumps of rock. Even after ten man years we still can't achieve a 0.5% level of accuracy. It has always been very hard in NMR to make accurate measurements of concentration, even in 5 mm NMR tubes, because of the signal to noise limitations. So if this is important enough, it can be done with a great investment of time and effort, but it will not be done using procedures similar to routine hospital scans.

Dieppe: How easy is it going to be to differentiate synovium edema with water from free synovial fluid?

Hall: This differentiation will not be possible from simple MRI scans. Additional experiments that provide T_1 and T_2 relaxation measurements are required. We now obtain complete three-dimensional data sets for every volume element, i.e., proton density, T_1, and T_2. It takes a long time to acquire these data, much more than is possible in clinical practice. What now takes 20 hours to do on a lump of rock, will be possible to do next year in less than 1 hour in man. Then we can begin to answer your question.

Hascall: Will it ever be feasible to use some of the techniques of two-dimensional NMR, or to tune to specific structures in glycosaminoglycan chains to get information about their mobility in cartilage?

Hall: I think it is impossible to do such experiments directly. We *can,* however, measure accurately proton relaxation from water. Then you can develop models to infer something about the microenvironment, but those models do not exist yet.

Pritzker: My comment is that even fuzzy data can be extremely valuable in imaging the joints. Unlike brine in rock, the water environment in joints changes over time, reflecting changes in molecular constituents. Even if we cannot define the interactions precisely, changes in water quality that are now measured may well be important to assess the conditions of cartilage.

Articular Cartilage and Osteoarthritis,
edited by K. Kuettner et al.
Raven Press, Ltd., New York © 1992.

46

Arthroscopy and Arthroplasty

Wolfhart Puhl

*Orthopädische Klinik und Querschnittgelähmtenzentrum/RKU Forschungs- und
Lehrbereich der Universität Ulm, 7900 Ulm, Germany*

An orthopedic surgeon invited to speak at an international workshop for articular cartilage and osteoarthritis to international experts in the field of basic research is in a fix. Are they really interested in the clinic routine of arthroscopy and arthroplasty? Of course we should not forget that the patient has a painful knee, but does it help if I tell them about the history and evaluation of our standard operation methods? Would they like to hear about risks or even bad results in surgery? Let me try to build a bridge between clinic and basic research work and provide some information about the clinical features of osteoarthrosis and their consequences for interpretating research data.

An orthopedic surgeon talking about osteoarthritis (OA) knows that it is easy to diagnose OA but very hard to tell anything about a patient's prognosis whether the disease is treated or not. It is also very difficult to form a clear picture of the disease in terms of basic research.

More precisely, if we discuss a case of gonarthrosis with a certain degree of arthrosis, for example, a varusgonarthrosis, we collect all clinical data before deciding treatment regimens. If the patient reports pain with only a little impairment of knee function in clinical examination and no pathological findings in x-rays, we can not be sure whether an osteotomy correcting his deformity will be successful or not. Tissue specimens collected from such an osteoarthrotic joint and examined in a basic laboratory would show various degrees of OA from nearly normal to severely changed specimens. In these cases, an arthroscopy enables us to see the extent and localization of the damaged cartilage and to take specimens for further study from various regions of the joint surface and joint capsula. In this way we may obtain more information about our patient's knee, and judge more accurately whether the patient's condition would improve after doing an osteotomy. If arthroscopy shows that only the medial parts of the joint are severely damaged, i.e., the joint surface denuded of cartilage and sclerotic bone visible, while next to this there are areas covered with white and deeply cleft or eburnized cartilage, we can help our patient by doing an osteotomy. But if we find that the lateral parts of the joint are severely damaged as well, than osteotomy would not help.

Macroscopic x-ray findings of these conditions reveal clear differences in the subchondral bone. Joint areas not covered with articular cartilage have a tremendous thickening and sclerosis of subchondral bone, typical signs of adaptation to stress due to cartilage damage.

HISTOLOGY AND CULTURE

Macroscopical and histological findings demonstrate that we should not focus on a whole joint, but rather on limited areas with certain degrees of OA. This implies that information shared between the orthopedic surgeon from the operating room and the basic research colleague in the laboratory should be extensive and intensive. Biochemical and ultrastructural studies should be clearly correlated.

In our laboratory we did histological examinations of biopsies taken from different areas of osteoarthrotic cartilage. Cell and tissue cultures were also established to study anabolic or catabolic parameters using radioisotopic precursors. Scintillation counting provides overall estimates for metabolic activity, and autoradiography allows some comparison between individual chondrocytes. The incorporation of radioactive proline and sulfate provides information about collagen and proteoglycan synthesis. These results demonstrate that there are not only enormous differences in the metabolic activity of different joints, but also within different regions of a single OA joint.

Chondrocytes in osteoarthrotic cartilage can synthesize normal matrix components, but there is a disregulation of the cell metabolism in OA cartilage. Increased cell metabolism is directly related to the histopathological grade of OA (1). Several systems have been developed in vitro and in vivo to study the pathogenic mechanism of OA (2–8). Studies in vitro with human and experimental OA cartilage explants showed an initial period of enhanced proteoglycan synthesis. At the same time, however, an increased loss of newly synthesized proteoglycan and proteoglycan subunits from the tissue was noted (9–11). Apparently the repair mechanism might be ineffective. Also, cell proliferation increases with increasing histopathological grades of OA. But in the most severe forms of OA, mitotic activity of chondrocytes is much reduced (9–12).

Currently we do not have any reliable, long-term culture system to help us study the changes in osteoarthrotic cartilage. Chondrocytes in cell culture systems are missing their natural matrix and are therefore of limited value in studying OA changes. Cartilage tissue can only be cultured for 4 to 8 weeks. We cultured cartilage tissue in Dulbecco's modified Eagles Medium with fetal bovine serum, -glutamine, and antibiotics. Our results show a decrease of metabolic activity of cartilage tissue in vitro that is clearly time-related. At an average of 6 weeks after incubation, the proline uptake reaches the metabolic level of an avital piece

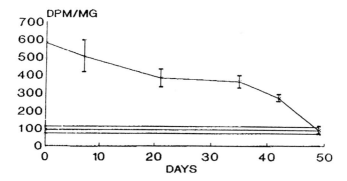

FIG. 1. 3-H-Proline incorporation in cartilage tissue cultures.

of cartilage (Fig. 1). Figure 1 shows the time-related uptake of 3-H-proline. It is measured by liquid scintillation counting and is indicated in disintegrations per minute. Six pieces of cartilage were measured at certain times. Further studies are necessary to prolong the vitality of cartilage tissue in culture.

ARTHROSCOPY'S ACTUAL SITUATION

Besides using arthroscopy for diagnostic reasons, there has been an encouraging development in arthroscopic operation techniques over the last few years. As head of a university hospital, it is especially interesting and important to me to introduce and evaluate these new techniques. One very promising method is laser surgery.

Conventional shaver systems are based on mechanical removal of osteoarthrotic cartilage by rotating cutting blades. Thus the cartilage debris is eliminated by reducing the osteoarthrotic cartilage up to the basal layers. However, the cartilage removed contains up to 80% of the vital chondrocytes, and although the rough joint surface is smoothed, precious biological material is wasted. In those desperate cases of osteoarthrosis we clinicians know all too well, these chondrocytes might still be very important. Here laser surgery might open up new horizons by enabling us to remove the cartilage debris responsible for the patient's osteoarthritis while saving a maximum of vital chondrocytes.

Laser therapy in medicine started in 1961 when Campbell et al. (13) introduced laser equipment to ophthalmology. His encouraging results and the development of new laser systems led to laser use in almost the whole range of medicine. Arthroscopic surgery, however, could not use this technique until energy transmission systems small enough for arthroscopic use were developed. In 1982 Whipple et al. (14) published the first results for CO_2 laser meniscectomies in which a small mirror system was used for energy transmission. Glick (15) used an yttrium aluminium garnet (YAG) laser for arthroscopic laser meniscectomies at about the same time.

Arthroscopic surgery today uses the CO_2 laser, the neodymium:YAG laser, or the holmium:YAG laser which emit light in the infrared range and work by thermal effects. The photon energy is partly absorbed in the various tissue layers. Depending on the power densities inside the tissue, this causes several thermal effects. Power densities below 150 W/cm² cause necrosis, and higher power levels lead to vaporization of intracellular water. Cutting tissue requires power densities between 10^4 and 10^6 W/cm² (Fig. 2). When energy from one of the laser systems is applied to joint cartilage, three typical zones are found (Fig. 3). Next to the cutting crater there is an area of complete carbonization of tissue. Adjoining this area there is a zone of tissue necrosis gradually changing into a zone of thermal damage with increasing distance from the vaporization zone. Modified pulse rate and pulse duration can decrease the zones of thermal damage, but side effect is always present when using these lasers.

In the early 1980s, so-called Excimer lasers (the word coming from *exci*ted di*mer*s) were developed. These laser systems emit energy in the far ultraviolet portion of the light. In contrast to the lasers mentioned above, photons produced by Excimer lasers are absorbed in the first few 10 μms of the tissue, thus reaching power densities between 10^9 and 10^{11} W/cm² over very short distances (see Fig. 2). Srinivasan (16) was the first to examine the effects on tissue caused by XeCl

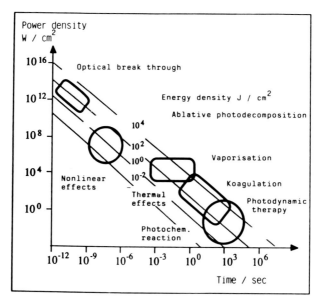

FIG. 2. Power density-pulse diagram. (Modified from Berlien, Müller, Angewandte Lasermedizin Ecomedverlag, 1989, [29] with permission.)

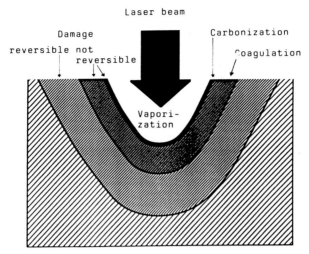

FIG. 3. Zones of injury after laser cut. (Modified from Berlien, Müller, Angewandte Lasermedizin Ecomedverlag, 1989, [29] with permission.)

Excimer lasers. The power densities achieved disintegration of molecular structures with almost no thermal side effects to the adjoining tissue. Srinivasan called this effect "ablative photodecomposition."

In several experiments *in vitro,* we have examined the effects of an XeCl Excimer laser on joint cartilage. Light microscopical examinations (Fig. 4) showed only small areas of tissue damage that were similar in morphology but not in

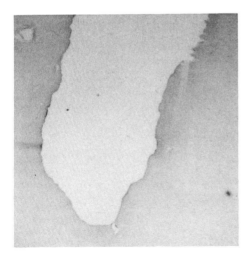

FIG. 4. Laser cut haematoxylin-eosin (HE) stained enlargement, 100×.

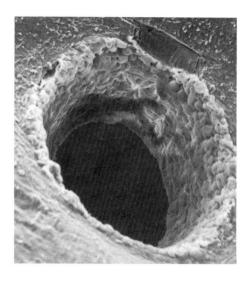

FIG. 5. Laser cut SEM examination.

extent to the zone of necrosis caused by a CO_2 laser. A small zone of thermal conductivity was also observed. In comparison to the damage caused by other laser systems, damage of surrounding cartilage is much reduced when an XeCl laser is used. The zone of carbonization was completely missing in all cases. Similar results were described by Hohlbach et al. (17), Kroitzsch et al. (18), and Kolbe et al. (19).

Scanning electron microscopy (SEM) examinations of XeCl laser cuts reveal a small area of uniform structure next to the sharply visible edge of the crater which gradually changes into normal appearing cartilage (Figs. 5, 6). Siebert et al. (20) compared the ability of different lasers to smooth the surface of osteoar-

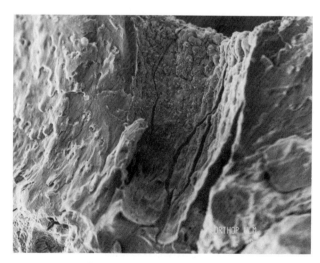

FIG. 6. Laser cut SEM examination.

throtic cartilage and found the best results using an XeCl Excimer laser. Similar to our clinical findings, he demonstrated that the XeCl laser creates a nearly smooth but hardened cartilage surface. SEM examinations of the surface of OA cartilage after use of an XeCl laser reveal a smooth surface, with the cartilage appearing to be almost sealed.

After 2 years of clinical experience, we now use this laser routinely in arthroscopic surgery of OA patients. Some clinical examinations have been undertaken to evaluate the follow-up of laser therapy in arthroscopic operations of OA patients (21), but convincing results are still missing. However, Excimer laser therapy appears to be an interesting and promising method for treating OA patients.

ARTHROPLASTY

Last but not least, we can restore function of the osteoarthrotic joint using joint replacements. With the help of this technique, we can achieve pain relief, an acceptable range of motion, and sufficient joint stability.

With knee arthroplasty, results have improved since the introduction of surface replacements instead of hinge prothesis with stems in femur and tibia in all cases where knee ligaments are intact. With this method, only the destroyed joint surfaces are replaced by metal, metal-backed polyethylene, or unbacked polyethylene components. The complex motion of the knee joint can be largely preserved which leads to a better outcome. Only in cases of severe deformity or lax knee ligaments can the hinge prosthesis be preferred to surface replacements.

The problem of whether to use cemented or uncemented components remains unresolved. There are as yet no convincing arguments against bone cement from either the orthopedic surgeon's point of view or from basic research (22). In our experience, the cement guarantees an immediate and close contact between the prothesis and the underlying bone, and therefore provides good transmission of pressure and tensile forces. Cystic defects of the femur condyles or the tibial plateau have to be filled with autologous or homologous bone grafts.

Total hip replacement presents a different situation. In this case, especially when using the femoral component, we constantly violate nature and this can be a main reason for aseptic loosening. In a normal hip joint, transmission of forces occurs from the acetabulum to the femoral head and neck. Within the femoral neck a complex system of bone trabeculae guarantees the distribution of tensile and pressure forces to the cortical bone of the metaphysis and diaphysis. Resecting the femoral head and neck and implanting a solid shaft prothesis means a complete change of force conduction, with a load maximum at the inner side of the proximal femur. This requires nature to be highly adaptable to force redistributions. To reduce the problems, we have attempted to adapt the femoral stems to the anatomical and biomechanical findings. We used cementless stems to exclude difficulties we suspected might occur with bone cement. The uncemented technique was considered to be the biological way of hip replacement (23,24). However, the best results so far are reported from cemented stems implanted with contemporary cementing patterns (25,26). This is reasonable because the bone cement makes the closest contact between the prosthesis and the trabecular bone. Thus, the contact area between the stem and the surrounding bone is as wide and as intensive as possible, a situation which will not be achieved using cementless components.

Looking at the socket the situation is less pronounced as we find comparable results on the short-term using cementless or cemented acetabular components (27,28).

I hope that this is what you wanted to hear from a clinician as a brief insight into our daily work. In my opinion some improvements in the treatment have already been achieved, but there are still more steps to go, not only for us, but also for the patient suffering from OA who should take his steps without pain.

REFERENCES

1. Bulstra SK, Buurman WA, Walenkamp GHIM. Metabolic characteristics of in vitro cultured human chondrocytes in relation to the histopathologic grade of OA. *Clin Orthop Rel Res* 1989;242: 294.
2. Amadio PC, Ehrlich MG, Mankin HJ. Matrix synthesis in high density cultures of bovine epiphyseal plate chondrocytes. *Connect Tissue Res* 1983;11:11ff.
3. Delbrueck A, Dresow B, Gurr E. In vitro culture of human chondrocytes from adult subjects. *Connect Tissue Res* 1986;15:155ff.
4. Fife RS, Palmoski MJ, Brandt KD. Metabolism of a cartilage matrix glycoprotein in normal and osteoarthritic canine articular cartilage. *Arthritis Rheum* 1987;29:1256ff.
5. Thonar EJ, Buckwalter JA, Kuettner KE. Maturation-related differences in the structure and composition of proteoglycans synthesized by chondrocytes from bovine articular cartilage. *J Biol Chem* 1986;261(5):2467.
6. Malemud CJ, Papay RS. Rabbit chondrocytes maintained in serum free medium. *Exp Cell Res* 1986;167(2):440.
7. van Kampen GPJ. Cartilage response to mechanical force in high density chondrocyte cultures. *Arthritis Rheum* 1985;28:419ff.
8. Weiss A, van der Mark K, Silbermann M. A tissue culture system supporting cartilage cell differentiation, extracellular mineralisation and subsequent bone formation, using mouse condylar progenitor cells. *Cell Differ* 1986;19:103.
9. Mankin HJ, Dorfman H, Lipiello MS, et al. Biochemical and metabolic abnormalities in articular cartilage from osteoarthritic human hips. *J Bone Joint Surg* 1971;58B:523ff.
10. Roughly PJ, White RJ. Age related changes in the structure of proteoglycan subunits from human articular cartilage. *J Biol Chem* 1980;255:217ff.
11. Verbruggen G, Luyten FP, Veys EM. Repair function in organ cultured human cartilage. Replacement of enzymatically removed proteoglycans during long term organ culture. *J Rheumatol* 1985;12:665ff.
12. Sandy JD, Barrach HJ, Flannery CR. The biosynthetic response of the mature chondrocyte in early osteoarthritis. *J Rheumatol* 1987;8:16ff.
13. Campbell CJ, Rittler MC, Koester CJ. The optical laser as a retinal coagulator; an evaluation. *Trans Am Acad Ophthalmol Otolaryngol* 1989;67:58–67.
14. Whipple TL, Caspari RB, Meyers JF. Arthroscopic meniscectomy by CO2 laser vaporisation in a gas medium. *Orthop Trans* 1982;6:136–142.
15. Glick J. YAG Laser meniscectomy. Presented at the Triannual Meeting of the International Arthroscopy Association of North America, Rio de Janeiro/Brazil, August 1981.
16. Srinivasan R. Ablation of polymers and biological tissues by ultraviolet lasers. *Science* 1986;234: 559–565.
17. Hohlbach G, Möller KO, Schramm U, Baretton G. Experimentelle Ergebnisse der Knorpelabrasio mit einem Excimer-Laser. Histologische und elektronenmikroskopische Untersuchungen. *Z Orthop* 1989;127:216–221.
18. Kroitzsch U, Laufer G, Egkher E, Wollenek G, Horvath R. Experimental photoablation of meniscus cartilage by excimer laser energy. *Arch Trauma Surg* 1989;108:44–48.

19. Kolbe T, Hibst R, Steiner R. Untersuchungen zu Parametern der Excimer-Laser-Angioplastie in Bezug auf Effizienz und Gewebeschäden. In: Steiner R. (Hrsg) Verhandlungsbericht der Deutschen Gesellschaft für Lasermedizin e.V. 5. Jahrestagung 28.–30.9.1989. München: EBM-Verlag 1990;36–47.
20. Siebert WE, Kohn D, Wirth CJ. Histologische und rasterelektronenmikroskopische Veränderungen an Knorpeloberflächen nach Bearbeitung mit verschiedenen Lasern im Vergleich zu mechanischen Instrumenten. In: Steiner R. (Hrsg) Verhandlungsbericht der Deutschen Gesellschaft für Lasermedizin e.V. 5. Jahrestagung 28.-30.9.1989. München: EBM-Verlag 1990;334–342.
21. Raunest J, Löhnert J. Arthroscopic cartilage debridement by excimer laser in chondromalacia of the knee joint. *Arch Orthop Trauma Surg* 1990;109:155–159.
22. Freeman MAR, Railton GT. Die zementlose Verankerung in der Endoprothetik. *Orthopäde* 1987;16:206–219.
23. Harris WH, Maloney WJ. Hybrid total hip arthroplasty. *Clin Orthop* 1989;249:21–29.
24. Maloney WJ, Harris WH. Comparison of a hybrid with an uncemented total hip replacement. *J Bone Joint Surg* 1990;72A:1349–1352.
25. Morscher E. Zukunft der Hüftendoprothetik mit oder ohne Knochenzement? *Swiss Med* 1987;9:27–44.
26. Rothman RH, Cohn JC. Cemented versus cementless total hip arthroplasty. *Clin Orthop* 1990;254:153–169.
27. Russotti GM, Coventry MB, Stauffer RN. Cemented total hip arthroplasty with contemporary techniques. *Clin Orthop* 1988;235:141–147.
28. Wilson-MacDonald J, Morscher E. Comparison between straight- and curved-stem Müller femoral protheses. *Arch Orthop Trauma Surg* 1989;109:14–20.
29. Berlien HP, Müller G. (Hrsg) Angewandte Lasermedizin. München: ecomed-Verlag 1989.

DISCUSSION

Kuettner: When you did a smoothening of the fibrillated arthrotic cartilage using a mechanical shaver during arthroscopy, the superficial layer was removed. One year later, when you looked in the joint, was there any evidence for replacement of the superficial layer?

Puhl: Doing control arthroscopy 1 year after the first operation we could find no repair or replacement of the superficial layer. The joint surface appeared stable without new fibrillated osteoarthrotic cartilage visible.

Kuettner: Does that mean that the intermediate zone may be able to take over the function of the superficial zone? Did it look normal?

Puhl: The intermediate zone took over the function of the superficial zone but it did not change macroscopically to look like the superficial zone. Obviously there was no progress of OA; either a steady-state was reached by the cartilage or there was no mechanical overuse of the cartilage.

Buckland-Wright: Some of your arthroscopic pictures of joints that were not inflamed showed pannus-like overgrowth or invasion. Is this seen often?

Puhl: In the beginning of the 1970s we started doing arthroscopies first in unclear situations in rheumatoid arthritis. There we saw pannus overgrowth as a typical sign of inflamed joints. We very soon learned that there is a pannus formation in many OA cases, too. Being interested in these mechanisms of joint reactions, we did animal experiments in which the femoropatellar joints of rabbits were subjected to various mechanical stresses, especially high-impulse overload. If the clearly localized damage was situated near the borderline between synovium and joint cartilage, the synovium formed pannus-like structures overgrowing and destroying the cartilage. If the damage was further away from the cartilage-synovium borderline, we did not see any pannus overgrowth.

Articular Cartilage and Osteoarthritis,
edited by K. Kuettner et al.
Raven Press, Ltd., New York © 1992.

47

Molecular Markers of Cartilage Turnover

A Role in Monitoring and Diagnosis of Osteoarthritis?

L. Stefan Lohmander

Department of Orthopedics, University Hospital, S-22185 Lund, Sweden

We currently diagnose osteoarthritis (OA) on the basis of combined clinical symptoms and radiological findings (1–3). Since the diagnosis is based on obligatory radiological signs, often including a decrease of the joint space, it is dependent on the actual destruction of joint cartilage. By definition, the diagnosis will thus be made only late in the disease process. However, the osteoarthritic process in the joint cartilage is initiated long before the radiological diagnosis can be made, and our inability to diagnose the disease at these earlier stages is a reflection of the lack of methods available to monitor the health of the joint cartilage *in vivo.* Even the commonly used radiological terminology of "joint space" or "joint gap" illustrates the power of the word over the mind: it tempts us to ignore the central issue of the disease, namely the joint cartilage. Our current methods for diagnosis and staging of OA are better suited for the preoperative planning by the orthopedic surgeon aiming for an osteotomy or a joint replacement, than for the diagnosis of the early stages of the disease process.

Treatment of the early, symptomatic stages of OA centers on the use of physiotherapy, oral nonsteroidal antiinflammatory drugs (NSAIDs), and sometimes intraarticular or intramuscular injections of steroids, hyaluronan, or other compounds. None of these treatments has been shown to influence the progress of the human disease or to retard the destruction of the joint cartilage in OA. On the other hand, high tibial valgus osteotomy used in early stages of medial compartment OA of the knee has been shown to delay the necessity for joint replacement for many years (4). Interestingly, postoperative regrowth of cartilage on the damaged joint surfaces has been observed in some patient series, although it is still unclear whether the good outcome of the procedure is in any way related to the observed cartilage regeneration (5,6). However, the fact that some regrowth of cartilage on damaged joint surfaces may take place at all is significant. If we are to utilize the apparent limited healing capacity of joint cartilage, it is of obvious advantage to diagnose the disease in its early phase.

Injury to the cruciate ligaments and menisci of the knee carries with it an increased risk of posttraumatic OA (7–9). Much effort is currently invested in improving the techniques for surgical repair or replacement of injured ligaments or menisci, with the aim of decreasing the short-term symptoms of the instability and the hope of decreasing the risk of future posttraumatic OA of the injured joint. However, the rationale for these efforts is often limited to the biomechanical aspects of the procedure and thoroughly ignores the biology of the cartilage and other tissues in the joint. At the present time, the situation with these surgical procedures is the same as with the pharmacological treatment of OA: the treatment sometimes diminishes the symptoms associated with the condition, but none of the procedures has been shown to decrease unequivocally the frequency or rate of development of posttraumatic OA. The overall situation in OA therapy is thus similar to that in rheumatoid arthritis, where current routine drug therapy or surgical synovectomy decreases the symptoms associated with the synovitis, but does not change the course of the joint destruction (10,11).

Although the rate of development of posttraumatic OA is often rapid compared to primary OA, it still stretches over years, and sometimes decades, before the diagnosis can be made with our current gold standard, namely the weight-bearing radiographs (1,3). As a consequence, patients in a clinical trial of OA treatment, be it surgical or pharmacological, must be followed for many years before the efficacy of the treatment can be evaluated with regard to its influence on the disease progression. This makes such trials very difficult and costly to perform. The development of improved methods to diagnose and monitor OA is thus of interest not only to the patient, orthopedic surgeon, and rheumatologist, but also to the pharmaceutical industry. Such new methods need to monitor the current state of health of the joint cartilage *in vivo,* not only to provide a historical record of past destructive disease.

The precise mechanisms involved in the disease process in OA are not known. Presumably the pathogenesis is multifactorial with genetics, joint malalignment, joint overload or trauma, obesity, and aging as some of the known or suspected general contributing factors. Even less well known is how these general factors are translated into disease mechanisms at the tissue and cell level. Since, undisputably, changes in the properties of joint cartilage and loss of matrix components are an integral part of the disease process, it may be argued that degradation of cartilage matrix is a key event at some time in the development of OA. During this process, matrix molecules or fragments thereof are released to the joint fluid and eventually to other body fluids. These molecules and fragments could be used as markers of cartilage matrix metabolism.

MECHANISMS OF MATRIX TURNOVER

The physiological turnover rate of adult joint cartilage matrix is slow, with average biological half-lives in the order of months and years. Several studies demonstrate, however, that the turnover of different matrix components is not homogeneous, and there are, for example, several pools of matrix proteoglycans turning over at different rates (12, see also van Kampen). Little or nothing is known about the turnover rates *in vivo* of the more recently characterized components of the cartilage matrix, such as the minor collagens, the cartilage matrix proteins, or the small proteoglycans (13).

The chondrocytes play a major role in both the physiological turnover of cartilage matrix in growth and development and in the pathological degradation which occurs in joint disease (Fig. 1). Degradative enzymes derived from synovial cells may be important in certain conditions. The role of enzymes derived from leukocytes in matrix degradation in arthritis may be questioned though, since joint destruction is not inhibited in neutropenic, arthritic animals, nor in arthritic animals genetically deficient in neutrophil elastase or cathepsin G (14–15). The degradative activity of the chondrocytes is greatly stimulated by cytokines such as interleukin-1 or tumor necrosis factor released from cells of the synovium (16,17), and this has been suggested to be an important disease mechanism in inflammatory joint disease. However, the significance of this signal pathway for the stimulation of cartilage destruction in OA has not been demonstrated.

The primary cleavage of the cartilage matrix molecules is extracellular and is mediated by proteinases, the majority of which are probably produced by the chondrocytes themselves. A central role in cartilage matrix degradation has been proposed for the metalloproteinase family, with stromelysin, collagenase, and gelatinase as its most prominent members (18). These enzymes are secreted in a latent proenzyme form and activated extracellularly, and the active forms are inhibited by strong binding to tissue inhibitors of metalloproteinase (TIMPs) or

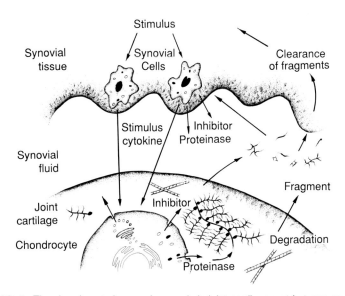

FIG. 1. The chondrocyte has a primary role in joint cartilage matrix turnover.

to alpha-2-macroglobulin. Several levels of regulation of cartilage matrix degradation therefore exist: gene expression and secretion of enzyme protein, extracellular activation of proenzyme, and inhibition of activated enzyme by TIMP and other inhibitors. The TIMP is also synthesized by the chondrocytes. The potential thus exists for a very close and local regulation of proteinase activity in the cartilage matrix, perhaps explaining some of the heterogeneity observed in the turnover of matrix components.

Collagenase primarily cleaves the native triple helix of types II and X cartilage collagens, while gelatinase cleaves denatured interstitial collagen, as well as type IV and V collagen. Stromelysin, on the other hand, has a broader specificity and cleaves not only the core protein of the large cartilage proteoglycan, but also types II, IX, X, and XI collagen and other components of the cartilage matrix (19). The chondrocyte thus produces a range of proteinases which can degrade most or all of the structural components of the cartilage matrix.

RELEASE OF MATRIX FRAGMENTS
TO BODY FLUID COMPARTMENTS

Fragments of cartilage matrix molecules produced by enzyme action are either taken up by the chondrocytes and further degraded by lysosomal enzymes, or are lost to the joint fluid by diffusion (Fig. 2). It is possible that in addition, small amounts of matrix components are lost from the tissue by diffusion, independent of enzyme action (20,21). The cartilage tissue does not, however, accumulate any appreciable amounts of diffusible matrix molecule fragments. In line with

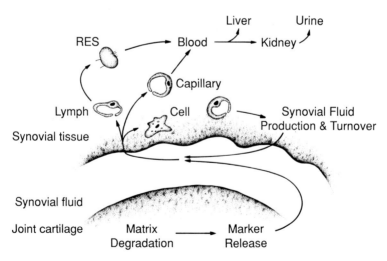

FIG. 2. Turnover of joint cartilage matrix fragments released to the joint fluid and other compartments.

these observations, even vigorous physical exercise does not markedly increase the concentration of proteoglycan fragments in human knee joint fluid (22).

Fragments of matrix molecules released to the joint fluid may be taken up by and further degraded in the synovial cells, or may be removed by bulk flow with the circulating synovial fluid to the lymph circulation (23). In addition, tissue fragments and collagen fibrils can be phagocytosed by cells of the joint fluid (24). A significant proportion of matrix molecule fragments removed by the lymphatic circulation are probably eliminated or at least further degraded in the regional lymph nodes (23,25). The majority of the remaining fragments which reach the blood stream are rapidly and within minutes removed from circulation, most likely by the liver cells (26–28). The collagen cross-links, however, survive the circulation and are found enriched in urine, as compared to other compartments (29,30).

It should be observed in this context that only a small proportion (<10%) of the body cartilage mass is located in the joints, the rest being found in ribs, airways, intervertebral disks, etc. (31). In addition, the concentration of a marker in, for example, joint fluid or serum can not be interpreted in a quantitative fashion unless the clearance rate for that fragment is also known (see Levick). Since the clearance rate of synovial fluid components has been shown to vary in different joint diseases (32), great caution should be exercised when attempting quantitative interpretations of data on cartilage markers in body fluids.

A RATIONAL CHOICE OF MARKERS AND MODELS?

Even if we at this time have to exercise care when translating cartilage marker data into quantitative disease terms, this area is developing rapidly, and results of current work should help us to identify disease mechanisms better and with time, to provide the means to monitor treatment. A sound basis for the rational development of effective treatment of OA would thereby be provided.

Markers

In the wide sense, markers of cartilage degradation in OA can be identified within several areas: cytokines, proenzymes, active proteinases, proteinase inhibitors, fragments of matrix molecules produced by enzymes, serum antibodies to cartilage components, and matrix molecules synthesized as an adaptive response to matrix degradation. Sensitive and specific assays are now available for several molecular species within each group:

1. Cytokines can be determined in synovial fluid (33,34).
2. Proteinases and their inhibitors can be assayed, either by enzyme activity or by enzyme protein content (35–38).
3. Matrix components and their fragments can be assayed in the form of glycosaminoglycans (39,40), hyaluronan (41), keratan sulfate (42), different forms

of chondroitin sulfate (43), proteoglycans (44–46), matrix proteins (47), collagen cross-links (29,48), and collagen propeptides (49,50).

4. Serum antibodies to cartilage collagen and chondrocyte membrane proteins have been detected in joint disease (51–54).
5. The availability of monoclonal antibodies to specific structures on the chondroitin sulfate chain allows the assay of proteoglycan subpopulations synthesized in increased amounts as a response to joint disease (43,55).

Compartments

The interpretation of data obtained with any of the above assays will depend on the compartment chosen for sampling. A joint fluid sample will mirror the condition of the cartilage contained within that joint, while both serum and urine samples will contain an integrated measure of cartilage turnover in all joints and potentially in all body cartilage. Although it may be argued that serum samples are easier to interpret on the basis of more straightforward clearance calculations, marker concentrations are much lower in serum than in synovial fluid, complicating assay techniques. Additionally, many joint cartilage markers may be degraded en route to the blood circulation, and they are also diluted by markers from healthy joints and nonarticular cartilage. The exception to this case so far seems to be the collagen cross-links, which survive endogenous metabolism and which are concentrated in urine compared to serum and joint fluid. In fact, the levels of type II collagen hydroxypyridinium cross-link in joint fluid are below the detection limit for current high-performance liquid chromatography based methods and are less than 1% of urine levels (Eyre & Lohmander, unpublished data).

On the basis of these arguments, it would seem that much speaks in favor of focusing on synovial fluid samples in the initial stages of marker investigations. When promising markers have been identified in joint fluid, a search can then be made in other body fluid compartments. Above all, efforts should be made to correlate marker levels in several compartments using the same assays and the same sample donors. Moreover, much can be gained by coordinating assays of more than one marker in one and the same sample set. It is very difficult to draw conclusions on the basis of data on different markers assayed in different patient series when patient selection criteria vary and are often ill-defined.

Stratification

All published reports on body fluid markers of cartilage turnover demonstrate a considerable range of values between individual patients within each diagnostic group. While a significant portion of this variability must be due to biological variation between individuals, it is also clear that many patient groups are heterogeneous, and sometimes ill-defined criteria are used for inclusion or exclusion of patients in a specific group. Suggested minimum requirements in a study on OA patients should be specified inclusion and exclusion criteria, age, sex, previous joint trauma and/or injury, duration of symptoms or time since joint trauma, previous joint surgery, medication for joint disease, arthroscopic or radiological data (or both), and staging of disease, if possible.

Several studies have demonstrated that a stratification of the patients within each diagnostic group will decrease the scatter of the assay data (42,45,46,56,57). For example, assays of proteoglycan fragments in knee joint fluids after injury demonstrate a great decrease in the average marker concentration within the first 6 months after trauma and a more-or-less level plateau after 6 months. Thus, a recent joint trauma will greatly influence synovial fluid marker concentration (Fig. 3). A stratification of OA patients according to disease stage further demonstrates an inverse relation between OA stage (as estimated by arthroscopy and radiology) and joint fluid proteoglycan concentration. Thus, the advanced radiological stages show lower concentrations than the early cases with only mild joint cartilage damage as observed in the arthroscope (Fig. 4).

Models

As remarked earlier in this chapter, human OA is of a heterogeneous pathogenesis, and the clinical diagnosis should probably not be regarded as a single

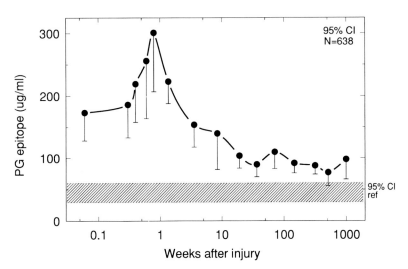

FIG. 3. Proteoglycan fragment concentration in knee joint fluid after injury. Joint fluid samples were obtained at different times after trauma from 638 patients (age 18–45 years) with injury of cruciate ligament either isolated or combined with additional meniscal and ligament injury or with isolated meniscus injury only. Proteoglycan fragments were quantified by immunoassay (46). *Bars* indicate 95% confidence intervals for the means. The *shaded area* indicates mean and 95% confidence interval for knee healthy controls. Note logarithmic time scale.

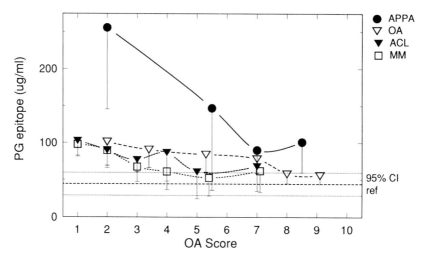

FIG. 4. Proteoglycan fragment concentration in joint fluid in relation to osteoarthritis staging. Joint fluid samples were obtained from patients with primary OA (OA), OA combined with pyrophosphate arthritis (APPA), or posttraumatic OA after injury to cruciate ligament isolated or combined with meniscus injury (ACL) or meniscus injury only (MM) (504 patients total, age 18–75 years). In the latter two groups, all samples were taken more than 6 months after trauma. Joint fluid proteoglycan fragment concentration was correlated to OA staging as obtained by arthroscopy and radiology (56,57). A score of 1 is normal joint cartilage by arthroscopy, scores 2–5 indicate increasing arthroscopic cartilage changes but normal weight-bearing x-ray films, and scores 6–10 indicate increasing radiological changes (1). *Bars* indicate 95% confidence intervals for the means. The *horizontal dashed and dotted lines* indicate mean and 95% confidence intervals for healthy controls. Immunoassay as in Fig. 3.

disease entity, but rather as a final common pathway of joint cartilage failure. The symptoms and radiological presentation in this end-stage are similar, irrespective of the origin of the condition. Important information on the disease mechanisms of OA has been gained by the use of a variety of animal models that mimic different aspects of the human disease (58). For example, naturally occurring OA in monkeys and mice have been used as models of human primary OA (59–61), while surgically induced ligament or meniscus lesions or blunt trauma of the knee in the rabbit or dog have been used to model the human posttraumatic OA (62–64).

Human Osteoarthritis and Cartilage Markers

In human studies, we need to select subgroups of patients in order to decrease scatter and to simplify the interpretation of marker data. The subpopulation of patients with posttraumatic OA of the knee offers an attractive model for the general disease. It has the distinct advantage in that the beginning of the disease process can be identified as the time of trauma, early and precise diagnosis of

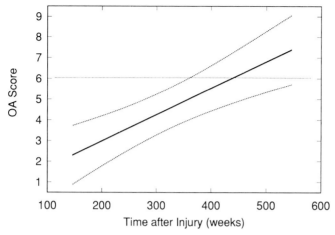

FIG. 5. Average time for development of osteoarthritic changes after knee trauma and injury to cruciate ligament and/or meniscus (372 patients). The time since trauma was plotted against the OA score (OA score as in Fig. 4). A least squares linear regression was performed; the *dashed lines* indicate the 95% confidence intervals for the mean. The *horizontal dotted line* indicates the lowest OA score with radiological OA (1).

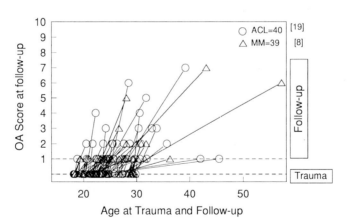

FIG. 6. Individual rates of progress of osteoarthritic changes after knee injury. A total of 79 patients who sustained an injury of cruciate ligament (ACL) or meniscus (MM) more than 6 months (average 4 years) before arthroscopy were selected from a pool of some 600 patients with joint injury. In all cases the trauma occurred between the ages of 18 and 30 years (average, 23 years). It was assumed that all these patients had a normal joint cartilage (OA score = 1) at the time of trauma. The age at trauma is marked (*bottom dashed line*) with a symbol and is connected with a line to a second symbol (*at or over top dashed line*) representing age and OA score at the time of arthroscopy and radiography. Each patient is thus represented by two symbols connected by a line. The steeper the rise of the line, the faster is the rate of OA progress for that patient. A total of 27 out of 79 patients had an OA score higher than 1 at the follow-up examination.

the injury can be made through arthroscopy, the osteoarthritic process can be followed from its early stages in prospective studies in a high-risk group, and finally the disease progress is comparatively rapid.

In our data of more than 600 patients with injury to the cruciate ligament or meniscus of the knee, the average time from injury to the appearance of radiological changes consistent with OA (1) is about 10 years (Fig. 5). Interestingly, the average rate of progression is about the same for the patients with cruciate ligament injury and for those with only meniscus injury. However, the rate of progression varies widely between individual patients, where some individuals acquire radiological OA within a couple of years after the injury, while the joints of others apparently survive for decades (Fig. 6). The underlying reasons for this wide difference in susceptibility are unclear, but continued joint abuse and inborn factors may have a role (7–9,65,66). Whichever is the case, such a patient group provides an important starting point for prospective studies on OA and markers of cartilage turnover (58,67,68). Retrospective studies on such patient groups demonstrate interesting temporal patterns of release of proteoglycan fragments to joint fluid (Fig. 7). A significant release of proteoglycan fragments occurs within the first day after trauma, with the highest average concentrations observed at 5 to 7 days after injury and with sustained and significantly elevated levels for up to 20 years after injury, as compared with a healthy control group. However, the proteoglycan release patterns in the time period from about 5 weeks to 1 to 2 years after trauma differ markedly between patients with either cruciate ligament or meniscus injury. The hemarthrosis commonly associated with cru-

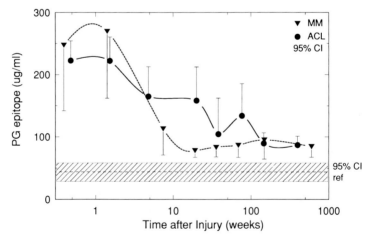

FIG. 7. Temporal patterns of release of proteoglycan fragments to joint fluid after knee trauma and injury to the cruciate ligament with or without associated meniscus injury (ACL), as compared to meniscus injury only (MM) (777 patients total). *Bars* indicate 95% confidence interval for the means. The *shaded area* indicates mean and 95% confidence interval for knee healthy controls. Immunoassay as in Fig. 3. Note logarithmic time scale.

ciate ligament injury may be one of several possible reasons for the different patterns of release in these two types of knee injury.

Work on animal posttrauma OA has demonstrated very early dramatic changes in joint cartilage composition and metabolism, showing the advantages of being able to monitor the earliest stages of the disease before secondary cascade phenomena complicate the picture (63,64,69). Indeed, if concentration of proteoglycan fragments in joint fluid mirrors disease activity in OA, then the peak of disease activity occurs well before the condition can be diagnosed by routine radiography (Fig. 4). Clearly, this should influence the strategies for both surgical and pharmacological interventions which aim at inhibiting joint cartilage destruction.

CONCLUSIONS

The area of osteoarthritis and cartilage marker research is still in the early stages of identifying useful markers, suitable disease models, and patterns of correlation. The published results of retrospective case-control studies can now serve as hypothesis-generating investigations which allow us to design relevant prospective studies to test our hypotheses. Such longitudinal, prospective studies will be necessary to answer with certainty questions on the relevance of cartilage markers for the prediction of disease outcome.

Meanwhile, ongoing work already has the potential to give us a better understanding of the disease mechanisms involved in OA at the cell and tissue level. Thus, we can correlate quantitative data on molecular fragments, proteinases, and inhibitors with each other. We are also able to obtain structural information on matrix molecule fragments released to joint fluid as well as on those remaining in the tissue. This allows us to draw conclusions about the identity of the enzymes active in the destruction of the joint cartilage, a central issue in OA. Together, these areas of investigation should offer the means for improved diagnostic and prognostic tools in OA, as well as to provide a basis for the rational development and monitoring of treatment with the aim of inhibiting cartilage destruction in osteoarthritis.

ACKNOWLEDGMENTS

This work was supported by grants from the Swedish Medical Research Council, the King Gustaf V 80-Year Birthday Fund, the Ax:son Johnson Foundation, the Kock Foundation, the Österlund Foundation, the Zoega Foundation, and the Medical Faculty of Lund University.

REFERENCES

1. Ahlbäck S. Osteoarthritis of the knee: a radiographic investigation. *Acta Radiol (Stockholm)* 1968;(Suppl.)277:7–72.

2. Altman R, Asch E, Bloch D, Bole G, Borenstein D, Brandt K, Christy W, Cooke TD, Greenwald R, Hochberg M, Howell D, Kaplan D, Koopman W, Longley SI, Mankin H, McShane DJ, Medsger TJ, Meenan R, Mikkelsen W, Moskowitz R. Development of criteria for the classification and reporting of osteoarthritis. *Arthritis Rheum* 1986;29:1039–1049.

3. Altman RD, Fries JF, Bloch DA, Carstens J, Cooke TD, Genant H, Gofton PGH, McShane DJ, Murphy WA, Sharp J, Spitz P, Williams CA, Wolfe F. Radiographic assessment of progression in osteoarthritis. *Arthritis Rheum* 1987;30:1214–1225.

4. Odenbring S, Egund N, Knutson K, Lindstrand A, Toksvig Larsen S. Revision after osteotomy for gonarthrosis. A 10–19-year follow-up of 314 cases. *Acta Orthop Scand* 1990;61:128–130.

5. Odenbring S, Egund N, Lindstrand A, Lohmander LS. Proteoglycan epitope in synovial fluid after tibial osteotomy for medial gonarthrosis. *Acta Orthop Scand* 1991;62:169–173.

6. Odenbring S, Egund N, Lindstrand A, Lohmander LS, Willén H. Cartilage regeneration after proximal tibial osteotomy for medial gonarthrosis: an arthroscopic, radiographic and histologic study. *Clin Orthop* 1991(in press).

7. Graham GP, Fairclough JA. Early osteoarthritis in young sportsmen with severe anterolateral instability of the knee. *Injury* 1988;19:247–248.

8. Sherman MF, Warren RF, Marshall JL, Savatsky GJ. A clinical and radiographical analysis of 127 anterior cruciate insufficient knees. *Clin Orthop* 1988;227:229–237.

9. Kannus P, Järvinen M. Posttraumatic anterior cruciate ligament insufficiency as a cause of osteoarthritis in a knee joint. *Clin Rheumatol* 1989;8:251–260.

10. Ianuzzi L, Dawson N, Zein N, Kushner I. Does drug therapy slow radiographic deterioration in rheumatoid arthritis? *N Engl J Med* 1983;309:1023–1028.

11. Doets HC, Bierman BTM, Soesbergen RM. Synovectomy of the rheumatoid knee does not prevent deterioration. 7-year follow-up of 83 cases. *Acta Orthop Scand* 1989;60:523–525.

12. Lohmander S. Turnover of proteoglycans in guinea pig costal cartilage. *Arch Biochem Biophys* 1977;180:93–101.

13. Heinegård D, Oldberg Å. Structure and biology of cartilage and bone matrix non-collagenous macromolecules. *FASEB J* 1989;3:2042–2051.

14. Pettipher ER, Henderson B, Moncada S, Higgs GA. Leukocyte infiltration and cartilage proteoglycan loss in immune arthritis in the rabbit. *Br J Pharmacol* 1988;95:169–176.

15. Schalwijk J, Joosten LAB, van den Berg W, van de Putte LBA. Experimental arthritis in C57 black/6 normal and beige (Chediak-Higashi) mice: in vivo and in vitro observations on cartilage degradation. *Ann Rheum Dis* 1988;47:940–946.

16. Saklatvala J, Sarsfield SJ, Townsend Y. Pig interleukin 1: purification of two immunologically different leukocyte proteins that cause cartilage resorption, lymphocyte activation and fever. *J Exp Med* 1985;162:1208–1222.

17. Saklatvala J. Tumor necrosis factor stimulates resorption and inhibits synthesis of proteoglycan in cartilage. *Nature* 1986;322:547–549.

18. Docherty AJP, Murphy G. The tissue metalloproteinase family and the inhibitor TIMP: a study using cDNAs and recombinant proteins. *Ann Rheum Dis* 1990;49:469–479.

19. Wu J-J, Lark MW, Chun LE, Eyre DR. Sites of stromelysin cleavage in collagen types II, IX, X, and XI of cartilage. *J Biol Chem* 1991;266:5625–5628.

20. Bolis S, Handley CJ, Comper WD. Passive loss of proteoglycan from articular cartilage explants. *Biochim Biophys Acta* 1989;993:157–167.

21. Sah RL-Y, Doong J-YH, Grodzinsky AJ, Plaas AHK, Sandy JD. Effect of compression on the loss of newly synthesized proteoglycans and proteins from cartilage explants. *Arch Biochem Biophys* 1991;286:20–29.

22. Dahlberg LRH, Ekblom B, Celsing F, Lohmander LS. Proteoglycan epitope in joint fluid after exercise. *Orthop Trans* 1991;16:334.

23. Fraser JRE, Kimpton WG, Laurent TC, Cahill RNP, Vakakis N. Uptake and degradation of hyaluronan in lymphatic tissue. *Biochem J* 1988;256:153–158.

24. Moreland LW, Stewart T, Gay RE, Huang GQ, McGee N, Gay S. Immunohistologic demonstration of type-II collagen in synovial fluid phagocytes of osteoarthritis and rheumatoid arthritis patients. *Arthritis Rheum* 1989;32:1458–1464.

25. Tzaicos C, Fraser JRE, Tsotsis E, Kimpton WG. Inhibition of hyaluronan uptake in lymphatic tissue by chondroitin sulphate proteoglycan. *Biochem J* 1989;264:823–828.

26. Engström-Laurent A, Hellström S. The role of liver and kidneys in the removal of circulating hyaluronan, an experimental study in the rat. *Connect Tissue Res* 1990;24:219–224.

27. Smedsröd B, Melkko J, Risteli L, Risteli J. Circulating C-terminal propeptide of type-I procollagen

is cleared mainly via the mannose receptor in liver endothelial cells. *Biochem J* 1990;271:345–350.

28. Maldonado BA, Williams JM, Otten LM, Flannery M, Kuettner KE, Thonar EJ-MA. Differences in the rate of clearance of different KS-bearing molecules injected intravenously in rabbits. *Orthop Trans* 1989;14:161.

29. Seibel MJ, Duncan A, Robins SP. Urinary hydroxy-pyridinium crosslinks provide indices of cartilage and bone involvement in arthritic diseases. *J Rheumatol* 1989;16:964–970.

30. Eyre DR, Dickson IR, Van Ness KP. Collagen cross-linking in human bone and articular cartilage. Age-related changes in the content of mature hydroxypyridinium residues. *Biochem J* 1988;252:495–500.

31. Attencia LJ, McDevitt CA, Nile WB, Sokoloff L. Cartilage content of an immature dog. *Connect Tissue Res* 1989;18:235–242.

32. Wallis WJ, Simkin PA, Nelp WB. Protein traffic in human synovial effusions. *Arthritis Rheum* 1987;30:57–63.

33. Feldmann M, Brennan FM, Chantry D, Haworth C, Turner M, Abney E, Buchan G, Barrett K, Barkley D, Chu A, Field M, Maini RN. Cytokine production in the rheumatoid joint: implications for treatment. *Ann Rheum Dis* 1990;49:480–486.

34. Bensouyad A, Hollander AP, Dularay B, Bedwell AE, Cooper RA, Hutton CW, Dieppe PA, Elson CJ. Concentrations of glycosaminoglycans in synovial fluids and their relation with immunological and inflammatory mediators in rheumatoid arthritis. *Ann Rheum Dis* 1990;49:301–307.

35. Martel-Pelletier J, Pelletier J-P, Malemud CJ. Activation of neutral metalloprotease in human osteoarthritic knee cartilage: evidence for degradation in the core protein of sulphated proteoglycan. *Ann Rheum Dis* 1988;47:801–808.

36. Henderson B, Pettipher ER, Murphy G. Metalloproteinases and cartilage proteoglycan depletion in chronic arthritis. Comparison of antigen-induced and polycation-induced arthritis. *Arthritis Rheum* 1990;33:241–246.

37. Cooksley S, Hipkiss JB, Tickle SP, Holmesievers E, Docherty AJP, Murphy G, Lawson ADG. Immunoassays for the detection of human collagenase; stromelysin; tissue inhibitor of metalloproteinases (TIMP) and enzyme-inhibitor complexes. *Matrix* 1990;10:285–291.

38. Walakovits LA, Moore VL, Bhardvaj N, Gallick GS, Lark MW. Detection of stromelysin and collagenase in synovial fluid from patients with rheumatoid arthritis and post-traumatic knee injury. *Arthritis Rheum* 1991(in press).

39. Carroll G. Measurement of sulphated glycosaminoglycans and proteoglycan fragments in arthritic synovial fluid. *Ann Rheum Dis* 1989;48:17–24.

40. Silverman B, Cawston TE, Thomas DPP, Dingle JT, Hazleman BL. The sulphated glycosaminoglycan levels in synovial fluid aspirates in patients with acute and chronic joint disease. *Br J Rheumatol* 1990;29:340–344.

41. Engström-Laurent A, Laurent UBG, Lilja K, Laurent TC. Concentration of sodium hyaluronate in serum. *Scand J Clin Lab Invest* 1985;45:497–504.

42. Sweet MB, Coelho A, Schnitzler CM, Schnitzer TJ, Lenz ME, Jakim I, Kuettner KE, Thonar EJ-MA. Serum keratan sulfate levels in osteoarthritis patients. *Arthritis Rheum* 1988;31:648–652.

43. Caterson B, Griffin J, Mahmoodian F, Sorrell JM. Monoclonal antibodies against chondroitin sulphate isomers: their use as probes for investigating proteoglycan metabolism. *Biochem Soc Trans* 1990;18:820–823.

44. Witter J, Roughley PJ, Webber C, Roberts NKE, Poole AR. The immunologic detection and characterization of cartilage proteoglycan degradation products in synovial fluids of patients with arthritis. *Arthritis Rheum* 1987;30:519–529.

45. Ratcliffe A, Doherty M, Maini RN, Hardingham TE. Increased concentrations of proteoglycan components in the synovial fluids of patients with acute but not chronic joint disease. *Ann Rheum Dis* 1988;47:826–832.

46. Lohmander LS, Dahlberg L, Ryd L, Heinegård D. Increased levels of proteoglycan fragments in knee joint fluid after injury. *Arthritis Rheum* 1989;32:1434–1442.

47. Fife R. Identification of cartilage matrix glycoprotein in synovial fluid in human osteoarthritis. *Arthritis Rheum* 1988;31:553–556.

48. Eyre DR, Koob TJ, Van Ness KP. Quantitation of hydroxypyridinium crosslinks in collagen by high-performance liquid chromatography. *Anal Biochem* 1984;137:380–388.

49. Madsen JS, Jensen LT, Strom H, Horslev-Petersen K, Svalastoga E. Procollagen type-III ami-

noterminal peptide in serum and synovial fluid of dogs with hip dysplasia and coxarthrosis. *Am J Vet Res* 1990;51:1544–1546.

50. Shinmei M, Ito K, Matsuyama S, Inamori Y, Matsuzawa K, Shimomura Y. Carboxy-terminal type II procollagen peptide levels in joint fluids as a marker of collagen biosynthesis of cartilage in joint diseases. *Ann Rheum Dis* 1992 (in press).
51. Niebauer GW, Wolf B, Bashey RI, Newton CD. Antibodies to canine collagen types I and II in dogs with spontaneous cruciate ligament rupture and osteoarthritis. *Arthritis Rheum* 1987;30: 319–327.
52. Mollenhauer J, von der Mark K, Burmester G, Glückert K, Lütjen-Drecoll E, Brune K. Serum antibodies against chondrocyte cell surface proteins in osteoarthritis and rheumatoid arthritis. *J Rheumatol* 1988;15:1811–1817.
53. Paróczai C, Németh-Csóka M. Estimation of serum anticollagen and the antibodies against chondrocyte membrane fraction: their clinical diagnostic significance in osteoarthritis. *Clin Biochem* 1988;21:117–121.
54. Choi EK, Gatenby PA, McGill NW, Bateman JF, Cole WGYJR. Autoantibodies to type II collagen: occurrence in rheumatoid arthritis, other arthritides, autoimmune connective tissue diseases, and chronic inflammatory syndromes. *Ann Rheum Dis* 1988;47:313–322.
55. Caterson B, Mahmoodian F, Sorrell JM, Hardingham TE, Bayliss MT, Carney SL, Ratcliffe A, Muir H. Modulation of native chondroitin sulphate structure in tissue development and disease. *J Cell Science* 1990;97:411–417.
56. Lohmander LS, Dahlberg L, Ryd L, Heinegård D. Joint cartilage markers in synovial fluid in human osteoarthritis. *Orthop Trans* 1990;15:212.
57. Lohmander LS, Dahlberg L. Proteoglycan epitope in joint fluid in human osteoarthritis. *Orthop Trans* 1991;16:227.
58. Lohmander LS. Osteoarthritis: man, models and molecular markers. In: Maroudas A, Kuettner K, eds. *Methods in cartilage research*. London: Academic Press, 1990;337–340.
59. Sokoloff L. Natural history of degenerative joint disease in small laboratory animals. *AMA Arch Pathol* 1956;62:118–128.
60. Walton M. Patella displacement and osteoarthrosis of the knee joint in mice. *J Pathol* 1979;127: 165–172.
61. Chateauvert JMD, Pritzker KPH, Kessler MJ, Grynpas MD. Spontaneous ostearthritis in Rhesus Macaques: I. Chemical and biochemical studies. *J Rheumatol* 1989;16:1098–1104.
62. Donohue JM, Buss D, Oegema TR, Thompson RC. The effects of indirect blunt trauma on adult canine articular cartilage. *J Bone Joint Surg* 1983;65-A:948–957.
63. Carney SL, Billingham MEJ, Muir H, Sandy JD. Demonstration of increased proteoglycan turnover in cartilage explants from dogs with experimental osteoarthritis. *J Orthop Res* 1984;2:201–206.
64. Carney SL, Billingham MEJ, Muir H, Sandy JD. Structure of newly synthesized (35S)-proteoglycans and (35S)-proteoglycan turnover products of cartilage explant cultures from dogs with experimental osteoarthritis. *J Orthop Res* 1985;3:140–147.
65. Doherty MWI, Dieppe P. Influence of primary generalised osteoarthritis on development of secondary osteoarthritis. *Lancet* 1983;2(8340):8–11.
66. Noyes FR, Mooar PA, Matthews DS, Butler DL. The symptomatic anterior cruciate-deficient knee. Part I: The long-term functional disability in athletically active individuals. *J Bone Joint Surg* 1983;65-A:154–162.
67. Lohmander S. Proteoglycans of joint cartilage: structure, function turnover and role as markers of joint disease. *Clin Rheumatol* 1988;2:37–62.
68. Lohmander LS. Cartilage markers in joint fluid in human osteoarthritis. In: Brandt K ed. *Cartilage changes in osteoarthritis*. Indiana University School of Medicine Press, 1990;98–104.
69. Hoch DH, Grodzinsky AJ, Koob TJ, Albert ML, Eyre DR. Early changes in material properties of rabbit articular cartilage after meniscectomy. *J Orthop Res* 1983;1:4–12.

DISCUSSION

Levick: The magnitude of differences you observed were moderate. Such shifts could easily reflect changes in hyaluronan concentrations. For example, inflammation may dilute the hyaluronate making more space available to proteoglycan fragments, then the joint improves, hyaluronate reconcentrates, and less space is available.

Lohmander: I certainly agree with you; this could be a problem. It may not be too serious, however. If the volume corrections are used with our concentration data converting them into mass per joint, the trends are almost identical.

Levick: That's not too surprising. It is the volume turnover rate that really matters. Have you measured hyaluronate concentrations?

Lohmander: Not yet. An important principle in these studies is that we need to build libraries of samples together with good data on who the sample came from and when. We can then go into these libraries from time to time to assay new parameters and test new hypotheses. However, we should try not to exhaust our samples by collecting non-critical data. That is why I am slow in using my samples on a new assay.

Dieppe: I want to make a point about synovial fluid samples that has not been made yet, and that is the problem of who we can get it from and when. We know the values of looking at synovial fluid as long as we pay attention to Rodney Levick's comments. Many patients have effusions only at certain times, and I am concerned about the influence of puncturing joints in persons who do not have effusions. Is it possible that puncturing a joint repeatedly may in itself produce changes?

Lohmander: We can now get synovial fluid from about eight out of ten normal healthy knee joints of our volunteers. In our longitudinal studies, patients have been supplying us with joint fluid samples from six times per year to once every second year, depending on the purpose of the study. At this time I cannot answer your question on whether this affects the joint *per se.*

Cooke: Dr. Lohmander, I want to comment on your point that x-ray analyses are always too late to define disease progression. I think that we can consider x-ray analyses of knees as a gold standard by which to look at progression. It is after all very important to have some way to follow the disease independently of markers.

Lohmander: We are using the Questor technology in Lund as a more precise way to measure joint alignment and other variables of the knee joint to improve assessment of radiological progression.

Brandt: We should regard radiographs with some caution. Conventional radiographic analyses were used to evaluate joint space narrowing in 160 knees, all of which were viewed by arthroscopy to visualize the cartilage directly with regard to patello-femoral narrowing. All patients showed early radiographic disease in terms of joint space narrowing. However, 30% were false positives based on the morphological appearance of the cartilage in arthroscopy.

Articular Cartilage and Osteoarthritis,
edited by K. Kuettner et al.
Raven Press, Ltd., New York © 1992.

Part XIII: The Impact of Basic Research on the Diagnosis, Understanding, and Management of Osteoarthritis

Jacques G. Peyron* (Panelists: Kenneth D. Brandt,**
David C. Howell,[†] Klaus E. Kuettner,[‡] Eric Vignon[§])

*Rhumatologue Qualifie, Neuilly sur Seine, France, **Rheumatology Division,
Indiana University School of Medicine, Indianapolis, Indiana 46223; [†]Department of
Medicine, University of Miami, Miami, Florida 33101; [‡]Departments of Biochemistry
and Orthopedic Surgery, Rush Medical College at Rush Presbyterian-St. Luke's
Medical Center, Chicago, Illinois 60612; [§]Hopital Edouard Herriot, Pavillon F,
Place d'Arsonval, 694437 Lyon, Cedex 03ne D8-7, France*

The final discussion is intended to be a free flowing session with prospective orientation fostering an exchange of views between the discussion participants so they can bring forth their main concerns. The panelists are there to spark the discussion.

Brandt: If you look at pathologic evidence of osteoarthritis in people over the age of 60 by simply examining joints at autopsy, it is virtually universal. If you do x-ray surveys of the same group, the data suggest that the incidence is lower, but still pretty high, maybe 50%. However, if we look at who has significant symptoms, not trivial aches and pains, it is a much lower percentage, although still significant in terms of the sheer numbers as a socioeconomic issue. Why? There has been very little discussion, apart from Paul Dieppe's paper, on risk factors for pain and for disability. He described one, namely quadriceps weakness, which his data seemed to indicate is important. It is doubly important if that is the case, because it is remediable. Even in people 80 and 85 years old, quadriceps can be built and sustained over a period of time with simple exercises. We have data which suggest that maybe hamstrings as well as quadriceps, or an imbalance in the ratio of strength between quadriceps and hamstrings may be a more significant factor than quadriceps alone. The interesting questions are not only how this relates to pain or why weakness predisposes to pain in people who have pathologic changes, but also, has it got anything to do with the pathology, and what is the association between muscle weakness and pathologic changes, at least as they are seen on the x-ray? We do have a study that shows very clearly that in people with moderately severe radiographic OA of the knee who have chronic pain, simply applying straight muscle exercise is effective in reducing pain (and the need for pain killers). So it is not just a long-term issue for pathology, but also for symptomatic relief.

Lust: In a dog with hip dysplasia, muscle weakness and muscle atrophy are among the very first signs that you see. These dogs lose tremendous amounts of muscle mass and when the veterinarian's advice is sought, they tend to have no muscle in the pelvic area. We have tried ways to build this up, but we haven't been successful.

Brandt: In this workshop there have been suggestions that OA is a systemic cartilage disease which may be expressed selectively in one, or two, or X number of joints. That is suggested by the data from Eugene Thonar showing that elevated KS epitope levels may be a reflection of systemic, excessive turnover of cartilage matrix. That may predispose this or that joint for local reasons to become symptomatic. Paul Dieppe presented data showing an association between knee OA and hand OA. It is important to think about drug therapy that would perhaps modify cartilage systematically, if that is feasible.

Dieppe: I look on osteoarthritis as a combination of some local mechanical risk factors and some systemic predisposition. The greater the mechanical abnormality, the less you need a systemic predisposition and vice versa. Some years ago, Mike Doherty and I looked at postmeniscectomy arthritis, which is quite a good model, though probably not as good as Stefan Lohmander's model of anterior cruciate ligament changes, because there is a rather lower incidence of osteoarthritis in the meniscectomy group. We compared the 20% of postmeniscectomy people who do get osteoarthritis with the 80% who don't, and we found that, in addition to factors such as the severity of the mechanical abnormality and age, there was another factor clearly associated with the first group. This was disease of the hand, which we consider a reasonable marker for systemic predisposition to OA. These data suggested that even in a situation where there is a clear mechanical abnormality of joints, the extent to which you will develop posttraumatic osteoarthritis is also dependent on a systemic predisposition which has yet to be defined.

Brandt: To emphasize the difficulties with regard to symptoms, socioeconomic status is also a risk factor for pain, given comparable degrees of pathology, at least as judged by x-ray. Women are more likely to be symptomatic and have more severe symptoms than men. People who are in disability are more likely to be symptomatic for comparable degrees of pathology than those who are not. When you look at this in clinic populations as opposed to the community, you have a very skewed population and are likely to draw some misleading conclusions.

Kuettner: How high a percentage in your general patient population would have a polyarticular osteoarthritis?

Dieppe: I think there are some misconceptions that are worth trying to clear up. I do not think that polyarticular OA is a useful differentiation. OA of the hip is a disease separate from everything else in osteoarthritis, and so is OA of the spine. Only OA of the hand and the knee have a strong association. How many joints are involved depends on when the disease is monitored, because new joints are slowly acquired. It will be mono-articular when the patient is 50, oligoarticular at 60, and polyarticular at 80. While that is an oversimplification, it is important to recognize. So the differentiation by number of joint sites or by the presence of hand disease is probably not very useful. It emphasizes, however, that OA can have a systemic predisposition involving those joints that are mechanically susceptible. In population studies of osteoarthritis, hand disease is much more frequent than hip disease. People with OA in several hand joints usually develop OA in both knees, and they make up the majority of OA in the community.

Peyron: Should we really discount hip osteoarthritis altogether? There are several pieces of evidence that hip OA is significantly associated with arthritis in other locations, especially in the hands. This tells us that there might be subsets in osteoarthritis within the same joint, which implicates different pathophysiological mechanisms.

Dieppe: I am not discounting hip OA at all. I am just trying to make the point that in looking for systemic predispositions such as biochemical factors, we may need to study them separately by joint site. I think our data show—and probably my orthopedic colleagues would agree—that in hip OA, there is a much higher incidence of predisposing mechanical factors than for knee OA. To what extent depends on the ability to detect them. Another point worth mentioning concerns the families that Sergio Jimenez and others have described. They have premature osteoarthritis with a major impact on the hip. That is a totally different ball park and they are very rare. However, they might provide additional clues to what is happening in the hip.

Cooke: Concerning systemic manifestations, we investigated 110 cases presenting for arthroplasty of the hip and knee. About 80% of the population had evidence of other joint involvement. Those patients allowed me to examine their asymptomatic cervical spine, hands, knees, and feet. Most showed a very high level of polyarticular involvement. The fascinating thing was that we found an association between hip and hand, and between knee and hand, but dissociation between hip and knee. I think it underscores the assumption that there are other factors involved in hip OA, but that it can also be part of an overall process. In Japan, the incidence of hip disease is very low. Almost 100% are due to dysplasia. In North America hip disease is much more poly-involved, and a significant percentage are central patterns of hip arthritis which go along with more generalized OA. Another minor point, the significance of which I cannot ascertain at the moment, is that in the patients with polyarticular patterns, we found IgA and IgG staining in the cartilage in over 60%. It was seldom seen in oligoarticular OA and, perhaps, is a manifestation of secondary OA.

Brandt: However, there are clearly local factors that are decisive. Epidemiological studies done by Norton Hadler, for example, show an increase in hand OA in people who worked in cotton mills, and the pattern of joint involvement was related to their specific tasks and how they used their hands. It is certainly attractive to speculate that the hand disease is a clue to a systemic problem, but it is not necessarily so. There may be local factors acting there. Some people may have local factors acting in the knees.

Tyler: If I remember correctly, the study of the cotton mill workers mainly showed that the overuse of the joint did not so much predispose to osteoarthritis. The incidence of OA in these women was about the same as in the overall population. It was primarily that the particular joint that was overused was the one which first developed symptoms.

Peyron: That is correct. However, there are several epidemiological population-based studies which tend to show that sheer overuse of supposedly normal joints is a risk factor for OA. This emerges from surveys of groups of professional sportsmen, and of a certain number of occupational groups as well, conducted in different countries and pertains mostly to knee OA. It is not an outstanding factor, but it has some importance. It is a slow-acting factor. Thus, it appears that chronic mechanical stress by itself is capable of inducing OA. Now, I suggest that we discuss this new approach to the natural history of OA.

Brandt: In knees of dogs opened 12 months after anterior cruciate ligament transection, femoral condyles of the unoperated knees contain much less cartilage (about 30% less) than the femoral condyles of the operated knees. This reflects a phenomenon of cartilage hypertrophy in the destabilized knees. The bone has remodeled as well. I want to emphasize how this kind of hypertrophy *in vivo* may be successful in the course of OA for a reasonable period of time, even though there is no restitution to normal cartilage. This is abnormal cartilage with increased bulk, but it is biomechanically inferior in comparison with pristine hyaline cartilage. However, it stays on the joint for relatively long periods of time in some cases. This description of thickening of the articular cartilage in the earlier stages of OA, sometimes with documented biochemical data showing an increase in proteoglycan concentration and fixed charge in density, is not a new observation. It was first made in 1937 by Eric Baywaters, and several investigators have reported comparable findings since then. Recently, Chris Buckland-Wright observed the same phenomenon in hand OA, where joint space widening may precede other changes. Dogs followed serially by MRI over a period of 3 years after cruciate transection retain hypertrophic changes. After a yet longer period of time, articular cartilage eventually falls apart with progressive ulceration of cartilage over the medial femoral condyle and the medial tibial plateau down to the bone.

Peyron: This has a bearing, of course, on the general management and the way we treat osteoarthritis over the years, particularly in the presymptomatic phase.

Vignon: This is a very simple diagram (Fig. 1) which summarizes what we think of the evolution of traumatic OA. On the left we have a normal cartilage. Then one does a destabilizing joint operation. This induces changes in the regulation of the cells, which leads to a hypertrophic state which is not progressive, but is rather in a steady-state and is probably a hypermetabolic stage. This will last for perhaps 3 or 4 years in the dog. It should be equivalent to 20 to 30 years in the human. And finally, there is a failure of the cartilage and destruction of the joint. We think that in man, there is a preradiological stage which may be very long—maybe 20 to 30 years—and it can be associated with mild or intermittent symptoms. Probably the patient at this stage will experience occasional pain flare, but no classical radiological signs of OA. The treatment of osteoarthritis will be quite different at this stage and at the time of cartilage failure. To begin with the end stage, the clinical and radiological stage, when our patients usually come to see us, is it possible to restore a damaged joint space to its normal state?

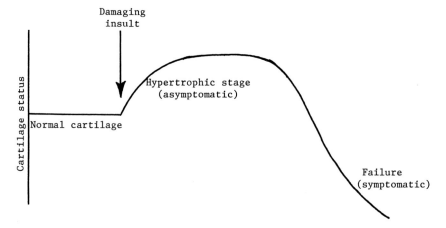

FIG. 1. Diagram of the evolution of osteoarthritis.

Cooke: If the lesion is a mechanical lesion, the treatment is to correct the mechanical lesion.

Vignon: Indeed, this can occur. We followed a 60-year-old patient who underwent osteotomy of the femoral neck for very severe OA. Four years after surgery, a new joint space was seen. Thus, I conclude that the treatment of advanced osteoarthritis is possible.

Muir: With regard to the thickening of the cartilage at the operated site, the increase is not largely from proteoglycans, nor from collagen. The total dry weight increases due to an increase of the other matrix proteins. With repair in advanced OA of the hip, there is obviously fibrocartilage production in resurfacing the joint and that can function normally. There have been reports of cases where this happened spontaneously. Once the collagen network of the preexisting cartilage is damaged, however, we have reached a point of no return. In this case, there may be repair by fibrocartilage, but this is not as good as the original.

Peyron: On this point, I would like to direct a question to Michel van der Rest: What is tissue repair at the level of the collagen network?

van der Rest: In adult cartilage, there is a type II collagen network with proteoglycans entrapped in it. We do not really know how the architecture of the matrix was made originally. To reform cartilage, we have to think about where the collagen fibrils are anchored. The fibrils observed in healing cartilage are probably missing the proper anchorage points. The original network of collagen fibrils in cartilage may be laid down by cells that would not be called chondrocytes and actually may contain collagens other than the classical collagens in mature cartilage. Chondrocytes may just deposit a matrix on the preexisting scaffold. Therefore, in order to return to the original cartilage, the original scaffold must first be reconstructed.

Maroudas: With regard to preexisting cartilage, first, the increase in bulk of the material in hypertrophy must be mostly water because even if there are any increases in proteoglycans or in proteins, this cannot be a 50% increase as there is not that much dry weight in the tissue. Secondly, if there has been any previous damage to the actual surface zone, then bulk analyses of the tissue may show an apparent increase in the proteoglycan content, because in the absence of the surface zone, the middle zone is richer in proteoglycans. Finally, an increase in water also means that the tissue is biomechanically less viable and that the collagen network has been damaged. From some recent work on the turnover of collagen using the racemization of aspartic acid, it appears that collagen is not readily replaced and actually appears to have a very long life.

Lohmander: Sections from punched biopsies taken from the loaded area of a patient's knee joint at the time of tibial osteotomy showed rather severe changes of the joint cartilage. Two years after osteotomy, similar analysis of a site immediately adjacent to the first biopsy revealed a high degree of overgrowth of something that looks like cartilage. We know nothing about the biomechanical properties of it, but there is something that indeed looks like cartilage.

Dieppe: Stabilization of joints, sometimes with increased joint space, is a very real phenomenon that occurs significantly often. It is certainly our impression that what happens to the subchondral bone is absolutely critical to the stabilization of the whole outcome of OA, not just the stabilization of the radiological changes, but also of the patient's problems.

Cooke: Treatment of anterior cruciate ligament (ACL) injuries in humans is an experimental model in surgery. The natural history of these injuries has been of intense interest to many clinicians all over the world. There is now a substantial body of data that has correlated ACL instability with progressive damage in the joint that leads to histopathology of OA. We do not know the natural history well enough, however, because many ACL disruptions occur without the patient coming to the clinician for treatment. Therefore, having an ACL injury does not necessarily develop into a clinical problem. With respect to the influence of surgery, it looks as though it may slow down some of the progressive factors of damage, especially if it is undertaken relatively early. I would submit that the ACL injury problem is exactly that, and only in a percentage of ACL injuries is there *clinical* manifestation of overt symptomatic OA. If I extrapolate that back to animal models, perhaps we should consider the ACL dog lesion as some kind of an injury model. If we are looking at injury models and their potential to develop osteoarthritis, it may be very important to categorize the mechanical factors involved. Clearly in ACL injury in man, antero-posterior, and to a certain extent medial-lateral shears, are induced by the loss of the ligament. In animals, the precise quantification of the type of imbalance—I'm not so sure it has been quantitated yet—may allow us to say, "it's this kind of imbalance which induces this kind of cartilage lesion." In exactly the same way, the damage of a blow on the patella, as in the model described by Ted Oegema, is analogous to a trauma of a fall on the knee that produces its own type of cartilage injury. Before we start categorizing all these things as OA, we should have a label for what kind of mechanism and situation induced it. In the animal model, it would be interesting to know what impact attempts to repair the ACL would have on outcomes with respect to the OA changes that are seen in the cartilage after the injury.

I also want to make a comment about osteotomy of joints in man. Certainly in many surgeons' hands, at least 50% of cases treated with osteotomy go on without having to undergo further surgery. This does suggest that realignment has an ameliorative effect on the clinical problem of osteoarthritis. That then brings back the whole issue of the role of mechanical factors. I do not think we have really addressed the role of mechanical factors in the etiopathogenesis of OA enough, but it is a terribly important one.

Lohmander: I am certainly happy to hear Derek Cooke plug for the human ACL injury as an OA model, because that is exactly the model we are using in our work.

As far as osteotomy is concerned, I again agree. I should, however, add a note of caution. In studies that we have done, we have studied osteotomies with preosteotomy and postosteotomy sampling of cartilage and second-look arthroscopies. We do find cartilage regrowth on the damaged joint surfaces in the medial compartment in about two-thirds of the patients. However, there is no clear correlation between the amount of cartilage regrowth and the outcome from the point of view of the patient, i.e., how satisfied the patient is with the procedure. In another study, a retrospective comparison of osteotomy and unilateral joint replacement was done which showed that a well-performed osteotomy on the right patient actually outlives a unilateral joint replacement. That is a point in favor of a biological solution.

Kuettner: The ultimate purpose of a meeting like this is to eliminate the subspecialty of orthopedic surgery. We want to step in earlier, to find treatment before it is necessary to replace the joint. I heard a nice phrase during the lunch break: "Orthopedic surgery is the failure of internal medicine." What do we want to accomplish in the next, let's say, 5 years is to indicate which way early treatment can or should be directed? Based on what Paul Dieppe just mentioned, maybe only bone, not cartilage, is involved. Once the cartilage is going downhill, then there is nothing more we can do. So we need to identify bone changes much earlier. Serum markers for earlier abnormal bone involvement may be very useful.

Robins: I am not sure about the possibility of bone markers revealing early changes. We have looked at the bone collagen cross-link markers in synovial fluid. Essentially we find very low levels, much lower levels than in serum. Furthermore, the cross-link levels only increase in late stages of OA. That is certainly the situation for synovial fluid. In serum, I think most of the cross-links are derived from general skeletal bone turnover. I think we would really have problems looking for local lesions by measuring serum levels of bone collagen cross-links.

Heinegård: We have been looking at another bone-specific molecule, namely bone sialoprotein, which appears to be a repair molecule more than anything else. It is increased in synovial fluid from OA patients more than it is in serum. There is clearly a gradient from the synovial fluid to serum in this case. That would indicate extra release in an affected joint, perhaps indicative of bone remodeling.

Kuettner: Ultimately, when developing drugs, we must find ways to monitor their efficacy. At the moment we do not even know where to begin looking. Should we decrease bone activity? Should we decrease cartilage degradation by using inhibitors? Is it worthwhile looking at treatment with protease inhibitors?

Vignon: A few years ago, basic researchers told us that cartilage degradation was not only a mechanical process, but an enzymatic process due to metalloprotease as well. Now, though, it looks as though there are some questions about the practicality of using enzyme inhibitors.

Roughley: Theoretically, it is possible to use these inhibitors in treatment. The problem is that it is difficult to get them to the joint without repeated intraarticular injections. I think that would be a very unwise thing to do. Applying this kind of inhibitor systemically would also present a real problem because all of these enzymes perform multiple functions in the body, and by inhibiting the joint enzymes causing the damage, you would probably inhibit the enzymes which control the tissue turnover elsewhere in the body. You may kill the arthritis and kill your patient as well!

Handley: I would like to support Peter Roughley on that. Certainly using recombinant TIMP in animals has been quite disastrous because you get quite drastic changes in the lungs.

Roughley: One exciting development I have heard here is that it now seems possible to take small cartilage samples from arthroscopy. That gives us a chance to look at early-stage OA, something we have not been able to do. Some of the new techniques, such as *in situ* hybridization or immunohistochemistry, can then really tell us a lot about what is actually taking place in the early stages of these disorders. One thing that may come is the development of specific inhibitors to specific proteinases that are implicated in causing the damage. There is also the possibility of targeting specific peptide agents which can inhibit interleukin-1 or other cytokines. Certain molecules do get targeted now. For example, cartilage contains a lot of lysozyme which is not made by the chondrocytes, but rather accumulates in the matrix in large amounts. It enters via the circulation and is concentrated there, probably because it is small and cationic. Perhaps in the near future it will be possible to make constructs of small peptides which will inhibit proteinases or cytokine action combined with positively charged proteins that will then concentrate in the joint. I think that is a very exciting subject.

Tyler: There have been quite a number of studies done over the past few years using *in situ* hybridization and immunolocalization for a range of metalloproteinases and TIMPS. I think it is quite clear that where there is rapid degradation, there is not much expression of these enzymes and inhibitors. However, they are present in remodeling and repair situations. Certainly stromelysin, gelatinase, and collagenase are very important enzymes that take part in reparative processes. This must be borne in mind when considering inhibition of general metalloproteinase activity. The relation between inflammation and degradation is very complex. In OA, we have to consider the joint as a whole. There are other tissues such as the synovium, and possibly even ligaments, that can be involved in inflammatory responses. Also, almost any trauma may initiate an inflammatory response. Allergy or mechanical injury can lead to transient inflammation. This will lead to local IL-1 expression and colony stimulator activation, which will bring effector cells to the site of injury. How long will such a cycle of inflammation last? From what we know about osteoarthritis, it is usually transient and secondary to the disease, but it does occur, and we really have no idea what role this plays in the overall progression of the disease.

Peyron: The signal symptom of osteoarthritis in patients is pain, and thus we prescribe antiinflammatory drugs which have proven to be the best pain relievers in most arthritic patients. What do we do when we apply this class of drugs? Does this only inhibit the synthesis of prostaglandin E2 or does it do something else? Are the effects of prostaglandin E2 linked to destructive processes? Does this kind of drug break a viscious circle of inflammation degradation or not?

Schleyerbach: Obviously not, if you look for a therapeutic effect of nonsteroidal antiinflammatory agents on the pathology of osteoarthritis. This is clear from the clinical trial described by Paul Dieppe. These drugs have no long-term effect. This suggests that they are either ineffective in controlling the complex inflammation in this condition, or that inflammation does not play a major role in the disease.

Lohmander: Is it not true that there are few if any studies which show that the destruction of the joint can be delayed with any of the treatments that are given today, antiinflammatory or otherwise?

Howell: Nothing conclusive, although McCarthy's study of rheumatoid arthritic fingers treated with low-dose corticosteroid at 3 years claimed that advancement of the disease had been retarded. This is an example of attempts in this direction.

Kuettner: Should we develop a hypothetical drug to stimulate repair?

Rosenberg: I think it is extremely misleading to equate the reparative process observed after an osteotomy of the hip with the problem confronting us when arthroscopy reveals fibrillation of articular cartilage in the knee of younger patients. Ken Pritzker, would you like to say something about this?

Pritzker: I agree that repair after osteotomy is quite different from fibrillation when cartilage is still present or if there is repair within that setting. But there are some similarities, such as clear changes in the subchondral bone plate. One of the problems at this meeting is that it has focused almost entirely on the cartilage in osteoarthritis. Early changes in osteoarthritis involve proliferative changes in the cartilage, in the synovial lining cells, and in the subchondral bone. We should be looking for drugs that control proliferation in all those areas, something that influences activation of the articular cartilage and bone, and also of the synovium. Whereas the synovium may be secondary, I am convinced that in the articular plate, both cartilage and bone are activated simultaneously and early on in the osteoarthritic process.

Rosenberg: Some studies show that the improvement seen by x-ray after osteotomy of the hip and sometimes after osteotomy of the knee is not the result of local repair of the lesion restricted to fibrillation of articular cartilage in the center, but is rather the formation of an osteophyte and of a mass of new cartilage and bone creeping over the surface from the periphery. I think the focus has to change from the patient with end-stage disease to the patient with early patello-femoral osteoarthris demonstrated by arthroscopy, the patient with extensive fibrillation. One of the basic questions that has to be answered is: Do a large percentage of these patients with extensive patello-femoral arthritis and fibrillation go on to classic patello-femoral osteoarthritis? If a significant proportion of these patients, say 50%, seen in arthroscopy at ages 30 to 50 are going to progress to OA, this can provide an opportunity to instigate new forms of treatment to elicit and stimulate repair of the fibrillated cartilage. This is where a strategy to remove the dermatan sulfate proteoglycans or other macromolecules which inhibit the adhesion of cells might be useful. The lack of cell migration and attachment is probably a fundamental part of this problem. Removing molecules which inhibit adhesion and perhaps adding ones that stimulate chemotaxis and cell migration will facilitate filling-in of defects.

Pritzker: I think it is a good idea to try to control the adhesiveness of cells at the surface of cartilage. However, perhaps the reason that the fibrillation does not fill relates to the point that Chris Buckland-Wright made in response to the question of visualization of the fibrillation in magnetic resonance imaging. When the cartilages are normally opposed to each other, the fibrillation probably does not exist in a physiological sense. In other words, the surfaces move together without these spaces which are seen histologically. They are squeezed together. Maybe cartilage does not repair that fibrillation because there is no physiological need to do so.

Kuettner: If there are really 20 or 30% of the population suffering from osteoarthritic lesions, how do we find a way to screen for them early enough?

Rosenberg: I've got an answer. There are thousands of arthroscopies being done now by orthopedic surgeons and sports medicine people. Half of these patients with symptomatic knee problems may have erosive lesions of cartilage and fibrillation of cartilage that ranges from moderate to more extensive. Suppose a biological method has been developed to elicit the repair of articular cartilage. The orthopedic surgeon arthroscopes a patient or does an arthrotomy and finds a large lesion that he believes, based on his experience (and hopefully published work!), will go on to patello-femoral arthritis. Then he has a series of vials in the operating room and injects three solutions, one to remove molecules that inhibit attachment, then two others that contain factors which elicit chemotaxis and differentiation of chondrocytes. So you don't screen, you treat the thousands of patients who are being seen in arthroscopy and show early lesions.

Puhl: We treat lots of patients with anterior cruciate ligament damage. This is a very interesting group of patients having very early stages of OA, and we can obtain specimens and take exact photographs. Thus we have macroscopic and microscopic findings from the very beginning.

Hunziker: You asked what may be realistic to develop in the next 5 years. We have heard several times that the etiology of osteoarthritis is not known and that it is probably multifactorial. As long as the etiology is not known precisely, we cannot develop a cure. No matter what we develop at this stage—inhibitors, modulators, etc.—it will remain symptomatic. What we need now are markers and refined imaging procedures to detect early lesions and thus be able to induce local repair. If healing of articular cartilage can be induced, healing that would endure some 20 or 30 years, this would be a great thing for the patient. But before we can go further and find a cartilage remodulator to cure OA, we need to know the etiology first.

van der Mark: In response to what Larry Rosenberg said about the hope for repair by cell migration, a chondrocyte normally is not a migrating cell. A chondrocyte simply does not migrate. Fibroblastic cells can migrate from the periphery. However, it has been shown from animal experiments that in this case, fibrocartilage is produced, and that is never the same as articular cartilage. Once there is surface fibrillation and chondrocyte clusters appear, it is no longer possible to effect repair. I think that repair can proceed from the bone. When there are deep lesions, new cartilage can be produced via the bone or osteophytes may produce true cartilage. But you never get repair of fibrillated cartilage from within the hyaline cartilage.

Rosenberg: We understand that. The chondrocytes and the chondrocyte clusters will not migrate into the fibrillated cartilage and fill in the clefts and fissues. But cells could be elicited from other loci which will fill the defects.

Vignon: I do not agree that chondrocytes are not able to migrate in the matrix, because in an experimental osteoarthritis, there is clear evidence that they are able to do that. In the first stage of osteoarthritis induced by joint instability, there are small clusters of cells. When the cartilage gets hypertrophic, there are no more clusters and the distribution of cells is quite normal. In the late stage, cell clusters become more and more prominent. We can postulate that cartilage failure in the late stage may be a defect of cell migration in the matrix. I agree then that a very important treatment would be to produce cells and induce them to migrate in the matrix. There should then be a possibility of repair.

Oegema: There are many new technologies for delivering drugs, for example, indwelling pumps. This provides a way to treat a single joint with a compound that cannot be given systemically. The method is being used for chemotherapy; we have tried it in dogs, both for discs and for knee joints. There has already been reported use of fibroblast growth factor with a pump delivery system to treat cartilage damaged by laceration. This did indeed promote repair.

Okyayuz-Baklouti: In other degenerative diseases, attempts have been made to inject cells directly into the site where repair is needed, such as myoblast transfer in some muscle diseases. Can this be done with chondrocyte cartilage defects?

Howell: Many investigators have implanted chondrocytes in different forms into joints with cartilage defects. It does not seem to have been successful in the long term, but maybe it could be done in more sophisticated ways.

Rosenberg: There have been attempts to embed chondrocytes in fibrin clots and introduce them into defects. However, almost every approach except for one or two has involved procedures that would not be appropriate for use in arthroscopy for a lesion restricted to cartilage. They normally make a lesion that penetrates into subchondral bone and introduce the fibrin clot into that crater, or make a periostal graft or something similar. That would not be appealing to the arthroscopist who wants to use a more limited procedure.

Puhl: Cartilage cell transplantation was done by colleagues in Ulm and it was stopped because of the bad results. It is much better to look for metaplasia of a tissue coming from the bone.

Maroudas: I am going to make a fanciful suggestion. Since we cannot repair the existing cartilage but can induce fibrocartilage to grow, could we not find something that will encourage the transformation of fibrocartilage into a biomechanically more viable tissue? Maybe that is one of the directions in which we should be looking.

Peyron: This requires a sizeable change in the collagen type and in fibrillogenesis. How can one influence the nature and structure of the collagen network?

Hunziker: It would be nice to fill a cartilage defect with fibrocartilage or another type of tissue and then transform it for competence and long-lasting resistance. But this is not what happens physiologically. When articular cartilage is formed, it is added by growth during the addition of the bone to the epyphysis. This is a growth process, not a transformation process. It will be very hard to induce something that physiologically does not occur in adult cartilage.

Cooke: My colleague, Dr. Ohno, has used electron microscopy to study patients with chondromalacia with defined mechanical problems in the soft, nonfibrillated part of the cartilage. He showed the presence of very nonspecific loosening of the collagen network in the subsurface areas and the presence of matrix streaks in the tissue which could represent an initial break in the three-dimensional organization of the collagen. Maybe if anything is to be done to repair the tissue, that is the right time to do it. Once the collagen network is fissured, it is too late. I think the point that Michel van der Rest raised is a really important one. It will be extremely difficult to reconstruct a network which has the normal anchorage of collagen fibers and to obtain the advantageous biomechanical features found in cartilage. If Larry Rosenberg is looking for a time to induce repair, the time would be when the cartilage is "soft" and the mesh is largely intact, when there is only a single change in one dimension that may be fixable. Indeed, there is some work on intraarticular repair of menisci in which holes have been healed with cells placed into the plugs along with growth factors. But there are as yet no outcome data in terms of the integrity of the tissue. I suspect in the long term it will be the same problem, because the repair tissue does not have the correct architecture.

Pritzker: With respect to regeneration of cartilage, there is a natural experimental model which we cannot yet replicate. That is synovial chondrometaplasia in which perfect hyaline cartilage forms in an abnormal way in a mature adult. Maybe the way to modulate the cells that form fibrocartilage so that they make hyaline cartilage is to control collagen formation. We have learned in this meeting that collagen formation around chondrocytes is extremely complex. If we could selectively regulate certain kinds of collagen formation, we might even be able to control the matrix.

van der Rest: I think there are still problems: It is not so much a matter of laying down the right collagen. A preexisting framework, or a template, is required for the chondrocyte to add type II, type IX, type XI collagen, or whatever. If that template is lost, there is no way to return to the original shape of the tissue unless we can provide an artificial template to give the cells the proper orientations for the fibrils, and to anchor them as well.

Tyler: I support everything that Larry Rosenberg said. This is the way it should go, but it is quite difficult to get these three test tubes for orthopedic surgeons to use. However, I think this notion of encouraging fibrillogenesis is really important. Almost nothing is known about fibrillogenesis in cartilage. The problem with all the animal models that involve implanting chondrocytes, implanting various carbon fibers, implanting all sorts of things into these holes, which can form quite good cartilage nodules, is that they fail after 1 or 2 years because there is no proper integration of the implant with the original tissue. It is also necessary to encourage the resident cells to migrate and integrate into this nodule and to get fibrillogenesis that spans across the lesion.

Howell: Acromegalics have more cartilage than normal, which is not just hydration, but rather actual addition of numbers of chondrocytes. Maybe they form a new collagen network of some sort that could be studied.

Pritzker: Acromegalic cartilage looks like superosteoarthritis—many more cells, much thicker cells—but, yes, it is hyaline cartilage.

van der Mark: I am more optimistic than Michel van der Rest as regards the formation of new hyaline cartilage. We looked at collagen types in many osteophytes at various stages, and they contain perfect hyaline cartilage with all the collagens necessary and with good morphological appearance. I would not be surprised if they can even span a normal cartilage defect without requiring a preexisting scaffold. This new cartilage is formed out of fibrous tissue, and it can cover a wide area with almost the same morphology as the original articular cartilage.

Hunziker: As Jenny Tyler said, tissue integration is a major problem in terms of transplantation of matrix. We have done experiments to remove superficial proteoglycans and expose the superficial collagen network. We take another piece of tissue and try to cross-link it to the exposed surfaces by using transglutaminases. This can yield clear mechanical gluing or adhesion within a short period of time. It is one possible approach for solving this problem.

Plaas: Maybe chondrocytes that produce repair cartilage are like chondrocytes in the growth plate, which is a natural remodeling system. So we need to understand how the different chondrocyte populations in such growing or remodeling tissues are kept under very tight control. Then maybe we could intervene in this sequence of a proliferative matrix-producing chondrocyte and then a hypertrophic chondrocyte.

Lohmander: I think we should set our goals in steps. We do not need to create a perfect hyaline cartilage. If any kind of treatment can delay joint arthroplasty by 10 years or so, like can be done by osteotomy, that would be a great step forward. This could serve as a point of departure for the next step.

Olsen: I wanted to add to what Anna Plaas said. We have just scratched the surface in understanding the mechanisms of chondrocyte differentiation and matrix synthesis. We need much better *in vitro* systems than have been described at this meeting. We can look at primary cell cultures almost to infinity and we would only be able to describe what happens, we would never be able to get to the mechanisms. We need to develop stable chondrocyte cell lines that would maintain their type and matrix production, at least to some extent. We need to determine what genetic transformations are required to do that, because with only primary cells, we would never be able to do the molecular biology necessary to identify the genes that control chondrocyte differentiation and maturation and really understand how they produce their matrix.

Kimura: I am not sure that normal hyaline cartilage is what is required in the osteoarthritic joint, where there is also considerable sclerosis of the bone. The permeability of normal hyaline cartilage is relatively low under high, rapid loading rates. In a hydrostatic system with normal cartilage, loads could be transmitted immediately to the bone without much dispersion. Maybe fibrocartilage would have a greater permeability and serve more to disperse the loading forces that the patient will be exposed to during normal limb function.

Heinegård: As Paul Dieppe said, we may be looking at the wrong place when we look at the cartilage. After a cruciate ligament tear, for example, the cartilage achieves some balance and starts repairing. This can last for a number of years and then some process fails. It may very well be that bone remodeling is changing the system. As Jim Kimura says, perhaps it would be better to have the fibrocartilage on top of the bone. Bone is not constant either, and can change any time.

Williams: There are several synovial joints which have fibrocartilage and function perfectly well. The medial end of the clavicle bearing the weight between the upper extremity and the axial skeleton has fibrocartilage. There is also fibrocartilage present in the temporal mandibular joint and the ankle joint of the chicken. I am interested in learning more about the mechanical properties of this cartilage and why it is found in particular joints where it functions the same way hyaline cartilage does in other synovial joints.

Peyron: I hate to interrupt such a lively discussion, but it is time for lunch. Klaus Kuettner expected this discussion to provide him with some kind of frame for the next meeting, and I think there have been many brilliant ideas put forward to this end. *Auf Wiedersehen!*

SUMMARY

Several highlights pointing to the main concerns of those engaged in osteo-arthritis and cartilage research have emerged clearly from this free discussion. The two-stage evolution of OA with early-stage hypertrophy, probably hyper-metabolic, during which the cartilage constituents, collagen(s), and proteoglycans are abnormal, seems to be widely accepted. Although they are imperfect, repair processes are already active during this early stage and involve bone as well as cartilage. Learning how to detect and characterize these early changes is crucial if one plans to influence the repair processes. Genetic engineering may be the safest means for controlling cell differentiation and the synthesis and organization of a proper matrix.

J.G.P.

Abstracts

48

Structural Differences Between Two Populations of Articular Cartilage Proteoglycan Aggregates (PGAs)

Joseph A. Buckwalter,* Julio C. Pita (deceased),†
and Francisco J. Müller†

*University of Iowa Department of Orthopedic Surgery and Veterans Medical Center,
Iowa City, Iowa 52242; †University of Miami Department of Medicine and Veterans
Medical Center, Coral Gables, Florida 33101

Centrifugation studies of articular cartilage proteoglycans (PGs) have shown a bimodal distribution consisting of: (a) a slow sedimenting population of aggregates (PGA-I) with a low chondroitin sulfate (CS) to hyaluronate (HA) ratio; and (b) a fast sedimenting population of aggregates (PGA-II) with a high CS to HA ratio. The purpose of this study was to determine the structural basis for these differences in sedimentation velocity and composition.

Articular cartilage from female greyhounds was digested with collagenase to extract PGs nondissociately. The extract was purified by equilibrium density centrifugation to isolate PG monomers and the PGA-I and PGA-II populations. Samples were studied by electron microscopy (EM) and the dimensions of the PGs were measured.

The PGA-I and PGA-II samples had average S values of 106 and 270 Svedbergs, respectively. EM showed that the monomer samples contained scattered monomer clusters that may represent small aggregates. The PGA-I and PGA-II aggregates both consisted of central HA filaments with multiple attached monomers, but differed significantly in HA length and in number of monomers per aggregate. They did not differ in monomer length or in spacing of monomers along the HA filaments. Table 1 shows the mean values for the EM measurements of all three samples.

The three-fold greater number of monomers per aggregate in the PGA-II samples agrees with the greater S value of these molecules. The significance of the threefold difference in HA length is less certain. It may reflect a true difference in HA length; but other studies have shown that increasing the number of monomers per aggregate and the concentration of link protein increase the mean length of aggregate HA filaments visible by EM, presumably because regions of HA that lack link proteins and monomers assume a less extended form. If this

TABLE 1. *Electron microscopic parameters*

Sample	HA length (nm)	# Monomers/ PGA	HA length/ # monomers (nm)	Monomer length (nm)
Monomer clusters	163 ± 95	5.4	34 ± 22	211 ± 81
PGA-I	400 ± 159	15.0	27 ± 5	211 ± 74
PGA-II	1162 ± 433	44.1	27 ± 6	211 ± 73

is so, then the two aggregate populations may have HA filaments with similar lengths and since the PGA-II aggregates contain more monomers, they would have a higher ratio of CS to HA. Whatever the explanation for the differences in HA lengths visible by EM, this study confirms the existence of significant structural differences between PGA-I and PGA-II aggregates of articular cartilage.

49

Comparative Sequence Information for Chicken Chondroitin Sulfate Proteoglycan

L. Chandrasekaran and Marvin L. Tanzer

Department of BioStructure and Function, School of Dental Medicine, University of Connecticut Health Center, Farmington, Connecticut 06030

The large aggregating chondroitin sulfate proteoglycan is a major structural component of cartilage. This proteoglycan binds to hyaluronic acid via an amino terminal globular domain and is extensively modified by chondroitin sulfate and keratan sulfate side chains. Complete cDNA sequences for this proteoglycan from rat chondrosarcoma and human cartilage have been reported. We have obtained about 80% of the coding sequence for the chicken cartilage proteoglycan core protein by a combination of cDNA and genomic DNA sequencing. An initial 1.2 Kb cDNA clone was isolated by screening a chicken embryo sternal cartilage cDNA library. The deduced amino acid sequence of this clone has 80% homology with the carboxyterminal lectin-binding domains of rat and human proteoglycan sequences, showing that this domain is the most highly conserved among sequences compared so far. Sequences 5' to this domain were obtained by a primer extension method and used to screen a chicken genomic library. The clone containing the large exon encoding the chondroitin sulfate domain was thus isolated and sequenced. The chondroitin sulfate domain of chicken cartilage proteoglycan has a 5' region which has discontinuous repeats of 10 amino acids and a 3' region which has a continuous 20 amino acid repeat sequence. Overall there is only about 50% homology between chicken and rat/ human sequences in this domain. The keratan sulfate domain which is 5' to the chondroitin sulfate domain shows only 37% homology with rat/human sequences, although there is 71% homology between the rat and human sequences themselves. The deduced amino acid sequence of the G2 domain which lies 5' to the keratan sulfate domain seems to be highly conserved (70%) among the different species compared in this study. These structural comparisons illustrate the similarities and differences between equivalent molecules of different animal species.

ACKNOWLEDGMENT

This work was supported in part by grant HD 22610 from the National Institutes of Health.

50

Immunological Detection of EGF-Like Domain of the Core Proteins of Large Proteoglycans from Human and Baboon Cartilage

Victor Stanescu, F. Chaminade, and T. Do

CNRS URA.584, Hôpital des Enfants-Malades, Paris, France

Recent data from the literature have shown that cDNA clones for the carboxy-terminal domain of the core protein of large proteoglycan monomers from human cartilage contain an EGF-like domain, which appears to undergo alternative splicing (1). In the present study, we have found, using immunoblotting and ELISA techniques, that this domain can be recognized by anti-EGF polyclonal antibodies in the core protein preparations of large proteoglycans (PGs) from baboon and human articular cartilage. Optimal working dilutions of antibodies and specificity were determined using a wide range of antibody dilutions and competitive inhibition assays. Preparations of large cartilage PGs were submitted to electrophoresis in agarose gels, transferred to membranes, digested with chondroitinase ABC on membranes, and reacted with anti-EGF antibodies (Fig. 1). The domain was detected in core preparations of both aggregating monomers from articular cartilages of young humans and baboons. It was also detected in core preparations of large monomers from human articular cartilage of various ages (fetal, newborn, young, and aged) and in PGs from cartilage of thanatophoric dysplasia and homozygous achondroplasia. Immunoblotting of trypsin fragments has shown that in the fetal monomer and in the two postnatal monomer cores

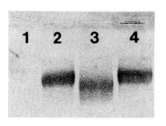

FIG. 1. The nitrocellulose membrane with transferred baboon PGs from slab gel electrophoresis was blocked with albumin-Tween 20, digested on the membrane with chondroitinase ABC, and reacted with polyclonal anti-EGF 1/1000. **1:** Digestion mixture; **2:** fetal PGs; **3:** young baboon PGs; **4:** fetal PGs.

from baboon articular cartilage, the EGF-like epitope is contained in a peptide with an apparent Mr of 68000. Immunological detection and quantitative analysis of the EGF-like domain could be useful for analysis of various PG samples.

REFERENCE

1. Baldwin CT, Reginato AM, Prockop DJ. A new epidermal growth factor-like domain in the human core protein for the large cartilage specific proteoglycan. *J Biol Chem* 1989;264:15747–15750.

51

Studies of the Biochemical Properties of Link Protein

Lawrence C. Rosenberg, H. U. Choi, T. Johnson,
L.-H. Tang, D. Lyons,* and T. M. Laue*

*Montefiore Medical Center, Bronx, New York 10467 and *University of New Hampshire, Durham, New Hampshire 03824*

Because of the apparent insolubility of link protein (LP), no studies have been carried out to examine the binding of intact LP to G1 in low ionic strength, physiologic solvents. Recently we defined conditions under which LP is readily soluble and functional in physiologic solvents. Studies involving metal chelate affinity chromatography demonstrate that link protein is a metalloprotein that binds Zn^{++}, Ni^{++}, and Co^{++}. Binding studies with ^{65}Zn indicate that LP has two high affinity binding sites for Zn^{++}, with $K_a = 3 \times 10^7$. Zn^{++} and Ni^{++} decrease the solubility of LP and result in its precipitation. However, LP is readily soluble and functional in low ionic strength solvents from which divalent cations have been removed with Chelex 100. These observations made it possible to study the oligomeric state of LP alone, the binding of LP to G1, and the transformation in the oligomeric state of LP which occurs when LP binds to G1 or HA in Chelex 100-treated physiologic solvents.

In Chelex 100-treated low ionic strength solvents, LP exists as hexamers. On binding HA_{10} or HA_{12}, LP dissociates to dimers. Studies were carried out of the binding of LP to G1 in the absence of HA. Relatively monodisperse G1 fractions (i.e., 71.8 kDa G1) were prepared. Binding studies were carried out by DEAE chromatography using a 0.15 M NaCl to 0.5 M NaCl gradient. LP does not bind to DEAE and is eluted quantitatively in the 0.15 M NaCl wash. 71.8 kDa G1 binds and is eluted at 0.5 M NaCl. When LP was combined with excess 71.8 kDa G1, all of the LP bound to G1, and the LP and G1 coeluted at 0.5 M NaCl. Similar studies were carried out using a molar excess of LP relative to G1, which made it possible to calculate the stoichiometry of binding of LP to G1. The results demonstrate that in the absence of HA, LP binds avidly to G1, and that in the LP/G1 complex, the molar ratio of LP to G1 is 1:1. Link protein hexamer dissociates to LP monomer when LP binds G1 in the absence of HA.

ACKNOWLEDGMENTS

This work was supported by National Institutes of Health grants AR21498 and AR34614, and National Science Foundation grants BBS-86-15815 and DIR 9002027.

52

Small Proteoglycans of Articular Cartilage

Hans Kresse, Petra Witsch-Prehm, Alfred Karbowski,
Birgit Ober, and Heinz Hausser

*Institute of Physiological Chemistry and Pathobiochemistry and
Orthopedic University Hospital, University of Münster, Germany*

Articular cartilage contains several species of chondroitin/dermatan sulfate proteoglycans. In addition to aggrecan, chondrocytes produce a large proteoglycan immunologically related to a large, heterodimeric proteoglycan from fibroblasts, tentatively named bisderman. Of the small proteoglycans, articular cartilage contains decorin and biglycan and a newly discovered proteoglycan, PG-100. Decorin is the most prominent species in adult human articular cartilage.

Considerable portions of decorin and biglycan are present in cartilage as glycosaminoglycan-free core proteins, as intact cores with shortened glycosaminoglycan chains, and as glycosaminoglycan chain-bearing core protein fragments. At least in the case of decorin, the proportion of core protein and of glycosaminoglycan fragments is greater in the superficial than in deeper zones of cartilage, and more fragments are found in knee than in hip joints. Preliminary data indicated a gonarthrosis-related increase in the proportion of decorin core protein fragments.

Rabbit knee-joint cartilage also contains decorin core protein fragments of 39, 23, and 18 kDa, each one amounting to about 5 to 6% of the intact core protein. Continuous infusion of interleukin (IL)-lα for 14 days (200 ng/day) into the knee-joint led in condylar cartilage to a 50% reduction in the amount of intact core protein. The concentration of all the core protein fragments became reduced to a similar extent. Additional fragments were not found. Patellar cartilage exhibited a smaller response than condylar cartilage with regard to the changes in decorin content.

Extracellular degradation is complemented by intracellular degradation occurring after receptor-mediated endocytosis. Articular chondrocytes maintained in alginate gels endocytose both decorin and biglycan and express an endocytosis receptor protein of 48 kDa which binds the core proteins of both proteoglycans.

PG-100 is barely internalized, suggesting the existence of different metabolic routes for different proteoglycans.

53

Mechanism of Catabolism of the Large Aggregating Proteoglycan by Explant Cultures of Articular Cartilage

Christopher J. Handley, Mirna Z. Ilic, Meng Tuck Mok, and H. Clem Robinson

Department of Biochemistry, Monash University, Clayton, Victoria 3168, Australia

Using metabolically active explant cultures of adult bovine articular cartilage, we have shown that degradation of the large, aggregating proteoglycan of the tissue involves cleavage of the core protein at a number of distinct sites. Eight polypeptide chains originating from this proteoglycan have been isolated from the medium of cultures. Partial characterization of these molecules has revealed that the largest two of these peptides (~Mr 300 and 250 kD) have a functional G1 domain and also contain a G2 domain as well as keratan sulfate and chondroitin sulfate attachment domains. These core proteins are derived from proteoglycan aggregate that is passively lost from the tissue. The six smaller fragments (~Mr 230, 200, 170, 130, 100, and 60 kD) represent core protein polypeptides that do not contain a functional G1 domain; three peptides (~Mr 230, 200 and 170 kD) contain the G2 domain as well as the keratan sulfate and chondroitin sulfate attachment regions, while the two smaller peptides (~Mr 130 and 100 kD) do not contain the G2 domain but do contain the keratan sulfate and chondroitin sulfate attachment domains. The smallest (60 kD) contains only the chondroitin sulfate attachment region. Amino acid sequencing of the core protein peptides of 130 and 100 kD indicate they have N-terminal sequences AGEGPXGILE and LGQRPPVTYT, respectively, and correspond to cleavage of the core protein at amino acid residues 183 and 283 in the partial sequence of the bovine core protein (2) or residues 1839 and 1939 in the complete sequence of the human core protein (1). Both these sites are within the chondroitin sulfate attachment domain 2 in regions of the core protein that are not glycosylated. N-terminal sequence data from peptides of 230, 200, and 170 kD suggest a common sequence AXGXVIL generated by cleavage of the core protein at amino acid residue 393 in the human core protein (1). This cleavage site is in the interglobular domain close to the G1 region. Analysis of the kinetics of appearance of radiolabeled core protein peptides with time in culture suggests the multipoint cleavage of the core protein of the large aggregating proteoglycan occurs throughout the 10-day culture period. Analysis of synovial fluid from the same joints used in the above work revealed that the same core protein peptides were present thus indicating the cleavage observed *in vitro* is the same as that observed *in vivo*. Examination of the amino acid sequences around these cleavage sites show a similar pattern TEGE ARGS (230–170 kD peptide), TAQE AGEG (130 kD peptide) and VSQE LGQR (100 kD peptide) suggesting a single proteinase may be involved in the catabolism of the large aggregating proteoglycan of cartilage, cleaving the core protein between glutamate and alanine/leucine residues.

ACKNOWLEDGMENTS

This work was supported by the National Health and Medical Research Council of Australia and the Arthritis Foundation of Australia.

REFERENCES

1. Doege KJ, Sasaki M, Kimura I, *et al.* Complete coding sequence and deduced primary structure of the human cartilage large aggregating proteoglycan, aggrecan. *J Biol Chem* 1991;266:894–902.
2. Oldberg Å, Antonsson P, Heinegård D. The partial amino acid sequence of bovine cartilage proteoglycan, deduced from cDNA clone, contains numerous ser-gly sequences arranged in homologous series. *Biochem J* 1987;243:255–259.

54

Effect of the Metalloproteinase Inhibitor, U27391, on the Degradation of Rat or Human Femoral Head Cartilage by Interleukin-1β

M. P. Seed,* S. Ismaiel,† T. A. Thomson,*
C. R. Gardner,* and C. J. Elson†

*Roussel Laboratories, Swindon, Wiltshire, United Kingdom; and
†Department of Pathology, University of Bristol, United Kingdom

The effect of the metalloproteinase inhibitor U27391, N-[2-[(2-hydroxyamino)-2-oxoethyl]-4-methyl-L-oxopentyl]-L-leucyl-L-phenylalaninamide, on cartilage degradation by rhIL1β was investigated. rhIL1β (1–100 ng/ml) induced a concentration-dependent decrease in proteoglycan synthesis (measured via $^{35}SO_4$ uptake) and a parallel increase in glycosaminoglycan (GAG) loss (measured with a dimethylmethylene blue assay) in rat femoral head cartilage (FHC). Intact cartilages were incubated for 48 hr at 37°C in Dubecco's modified Eagles medium. rhIL1β (100 ng/ml) was then added and the tissues were incubated for 5 days. On day 4, a 0.25 μCi pulse of $^{35}SO_4$ was added, and the experiments were stopped 16 hr later. Tissues were digested with papain prior to assay.

U27391 (3–100 μM) induced concentration-dependent inhibition of both actions of rhIL1β. Enhanced GAG loss was totally reversed at 30–100 μM and was significantly inhibited by lower concentrations than are required to decrease sulfate uptake, which was not fully reversed. U27391 had no effect on sulfate uptake in the absence of IL1β, although basal GAG loss was slightly decreased. Although similar 5-day incubations of normal human FHC with rhIL1β had no effect, an increase in GAG loss was induced using 14-day incubations with 10 ng/ml rhIL1β. Under these conditions, U27391 (10–100 μM) inhibited the decrease in cartilage GAG induced by rhIL1β. These data suggest that metalloproteinase enzymes play a part in rhIL1β-induced FHC degradation.

55

Mechanisms of Cartilage Degradation in Arthritic Disease

S. Ismaiel, M. F. Pearse, R. Atkins,
Paul A. Dieppe, and C. J. Elson

*Departments of Pathology, Orthopaedic Surgery and Rheumatology,
University of Bristol, Bristol BS8 1TD, United Kingdom*

Cartilage loss is a feature of both rheumatoid arthritis (RA) and osteoarthritis (OA), although the anatomical distribution of such loss differs between the two diseases. If a substance is a mediator of cartilage loss in these diseases, then inhibitors of the mediator should inhibit degradation in models of the disease, and pure preparations of the mediator should degrade human articular cartilage. These predictions were examined for human cartilage biopsies by culturing them with and without test substances. For each experiment, ten biopsy specimens were taken from cartilage slices and cut in half. At the end of the culture period, the sulfated glycosaminoglycan contents of the biopsies were measured (by a colorimetric method) and compared. The results revealed that both RA and OA synovial fluids (SFs) can rapidly (2 days) degrade the cartilage explants. Neutralizing antisera to interleukin (IL)-1α, IL-1β, and tumor necrosis factor (TNF) inhibited the degradative effect of RA SFs, although different antisera were effective with different SFs. By contrast, recombinant IL-1α, IL-1β, and TNF either alone or in combination had no degradative effect over 2 days on human cartilage explants. The IL-1α and IL-1β effectively degraded cultures of rat cartilage explants over 5 days, but RA SF had no degradative effect, demonstrating that human and rat cartilage differ in their responses to degrading stimuli. IL-1α and IL-1β also degraded a proportion (30%) of normal human cartilage over 14 days. Both SFs and IL-1 (α and β) degraded all OA cartilage with high efficacy, and similar results were obtained with the RA cartilage tested. It is considered that SFs degrade cartilage by cytokines acting in concert with another component of SF and that OA cartilage is more susceptible than normal cartilage to degradation.

56

Degradation of Cartilage Collagens Types II, IX, X, and XI by Collagenolytic Enzymes Derived from Human Articular Chondrocytes

Suresh J. Gadher,* David R. Eyre,** S. F. Wotton,†
T. M. Schmid,‡ and D. E. Woolley*

*University Hospital of South Manchester, Manchester, United Kingdom; **University
of Washington, Seattle, Washington, 98195; †A.F.R.C. Institute of Food Research,
Bristol, United Kingdom; ‡Rush Presbyterian, St. Luke's Medical Center,
Chicago, Illinois 60612

Loss of articular cartilage in both osteoarthritis and rheumatoid arthritis may involve the action of degradative enzymes derived from various synovial cells and/or chondrocytes. Collagen is one of the skeletal components of hyaline cartilage. Type II collagen fibrils predominate and smaller amounts of collagen types VI, IX, X, and XI also exist. These collagens probably have different functional roles, and their distribution and possible interaction with collagen type II and various proteoglycans determine the unique properties of articular cartilage. Synovial collagenase and polymorphonuclear leukocyte elastase have specific and restricted capacities to degrade the various cartilage collagen species. However, chondrocyte-derived collagenolytic activity is probably more relevant than other enzyme sources for chondrolysis in normal and diseased states, and hence we have examined the activity of chondrocyte-derived enzymes on cartilage collagen types II, IX, X, and XI.

Human articular chondrocytes were cultured in serum-free Dulbecco's modified Eagles medium supplemented with human recombinant interleukin-1 alpha. Conditioned medium from these cultures contained collagen- and proteoglycan-degrading activities. Preparations of soluble type I collagen and the cartilage collagen types II, IX, X, and XI were all degraded when incubated with the conditioned culture medium at 35°C. Fractionation of the enzymic activities using Ultragel AcA 34 and heparin-sepharose allowed the separation and identification of neutral proteinase, and collagenolytic and proteoglycan-degrading activities. Eluant fractions which contained type I collagenase activity effectively degraded collagen type II, but these fractions did not correspond precisely with those which degraded the collagen types IX, X, and XI. These observations indicate that IL-1–activated chondrocytes have the potential to produce a conventional interstitial type II collagenase together with other enzymes having some specificity for the other cartilage collagens. Thus IL-1–activated chondrocytes produce a range of collagenolytic and proteoglycan-degrading enzymes which can process most of the structural components of the cartilage matrix.

57

Correlation Between Proteoglycan and Collagen Synthesis and Actin Organization in Dedifferentiating Chondrocytes

Frédéric Mallein-Gerin, Robert Garrone, and
Michel van der Rest

*Laboratoire de Cytologie Moléculaire UPR CNRS 412, Institut de Biologie
et Chimie des Protéines, 69622 Villeurbanne Cedex, France*

Chondrocyte dedifferentiation in culture is associated with a transition from a rounded to a spread morphology. We have previously shown that the loss of the expression of the genes of cartilage sulfated proteoglycan (CSPG) and of type II collagen, used as markers of the differentiated chondrocyte, does not correlate with cell shape changes during long-term chondrocyte cultures (1). Furthermore, the work of Benya *et al.* (2) and of Brown and Benya (3) has demonstrated that dedifferentiated chondrocytes can reexpress type II collagen and proteoglycan if treated by dihydrocytochalasin B without a return to the spherical shape, suggesting that changes in actin organization rather than cell shape are involved in the reexpression of the chondrogenic phenotype.

Here we have investigated whether the synthesis of CSPG type I and type II collagens by chick chondrocytes undergoing dedifferentiation in low density cultures correlates with actin organization. Chondrocytes were analyzed in double-staining experiments (rhodamin-conjugated antibodies and fluorescein-conjugated phalloidin) at 2, 16, and 30 days of culture. At 2 days of culture, all the cells were spherical, stained with anti-CSPG or anti-type II collagen antibodies, and did not contain actin cables. At 16 and 30 days, cultures were heterogenous in morphology, consisting of a mixture of rounded and spread cells. Our data show that the loss of CSPG and type II collagen synthesis occur in cells exhibiting actin cables, independently of the cell shape. Type I collagen synthesis, characteristic of chondrocyte dedifferentiation, is mainly associated with spread cells showing prominent actin cables. Together with other studies, these results suggest that the stress fiber-like organization of actin could play a signal role in the modulation of the chondrogenic phenotype, at least *in vitro.*

REFERENCES

1. Mallein-Gerin F, Ruggerio F, Garrone R. Proteoglycan core protein and type II collagen gene expression are not correlated with cell shape changes during low density cultures. *Differentiation* 1990;43:204–211.
2. Benya PD, Brown PD, Padilla SR. Microfilament modification by dihydrocytochalasin B causes retinoic acid-modulated chondrocytes to reexpress the differentiated collagen phenotype without a change in shape. *J Cell Biol* 1988;106:161–170.
3. Brown PD, Benya PD. Alterations in chondrocyte cytoskeletal architecture during phenotype modulation by retonoic acid and dihydrocytochalasin B-induced reexpression. *J Cell Biol* 1988;106:171–179.

58

Alginate Beads: A New Culture System for Articular Chondrocytes

Hans J. Häuselmann,* Margaret B. Aydelotte,*
Eugene J-M. Thonar,*† Steven H. Gitelis,†
and Klaus E. Kuettner*†

*Departments of Biochemistry, †Internal Medicine, and ‡Orthopedic Surgery,
Rush Medical College at Rush-Presbyterian–St. Luke's Medical Center,
Chicago, Illinois 60612

Cultures of chondrocytes in agarose gel offer several advantages over those grown in monolayer culture. The cells exhibit the typical spherical morphology of chondrocytes and deposit a characteristic matrix. Because of the difficulties in recovering the cells and further processing them with time in culture, we used the new alginate bead system which has recently been used by Jourdian and colleagues (1) to study the metabolism of proteoglycans (PGs) by human articular chondrocytes. Alginate is a naturally occurring negatively charged, unsulfated copolymer of L-glucuronic acid and D-mannuronic acid. ^{35}S-sulfate–labeled molecules extracted from the agarose gel and alginate beads yielded identical profiles on Sepharose CL-2B chromatography. PGs of large size (average partition

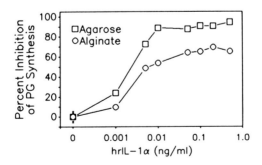

FIG. 1. Biosynthetic response (proteoglycan synthesis) of human articular chondrocytes (22-year-old male, knee joint) in agarose and alginate. Cultures were treated over three days with hrIL-1α, starting on day six. Note the only slight difference in IL-1α response of chondrocytes in agarose and alginate.

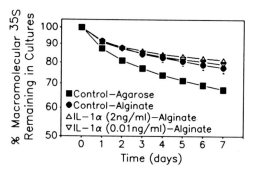

FIG. 2. Rate of loss of proteoglycans. Cultures prelabeled with ^{35}S were treated with or without hrIL-1α from day six to 13 of culture. Graph shows percentage of macromolecular ^{35}S remaining in agarose and in alginate cultures of human articular chondrocytes (63-year-old male, knee joint). Notice the significant difference of IL-1α response in chondrocytes between agarose and alginate.

coefficient = 0.36–0.40) predominated, but small amounts (10–15%) of smaller PGs were also present (average partition coefficient = 0.70). Long-term culture experiments revealed that ^{35}S-labeled keratan sulfate (KS) made up a significant proportion of the ^{35}S-sulfate incorporated on day 35 (medium: KS = 19%; extract: KS = 13%). The half-lives of PGs in cultured chondrocytes were ≈25 days in the alginate bead system and ≈15 days in the agarose gel system. hrIL-1α was extremely effective in inhibiting PG synthesis in both culture systems; the IC-50 was approximately 0.002 ng/ml in the agarose system and 0.008 ng/ml in the alginate beads (Fig. 1). In contrast, hrIL-1α, even at high concentrations (2 ng/ml), had little effect on the rate of PG loss, especially in the alginate bead system (Fig. 2). These data strongly suggest that hrIL-1α is much more effective in inhibiting PG synthesis by adult human articular chondrocytes than in promoting PG catabolism (measured as PG loss). This observation that hrIL-1α had almost no effect on PG catabolism, especially in the alginate bead system, agrees with published reports of others, which showed the same results in organ cultures of human articular cartilage. This suggests that isolated articular chondrocytes cultured in alginate beads may react very similarly to chondrocytes in their natural surrounding.

REFERENCE

1. Guo J, Jourdian GW, MacCallum DK. Culture and growth characteristics of chondrocytes encapsulated in alginate beads. *Connect Tissue Res* 1989;18:277–299.

59

Characterization of the Response of Chondrocytes to Mechanical Deformation

James H. Kimura,* P. M. Freeman,† R. N. Natarajan,†
and T. P. Andriacchi†

*The Bone & Joint Center, Henry Ford Hospital, Detroit, Michigan 48202, and
†Departments of Biochemistry and Orthopedic Surgery, Rush-Presbyterian–St. Luke's
Medical Center, Chicago, Illinois 60612

Chondrocytes exist in an active mechanical environment which exposes them to periodic alterations in hydrostatic pressure, electrical potential, and compressive strain. Such alterations in the physical environment can modulate their metabolic activity to modify the composition of cartilage to accommodate changing mechanical demands on the tissue. It is not yet possible to assign a relative importance to any of the environmental changes as signals to chondrocytes. In cartilage, the relative contributions of each type of physical change are difficult to assess because of the coupling of electrical and mechanical events. By substituting an uncharged agarose gel for the highly charged matrix of cartilage, we were able to study the individual effects of mechanical and electrical perturbations on the cells. We report here on the effect of uniaxial mechanical compression of agarose-cell composites on the mechanical behavior of individual chondrocytes from a rat chondrosarcoma. Five $\times$ 10^6 cells/ml in 2% agarose were exposed to compressive strains of 5, 10, or 15%, and alterations in cellular morphology were followed for 15 min after application by video recording of microscopic fields. The cellular dimensions in two principal axes were obtained by analysis of digitized images. The results indicated that the cells became ellipsoidal upon compression with an initial axial ratio of 1.2, 1.4 and 1.6 at 1 min, for 5, 10 and 15% strains, respectively. At the end of 15 min, the cells became more circular in cross-section, relaxing to a ratio of 1.1, 1.3, and 1.4, approximately in conformance to stress relaxation in the agarose, although it did appear that the addition of cells to the agarose resulted in an increase in the relaxation time constant without dramatic changes in the relaxed elastic modulus when compared to agarose alone. The relaxed cross-sectional area of the cell was calculated assuming an ellipse for the cell shape. At 5% compression the cell area decreased by 2%, at 10% compression by 5%, and at 15% compression by 7%.

The geometry of the compression device did not permit expansion of the agarose in the third dimension. Thus, the cell area can be regarded as proportional to cell volume as defined by the formula for the volume of an ellipsoid. The decrease in cellular volume at each strain was more than could be accounted for solely by an increase in the physical pressure to the cells. The peak pressures as measured by a force transducer attached to the compression arm were 3, 7 and 14 kPa, respectively. Such a change in volume in the absence of an activation of ion transport systems would have required pressures of 13, 34 and 49 kPa. The results therefore suggested that the cells responded actively to the mechanical perturbation of their shape.

60

Interactions of Immunoglobulins and Chondrocytes

Derek Cooke,* Ryuichi Saura,† Shinichi Satsuma,*
and Allan Scudamore*

*Department of Surgery, Orthopaedic Division, Queen's University,
Kingston, Ontario, Canada, K7L 3N6; †Orthopaedic Surgery,
Kobe University School of Medicine, Chuo-ku, Kobe 650, Japan

The study relates to damage of articular cartilage by deposition of immune complexes. Addition of IgG to cultured chondrocytes affected their metabolism by boosting metalloprotease synthesis, generating superoxide anion (O_2^-), and reducing the synthesis of sulfated glycosaminoglycans (S-GAG). Heat-aggregation of the IgG enhanced its effect on O_2^- and S-GAG. Some interleukin-1β (38 pg/ml) was detected by ELISA after exposure to heat-aggregated IgG. There was no cytotoxic effect due to IgG alone, but addition of complement (5% bovine serum) caused significant loss of intracellular ^{51}Cr, which was further increased by addition of heat-aggregated IgG. Similar responses of chondrocytes *in vivo* might account for immune complex mediated damage of cartilage.

61

Complement and Complement Receptors in Human Articular Chondrocytes

Monika Oestensen, R. Stiansen, G. Hetland, and P. Garred

Institute of Immunology and Rheumatology, Rikshospitalet, Oslo, Norway

Deposits of immunoglobulin and C3 have been detected by immunohistochemistry in cartilage from patients with rheumatoid arthritis (RA) and osteoarthritis (OA). Activation of chondrocytes by immune complexes may stimulate chondrocytic chondrolysis. The ability of human articular chondrocytes to secrete complement factors and to express complement receptors was investigated.

METHODS

Chondrocytes were isolated by enzymatic digestion from human articular cartilage obtained from healthy individuals and from patients with RA and OA. Cells were grown in monolayer culture in Ham's F12 medium supplemented with 10% FBS for 10 days. Cultures for assays of complement factors were continued in serum-free medium for 1 to 3 days. Subsequently, complement factors C3, C5, C9, and C3-activation products were measured by radioimmunoassay or ELISA techniques. Complement receptors CR1 and CR3 were assayed by staining with monoclonal antibodies and flow cytometry on freshly isolated chondrocytes and chondrocytes grown in monolayers. An isotype-specific unrelated monoclonal antibody served as control.

RESULTS

C3 was secreted by all chondrocyte cultures, with RA chondrocytes producing the highest amount. C5 and C3 activation products were exclusively found in supernatants from RA chondrocytes. Analysis of chondrocytes staining positively for complement receptors showed the following: Chondrocytes from healthy individuals did not express CR1 or CR3, neither immediately after isolation nor after 10 days in culture. CR1 and CR3 were not detected on freshly isolated RA chondrocytes, but were expressed on chondrocytes grown for 10 days in monolayers. The degree of positively staining cells varied from 30 to 66%.

COMMENT

The results show that human articular chondrocytes can be activated by inflammatory rheumatic disease to secrete complement factors and to express complement receptors. The presence of the multifunctional complement receptors on chondrocytes could indicate not only complement binding, but also cell-to-cell interactions during synovitis. As the complement system is an important component of inflammation, chondrocytes may contribute to key events of joint damage.

62

Autoantibodies to Chondrocyte Membrane Proteins in Osteoarthritis and Experimental Animal Arthritis

J. Mollenhauer,* C. Franzelius,* A. Schulmeister,*
Eugene J-M. A. Thonar,† James M. Williams,* and Kay Brune*

*Institute für Pharmakologie und Toxikologie, Universität Erlangen-Nürnberg 22,
8520 Erlangen, Germany; †*Departments of Biochemistry and Anatomy,
Rush-Presbyterian–St. Luke's Medical Center, Chicago, Illinois 60612

Recently we described the occurrence of an immune reaction against cartilage cell membrane components in patients with rheumatic diseases, osteoarthritis and rheumatoid arthritis. This reaction could be defined in a quantitative manner by ELISA using cell membranes as the antigen source and patients' sera. In Western blots, a number of proteins, especially a 65 KD polypeptide, biochemically and immunologically distinct from the 60 KD heat shock protein, could be detected and gave a prominent reaction with the sera (1). In addition, a T cell proliferation assay with peripheral leukocytes from patients and chondrocyte membranes showed corresponding results (2). To elucidate the role of the chondrocyte membrane proteins during onset and development of the arthritis, two animal models were investigated; rat adjuvant arthritis and the less inflammatory papain-induced arthritis in the rabbit. In both forms of arthritis, the 65 KD protein appeared to be a dominant autoantigen. The antibody titers against chondrocyte membranes rose during the first week after arthritis induction and remained stable for as long as 6 months. In rabbits and humans, the antibody titers correlated with the release of cartilage-specific keratan sulfate into the blood. Treatment of the rats with immune modulating drugs (dexamethasone, cyclosporin A, leflunomide) reduced antibody titers and joint swelling. Indomethacin and other nonsteroidal antiinflammatory drugs did not influence autoantibody production or paw swelling.

ACKNOWLEDGMENTS

This work was supported by the Bundesministerium fuer Forschung und Technologie [BMFT], grant #01VM88072, and by the DFG-SFB 1392.

REFERENCES

1. Mollenhauer J, et al. Serum antibodies against chondrocyte cell surface proteins in osteoarthritis and rheumatoid arthritis. *J Rheumatol* 1988;15:1811–1817.
2. Alsalameh S, et al. Cellular immune response toward human articular chondrocytes. *Arthritis Rheum* 1990;33:1477–1496.

63

Mapping of Age-Related and "Arthritogenic" Epitopes of Proteoglycans in Normal and Pathological Cartilage Samples

Tibor T. Glant,*†‡ K. Mikecz,*† Cs. Fülöp,*‡ D. A. Dossing,*
E. Buzás,‡ G. Cs-Szabó,§‖ Michael T. Bayliss,‖
Vincent C. Hascall,# and Klaus E. Kuettner*†

*Departments of *Biochemistry and †Orthopedic Surgery, Rush-Presbyterian–St. Luke's
Medical Center, Chicago, Illinois 60612; Institutes of ‡Anatomy and §Biochemistry,
University of Medicine, Debrecen, Hungary, ‖Biochemistry Division,
Kennedy Institute of Rheumatology, London, England; and
#National Institutes of Health, NIDR, Bethesda, Maryland 20892*

High density proteoglycan (aggrecan) of articular cartilage displays several antigenic sites which may provoke cellular (T cell mediated) and/or humoral (antibody) immune responses in heterologous or, occasionally, in autologous systems. Protein structures of globular domains are highly conserved in phylogeny. Thus, the major "immunodominant" regions of aggrecan are likely to be located in the glycosaminoglycan-rich regions of the core protein in different species. Although a large number of analogous sequences are present in the chondroitin sulfate attachment region of the core protein in different species, the variability detected either by biochemical or immunochemical methods is frequent in this domain. Differences may be either (a) related to the amino acid sequences expressed as conformation-dependent or conformation-independent protein epitopes, (b) associated with the keratan sulfate structure, (c) dependent on the isomer structure and stereoscopic orientation of chondroitin sulfate side chains, or (d) the combination of peptide-carbohydrate structures. These variabilities in cartilage proteoglycans can induce different immune responses in different species or in different (murine) strains. On the other hand, (monoclonal) antibodies can detect fine specificities between aggrecan molecules from different sources, ages, and animal species.

We compared the expression of epitopes and the chemical composition of fetal, newborn, and adult cartilage proteoglycans from 9 species (human, bovine, sheep, pig, rabbit, chicken, canine, guinea pig, and mouse) using 36 monoclonal antibodies raised to human (29 antibodies) or mouse (7 antibodies) articular cartilage proteoglycans. The basic chemical compositions varied primarily with the developmental age of the tissue as shown for human or bovine tissues (i.e., less protein and keratan sulfate and more chondroitin-4-sulfate were detected in immature cartilages) and not with different species of the same developmental stage. Proteoglycans of mouse cartilage resemble those from osteophytes (chondrophytes) formed at the margins of human osteoarthritic cartilage and also those from fetal human articular cartilage. Proteoglycans from human osteophytes cross-react with monoclonal antibodies to fetal human cartilage, but do not, or very weakly react, with antibodies to adult proteoglycans. Moreover, several monoclonal antibodies raised against denatured human cartilage proteoglycans, which did not react with native aggrecan, detected epitope(s) on proteoglycans isolated from osteoarthritic cartilages.

Intact and chondroitinase ABC-digested proteoglycans from the 9 species were also used to immunize Balb/c mice to reveal their arthritogenic potential. Intact, nondegraded proteoglycans never produced arthritis. Chondroitinase-digested proteoglycans of human fetal and newborn articular cartilages, human osteophyte, fetal pig, newborn, and adult canine articular cartilages and human chondrosarcoma were the only ones able to induce arthritis consistently. The arthritogenic domain(s) are probably common in all proteoglycans which can generate an autoimmune response in Balb/c mice.

64

Genetically Induced Mouse Models of Rheumatic Diseases

Effects of Leflunomide on Articular Manifestations

Ruth X. Raiss, Robert R. Bartlett, and Rudolf Schleyerbach

*Pharmacologic Research Vasotherapeutics/Antirheumatics,
Hoechst AG Werk Kalle-Albert Wiesbaden, Germany*

For the preclinical evaluation of therapeutic concepts in rheumatic diseases, two genetically induced animal models were chosen to reflect the variability and complexity of the human diseases. Both mouse models are well established. The MRL lpr/lpr strain resembles systemic lupus erythematosus (SLE) and rheumatoid arthritis (RA), and the STR 1N strain is similar to osteoarthritis (OA). Leflunomide (HWA 486) is an immunomodulating drug designed for the treatment of SLE and RA, and has been found effective in a variety of parameters measured in animal models of rheumatic diseases. To investigate its effect upon joint manifestations, a semiquantitative histological score has been developed for the disease progression in both models. As an additional parameter, reflecting the individual impairment caused by the disease, proteinurea has been chosen for the MRL lpr/lpr model, and, for the STR 1N model, spontaneous overnight activity of the animals.

Leflunomide and cyclophosphamide were administered systemically to adult mice five times a week over a period of 2 or 3 months, respectively. During treatment, noninvasively, proteinurea was measured in MRL mice, and the spontaneous overnight activity was recorded in STR 1N mice. At the end of the experiment, histological sections of demineralized and paraffin-embedded whole knee joints were stained with hematoxylin-eosin, azan, and aldehydefuchsin-fast green. Sections of five animals per group were examined for histological grading.

In the MRL lpr/lpr mouse, the joint pathology involves swelling, pannus formation, and proliferation of synovial tissue. This was modified by treatment with leflunomide to an almost normal condition, shifting the histopathological score from 12 to 1.5 (median value). Especially the synovial proliferation and changes in vascularization were reduced. Cyclophosphamide, in contrast, did not alter the joint pathology. Proteinurea was improved by both drugs. Male STR 1N mice exhibit progressive cartilage degradation, subchondral bone re-modeling, and intermittent inflammational episodes in the joints, and the spon-taneous activity is reduced. Treatment of STR 1N mice with leflunomide had no measurable effect on the histopathological score of articular manifestations (17 compared to 20 in untreated diseased mice). Surprising, however, was an increase of the spontaneous activity of the diseased animals under leflunomide, which reached significance at the third week. This improvement may be of mul-tifactorial origin, but reflects a condition not unlike the subjective scores of patients in clinical trials. Combined with noninvasive disease parameters, a de-tailed histological examination helps in understanding a complex disease course in such genetic animal models, and in the evaluation of their therapeutic modification.

65

Immunohistochemical Localization of Chondroitin Sulfate Isomers in the Knee Joint of Osteoarthritic Mice

Ruth X. Raiss and Bruce Caterson*

*Pharmacologic Research, Hoechst AG Werk Kalle-Albert, Wiesbaden, Germany, and *Orthopaedic Surgery, University of North Carolina, Chapel Hill, North Carolina 27599*

The mouse strain STR 1N is known to develop spontaneously a focal osteoarthritis (OA) in the knee joint. Prior to lesions in the articular surface, the intensity of staining for proteoglycans (PG) is decreased in cartilage, indicating changes in matrix metabolism. In order to determine whether subtle changes in cartilage PG structure may be involved in that process, the distribution of different chondroitin sulfate (CS) isomers was assessed by immunolocation in histological sections of the whole knee joint. For this study, STR 1N mice were compared with two other mouse strains to detect possible strain-specific differences. Mice were examined at different ages to determine if changes in PG diversity played a role in aging with respect to development of the disease in the STR 1N strain. Histological sections of demineralized whole knee joints were deparaffinized, and, after chondroitinase digestion in some cases (+), were incubated with the following monoclonal antibodies (MABs): 2-B-6+ and 3-B-3+, which recognize nonreducing terminal disaccharides containing an unsaturated hexuronic acid residue adjacent to 4- and 6-sulfated N-acetylgalactosamine, respectively, on the chondroitinase-treated CS chain. MABs used without prior digestion were 3-B-3, 4-C-3, 6-C-3, and 7-D-4, which recognize different sulfation patterns of "native" epitopes on the CS chains. Biotinylated rabbit-anti-mouse immunoglobulin was used as a second antibody with DAB as a substrate for immunolocation. Immunoreactivity was assessed in nine areas of the joint and differentiated between intracellular, pericellular, and matrix staining. Sections of at least five animals per group were studied.

In mice of the same age, sex, and strain, the tissue distribution of the six epitopes was distinct from each other. Comparison of STR 1N mice with two other mouse strains (MRL++ and NMRI) of the same age revealed no differences in the distribution pattern of the chondroitinase-generated epitopes and two of the native ones, but articular cartilage and menisci staining differed for native epitopes recognized by 3-B-3 and 7-D-4; i.e., the STR 1N strain which develops OA differs from other strains in the expression of the 3-B-3 and 7-D-4 epitopes. The examination of male STR 1N mice at the age of 2–3, 4–5, and 6–7 months resulted in age-related changes in the staining pattern of at least four epitopes in articular cartilage, menisci, and patella, and, for one also in the growth plate. Osteophytes, including those at very early stages, stained intra- and pericellularly for all six epitopes, apparently expressing the largest array of different CS isomers. These studies indicate that differential expression of CS isomers is involved in aging and/or disease progression, and that native epitopes recognized by 3-B-3 and 7-D-4 may serve as diagnostic markers in the STR 1N model of OA.

66

Possible Role of Calcification in the Progression of Osteoarthritis in STR Mice

C. Collins,* C. J. Elson,* R. G. Evans,*
Peter Miller† and F. M. Ponsford*

*Department of Pathology, University of Bristol, United Kingdom;
and †Roussel Laboratories Ltd., Swindon, United Kingdom

Osteoarthritis (OA) is the most common of the rheumatic diseases. Animal models of this disease have proved useful for testing potential therapeutic drugs and for elucidating possible disease mechanisms. One such model is the STR mouse, where male animals spontaneously develop an OA-like disease. There have been several studies of the disease, but these have been descriptive, and the cause of the OA remains obscure. The purpose of our study was to quantify the progressive changes observed in these animals with the aim of identifying the primary pathological event(s). Patellar glycosaminoglycan (GAG) levels were measured by a colorimetric assay. In addition, we made quantitative assessments of radiological and histological changes in the knee and ankle joints and measured bone volume and density in the knees. Analysis of the chronology of these changes focused attention on the possible role of tendon calcification as a primary event in the progression of OA in this model. GAG levels in both males and females rose steadily with age. However, the increase was more marked in males where the slope value was 0.65 as compared with only 0.17 in females. When the total radiological scores for arthritic changes in the knee were compared, these were similar for male and female mice until 5 months. Subsequently, the score in males increased at a greater rate than in females, reaching a final value at 11 months of age of nearly twice that observed in female animals. However, when only calcified structures in the knee were considered, the radiological scores for both male and female mice rose in parallel until 3 months of age. Thereafter the value in females plateaued, whereas the score in males continued to increase, reaching a value almost three times that of females by 11 months. With regard to changes observed in the ankles of these animals, calcification of the Achilles tendon was observed as early as 2 months of age in some male mice.

67

Morphometric Analyses of Articular Cartilage, Tidemark Region, and Subchondral Bone Remodeling After Strenuous Training of Beagle Dogs

R. Oettmeier,* A. J. Roth,* K. Abendroth,*
H. J. Helminen,† J. Arokoski†

*Orthopaedic Clinic and Clinic of Internal Medicine, University of Jena,
0-6900 Jena, Germany; †Department of Anatomy, University of Kuopio,
F-70211 Kuopio, Finland

Many studies which try to investigate pathogenesis of osteoarthritis (OA) have the disadvantage of analyzing hyaline cartilage only. But all tissues of the complex joint system are affected in some way in OA as the joint is an interactively functioning unit. In understanding preosteoarthritic processes, it is useful to investigate the complex response of the joint system to exercise on the borderline of the physiologic range.

Twenty female beagle dogs were divided into runners (EXP) and controls [CON]. After a training period, the dogs were accustomed to run 40 km/day in a treadmill with a 15 degree uphill inclination (each working day for 15 weeks). The samples for histology were taken from 11 different locations of the knee joint; undecalcified sections were prepared and stained by LADEWIG. The thickness of hyaline (*hyc*) and calcified cartilage (*cc*) as well as subchondral bone plate (*sbp*) was measured in the central, intermedial, and peripheral zones of each specimen with a QUANTIMED 720 image analyzing computer. An eyepiece gradicule (described by Merz) was used to evaluate subchondral bone parameters.

Despite intact cartilaginous surfaces, direct contact areas between *hyc* and bone marrow ("gaps"), basal cystic degeneration of *cc* and *hyc*, hyaline plugs, and vascular invasions into the tidemark and *hyc* were observed, especially in peripheral zones. Occurrence of "gaps" and "plugs" was mostly combined with vessel contacts (R = 0.26, $p < 0.05$). Only in the retropatellar joint was the thickness of *hyc* and *sbp* significantly increased. Thickening of *cc* was observed in the peripheral and central zones of the medial portion of the joint. In all regions of the knee joint, bone formation (i.e., active osteoblastic surface and osteoid surface) as well as bone resorption was significantly increased. This high turnover remodeling dominated again in the central and peripheral zones. Only in the patellar surface of the femur was trabecular bone volume increased. Correlations were found between trabecular bone volume and thickness of cc (R_{EXP} = 0.45, R_{CON} = 0.81, $p < 0.01$) and sbp (R_{EXP} = 0.37, R_{CON} = 0.50, $p < 0.05$).

The enlarged bone turnover seems to be a primary answer of the joint to overloading. The increased bone formation provides more and stiffer subchondral bone which may impair the subchondral shock-absorbing capacity in OA.

68

Synthesis of Hyaluronate in Canine Normal and Osteoarthritic Cartilage

Daniel H. Manicourt

Arthritis Division and ICP Connective Tissue Group, University of Louvain in Woluwe, 1200 Brussels, Belgium

Osteoarthritis (OA) was induced in dogs (Pond-Nuki model) and articular cartilage was sampled from the different topographical areas of the operated OA knee and nonoperated normal contralateral knee. In OA cartilage, the total amount of hyaluronate (HA), as measured by enzyme-linked–immunosorbent assay, was about 60% of the values found in normal control cartilage. In contrast, the total hexuronate content, and thus the total proteoglycan (PG) content, was similar in both normal and OA cartilages.

To investigate further this significant depletion of HA in OA cartilage, normal and OA cartilage tissues were incubated in short-term explant culture with ^{3}H-glucosamine as precursor. After incubation, tissue and medium were digested with papain (neither cysteine, nor EDTA were added to the digestion mixture) and the glycosaminoglycans (GAGs) were isolated by ion-exchange chromatography.

In normal articular cartilage, ^{3}H-HA represented less than 10% of the total ^{3}H-GAG synthetized over the culture period. However, the distributions of ^{3}H-HA and ^{3}H-sulfated GAGs (S-GAG) were different: 30 to 40% of ^{3}H-HA appeared in the medium compared with 5 to 10% of ^{3}H-S-GAGs. Further, in the tissue, the ratio of ^{3}H-HA/^{3}H-S-GAGs was similar to that found for nonlabeled HA-hexosamine/nonlabeled S-GAG-hexosamine.

In OA cartilage, the total GAG synthesis was doubled and ^{3}H-HA represented 15 to 20% of the total ^{3}H-GAGs being synthesized. Fifty to sixty percent of ^{3}H-HA was recovered in the medium whereas 15 to 20% of ^{3}H-S-GAG was lost from the tissue. Further, the ratio of ^{3}H-HA/^{3}H-S-GAG present in OA cartilage was almost twice that found in normal cartilage.

In both normal and OA cartilage, the ^{3}H-HA molecules had a very similar size (Mr = 6–7 × 10^5) that was greater than that of nonlabeled HA molecules purified from the same tissues (Mr = 4–5 × 10^5). Both normal and OA media contained small ^{3}H-HA molecules (Mr = 5 × 10^5), whereas an additional population of ^{3}H-HA of higher size was detected only in OA media.

The observation that in normal articular cartilage, the ^{3}H-HA and ^{3}H-S-GAGs had a ratio that was similar to that existing between the total chemical amounts of these two components, supports the novel hypothesis that the metabolism of both HA and PGs are highly coordinated. The data also suggest that HA is synthesized in excess of PGs and that the newly synthesized HA molecules might undergo some extracellular cleavage and/or modification before their incorporation into PG aggregates. The low HA content of OA cartilage contrasts with the considerable increase in the synthesis of this GAG. The data suggest that HA catabolism is even more accelerated than PG catabolism and that some extracellular events are responsible for the depletion of HA in canine experimental OA.

69

Pharmacological Influence on Fibronectin and Keratan Sulfate Synthesis by Cultured Canine Articular Cartilage Chondrocytes

Juergen Steinmeyer,* Nancy Burton-Wurster,†
and George Lust†

*Institut für Pharmakologie und Toxikologie der Universität Bonn,
5300 Bonn, Germany; †James A. Baker Institute for Animal Health,
Cornell University, Ithaca, New York 14853

Several studies disclosed that osteoarthritic cartilage of several species including human, dog, rabbit, and horse contain increased amounts of fibronectin and that osteoarthritic canine articular cartilage explants synthesize three to five times more fibronectin than control. Since articular chondrocytes are potential targets of drugs which can influence the integrity of cartilage, we investigated the effect of three antiarthritic drugs: glycosaminoglycan polysulfate, diclofenac-Na, and S-adenosylmethionine sulfate p-toluenesulfonate on fibronectin, total protein, and DNA synthesis as well as on extra domain-A (ED-A) fibronectin and keratan sulfate content of chondrocyte cultures.

METHODS

Chondrocytes were isolated from adult canine articular cartilage and cultured in Ham F12 medium supplemented with 25 mM HEPES buffer (pH 7.2), ascorbic acid, L-glutamine, α-ketoglutarate, penicillin, streptomycin, and 10% fibronectin depleted fetal bovine serum. At the initial seeding, glycosaminoglycan polysulfate or diclofenac-Na was added to the cultures at concentrations of 10^{-7}, 10^{-6}, or 10^{-5} mol/L, whereas S-adenosylmethionine sulfate p-toluenesulphonate was added to the chondrocytes at concentrations of 10^{-6}, 10^{-5}, or 10^{-4} mol/L. The cultures were maintained at 37°C, 5% CO_2, and 95% humidity. After 3 days the culture media were harvested, and after adding 10% volume of protease inhibitor solution, stored frozen at -20°C until assayed. The cells were fed in the same media and cultured for another 3 days. On day 6, chondrocytes were labeled with 10 μCi/ml ^{35}S-methionine for 4.5 hr or with 2.5 μCi/ml ^{3}H-thymidine for

11 hr. ^{35}S-methionine labeled fibronectin was purified from the incubation media and cell layer extracts by affinity chromatography. Total protein synthesis was determined by precipitation of ^{35}S-methionine–labeled proteins from the cell layer extracts and incubation media with perchloric acid. DNA synthesis was estimated by precipitation of ^{3}H-thymidine–labeled DNA with trichloroacetic acid. The amounts of total fibronectin, ED-A fibronectin, and keratan sulfate in the incubation media and cell layer extracts were determined with ELISA.

RESULTS AND DISCUSSION

S-Adenosylmethionine sulfate *p*-toluenesulfonate decreased dose dependency the synthesis of fibronectin as well as the content of fibronectin and keratan sulfate of chondrocyte cultures. At the highest concentration of this drug tested, data suggest that cell viability was impaired as assessed by loss of DNA and protein synthesis and the release of lactate dehydrogenase into the incubation media. Fibronectin and DNA synthesis as well as ED-A fibronectin and keratan sulfate content of chondrocyte cultures were unaffected by diclofenac-Na. Our study confirmed that diclofenac-Na does not affect the anabolic activity of chondrocytes in contrast to some other nonsteroidal antiinflammatory drugs. Glycosaminoglycan polysulfate stimulated dose dependency incorporation of ^{35}S-methionine into fibronectin and protein whereas incorporation of ^{3}H-thymidine into DNA was unaffected. Total fibronectin, ED-A fibronectin, and keratan sulfate content were elevated in chondrocyte cultures treated with glycosaminoglycan polysulfate. It remains to be determined whether glycosaminoglycan polysulfate treatment has a deleterious effect on chondrocyte metabolism via an elevated fibronectin synthesis which is abnormal for chondrocytes *in vivo.*

70

Bovine Articular Cartilage Explant Cultures for Drug Evaluation

Roger M. Mason and Daphne C. L. Goh

Department of Biochemistry, Charing Cross and Westminster Medical School, London, W6 8RF, United Kingdom

Explant cultures of bovine articular cartilage have several advantages for investigating drug effects and can be cultured over a period of weeks in Dulbecco's modified Eagle's (DME) medium plus 20% fetal calf serum (FCS). The cartilage contains $11.0 \pm 1.0 \times 10^6$ chondrocytes per gram of wet tissue, and these depend almost exclusively on anaerobic metabolism of glucose for their energy requirement. Lactate production (~ 7.5 μmoles g^{-1} h^{-1}) was the same in initial and 5-week cultures. ^{35}S-Proteoglycan synthesis also remains relatively constant in this period following an initial rise during the first 24 hr of culture. Treatment with an NSAID of the phenylacetic acid class over a 5-week period had no effect on glycolysis, but inhibited proteoglycan synthesis by 25%.

Sodium iodoacetate, an inhibitor of SH-dependent enzyme activities including glyceraldehyde-3-phosphate dehydrogenase, induces an osteoarthrotic-like syndrome when injected into the knee joint of hens or rats. A 1 hr exposure of bovine articular cartilage explant cultures to 0.05 mM iodoacetate inhibited ^{35}S-proteoglycan synthesis (terminal 15 min) and lactate production (cumulative) by 90% and 50%, respectively. 0.01 mM Iodoacetate had no effect. After exposure to 0.1 mM iodoacetate for 30 min (PG synthesis and lactate, 32% and 64% of controls, respectively), cultures were maintained for a further week without iodoacetate. ^{35}S-Proteoglycan synthesis and lactate production recovered to 146% and 124% of untreated control levels. This is noteworthy since elevated proteoglycan synthesis occurs in early and experimental osteoarthrosis. It will be of interest to investigate whether drugs can modulate this effect in explant cultures.

71

A Biochemical Joint Function Test for Diagnosis of Osteoarthritis

Hans-Hubert Heilmann and Klaus Lindenhayn

*Humboldt University of Berlin, Medical School Charité,
Department of Orthopedic Surgery, Berlin, Germany*

The laboratory diagnosis of osteoarthritis (OA) is as yet not relevant for the physician since the use of serum or plasma as material for diagnostic trials have given no valid results in the single patient. Synovial fluid would be better but the latter cannot be obtained routinely in human beings since patients with osteoarthritis commonly have no joint effusion. To obtain defined material for biochemical investigations, we injected a defined volume of isotonic saline containing 0.5% of a high molecular weight physiological inert additive (e.g., hydroxyethyl starch) into the joint (e.g., 35 ml into the human knee joint or 200 μl into the knee joint of the guinea pig). After passive motion of the joint for 10 min, the resulting mixture with the synovial fluid is aspirated and the decrease in concentration of the additive is determined, as are the concentrations or activities of synovial proteins, glycoproteins, proteoglycans, hyaluronic acid, enzymes, and enzyme inhibitors. The volume of the synovial fluid prior to the test is calculated from the decrease of the concentration of the additive in the mixture caused by the synovial fluid. The concentrations or activities of the synovial parameters can be converted to their respective concentrations or activities in the synovia prior to the test, since the dilution factor is known. Using this method, we found the mean volume of the synovia to be 7.0 ml in healthy adult human knee joints and 55 μl in healthy adult knee joints of guinea pigs. The concentrations of low molecular weight compounds change by diffusion during the test. In the case of glucose, this change, estimated as corrected glucose influx, is of diagnostic value. In painful OA with necessary drug treatment, the activity of plasminogen activator is of diagnostic value (mean values: control 21 IU/L, latent OA 35 IU/L, active OA 66 IU/L). The necessity of antiinflammatory

724

treatment and the success of therapy can be evaluated with the biochemical joint function test.

REFERENCE

1. Lindenhayn K, Heilmann H-H, Regling G, Haupt R. Die Plasminogenaktivator-Aktivität der Synovialflüssigkeit als Indikator für Aktivierungsphänomene bei degenerativen Gelenkerkrankungen. *Z Rheumatol* 1989;48:246–253.

72

Distribution of Subchondral Bone as a Morphological Parameter of Stress in the Hip Joint of the Living

M. Müller-Gerbl, R. Putz, and R. Kierse

Anatomische Anstalt der Ludwig-Maximilians-Universität, 8000 München 2, Germany

It has been repeatedly discussed that the distribution of subchondral bone density may be regarded as the expression of the long-term effective stress in a joint. Our own results clearly indicate the regularity of the distribution of subchondral bone density as a function of the passing demands made upon a joint. We therefore developed CT osteoabsorptiometry, a method which allows one to visualize the area distribution of subchondral mineralization in the major joints *in the living*. The purpose of this study was to display the distribution of subchondral bone density in the acetabular cup of patients of different ages.

Computerized tomography data files of hip joints of 20 patients (18–89 years of age) were used. Density ranges, image analysis, and area presentation of the distribution of subchondral mineralization were determined.

Our results reveal that in 11 of 12 persons younger than 60 years, zones of maximum density are located in both the ventral and dorsal parts of the acetabular roof. In six of eight persons older than 60 years, however, the densest areas are most often found at the zenith of the acetabulum.

These morphological results reflect the distribution of the long-term stress within a joint surface. In normal, everyday loading of the hip joint, an incongruity is found. Under light load the contact areas are at the front and back of the acetabulum. This situation is predominantly the case throughout life and has its equivalent in the distribution of subchondral bone density. As the load increases, however, a point is reached where the dome of the acetabulum comes into contact with the femoral head. This increased stress is in the dome of the acetabulum, i.e., in *exactly* that area where degenerative changes are most often found. There is then a corresponding morphological reaction with a density maximum in the dome. This higher stress on the acetabular roof with subsequent osteoarthrosis could possibly be aggravated by a changed loading pattern. Our results clearly show that the mechanical situation differs in younger and older persons and this should be taken into consideration in designing therapy concepts (e.g., hip endoprothesis).

73

Joint Space Loss in Osteoarthritic Knees Using High Definition Macroradiography: Comparison of Weight Bearing Standing and Tunnel Views

J. C. Buckland-Wright,* D. G. Macfarlane,†
M. K. Jasani,‡ and J. A. Lynch*

*Division of Anatomy, UMDS (Guy's Hospital), London, United Kingdom;
†Rheumatology Department, Kent & Sussex Hospital,
Tunbridge Wells, Kent, United Kingdom;
‡Ciba-Geigy, Summit, New Jersey 07901

High definition microfocal radiography $\times 5$ of OA knee joints permitted direct measurement of the change in interbone distance from the standing loaded and partial weight bearing tunnel view of the tibio-femoral compartment in 39 patients, 11 male, 28 female (mean age, 59.5 ± 8.8 years, and disease duration, based on the duration of pain in the worst knee, of 5.5 ± 6.6 years, range 10 months to 30 years). All were selected on the basis of clinical assessment and the presence of joint space narrowing and subchondral sclerosis on conventional radiography. All patients had medial tibio-femoral compartment involvement. The results were compared with data from 15 nonarthritic controls (mean age, 31.3 ± 8.0 years). A crosswire cursor, linked to a MOP Videoplan (Zeiss Ltd.) was used to measure (in mm) the joint space width across the narrowest part of the medial tibio-femoral compartment. Subchondral sclerosis was measured as bone thickening (in mm) at the same point as was used for joint space width measurements. The number and size of osteophytes at the joint margins were measured.

OA patients had joint space width significantly narrower in standing ($p < 0.001$) and tunnel ($p < 0.0001$) views, and subchondral cortical thickness significantly greater in the tibia and femur in both knee positions ($p < 0.0001$) compared to the controls. Five OA subgroups were identified: (a) 53% of the OA knees had joint space width similar to the controls in both views, (b) 23% of the OA knees had moderate but significant ($p < 0.0001$) joint space width loss in both views compared to the controls, (c) 7% of the OA knees had very marked joint space loss ($p < 0.0001$) compared to the knees in (b), (d) 8% of the OA knees had very marked joint space loss on the standing view only ($p < 0.01$) compared to the knees in group (b), (e) 9% of the OA knees had very marked joint space loss on the tunnel view only ($p < 0.01$) compared with the knees in (b). Subchondral sclerosis and osteophytes were present in all groups. Osteophyte size correlated inversely with joint space width.

Measurement of joint space width identified five OA subgroups; one with early bone but without cartilage changes, one with early bone and cartilage changes, and the rest with advanced changes in both cartilage and bone at three different sites. The presence of bony changes without joint space loss in (a) confirms earlier findings in OA of the hand: that bony changes precede articular cartilage loss (1). Longitudinally studied over 18 months, all groups showed progressive cartilage loss.

REFERENCE

1. Buckland-Wright JC, Macfarlane DG, Lynch JA, *et al.* Quantitative microfocal radiographic assessment of progression in osteoarthritis of the hand. *Arthritis Rheum* 1990;33:57–65.

74

Ultrastructural Alterations of Articular Chondrocytes in the Precocious Osteoarthritis of Osteochondrodysplasias

Ritta Stanescu, Victor Stanescu, and P. Maroteaux

CNRS URA.584, Hôpital des Enfants-Malades, Paris, France

We have studied the ultrastructural appearance of femoral head chondrocytes in 12 cases of precocious osteoarthritis (hip replacement between the age of $14\frac{1}{2}$ and 48 years). In nine cases, osteoarthritis developed in patients with osteo-chondrodysplasias recognized at birth or during adolescence: multiple epiphyseal dysplasia, Fairbank type; Kniest disease; spondyloepiphyseal and spondyloepi-physeometaphyseal dysplasias; and Dyggve-Melchior-Clausen disease. In one case the osteoarthritis was the first clinical manifestation, but a careful examination showed skeletal signs of mild spondyloepiphyseal dysplasia. The last two patients presented precocious osteoarthritis without evident signs of osteochondrodysplasia or other known causes of secondary osteoarthritis. In patients with osteochondrodysplasias, the ultrastructural alterations of chondrocytes were of

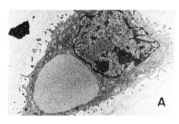

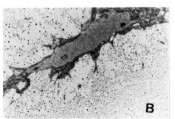

FIG. 1. A: Articular cartilage chondrocyte, polyepiphyseal dysplasia (PED), aged 48 years. **B:** Growth cartilage chondrocyte, PED aged 12 years, daughter of the first patient.

the same type as those we already found in the growth cartilage chondrocytes of the same syndromes and different from those of the "common" type of osteoarthritis. In two cases, we had the opportunity to compare the articular chondrocytes of the patients with the growth chondrocytes of their own children affected by the same disease, and we found a similar type of lesion (Fig. 1). In the last two patients with apparently normal skeletal growth and development, we found in one case balloon-shaped chondrocytes with many smooth membrane-bound vesicles containing granular and lamellar material, and in the other one a significant increase in the number of cytolysosomes of unknown origin. Defects common to growth and articular cartilage probably play a role, in addition to mechanical factors in the precocious osteoarthritis of the cases studied. In some of them the articular cartilage seems to be affected predominantly.

75

Clinical and Diagnostic Importance of the Determination of Glycosaminoglycan in Patients with Rheumatoid Arthritis and Osteoarthrosis

Alexander B. Zborovsky, Petr Issaev, Vladislav F. Martemjanow

Institute of Rheumatology Branch, USSR-AMS, Volgograd, USSR

In rheumatoid arthritis and osteoarthrosis, pathological processes cause marked changes in the connective tissue of the joint. These alterations affect the interrelationship of the cells, collagen fibers, and ground substance, and lead to quantitative and qualitative aberrations of the proteoglycans. Others have shown that glycosaminoglycans present in biological fluids reflect the degree of connective tissue damage. Our work, which is based on these premises, focuses on the content and composition of serum glycosaminoglycans as a tool to assess disease activity in arthridites and to differentiate between rheumatoid arthritis and osteoarthritis.

We have developed fast and uncomplicated methods for determining glycosaminoglycans in serum. Eighty-two patients with rheumatoid arthritis, 50 patients with osteoarthrosis, and 30 normal controls entered the study. We used disc electrophoresis in polyacrylamide gels to identify five different glycosaminoglycan fractions in normal control sera. The first represents chondroitin sulfate, the second dermatan sulfate, the third and fourth heparan sulfate and the fifth hyaluronate. In sera of hospitalized patients with rheumatoid arthritis with grade 1 disease activity, there was an overall increase in the concentration of total glycosaminoglycans. The level of chondroitin sulfate was markedly elevated, but those of dermatan sulfate and hyaluronate were lower. Rheumatoid disease activity correlated positively with the glycosaminoglycan concentration. After 2 weeks of treatment, glycosaminoglycan contents decreased, but the values returned to normal only in patients with minimal disease activity. In patients with grade 2 or 3 disease activity, the glycosaminoglycan contents were higher than in normal controls. Following treatment, the concentration of total glycosaminoglycans decreased. The values for chondroitin sulfate, dermatan sulfate, and hyaluronate varied. In patients with fast, progressive disease, the decrease in dermatan sulfate was more pronounced than in patients with slowly progressing disease. No correlation between the glycosaminoglycan data and the degree of joint destruction could be observed. Patients hospitalized for osteoarthrosis had higher serum levels of chondroitin sulfate but lower levels of dermatan sulfate and heparan sulfate than did controls. The overall concentrations of glycosaminoglycans, however, were not significantly higher than in controls, and were lower than in rheumatoid patients. Synovitis in osteoarthrotic patients was accompanied by a marked decrease in the level of dermatan sulfate. Treatment of the osteoarthrosis caused levels of all glycosaminoglycans to return to more normal values. Abnormalities in glycosaminoglycan metabolism in rheumatoid arthritis and osteoarthrosis appear to reflect a number of interrelated abnormal processes which contribute to the destruction of tissues in the joints. However, it is currently difficult to determine what are primary and secondary effects.

76

Keratan Sulfate Content of Synovial Fluid After Knee Injury

Dennis R. Ongchi, Eugene J-M. A. Thonar, C. Johnson,
James M. Williams, B. Bach, Jr., and Thomas J. Schnitzer

*Departments of Internal Medicine, Section of Rheumatology, Biochemistry, Anatomy &
Orthopedic Surgery, Rush Medical College at Rush-Presbyterian–
St Luke's Medical Center, Chicago Illinois 60612*

The rupture of a ligament or meniscus in the knee causes an increase in proteoglycan catabolism in articular cartilage. This results in a large rise in the level of proteoglycan fragments in synovial fluid. We have measured the level of a keratan sulfate (KS) epitope in synovial fluid lavage of the knee at various times after injury and have related changes to pathologic findings.

METHODS

Synovial fluid lavage was obtained at arthroscopy from 84 patients with subjective complaints of knee pain and a history of knee injury. The level of KS epitope was measured by an ELISA, using an antibody (1/20/5-D-4) against a highly sulfated epitope on KS and is reported as equivalents of a standard of KS purified from human costal cartilage. Patients were divided into four subgroups based on diagnosis at arthroscopy [group 1: rupture of cruciate ligament and/or meniscus only (N = 21); group 2: rupture of cruciate ligament and/or meniscus and chondromalacia patellae (N = 26); group 3: no evidence of ligament/meniscus injury but presence of chondromalacia (N = 25); group 4: symptomatic knee pain with no evidence of ligament injury or chondromalacia (N = 12)]. Patients were also divided into subgroups based on the time elapsed after injury.

RESULTS

The mean of KS levels ± standard error in groups 1, 2, and 3 was, in each case, higher during the first 5 weeks (group 1 = 9.18 ± 1.13; group 2 = 7.68 ± 2.46; group 3 = 6.48 ± 0.55 μg KS/ml, respectively) than in group 4 (0.30 ±

0.21), p = <0.001. However, the mean value in these patients did not differ from group to group, p > 0.05. The mean of KS levels in groups 1, 2, and 3 was in each case also higher during the first 5 weeks than between weeks 5 and 15 or at later times, p = <0.001.

DISCUSSION

The synovial fluid level of a KS epitope rises rapidly following rupture to a ligament or meniscus. It decreases during the weeks that follow but may remain slightly elevated in some patients. Levels were also elevated during the first 5 weeks after injury in patients with chondromalacia alone and showed a similar return to more normal values with time. Measurement of KS epitope in synovial fluid following knee injury thus provides important information about changes in the metabolism of cartilage proteoglycans. Longitudinal studies will help determine if the magnitude of the rise in the level of KS epitope in synovial fluid after injury correlates with the subsequent development of degenerative changes in articular cartilage in some patients.

77

Paired Serum and Synovial Fluid (SF) Levels of Keratan Sulfate (KS) in Osteoarthritis (OA)

Giles V. Campion,* F. McCrae,† Dennis R. Ongchi,‡
Paul A. Dieppe,† Eugene J-M. A. Thonar‡

*Rheumatology Section, Clinical Research, Hoechst AG Werk Kalle-Albert,
6200 Weisbaden, Germany; †Rheumatology Unit, Bristol Royal Infirmary,
Bristol BS2 8HW, England; ‡Departments of Biochemistry and Internal Medicine,
Rush-Presbyterian-St. Luke's Medical Center, Chicago, Illinois 60612

Serum levels of a highly sulfated KS epitope have been proposed as a marker of proteoglycan (PG) catabolism in cartilage. As cartilage loss is a prominent feature of OA, we have measured paired serum and synovial fluid (SF) samples and related them to features of disease in 24 patients with OA knee. In five additional patients, we have examined the effect of intraarticular corticosteroids (CS) on serum and SF KS.

METHODS

Group 1: Twenty-four patients (6 M, 18 F; mean age, (±SD) 68.9 ± 10.5; range, 42–85 years; disease duration, 22 ± 17 years) with knee OA from whom SF could be aspirated to dryness from one or both knees were studied. A clinical history and examination, and standing antero-posterior and lying lateral radiographs were obtained and scored by an independent observer. An aliquot of the SF was examined for cells and crystal content. The rest was stored with a serum sample at $-70°C$ prior to analysis for concentration of KS epitope by ELISA using the 1/20/5-D-4 monoclonal antibody. Results are reported as equivalents of a KS standard from human costal cartilage. Group 2: A separate group of 5 OA patients (4 F, 1 M,) requiring therapeutic intraarticular injection of CS had the respective joint aspirated to dryness. The SF examined together with serum taken pre- and 1 week postinjection were analyzed by the ELISA. Values obtained were compared by using parametric or nonparametric tests as appropriate.

RESULTS

Group 1: KS levels were much higher in SF than in serum (4.04 ± 2.56 vs. 0.38 ± 0.18, μg/ml, $p < 0.0001$), with no correlation between them. However, there was an inverse correlation between the radiographic assessment of joint space and levels of SF KS (r = −.36, p = .04). Group 2: The mean SF KS fell in all cases from a mean of 7.83 ± 4.43 to 4.56 + 3.55 μg/ml and the estimated total KS in the joint space fell over fivefold. Concurrently, serum levels fell from 0.29 ± 0.07 to 0.19 + 0.05 μg/ml, p = 0.059.

CONCLUSIONS

(a) SF KS levels are much higher than serum KS and there is little correlation between them. (b) There is a negative correlation between cartilage mass as measured by joint space narrowing and SF KS levels. (c) SF KS levels fall markedly after intraarticular injection of CS. (d) This fall is also seen in serum. (e) Levels of SF KS may aid monitoring of the joint in disease and during therapy.

Pyridinium Cross-link Measurements in Serum and Synovial Fluid of Patients with Osteoarthritis

Simon P. Robins,* Alison M. McLaren,* Phyllis Nicol,*
and Markus J. Seibel†

*Rowett Research Institute, Bucksburn, Aberdeen, Scotland; and †Bone Research
Laboratories, Department of Internal Medicine, University of Heidelberg, Germany

The pyridinium cross-links of collagen, pyridinoline (Pyd) and deoxypyridinoline (Dpd) have been developed as urinary markers of collagen degradation. High-performance liquid chromatography (HPLC) techniques (1) applied in studies of patients with osteoarthritis (OA) or rheumatoid arthritis (RA) have shown that in both diseases the urinary concentrations of both cross-links are elevated compared with healthy controls and that these changes reflect primarily increased rates of bone resorption. The purpose of the present study was to ascertain the feasibility of measuring the cross-links in serum and synovial fluid in order to gain more detailed knowledge of disease progression in particular joints.

Fifteen patients (F/M; 10/5) aged 36 to 76 years having OA of the knee were studied, with full clinical assessments and measurements of biochemical parameters and joint indices. For analyses of pyridinium cross-links, serum and synovial fluid were hydrolyzed in 6 M HCl at 107°C for 18 hr and were prefractionated on cellulose CF1 for HPLC analysis of cross-links as described previously (1). Diastereoisomers of pyridinoline were partially separated by ion-exchange chromatography using 67 mM sodium citrate buffer, pH 4.30. An inhibition ELISA for Pyd was developed using an antiserum raised in rabbits against the cross-link isolated from a bone hydrolysate (2). This assay showed 50% inhibition with 0.12 ng (0.28 pmol) of hydrolyzed Pyd, but the antiserum exhibited less than 15% cross-reaction with the analogue, Dpd. Measurements of Pyd in hydrolysates of serum and synovial fluid were made after fractionation by CF-cellulose chromatography using aliquots corresponding to between 5 and 200 μl of the original samples.

In hydrolysates of normal human serum, pyridinium cross-links could not be detected unequivocally by HPLC, but monitoring the fractions by ELISA showed only a single peak of activity in the position of Pyd. Analysis of serum or synovial fluid with added Pyd showed changes during hydrolysis in the pattern of diastereoisomers which reacted differently with the antiserum, giving an apparent increase in concentration of about 30%. The amounts of Pyd detected by the ELISA are therefore dependent to some extent on the conditions of hydrolysis.

The mean value ($\pm$SD) for Pyd concentrations in serum of the OA patients was 8.7 ± 3.4 (range, 4.5 to 15.4) pmol/ml. In synovial fluid of these patients, the mean Pyd concentration was 0.8 ± 0.6, but the cross-link was undetectable in two patients. The ratio between the Pyd concentrations in serum and synovial fluid varied from 3.5 to 39 (mean, 17.2). There was no correlation between Pyd concentration in serum and in synovial fluid. There were also no correlations between Pyd values and other biochemical parameters.

These results suggest that very little of the Pyd in serum is derived from collagen degradation within the joint. The very low levels of Pyd in synovial fluid indicate that this assay appears to have limited application in synovial fluid as an early indication of cartilage loss in OA.

ACKNOWLEDGMENT

We thank the Arthritis & Rheumatism Council, UK, for financial support.

REFERENCES

1. Black D, Duncan A, Robins SP. Quantitative analysis of the pyridinium crosslinks of collagen in urine using ion-paired HPLC. *Anal Biochem* 1988;169:197–203.
2. Robins SP. An enzyme-linked immunoassay for the collagen crosslink, pyridinoline. *Biochem J* 1982;207:617–620.

Subject Index